Pocket Companion to Neurology in Clinical Practice

Pocket Companion to Neurology in Clinical Practice

FOURTH EDITION

Walter G. Bradley, D.M., F.R.C.P.

Professor and Chairman, Department of Neurology, University of
Miami School of Medicine; Chief, Neurology Service, University of
Miami-Jackson Memorial Medical Center, Miami, Florida

Robert B. Daroff, M.D.

Professor of Neurology;
Interim Vice Dean for Education and Academic Affairs,
CASE School of Medicine, Cleveland, Ohio

Gerald M. Fenichel, M.D.

Professor of Neurology and Pediatrics, Vanderbilt University School
of Medicine; Director, Division of Pediatric Neurology;
Neurologist-in-Chief, Vanderbilt Children's Hospital,
Nashville, Tennessee

Joseph Jankovic, M.D.

Professor of Neurology; Director, Parkinson's Disease Center and
Movement Disorders Clinic, Baylor College of Medicine,
Houston, Texas

ELSEVIER
BUTTERWORTH
HEINEMANN

ELSEVIER
BUTTERWORTH
HEINEMANN

An Imprint of Elsevier

The Curtis Center
170 S Independence Mall W 300E
Philadelphia, Pennsylvania 19106

NOTICE

Medicine is an ever-changing field. Standard safety precautions
must be followed, but as new research and clinical experience
broaden our knowledge, changes in treatment and drug therapy
may become necessary or appropriate. Readers are advised to
check the most current product information provided by the
manufacturer of each drug to be administered to verify the
recommended dose, the method and duration of administration,
and contraindications. It is the responsibility of the treating
physician, relying on experience and knowledge of the patient,
to determine dosages and the best treatment for each individual
patient. Neither the publisher nor the editors assume any liability
for any injury and/or damage to persons or property arising from
this publication.

The Publisher

International Standard Book Number 0-7506-7468-7

Printed in the United States of America

Last digit is the print number: 9   8   7   6   5   4   3   2   1

Preface

The editors have extracted the salient points of *Neurology in Clinical Practice (NICP)* to provide a compressed, more portable, print format for the clinician away from the office. This companion volume complements the Web site. *NICP* has become one of the most frequently read textbooks in the field of neurology. The contributors are not only experts in their field but are also teachers who express themselves well. Butterworth-Heinemann has provided the editors a unique opportunity to bring the science and practice of neurology to our readers in more than one format to meet individual needs.

The Editors

Contents

Episodic Impairments of Consciousness, Falls, and Drop Attacks

1

IMPAIRMENTS OF CONSCIOUSNESS

Temporary loss of consciousness may be caused by impaired cerebral perfusion (syncope, fainting), cerebral ischemia, migraine, epileptic seizures, metabolic disturbances, sudden increases in intracranial pressure, or sleep disorders. Anxiety attacks, psychogenic seizures, and malingering may be difficult to distinguish from these conditions. In patients with episodic impairment of consciousness, the diagnosis relies heavily on the clinical history described by the patient and observers. Laboratory investigations may provide useful information, but in some patients a cause may not be established.

Syncope

Any condition that reduces cerebral blood flow may cause syncope. The pathophysiological basis of syncope is a failure of cerebral perfusion with reduction in cerebral oxygen availability.

Clinical Features
Lightheadedness, generalized muscle weakness, giddiness, visual blurring, tinnitus, and gastrointestinal symptoms characterize the symptom complex. The patient appears pale and feels cold and clammy. Loss of consciousness is generally gradual except when syncope is associated with cardiac arrhythmia. The gradual onset may allow patients to protect themselves from falling and injury. Emotional stress, unpleasant visual stimuli, prolonged standing, and pain are common precipitants of syncope. The duration of unconsciousness is brief, usually seconds to minutes. During the faint, the patient may be motionless or may stiffen and tremble (myoclonic jerks). Urinary incontinence is uncommon. The pulse is weak and often slow. Breathing may be shallow and the blood pressure barely obtainable. As the fainting

Table 1.1: Causes of syncope

Cardiac arrhythmias
  Bradyarrhythmias
  Tachyarrhythmias
  Reflex arrhythmias
Decreased cardiac output
Cardiac outflow obstruction
Inflow obstruction
Cardiomyopathy
Hypovolemia
Hypotension
Drug use
Dysautonomia
Carotid sinus
Vertebrobasilar disease
Vasospasm
Takayasu's arteritis
Metabolic
Hypoglycemia
Anemia
Anoxia
Hyperventilation
Vasovagal (vasodepressor; neurocardiogenic; neural mediated)
Cardiac syncope
Cough, micturition
Multifactorial

episode ends, color returns, breathing becomes more regular, and the pulse and blood pressure normalize. Afterwards, some residual weakness is noted, but drowsiness is uncommon. Table 1.1 classifies the causes of syncope.

Diagnosis
A careful history establishes the cause. The patient's own description often establishes the diagnosis. Emphasis is placed on precipitating factors, including posture, whether the onset was abrupt or gradual, position of head and neck, the presence and duration of preceding and associated symptoms, duration of loss of consciousness, rate of recovery, and sequelae. Examination is most informative when specific maneuvers reproduce the fainting. The examination is focused on the cardiovascular system.

Laboratory Studies
Studies are unnecessary when the cause is clear. In most patients, indicated laboratory studies include measurements of the

hematocrit and blood glucose concentrations and electrocardiographic (ECG) monitoring. Patients with suspected cardiac syncope may need a chest radiograph, tests of valvular function, and a Holter monitor. Exercise testing is useful in detecting coronary artery disease, and exercise-related syncopal recordings may localize conduction disturbances. The suspicion of cerebrovascular disease requires Doppler flow studies of the cerebral vessels and sometimes magnetic resonance angiography (MRA). The use of an electroencephalogram (EEG) is only to diagnose a seizure disorder.

Seizures

An epileptic seizure is a transitory disturbance of brain function resulting from an abnormal electrical discharge of cerebral neurons. The clinical and EEG features are the basis for classifying epileptic seizures. Alterations of consciousness occur in generalized (absence and tonic-clonic) and complex·partial seizures.

Clinical Features
The description by a witness is the usual basis for diagnosis. When this is inadequate, urge family members to videotape the event at home. Important elements of the history include a complete description of the seizure, particularly its onset, family history, prior neurological disturbances that may predispose to epilepsy, and precipitating events. An abnormal neurological examination usually indicates symptomatic epilepsy, and a normal examination suggests a primary (genetic) epilepsy. Table 1.2 compares clinical features of syncope with those of seizures.

Laboratory Studies
New-onset seizures are usually investigated with a complete blood cell count, urinalysis, measurement of blood electrolytes and glucose and calcium concentrations, an EEG, and a brain imaging study. Magnetic resonance imaging (MRI) is usually preferable to computed tomography (CT). Children with simple febrile seizures and absence do not require studies. Cerebrospinal fluid examination is imperative whenever suspicion exists of an underlying infection of the nervous system.

Psychogenic or Pseudoseizures (Nonepileptic Seizures)

Pseudoepileptic seizures are paroxysmal episodes of altered behavior that superficially resemble epileptic seizures but lack the expected EEG epileptic changes. However, approximately

Table 1.2: Comparison of clinical features of syncope and seizures

Features	Syncope	Seizure
Relation to posture	Common	No
Time of day	Diurnal	Diurnal or nocturnal
Precipitating factors	Emotion, injury, pain, crowds, heat	Sleep loss, drug/alcohol withdrawal
Skin color	Pallor	Cyanosis or normal
Aura or premonitory symptoms	Long	Brief
Convulsion	Rare	Common
Injury	Rare	Common (with convulsive seizures)
Urinary incontinence	Rare	Common
Postictal confusion	Rare	Common
Postictal headache	No	Common
Focal neurological signs	No	Occasional
Cardiovascular signs	Common (cardiac syncope)	No
Abnormal electroencephalogram recording	Rare (may show generalized slowing during the event)	Common

40% of patients with pseudoseizures or nonepileptic seizures also experience true epileptic seizures.

Breath-Holding Spells

Breath-holding spells occur in 2–5% of infants and young children. They are a hereditary, involuntary vagal reflex, reproduced in the laboratory by pressure on the globe of the eye. The usual age at onset is between 6 and 28 months but may be as early as the first month. They usually disappear by 5 or 6 years of age. The spells are either cyanotic or pallid; most children have one or the other.

Clinical Features
The trigger for cyanotic breath-holding spells can be fright, anger, or frustration. The child cries vigorously for a few breaths and then stops breathing in expiration. Cyanosis is rapid and intense. Consciousness is lost because of hypoxia, and recovery is complete within a few minutes. Stimuli that provoke pallid spells include a minor painful injury or startle. The child does not cry. Asystole occurs, and the child becomes pale and lifeless. Recovery is complete within minutes. During both cyanotic and pallid spells, the child often stiffens and trembles, but the EEG at this time is flat.

Diagnosis
The clinical features alone establish the diagnosis.

FALLS AND DROP ATTACKS

Everyone occasionally falls, but suspect a neurological disorder when falls occur repeatedly or without a prior sense of imbalance. An associated loss of consciousness implies syncope or seizures. The words *falls* and *drops* are used interchangeably, but the term *drop attacks* describes sudden falls occurring without warning. These result from intracranial causes, such as midline tumors and transient ischemic attacks (TIAs). Table 1.3 summarizes the causes of falls and drop attacks.

The medical history is essential in evaluating falls and drop attacks. The situational and environmental circumstances worth exploring are loss of consciousness; lightheadedness or palpitations that precede the event; and a history that suggests any of the following conditions: epilepsy, transitory cerebral ischemia, peripheral neuropathy, narcolepsy, or impairment of special senses. An abnormal neurological examination usually indicates a specific cause.

Table 1.3: Causes and types of falls and drops

Loss of consciousness
  Syncope
  Seizures
Transient ischemic attacks (drop attacks)
  Vertebrobasilar
  Anterior cerebral
Third ventricular and posterior fossa tumors (drop attacks)
Motor and sensory impairment of lower limbs
  Basal ganglia disorders
  Parkinson's disease
  Progressive supranuclear palsy
  Neuromuscular disorders (myopathy and neuropathy)
  Myelopathy
  Cerebral or cerebellar disorders
Cataplexy
Vestibular disorders
Cryptogenic falls in middle-aged women
Aged state

Unexplained Falls in Middle-Aged Women

A falling tendency exists in more than 3% of women older than 40 years. Twenty percent have at least one close relative (mother, aunt, or sister) with the same condition.

Clinical Features
The fall is usually forward and occurs without warning while walking. Loss of consciousness, dizziness, or even a sense of imbalance does not occur. Patients are convinced that they have not tripped but that their legs suddenly gave way. Walking continues normally upon rising. Falling often occurs between 2 and 12 times per year. Only one fourth of patients fall more than once per month or have clusters of frequent falls with prolonged asymptomatic intervals. Causal factors are not established.

Diagnosis
The clinical features establish the diagnosis.

Falls in the Elderly

Most patients presenting with falls are the chronically impaired elderly. After hip fracture, falls are the single most disabling condition leading to nursing home admission. Normal aging is associated with a decline in multiple physiological functions. Several factors interfere with the ability to compensate for external factors that challenge standing. These include decreased proprioception, loss of muscle bulk, arthritis of the leg joints, cardiovascular disturbances, deteriorating vision and ocular motor functions, cognitive impairment, and failing postural reflexes (*presbyastasis*). Even the healthy elderly have a pronounced age-related decline in the ability to compensate for simulated forward falling. Elderly patients with cardioinhibitory ("sick") sinus syndrome often describe dizziness and falling, rather than faintness. Orthostatic hypotension conveys a markedly increased risk of falling in the elderly and confounds other factors contributing to falls. Hypotension is usually associated with a presyncopal syndrome of progressive light-headedness, faintness, dimming of vision, and rubbery legs before consciousness is lost. Orthostatic hypotension is particularly problematic in the frail elderly, who have many other risk factors for falling.

Clinical Features
Most of the elderly patients who fall have one or more pre-disposing conditions. The chance of falling increases with the number of identified risk factors. Most falls are accidental, suggesting an interaction between a debilitated patient and potential environmental hazards. The important conditions associated with falls are dementia, metabolic and toxic encephalopathies, depression, cerebral infarcts, parkinsonism, neuropathy, arthritis, and gait disorders. Compared to healthy elderly people, patients with Alzheimer's disease have slower walking speed, more difficulty clearing obstacles, and further deterioration of gait properties, leading to falls. Performing a simultaneous cognitive task, such as talking when walking, has a high predictive value for falling.

Diagnosis
The clinical evaluation should aim at identifying predisposing conditions and differentiating accidental from endogenous falls. A detailed medication history is essential. Commonly used drugs such as antidepressants, antihypertensives, and tranquilizers increase the risk of falls. Finally, obtain a description of contributing environmental factors. Poorly lit staircases with variable step height, loose carpeting, cluttered room arrangements, and lack of sturdy furniture or handrails for support are a few examples of environmental hazards.

Laboratory Studies
Brain abnormalities on MRI scans correlate with postural instability in the elderly.

Management
Therapeutic and risk-reduction intervention include (1) treatment of correctable conditions, (2) provision of rehabilitative services and assistive devices, and (3) prevention by controlling environmental hazards.

For a more detailed discussion, see Chapters 2 and 3 in Neurology in Clinical Practice, 4th edition.

Stupor and Coma

2

Consciousness is a state of awareness of self and surroundings. This chapter deals with disturbances in arousal. Disturbances of cognitive and affective mental function include dementia, delusions, confusion, and inattention. These do not affect the level of arousal. Sleep is the only normal form of altered consciousness. The term *delirium* describes a clouding of consciousness with reduced ability to sustain attention to environmental stimuli. Four points on the continuum of arousal describe the clinical state of a patient: *alert, lethargic, stuporous,* and *comatose*. *Alert* is a normal state of arousal. *Stupor* is unresponsiveness from which the subject can be aroused by vigorous and repeated stimuli. *Coma* is unarousable unresponsiveness. *Lethargy* lies between alertness and stupor.

Several behavioral states may appear similar to coma or may be confused with it (Table 2.1). Further, patients who survive initial coma may progress to one of these syndromes. Coma is over once sleep-wake cycles reappear.

APPROACH TO COMA

Table 2.2 lists many of the common causes of coma. More than half of all cases are caused by diffuse and metabolic brain dysfunction. Three categories of diseases can cause coma: structural lesions, metabolic and toxic causes, and psychiatric causes. The history and physical examination determine the presence or absence of a structural lesion and differentiate the general categories to determine further diagnostic testing.

Rapid Initial Examination and Emergency Therapy

A relatively quick initial assessment of the comatose patient is important to ensure the patient is not in immediate need of

Table 2.1: Behavioral states confused with coma

Behavioral State	Definition	Lesion	Comments
Locked-in syndrome	Alert and aware, quadriplegic with lower cranial nerve palsy	Bilateral anterior pontine	A similar state may be seen with severe polyneuropathies, myasthenia gravis, and neuromuscular blocking agents
Vegetative state	Absent cognitive function but retained "vegetative" components	Extensive cortical gray or subcortical white matter with relative preservation of brainstem	Synonyms include apallic syndrome, coma vigil, and cerebral-cortical death
Abulia	Severe apathy, patient neither speaks nor moves spontaneously	Bilateral frontal medial	Severe cases resemble akinetic mutism, but patient is alert and aware
Catatonia	Mute, with marked decrease in motor activity	Usually psychiatric	May be mimicked by frontal lobe dysfunction or drugs
Pseudocoma	Feigned coma		

Table 2.2: Causes of coma

I. Symmetrical nonstructural

Toxins	Metabolic	Infections
Lead	Hypoxia	Bacterial meningitis
Thallium	Hypercapnia	Viral encephalitis
Mushrooms	Hypernatremia	Postinfectious encephalomyelitis
Cyanide	Hyponatremia*	Syphilis
Methanol	Hypoglycemia*	Sepsis
Ethylene glycol	Hyperglycemic nonketotic coma	Typhoid fever
Carbon monoxide	Diabetic ketoacidosis	Malaria
	Lactic acidosis	Waterhouse-Friderichsen syndrome
Drugs	Hypercalcemia	Psychiatric
Sedatives	Hypocalcemia	Catatonia
Barbiturates*	Hypermagnesemia	Other
Other hypnotics	Hyperthermia	Postictal*
Tranquilizers	Hypothermia	Diffuse ischemia (myocardial
Bromides	Reye's encephalopathy	infarction, congestive heart
Alcohol	Aminoacidemia	failure, arrhythmia)
Opiates	Wernicke's encephalopathy	Hypotension
Paraldehyde	Porphyria	Fat embolism*
Salicylate	Hepatic encephalopathy*	Hypertensive encephalopathy
Psychotropics	Uremia	Hypothyroidism
Anticholinergics	Dialysis encephalopathy	
Amphetamines	Addisonian crisis	
Lithium		
Phencyclidine		
Monoamine oxidase inhibitors		

Continued

Table 2.2: (continued)

II. Symmetrical, structural

Supratentorial
Bilateral internal carotid occlusion
Bilateral anterior cerebral artery occlusion

Subarachnoid hemorrhage
Thalamic hemorrhage*
Trauma—contusion, concussion*
Hydrocephalus

Infratentorial
Basilar occlusion*
Midline brainstem tumor
Pontine hemorrhage*

III. Asymmetrical, structural

Supratentorial
Thrombotic thrombocytopenic purpura
Disseminated intravascular coagulation
Nonbacterial thrombotic endocarditis (marantic endocarditis)
Subacute bacterial endocarditis
Fat emboli
Unilateral hemispheric mass (tumor, bleed) with herniation

Subdural hemorrhage bilateral
Intracerebral bleed

Pituitary apoplexy

Massive or bilateral supratentorial infarction

Multifocal leukoencephalopathy
Creutzfeldt-Jakob disease
Adrenal leukodystrophy
Cerebral vasculitis
Cerebral abscess

Subdural empyema
Thrombophlebitis

Multiple sclerosis

Leukoencephalopathy associated with chemotherapy

Acute disseminated encephalomyelitis
Infratentorial
Brainstem infarction
Brainstem hemorrhage

*Relatively common asymmetrical presentation.

Source: Data from Plum, F. & Posner, J. B. 1995, *The Diagnosis of Stupor and Coma*, 4th ed, FA Davis, Philadelphia; and Fisher, C. M. 1969, "The neurological evaluation of the comatose patient," *Acta Neurol Scand*, vol. 45 [Suppl. 36].

medical or surgical intervention. Urgent empirical therapy to prevent further brain damage is justified. These may include supplemental oxygen, thiamine (at least 100 mg), and intravenous 50% dextrose in water (25 g). Measure the serum glucose concentration before administering glucose.

An initial examination includes a check of general appearance, blood pressure, pulse, temperature, respiratory rate, breath sounds, best response to stimulation, pupil size and responsiveness, and posturing or adventitious movements. Stabilize the neck in all instances of trauma until after excluding cervical spine fracture or subluxation. Protect the airway in all comatose patients and place an intravenous line. Abdominal rigidity is a feature of peritonitis or perforated viscus. In coma, the signs of an acute condition in the abdomen may be subtle or nonexistent. Hypotension, marked hypertension, bradycardia, arrhythmias causing depression of blood pressure, marked hyperthermia, and signs of herniation mandate immediate therapeutic intervention. Hyperthermia or meningismus leads to consideration of urgent lumbar puncture. Perform a computed tomography (CT) scan of the brain *before* lumbar puncture in all comatose patients. Intravenous access and intravenously administered mannitol should be ready in case unexpected herniation begins after the lumbar puncture. If focal signs develop during or after the lumbar puncture, immediate intubation and hyperventilation may also be necessary.

Common Presentations

Coma usually presents in one of three ways. Most commonly, coma occurs as an expected or predictable progression of an underlying illness. Second, coma occurs as an unpredictable event in patients with known medical conditions, and finally, coma can occur in a patient who is totally unknown to the physician.

History

Once the patient is relatively stable, seek clues to the cause of the coma by briefly interviewing relatives, friends, bystanders, or medical personnel who may have observed the patient before or during the decrease in consciousness. Examine the patient's wallet or purse for lists of medications, a physician's card, or other information.

NEUROLOGICAL EXAMINATION

The neurological examination of a comatose patient serves three purposes: (1) to aid in determining the cause of coma, (2) to provide a baseline assessment of state, and (3) to help determine the prognosis of coma. For prognosis and localization of a structural lesion, the most helpful parts of the examination are as follows: (1) state of consciousness, (2) respiratory pattern, (3) pupillary size and response to light, (4) spontaneous and reflex eye movements, and (5) skeletal muscle motor response.

State of Consciousness

Record the exact stimulus and the patient's specific response. Use several modes of stimulation, including auditory, visual, and noxious, and apply stimuli with progressively increasing intensity. Ask all patients in apparent coma to open their eyes and look up and down to avoid the possibility of mistaking the locked-in syndrome. The Glasgow Coma Scale (see Table 2.3) is widely used to assess the initial severity of traumatic brain injury.

Respiration

Normal breathing is quiet and unlabored. The presence of any respiratory noise implies airway obstruction, which requires

Table 2.3: The Glasgow Coma Scale

Best motor response	
Obeys	M6
Localizes	5
Withdraws	4
Abnormal flexion	3
Extensor response	2
Nil	1
Verbal response	
Oriented	V5
Confused conversation	4
Inappropriate words	3
Incomprehensible sounds	2
Nil	1
Eye opening	
Spontaneous	E4
To speech	3
To pain	2
Nil	1

immediate correction to prevent hypoxia. Respiratory patterns that are helpful in localizing level of involvement include Cheyne-Stokes respiration, central neurogenic hyperventilation, apneustic breathing, cluster breathing, and ataxic respiration. *Cheyne-Stokes respiration* is a respiratory pattern that slowly oscillates between hyperventilation and hypoventilation. It is usually associated with bilateral hemispheric or diencephalic injury. A stable pattern of Cheyne-Stokes respiration implies that permanent brainstem damage has not occurred. *Central neurogenic respiration* refers to rapid breathing, from 40–70 breaths per minute, usually caused by central tegmental pontine lesions just ventral to the aqueduct or fourth ventricle. *Kussmaul breathing* is a deep, regular respiration observed with metabolic acidosis. *Apneustic breathing* is a prolonged inspiratory gasp with a pause at full inspiration caused by lesions of the dorsolateral lower half of the pons. *Cluster breathing*, which results from high medullary damage, involves periodic respirations that are irregular in frequency and amplitude, with variable pauses between clusters of breaths. *Ataxic breathing* is irregular in rate and rhythm and is usually caused by medullary lesions. Ataxic and gasping respirations indicate lower brainstem damage and are often preterminal.

Pupil Size and Reactivity

Normal pupil size in the comatose patient depends on the level of illumination and the state of autonomic innervation. Afferent input depends on the integrity of the optic nerve, optic chiasm, optic tract, and projections into the midbrain tectum and efferent fibers through the Edinger-Westphal nucleus and oculomotor nerve. Abnormalities in pupil size and reactivity help delineate structural damage between the thalamus and pons, act as a warning sign heralding brainstem herniation, and help differentiate structural causes of coma from metabolic causes.

Ocular Motility

Preservation of normal ocular motility implies that a large portion of the brainstem from the vestibular nuclei at the pontomedullary junction to the oculomotor nucleus in the midbrain is intact. Evaluation of ocular motility consists of three main elements: (1) observation of the resting position of the eyes, including eye deviation; (2) notation of spontaneous eye movements; and (3) testing of reflex ocular movements. Examination of ocular movement is not complete in the comatose patient without assessment of reflex ocular movements, including the oculocephalic reflex (doll's eye phenomenon) and, if necessary, the vestibulooculogyric reflex, by caloric (thermal) testing.

Motor System

Examination of the motor system of a stuporous or comatose patient begins with a description of the resting posture and adventitious movements. *Decerebrate posturing* is bilateral extensor posture, with extension of the lower extremities and adduction and internal rotation of the shoulders and extension at the elbows and wrist. Bilateral midbrain or pontine lesions are usually responsible for decerebrate posturing. *Decorticate posturing* is bilateral flexion at the elbows and wrists, with shoulder adduction and extension of the lower extremities. It may result from lesions in many locations, although usually above the brainstem.

Tonic-clonic or other stereotyped movements signal seizure as the probable cause of decreased alertness. *Myoclonic jerking*, nonrhythmic jerking movements in single or multiple muscle groups, occurs with anoxic encephalopathy or other metabolic comas, such as hepatic encephalopathy. *Rhythmic myoclonus* is usually a sign of brainstem injury. Tetany occurs with hypocalcemia. *Cerebellar fits* result from intermittent tonsillar herniation. Their characteristics are a deterioration of level of arousal, opisthotonos, respiratory rate slowing and irregularity, and pupillary dilation. Acute structural damage above the brainstem usually results in decreased or flaccid tone.

BRAIN HERNIATION

Traditional signs of herniation caused by supratentorial masses are usually variations of either an uncal or a central pattern. In the former, the early signs are of third nerve and midbrain compression. The pupil initially dilates from third nerve compression but later returns to the midposition with midbrain compression that involves the sympathetic and the parasympathetic tracts. In the central pattern, the earliest signs are mild impairment of consciousness, with poor concentration, drowsiness, or unexpected agitation. The pupils are small but reactive, reflex vertical gaze is poor or absent, and bilateral corticospinal tract signs appear. Increased intracranial pressure invariably accompanies brainstem herniation and may be associated with increased systolic blood pressure, bradycardia, and sixth nerve palsies. These signs, however, and many of the traditional signs of herniation described previously, actually occur relatively late. Earlier signs of potential herniation include decreasing level of arousal, slight change in depth or rate of respiration, and the appearance of an extensor-plantar response.

DIFFERENTIATING TOXIC-METABOLIC COMA FROM STRUCTURAL COMA

Generally, structural lesions have a more abrupt onset, whereas metabolic or toxic causes are more slowly progressive. Multifocal structural diseases such as vasculitis or leukoencephalopathy are the exception. They may exhibit slow progression, usually in a stepwise manner. Supratentorial or infratentorial tumors characterized by slow growth and surrounding edema may also mimic metabolic processes. In general, structural lesions have focal features or at least asymmetry on neurological examination. Toxic, metabolic, and psychiatric diseases show symmetrical disturbances.

Many features of the neurological examination differentiate metabolic or toxic causes from structural lesions:

1. *State of consciousness*. Patients with metabolic problems often have milder alterations in arousal and tend to have waxing and waning of the behavioral state. Patients with acute structural lesions tend to stay at the same level of arousal or progressively deteriorate. Toxins may also cause progressive decline in level of arousal.
2. *Respiration*. Deep, frequent respiration is usually due to metabolic abnormalities.
3. *Funduscopic examination*. Subhyaloid hemorrhage or papilledema are almost diagnostic of structural lesions. Papilledema does not occur in metabolic diseases except hypoparathyroidism, lead intoxication, and malignant hypertension.
4. *Pupil size*. The pupils are usually symmetrical in coma from toxic-metabolic causes.
5. *Pupil reactivity*. Pupillary reactivity is relatively resistant to metabolic insult and usually spared in coma from drug intoxication or metabolic causes, even when other brainstem reflexes are absent.
6. *Ocular motility*. Asymmetry in oculomotor function is typically a feature of structural lesions.

7. *Spontaneous eye movements.* Roving eye movements with full excursion most often suggest metabolic or toxic abnormalities.
8. *Reflex eye movements.* Reflex eye movements are usually intact in toxic-metabolic coma, except rarely in phenobarbital or phenytoin intoxication or deep metabolic coma from other causes.
9. *Adventitious movement.* Coma punctuated by periods of motor restlessness, tremors, or spasm is often caused by drugs or toxins such as chlorpromazine or lithium. Brainstem herniation or intermittent central nervous system (CNS) ischemia may also produce unusual posturing movements. Myoclonic jerking is generally metabolic and often anoxic in origin.
10. *Muscle tone.* Muscle tone is usually symmetrical and normal or decreased in metabolic coma. Structural lesions cause asymmetrical muscle tone. Tone may be increased, normal, or decreased by structural lesions.

LABORATORY STUDIES

Table 2.4 lists laboratory tests that are extremely helpful in evaluating the comatose patient.

CLINICAL APPROACH TO PROGNOSIS

The current state of knowledge does not reliably predict outcome in any comatose patient, unless that patient meets the criteria for brain death.

Nontraumatic Coma

Only about 15% of patients in nontraumatic coma make a satisfactory recovery. Functional recovery relates to the cause of coma. Diseases causing structural damage, such as cerebrovascular disease including subarachnoid hemorrhage, have the worst prognosis; coma from hypoxia-ischemia due to such causes as cardiac arrest has an intermediate prognosis; coma due to hepatic encephalopathy and other metabolic causes has the best ultimate outcome. Age is not predictive of recovery. The longer a coma lasts, the less likely the patient is to regain independent functioning.

Table 2.4: Laboratory tests helpful in coma

Laboratory Study	Result	Associated Disorders
Electrolytes (Na, K, Cl, CO_2)		See Chapters 55A and 62 in *Neurology in Clinical Practice*, 4th edition for discussion of disorders associated with abnormalities of electrolytes, glucose, blood urea nitrogen, calcium, and magnesium
Glucose		
Blood urea nitrogen		
Creatinine		
Calcium		
Magnesium		
Complete blood cell count with differential	Hematocrit:	
	Increased	Volume depletion, underlying lung disorder, myeloproliferative disorder, cerebellar hemangioblastoma; may be associated with vascular sludging (hypoperfusion)
	Decreased	Anemia, hemorrhage
	White blood cell count:	
	Increased	Infection, acute stress reaction, steroid therapy, after epileptic fit, myeloproliferative disorder
	Decreased	Chemotherapy, immunotherapy, viral infection, sepsis

Continued

Table 2.4: (continued)

Laboratory Study	Result	Associated Disorders
	Lymphocyte count: Decreased	Viral infection, malnutrition, acquired immune deficiency syndrome
Platelet count	Decreased	Sepsis, disseminated intravascular coagulation, thrombotic thrombocytopenic purpura, idiopathic thrombocytopenic purpura, drugs; may be associated with intracranial hemorrhage
Prothrombin time	Increased	Coagulation factor deficiency, liver disease, anticoagulants, disseminated intravascular coagulation
Partial thromboplastin time	Increased	Heparin therapy, lupus anticoagulant
Arterial blood gases		See *Neurology in Clinical Practice*, 4th edition
Creatine phosphokinase		See *Neurology in Clinical Practice*, 4th edition
Liver function studies		See *Neurology in Clinical Practice*, 4th edition
Thyroid function studies		See *Neurology in Clinical Practice*, 4th edition
Plasma cortisol level		See *Neurology in Clinical Practice*, 4th edition
Drug and toxin screen		See *Neurology in Clinical Practice*, 4th edition
Serum osmolality		See *Neurology in Clinical Practice*, 4th edition

Traumatic Coma

The prognosis for traumatic coma differs from that for nontraumatic coma. First, many patients with head trauma are young. Second, prolonged coma of up to several months does not preclude a satisfactory outcome. Third, in relationship to their initial degree of neurological abnormality, patients with traumatic coma do better than those with nontraumatic coma.

CLINICAL APPROACH TO BRAIN DEATH

A thorough knowledge of the criteria for brain death is essential for the physician whose responsibilities include evaluation of comatose patients. Despite differences in state laws, the criteria for the establishment of brain death are standard within the medical community. These criteria include the following:

1. *Coma.* The patient should exhibit an unarousable unresponsiveness. There should be no meaningful response to noxious, externally applied stimuli. The patient should not obey commands or demonstrate any verbal response, reflexively or spontaneously. Spinal reflexes, however, may be retained.
2. *No spontaneous respirations.* The patient should be removed from ventilatory assistance, and carbon dioxide should be allowed to build up because of the respiratory drive that hypercapnia produces. The diagnosis of absolute apnea requires the absence of spontaneous respiration at a carbon dioxide tension of at least 60 mm Hg. A safe means of obtaining this degree of carbon dioxide retention involves the technique of apneic oxygenation, in which 100% oxygen is delivered endotracheally through a thin sterile catheter for 10 minutes. Arterial blood gas levels should be obtained to confirm the arterial carbon dioxide pressure.
3. *Absence of brainstem reflexes.* Pupillary, oculocephalic, vestibulooculogyric on cold calorics, corneal, and gag reflexes must all be absent.
4. *Electrocerebral silence.* An isoelectric electroencephalogram (EEG) should denote the absence of cerebrocortical function. Some authorities do not regard obtaining an EEG mandatory in assessing brain death, and instances of preserved cortical function, despite irreversible and complete brainstem disruption, have been reported.
5. *Absence of cerebral blood flow.* Cerebral contrast angiography or radionuclide angiography can substantiate the absence of cerebral blood flow, which is expected in brain

death. These tests are considered confirmatory rather than mandatory. On rare occasions in the presence of supratentorial lesions with preserved blood flow to the brainstem and cerebellum, cerebral angioscintigraphy may be misleading.

6. *Absence of any potentially reversible causes of marked CNS depression.* This includes hypothermia, drug intoxication, and severe metabolic disturbance.

For a more detailed discussion, see Chapter 5 in Neurology in Clinical Practice, 4th edition.

Intellectual and Memory Impairments

3

The term *intellect* designates the totality of the mental or cognitive operations that human thought is composed of, the higher cortical functions that make up the human mind. The intellect and its faculties, the subject matter of human psychology, are the qualities that most separate human beings from other animals. Memory is a specific cognitive function: the storage and retrieval of information. As such, it is the prerequisite for learning, the building block of all human knowledge.

NEURAL BASIS OF COGNITION

Cerebral Cortex

Cognition takes place among a large network of cortical cells and connections, the neural switchboard that gives rise to conscious thinking. The cortical mantle contains more than 14 billion neurons. Within the cortical mantle, the areas that have expanded the most from animal to human are the "association cortices," cortical zones that do not have a primary motor or sensory function but interrelate the functions of the primary motor and sensory areas. Higher cortical functions, with few exceptions, take place in the association cortex.

Each of the primary sensory cortices receives signals in only one modality (vision, hearing, or sensation) and has cortical-cortical connections only to adjacent portions of the association cortex also dedicated to this modality, called *unimodal association cortex*. The processing of sensory information is sequential, in increasingly complex fashion, leading from raw sensory data to a unified percept. Within each cortical area are columns of cells with similar function, called *modules*. Unimodal association cortices communicate with each other by complex connections to the heteromodal association cortex. The heteromodal association cortex has two main areas. The posterior heteromodal association cortex involves the posterior inferior parietal lobe, especially the angular gyrus, and makes it possible to perceive an analogy between an association in one modality (e.g., a picture of a boat in the visual modality) with a percept in a different modality (e.g., the sound of the spoken word *boat*). The second heteromodal association cortex, in the lateral prefrontal region, is involved with attention or working memory and with sequential processes, such as storage of temporally ordered stimuli and the planning of motor activities. This temporal sequencing of information and of motor planning is also important to the executive function of the brain. A determination must be made of which of the many sensory stimuli reaching the brain merit attention and which motor outputs to activate at a given time. This part of the brain brings specific cognitive processes to conscious awareness and may be responsible for consciousness and self-awareness.

Consciousness

Understanding of the neural basis for *conscious awareness* and *sense of self* is poor. The best model for the study of consciousness is visual awareness. Neurons in the primary visual cortex are unlikely to have access to conscious awareness. Stated another way, we do not pay attention to much of what our eyes see and our visual cortex analyzes. A perceived object excites neurons in several areas of the visual association cortex, each with associations that enter consciousness or are stored in short-term memory. Conscious visual perception involves interactions between the visual parts of the brain and the prefrontal systems for attention and working memory. Neurons in the orbitofrontal cortex integrate interoceptive stimuli with exteroceptive sensory inputs, such as vision. This interaction between attention to external stimuli and internal stimuli underlies conscious awareness.

Several clinical examples of "unconscious" mental processing involve vision. Patients with cortical blindness sometimes show knowledge of items they cannot see, a phenomenon called *blindsight*. A familiar example of unconscious visual processing is the drive home from work; most individuals can remember very little of what they saw on the trip, yet they drove without accidents. Recent research links the right frontal cortex to the sense of self. Patients who develop a major change in self-concept during illness have predominant atrophy in the nondominant frontal lobe.

The functioning of the awake mind requires the ascending inputs of the *reticular activating system*, with its way stations in the brainstem and thalamus, as well as an intact cerebral cortex. Bilateral lesions of the brainstem or thalamus produce coma. Diffuse lesions of the hemispheres produce an "awake" patient who shows no responsiveness to the environment, a state called *coma vigil*. Less severe, diffuse abnormalities of the association cortex produce encephalopathy, delirium, or dementia. Focal lesions of the cerebral cortex generally produce deficits in specific cognitive systems.

The frontal lobes are involved in integration of the functions provided by other areas of cortex. Frontal lobe lesions may affect personality and behavior in the absence of easily discernible deficits of specific cognitive, language, or memory function. After commissurotomy, each hemisphere seems to have a separate consciousness. The left hemisphere has the capacity for speech and language. The right hemisphere cannot produce verbal accounts of items seen in the left visual field, but the subject can choose the correct item by pointing with the left hand.

MEMORY

Memory Stages

Memory refers to the ability of the brain to store and retrieve information. Clinical neurologists divide memory into three temporal stages. The first stage, *immediate memory span*, corresponds to *working memory*. *Immediate memory* refers to the amount of information a subject can keep in conscious awareness without active memorization. The normal human being can retain seven digits in active memory span. The second stage of memory, *short-term* or *recent* memory, involves the ability to register and recall specific items after a delay of minutes or hours. This second stage of memory requires the function of the hippocampus and parahippocampal areas of the medial temporal lobe for both storage and retrieval. *Long-term* or *remote memory* refers to long-known information, such as where one grew up, who was one's first-grade teacher, or the names of grandparents. Remote memory resists the effects of medial temporal damage; once memory is well stored, probably in the neocortex, retrieval does not use the hippocampal system.

Amnestic Syndrome

The *amnestic syndrome* refers to profound loss of the second stage of recent or short-term memory. These patients, most of whom have bilateral hippocampal damage, have normal immediate memory span and largely normal ability to recall remote memories, such as their childhood upbringing and education.

Syndromes of Partial Memory Loss

In contrast to the global amnesia seen in the amnestic syndrome, some patients have memory loss for selected classes of items. Patients who have undergone left temporal lobectomy for intractable epilepsy usually have detectable impairment of short-term verbal memory, whereas those who have undergone right temporal resection have impairment only of nonverbal memory. Isolated sensory-specific memory loss syndromes, such as pure visual or tactile memory loss, occur as well.

Transient Amnesia

Transient amnesia is a temporary version of the amnestic syndrome. The most striking example is the syndrome of transient global amnesia, lasting from several hours to 24 hours. An otherwise cognitively intact individual suddenly loses memory for recent events, asks repetitive questions about the environment, and sometimes confabulates. During the episode, the patient has both anterograde and retrograde amnesia, as in the permanent amnestic syndrome. As recovery occurs, the retrograde portion "shrinks" to a short period, leaving a permanent gap in memory of the brief retrograde amnesia before the episode and the period of no learning during the episode. The cause of the syndrome is unknown.

Bedside Tests of Memory and Cognitive Function

The most widely used bedside test is the Mini-Mental State examination (MMSE). The MMSE consists of 30 points:

    5 for orientation to time (year, season, month, date, and day)
    5 for orientation to place (state, county, town, hospital, and floor)
    5 for attention (either serial 7s with 1 point for each of the first five subtractions or "spell *world* backward")
    3 for registration of three items
    3 for recall of three items after 5 minutes
    2 for naming a pencil and a watch
    1 for repeating "no ifs, ands, or buts"

3 for following a three-stage command
1 for following a printed command "close your eyes"
1 for writing a sentence
1 for copying a diagram of two intersecting pentagons

For a more detailed discussion, see Chapter 6 in Neurology in Clinical Practice, 4th edition.

Behavior and Personality Disturbances, Depression, and Psychosis

4

Behavioral and personality disturbances are common in individuals with neurological disease, traumatic brain injury, and stroke. Identification and treatment of behavioral disturbances are critical because they are associated with reduced functional capacity, decreased quality of life, greater economic cost, larger care burden, and increased morbidity.

DEMENTIA

Alzheimer's Disease

The behavioral disturbances in patients with Alzheimer's disease (AD) include affective symptoms, agitation, aggression, and psychosis. These disturbances are associated with increased care, patient and caregiver abuse, greater use of psychotropic medications, more rapid cognitive decline, and earlier institutionalization. Once psychiatric symptoms are present, they often recur. Early identification and intervention may help alleviate the psychiatric disturbance in AD and may contribute to improved outcomes.

The true prevalence of depression in AD is unknown. The probability of depression in AD appears to be greater if there is a history of depression either in the patient or in the family. Selective serotonin reuptake inhibitors (SSRIs) are the preferred treatment for depression. *Apathy*, defined as diminished motivation not attributable to decreased level of consciousness, cognitive impairment, or emotional distress, is the most common behavioral change noted in AD and may occur in up to 92% of patients. Aggressive verbalizations and acts occur in 25–67%. Verbal aggression is more common in men and in individuals with delusions or agitation. The response rate of sertraline is 38% for the treatment of aggression and irritability in AD. The cumulative 4-year incidence of new-onset psychosis of AD is 51%. The most common psychotic symptoms in patients with AD are delusions and hallucinations. The delusions are typically paranoid type, nonbizarre, and simple. The hallucinations in AD are more often visual than auditory; the reverse is true for schizophrenia. Atypical antipsychotics are the preferred method of treatment.

Frontotemporal Dementia

Frontotemporal dementia (FTD), previously called *Pick's disease*, is composed of at least three syndromes: semantic dementia, progressive nonfluent aphasia, and frontal lobe degeneration of non-Alzheimer's type. Individuals with FTD exhibit symptoms of orbitofrontal syndrome, such as disinhibition, poor impulse control, tactlessness, and poor judgment. Loss of empathy, mental inflexibility, and stereotyped behaviors are common. Social relationships are inappropriate. Approximately 20% of patients exhibit delusions and 7% hallucinations.

Vascular Dementia

Vascular dementia primarily disrupts frontal-subcortical circuits. Behavioral disturbances are common and result in challenges to health care providers and caregivers, apathy, and depression. Those with depression are less likely to have had a stroke and more likely to have a history of depression. Apathy is associated with increased impairment in both basic and instrumental activities of daily living. Delusions (33%) and visual hallucinations (13–25%) are associated with impaired cognitive functioning. Nineteen percent are anxious. Generalized anxiety disorder is more common than panic disorder. Anxiety is not associated with severity of cognitive impairment or changes in functional abilities.

Dementia with Lewy Bodies

Psychotic symptoms, particularly hallucinations, are a hallmark of dementia with Lewy bodies. Most individuals experience visual hallucinations. Insight is usually poor. The observed psychotic symptoms are similar to those seen in l-dopa–induced psychosis. Mania is unusual. Avoid typical neuroleptics because individuals may experience severe parkinsonian symptoms. Neuroleptics, such as clozapine and quetiapine, as well as cholinesterase inhibitors, improve cognition and decrease psychotic symptoms.

Human Immunodeficiency Virus Disease

The lifetime rate of major depression in individuals infected with human immunodeficiency virus is approximately 50%. Approximately 25% meet criteria for an anxiety disorder.

MOVEMENT DISORDERS

Parkinson's Disease

Depression is the most common psychiatric disturbance in persons with Parkinson's disease (PD). The overall frequency is 70%. Risk factors for depression in PD include greater cognitive impairment, earlier disease onset, and family history of depression. SSRIs are first-line therapy for depression but may worsen motor symptoms. In such cases, tricyclic antidepressants are an effective alternative. Paroxetine decreases depressive symptoms in PD. Hallucinations occur in 40% and delusions in 16% of patients. The prevalence of psychotic symptoms is greatest in patients with greater cognitive impairment, longer duration of illness, greater daytime somnolence, older age, and institutional care.

Progressive Supranuclear Palsy

Psychiatric and behavioral symptoms are common in progressive supranuclear palsy. Nearly all patients are apathetic, about half exhibit a change in personality, and less than half suffer from depression. Disinhibition, or loss of emotional control, occurs in one third.

Huntington's Disease

Psychiatric and behavioral symptoms are common in Huntington's disease (HD) and may be the presenting features of disease. Depression occurs in up to 63% of patients and often precedes the onset of neurological symptoms. Mania occurs in 2–12% of patients. Suicide is more common in HD than in other neurological disorders with high rates of depression. The critical periods are when neurological signs first appear and again later in the disease. Psychosis associated with HD is more resistant to treatment than psychosis in schizophrenia. Early signs of HD may include withdrawal from activities and friends, decline in personal appearance, lack of behavioral initiation, decreased spontaneous speech, and constriction of emotional expression.

Tourette's Syndrome

Psychiatric comorbidity is common. Attention-deficit/hyperactivity disorder (ADHD), obsessive-compulsive disorder (OCD), and oppositional defiant disorder (ODD) are estimated to co-occur in 40–70% of individuals with Tourette's syndrome (TS). ADHD symptoms may precede the onset of TS by 2–3 years. Approximately 30% of individuals with TS meet criteria for OCD.

MULTIPLE SCLEROSIS

The rate of depression in multiple sclerosis (MS) is 37–54%. Many experience depression before disease onset. Some report symptoms of depression even with outward signs of euphoria. Additionally, 73% report difficulty in controlling their emotions and 57% report increased irritability. Depression in MS is *not* associated with increased rates of stressful events, disease duration, MS type, age, gender, or socioeconomic status. The rate of depression is higher than with other chronic disabling disorders. Anxiety occurs in 25% of individuals with MS. The combination of anxiety and depression is strongly associated with somatic complaints, social difficulties, and suicidal ideation. The prevalence of euphoria is 25%. Such individuals are more likely to have cerebral involvement, enlarged ventricles, poorer cognitive and neurological function, and increased social disability.

AMYOTROPHIC LATERAL SCLEROSIS

Eleven percent of individuals with amyotrophic lateral sclerosis (ALS) meet criteria for major depressive disorder. Depression in ALS is associated with increased physical impairment.

EPILEPSY

Behavior and personality disturbances occur in up to 50% of individuals with epilepsy. Specific risk factors include additional brain injury, type and severity of epilepsy syndrome, and medication effects. Depression is the most common psychiatric disorder in epilepsy (8–63%). Depression in epilepsy typically runs a chronic course, with periods of major depression separated by periods of dysthymic mood. The suicide rate in epilepsy is four times that of the general population. The suicide rate in temporal lobe epilepsy is 25 times that of the general population. Risk factors include history of self-harm, family history of suicide, stressful life situations, poor morale, stigma, and psychiatric disorders.

STROKE

Within the first year after stroke, one third of individuals experience depression. Most occur within the first month. Depression is associated with longer hospital stays, poorer recovery, and increased morbidity. Left-sided lesions closer to the frontal pole are associated with depression immediately after stroke. At 1–2 years after stroke, depression is associated with nearness of the lesion to the frontal pole in the right hemisphere. Nortriptyline is more effective in the treatment of depression than either placebo or fluoxetine.

For a more detailed discussion, see Chapters 8 and 9 in Neurology in Clinical Practice, 4th edition.

Apraxia and Agnosias

5

APRAXIA

The motor system requires at least two major types of programs to deal effectively with the environment. One is *praxis* and the other is *intentional*. The praxis programs provide the knowledge of *how* to make learned skilled movements, whereas the intentional programs provide the knowledge of *when* to move.

Praxic (How) Disorders

The "how," or praxis, programs provide several types of instructions:

1. How to position one's limb when performing skilled movements.
2. How to move one's limbs in space.
3. How to orient a limb toward a target.
4. How rapidly to move a limb in space.
5. How to imitate a movement.
6. How to solve mechanical problems.
7. How to order components of an act to achieve a goal.

Disorders of this praxic system are called *apraxias*. A loss of the ability to make precise and independent movement (i.e., a loss of deftness) is called *limb-kinetic apraxia*. The term for failure to position, move, or orient a limb correctly in space is *ideomotor apraxia* (IMA). Patients with IMA also make temporal errors. Patients who perform imitation worse than gesture to command have *conduction apraxia*. Patients with *disassociation apraxia* may be impaired when attempting to perform skilled movements in response to stimuli in one modality (e.g., verbal command) but able to correctly perform movements in response to stimuli in a different modality (e.g., seeing a tool). The inability to solve mechanical problems is termed *conceptual apraxia*. Lastly, the inability to order correctly a series of movements is termed *ideational apraxia*. In the following sections we discuss each of these disorders.

Limb-Kinetic Apraxia
Patients with limb-kinetic apraxia demonstrate a loss of deftness or the ability to make finely graded, precise, independent finger movements.

Ideomotor Apraxia
Ideomotor apraxia is probably the most common type of apraxia. When patients with IMA perform learned skilled movements, including pantomimes, imitations, and use of actual objects, they make spatial and temporal errors.

Conduction Apraxia
Patients with conduction apraxia, unlike patients with IMA who improve with imitation, are more impaired when imitating than when pantomiming to command.

Disassociation Apraxia
When asked to use pantomime, patients with disassociation apraxia look at their hand but are unable to perform any recognizable actions. Their imitation and use of objects are flawless.

Ideational Apraxia
When performing a task that requires a series of acts, patients with ideational apraxia have difficulty sequencing the acts in the proper order.

Conceptual Apraxia
Patients with conceptual apraxia may not recall the type of actions associated with specific tools, utensils, or objects (tool-object action knowledge) and therefore make content errors.

Clinical Pathology
The different forms of limb apraxia discussed in this chapter are most commonly associated with strokes and degenerative dementia of the Alzheimer's and Pick's types. Apraxia occurs with many other diseases of the central nervous system, including tumors and trauma. Certain forms of apraxia (i.e., limb-kinetic and ideomotor) may be the presenting symptom of basal ganglia disorders such as corticobasal degeneration.

Intentional (When) Disorders

Four types of intentional instructions exist: (1) when to start a movement, (2) when not to start a movement, (3) when to continue or sustain a movement or posture, and (4) when to stop or complete a movement. The inability to initiate a movement in the absence of a corticospinal or motor unit lesion is termed *akinesia. Hypokinesia* is a delay in initiating a response. Inability to withhold a response to a sensory stimulus is *defective response inhibition.* Inability to sustain a movement or posture is *motor impersistence,* and the inability to stop a movement or an action program is *motor perseveration. Hypometria* refers to movements of decreased amplitude. *Motor impersistence* is the inability to sustain a motor act.

Defective Response Inhibition
Defective response inhibition is responding when no response of that body part is required. Defective response inhibition occurs in the eyes, head, or limbs.

Motor Perseveration
Perseveration is the incorrect repeating of a prior response.

Pathophysiology of Intentional or "When" Disorders
The frontal lobes play a central role in a human's intentional network. Any neurological disease that impairs the frontal lobes and the cingulate corpus callosum region can cause intentional disorders.

AGNOSIA

The word *agnosia* is Greek for "not knowing" and refers to a class of neuropsychological disorders in which patients fail to recognize familiar objects despite seemingly adequate perception, memory, language, and general intellectual ability.

Visual Agnosia

Apperceptive-Associative Distinction
Disorders of visual recognition can be divided into two types, apperceptive agnosia and associative agnosia. Apperceptive agnosics have a disorder of complex visual perceptual processes. They can describe their visual experience but do not have sufficient higher level visual perception to enable object recognition. In contrast to apperceptive agnosia, patients with associative agnosia have difficulty associating a perceptual representation with more general knowledge. A normal percept is stripped of its meaning.

Apperceptive Visual Agnosia
Patients with apperceptive visual agnosia are not cortically blind. They have conscious visual experience, yet their visual

perceptual processes are abnormal and cause impairment in object recognition. The brain damage in most cases of apperceptive agnosia is diffuse and posterior.

Associative Visual Agnosia
Associative visual agnosia refers to an impairment of visual object recognition not due to a more basic perceptual deficit, as seen in apperceptive visual agnosia, or to a higher order disorder of language, communication, intellectual impairment, or other deficits. Patients with associative visual agnosia are able to make good copies of objects that they cannot recognize.

Prosopagnosia
Prosopagnosics cannot recognize familiar people by their faces alone and must rely on other cues for recognition, such as voice, distinctive clothing, or hairstyle. The impairment of facial recognition represents damage to a distinct system for face recognition.

Pure Alexia
Pure alexia is an impairment of visual word recognition, in the context of intact auditory word recognition and writing ability. Pure alexia occurs alone or in association with visual object agnosia.

Auditory Agnosia

Auditory agnosia is a group of disorders characterized by a failure to recognize verbal or nonverbal sounds. They may be thought of as a spectrum of disorders, bounded by cortical deafness on one end and disorders of language and thought at the other.

Nonverbal Auditory Agnosia
Patients with nonverbal auditory agnosia fail to recognize common objects and events by their sounds, such as a dog barking, keys jingling, or a door slamming. Although the patients are not cortically deaf, most present with the clinical picture of cortical deafness.

Pure Word Deafness
Pure word deafness (*auditory agnosia for speech* or *verbal auditory agnosia*) is characterized by a disturbance in comprehension of spoken language not explainable by the more generalized auditory processing defects seen in cortical deafness or the broader linguistic impairments typical of Wernicke's aphasia or transcortical sensory aphasia.

Tactile Agnosia
Tactile agnosia refers to a disorder of object recognition via the tactile modality that cannot be attributed to a more basic somatosensory impairment, language dysfunction, hemispatial neglect, or generalized intellectual impairment.

For a more detailed discussion, see Chapters 10 and 11 in Neurology in Clinical Practice, 4th edition.

Language Disorders

6

APHASIA

Aphasia is an acquired disorder of language secondary to brain damage. This definition separates aphasia from congenital or developmental language disorders, called *dysphasias*. Aphasia is a disorder of language rather than speech. *Speech* is the articulation and phonation of language sounds; *language* is a complex system of communication symbols and rules for their use. Aphasia is distinguished from motor speech disorders, which include dysarthria, dysphonia (voice disorders), stuttering, and speech apraxia. *Dysarthrias* are disorders of articulation of single sounds that may result from mechanical disturbance of the tongue or larynx or from neurological disorders. *Apraxia of speech* is a syndrome of misarticulation of phonemes, especially consonant sounds. Unlike dysarthria, in which certain phonemes are consistently distorted, apraxia of speech contains inconsistent distortions and substitutions of phonemes.

Symptoms and Differential Diagnosis of Disordered Language

Muteness, a total loss of speech, may represent severe aphasia. A good rule is that if the patient can write or type and the language form and content are normal, the muteness is probably not aphasic in origin. Hesitant speech is a symptom not only of aphasia but also of motor speech disorders (dysarthria or stuttering), and of a psychogenic disorder. A second rule is that if one can transcribe the utterances of a hesitant speaker into normal language, the patient is not aphasic. *Anomia*, or inability to produce a specific name, is generally a reliable indicator of language disorder, although it may also reflect memory loss. *Paraphasic errors* are divided into literal or phonemic errors, characterized by substitution of an incorrect sound (e.g., *shoon* for *spoon*), and verbal or semantic errors, characterized by

41

substitution of an incorrect word (e.g., *fork* for *spoon*). A related language symptom is *perseveration*, the inappropriate repetition of a previous response. Occasionally, aphasic utterances involve nonexistent word forms called *neologisms*. A pattern of paraphasic errors and neologisms that contaminate speech so the meaning cannot be discerned is called *jargon speech*. Another cardinal symptom of aphasia is the failure to comprehend the speech of others.

Bedside Language Examination

The six-part bedside-language examination provides useful localizing information about brain dysfunction.

1. *Spontaneous speech*: A speech sample is elicited by asking the patient to describe the weather or the reason for coming to the doctor. The most important variable in spontaneous speech is fluency: Fluent speech flows rapidly and effortlessly; nonfluent speech is uttered in single words or short phrases, with frequent pauses and hesitations. The content of speech utterances should be analyzed in terms of the presence of word-finding pauses, circumlocutions, and errors such as paraphasias and neologisms.

2. *Naming*: The patient is asked to name objects, object parts, pictures, colors, or body parts to confrontation. The examiner should ask questions to be sure that the patient recognizes the items or people that cannot be named by the patient.

3. *Auditory comprehension*: The patient is asked to follow a series of commands of one, two, and three steps. Successful following of commands ensures adequate comprehension, but failure to follow commands does not establish loss of comprehension. The patient must hear the command, understand the language the examiner speaks, and possess the motor ability to execute it.

4. *Repetition of words and phrases*: Dysarthric patients have difficulty with rapid sequences of consonants, such as *Methodist Episcopal*, whereas aphasics have special difficulty with grammatically complex sentences. The phrase "no ifs, ands, or buts" is especially challenging.

5. *Reading*: Reading should be tested both aloud and for comprehension. The examiner should carry a few printed commands to facilitate a rapid comparison of auditory to reading comprehension.

6. *Writing*: Writing not only provides a further sample of expressive language but also allows an analysis of spelling. A specimen of writing may be the most sensitive indicator

of mild aphasia, and it provides a permanent record for comparison.

Differential Diagnosis of Aphasic Syndromes

Broca's Aphasia

The speech pattern in Broca's aphasia is nonfluent, mute, or telegraphic. Naming is impaired. Auditory comprehension is intact with some deficiency in the comprehension of complex syntax. Repetition, reading, and writing are impaired. Associated signs are right hemiparesis, hemisensory loss, apraxia of the oral apparatus and the nonparalyzed left limbs, and depression. *Aphemia*, a rare variant of Broca's aphasia, is a nonfluent syndrome in which the patient is initially mute and then able to speak with phoneme substitutions and pauses. All other language functions are intact, including writing. Aphemia is usually a transitory syndrome and results from small lesions of Broca's area, its subcortical white matter, or the inferior precentral gyrus.

Wernicke's Aphasia

Spontaneous speech in Wernicke's aphasia is fluent, with paraphasic errors. Naming is impaired, often with bizarre paraphasic misnaming. Comprehension, repetition, and reading for comprehension are impaired. Writing is well formed but usually as impaired as spontaneous speech. Right hemianopia is sometimes associated, but motor and sensory functions in the limbs are usually normal. Depression is less common than in Broca's aphasia. The brain lesions associated with Wernicke's aphasia are usually in the posterior portion of the superior temporal gyrus, sometimes extending into the inferior parietal lobe.

Pure Word Deafness

Pure word deafness is a rare but striking syndrome of isolated loss of auditory comprehension and repetition, without any abnormality of speech, naming, reading, or writing. Hearing for pure tones and for nonverbal noises, such as animal cries, is intact. Most cases have mild aphasic deficits, especially paraphasic speech. The anatomical substrate is a bilateral lesion, isolating Wernicke's area from input from both Heschl's gyri.

Global Aphasia

Global aphasia is the summation of Broca's and Wernicke's aphasia. Speech is nonfluent or mute, but comprehension is also poor, as are naming, repetition, reading, and writing. Most patients have a dense right hemiparesis, hemisensory loss, and often hemianopia. The lesions are usually large, involving both the inferior frontal and the superior temporal regions and often much of the intervening parietal lobe.

Conduction Aphasia

Repetition is the main difficulty in conduction aphasia. Spontaneous speech is usually normal, except some patients make paraphasic errors and hesitate frequently for self-correction. Naming may be impaired, but auditory comprehension is preserved. Repetition is so disturbed that even single words cannot be repeated. Hemianopia and hemisensory loss are sometimes associated, but motor ability is normal. The lesions are usually in either the superior temporal or the inferior parietal region.

Anomic Aphasia

Naming, access to the internal lexicon, is the principal deficit of anomic aphasia. Spontaneous speech is normal except for the pauses and circumlocutions produced by the inability to name. Comprehension, repetition, reading, and writing are intact. Isolated, severe anomia may indicate focal left hemisphere pathology.

Transcortical Aphasias

Lesions that disrupt connections from other cortical centers into the language circuit cause transcortical aphasias. The three syndromes of transcortical aphasia are analogues of global, Broca's, and Wernicke's aphasias, with intact repetition.

Subcortical Aphasias

Lesions in the basal ganglia or deep cerebral white matter define the subcortical aphasias. Left thalamic hemorrhages often produce a Wernicke-like fluent aphasia in which comprehension is better than in cortical Wernicke's aphasia. The patient's state may alternate between alert with nearly normal language and drowsiness with paraphasic mumbling and poor comprehension. Lesions of the left basal ganglia and deep white matter cause an "anterior subcortical aphasia syndrome" involving dysarthria, decreased fluency, mildly impaired repetition, and mild comprehension disturbance. More posterior lesions involving the putamen and deep temporal white matter are associated with fluent, paraphasic speech, and impaired comprehension resembling Wernicke's aphasia. In general, subcortical aphasias produce atypical aphasias that are difficult to classify and are often associated with dysarthria and right hemiparesis.

Pure Alexia without Agraphia

Patients with pure alexia without agraphia can write but cannot read their own written productions. Speech, auditory comprehension, and repetition are normal. Naming may be deficient, especially for colors. A right hemianopia or right upper quadrant defect is almost always associated. The causative lesion in pure alexia is nearly always a stroke in the territory of the left posterior cerebral artery, with infarction of the medial occipital lobe, the splenium of the corpus callosum, and often the medial temporal lobe. It is a disconnection syndrome, with one intact right visual cortex disconnected from the left hemisphere.

Alexia with Agraphia

Alexia with agraphia may be thought of as an acquired illiteracy, in which a previously educated patient becomes unable to read or write. Associated deficits include right hemianopia and elements of the Gerstmann syndrome: agraphia, acalculia, right–left disorientation, and finger agnosia. The lesions are typically in the inferior parietal lobule, especially the angular gyrus.

Agraphia

Writing may be affected in isolation (*pure agraphia*) or in association with aphasia (*aphasic agraphia*). In addition, writing can be impaired by motor disorders, by apraxia, and by visuospatial deficits. Isolated agraphia has been described with left frontal or parietal lesions.

Aphasic Alexia

In addition to the two classic alexia syndromes, many patients with aphasia have associated reading disturbance. Four patterns of alexia are recognized: (1) *Letter-by-letter dyslexia* is equivalent to pure alexia without agraphia; (2) *deep dyslexia* is a severe reading disorder in which patients recognize and read aloud only familiar words, especially concrete, imaginable nouns and verbs; (3) *phonological dyslexia* is similar to deep dyslexia, with poor reading of nonwords, but single nouns and verbs are read in a nearly normal fashion, and semantic errors are rare; and (4) *surface dyslexia* involves spared ability to read laboriously by grapheme-phoneme conversion but inability to recognize words at a glance.

Agraphia

Like reading, writing may be affected either in isolation (pure agraphia) or in association with aphasia (*aphasic agraphia*). In addition, writing can be impaired by motor disorders, by apraxia, and by visuospatial deficits. Isolated agraphia has been described with left frontal or parietal lesions.

Language in Right Hemisphere Disorders

Left-handed patients may have right hemisphere language dominance and may develop aphasic syndromes from right hemisphere lesions. Right-handed patients occasionally become aphasic after right hemisphere strokes (*crossed aphasia*). These patients presumably have crossed or mixed dominance. Even in right-handed persons with left hemisphere dominance, right hemisphere damage may impair the affective aspects of language, making it sound flat and unemotional. Syndromes of loss of emotional aspects of speech are termed *aprosodias.*

Language in Dementing Diseases

Two patterns of language impairment occur in patients with dementia. Early Alzheimer's disease shows impairments in naming and discourse, impoverished language content, and loss of abstraction and metaphor. Grammatical construction of sentences, receptive vocabulary, auditory comprehension, repetition, and oral reading tend to remain preserved until later stages. The second pattern is one of gradual progressive aphasia, often without other cognitive deterioration. The pathology of primary progressive aphasia may show frontotemporal atrophy, lobar atrophy of Pick's disease, or spongiform degeneration.

Recovery and Rehabilitation of Aphasia

Patients with aphasia from acute disorders, such as stroke, generally show spontaneous improvement over days, weeks, and months. In general, the greatest recovery occurs during the first 3 months, but improvement may continue over a prolonged period, especially in young patients and in global aphasics. Speech therapy, provided by speech-language pathologists, attempts to facilitate language recovery by a variety of techniques and to help the patient compensate for lost functions. Other techniques include melodic intonation therapy, which uses melody to involve the right hemisphere in speech production; visual action therapy, which uses gestural expression; and treatment of aphasic perseveration, which aims to reduce repetitive utterances. Large randomized trials have clearly indicated that patients who undergo formal speech therapy recover better than untreated patients.

A new approach to language rehabilitation is the use of pharmacological agents to improve speech. The dopaminergic drug bromocriptine promotes spontaneous speech output in transcortical motor aphasia. Other studies support use of the drug in nonfluent aphasias.

DYSARTHRIA AND APRAXIA OF SPEECH

Motor Speech Disorders

Motor speech disorders are syndromes of abnormal articulation, the motor production of speech, without abnormalities of language. A patient with a motor speech disorder should be able to produce normal expressive language in writing and to comprehend both spoken and written language. Motor speech disorders include *dysarthrias*, disorders of speech articulation, *apraxia of speech*, a motor programming disorder for speech, and five rarer syndromes: *aphemia*, *foreign accent syndrome*, *acquired stuttering*, *primary progressive anarthria*, and the *opercular syndrome*.

Dysarthrias
Dysarthria is the abnormal articulation of sounds or phonemes because of abnormal activation of the oromandibular pharyngeal muscles. The speed, strength, timing, range, or accuracy of speech may be affected. Dysarthria is generally related to dysfunction of the central nervous system, nerves, neuromuscular junction, or muscles. Dysarthria can affect articulation, phonation, breathing, or prosody (emotional tone) of speech. Total loss of ability to articulate is called *anarthria*, whereas dysarthria usually involves the distortion of consonant sounds.

The Mayo Clinic classification of dysarthria includes six categories: (1) flaccid, (2) spastic and "unilateral upper motor neuron," (3) ataxic, (4) hypokinetic, (5) hyperkinetic, and (6) mixed dysarthria. *Flaccid* dysarthria is associated with disorders involving lower motor neuron weakness of the bulbar muscles. The speech pattern is breathy and nasal, with indistinctly pronounced consonants. *Spastic* dysarthria occurs in patients with bilateral lesions of the motor cortex or corticobulbar tracts, such as bilateral strokes. The speech is harsh or a "strain strangle" in vocal quality, with reduced rate, low pitch, and consonant errors. A milder variant of spastic dysarthria, *unilateral upper motor neuron* dysarthria, is associated with unilateral upper motor neuron lesions. This dysarthria is similar to spastic dysarthria, only less severe. Unilateral upper motor neuron dysarthria is one of the most common types of dysarthria, occurring in patients with unilateral strokes. *Ataxic* dysarthria associated with cerebellar disorders is characterized by one of two patterns: irregular breakdowns of speech with explosions of syllables interrupted by pauses or a slow cadence of speech with excessively equal stress on every syllable. The second pattern of ataxic dysarthria is referred to as *scanning speech.* Hypokinetic dysarthria, the typical speech pattern in Parkinson's disease, is notable for decreased and monotonous loudness and pitch, rapid rate, and occasional consonant errors. *Hyperkinetic* dysarthria, a pattern in some ways opposite to hypokinetic dysarthria, is characterized by marked variation in rate, loudness, and timing, with distortion of vowels, harsh voice quality, and occasional sudden stoppages of speech. This speech pattern is seen in hyperkinetic movement disorders such as Huntington's disease. *Mixed* dysarthria involves combinations of the other five types. One common mixed dysarthria is a spastic-flaccid dysarthria seen in amyotrophic lateral sclerosis.

The management of dysarthria includes speech therapy techniques to strengthen muscles, training of more precise articulations, slowing the rate of speech to increase intelligibility, and teaching the patient to stress specific phonemes. Devices such as pacing boards to slow articulation, palatal lifts to reduce hypernasality, amplifiers to increase voice volume, communication boards for patients to point to pictures, and augmentative communication devices and computer techniques can be used when the patient is unable to communicate in speech. Injections of collagen into the vocal folds and surgical procedures such as a pharyngeal flap to reduce hypernasality or vocal fold transposition to increase loudness may help the patient speak more intelligibly.

Apraxia of Speech

Apraxia of speech is a disorder of the programming of articulation of sequences of phonemes, especially consonants. The motor speech system makes errors in the selection of consonant phonemes, in the absence of any weakness, slowness, or incoordination of the muscles of speech articulation. The term *apraxia of speech* implies that the disorder is one of a skilled sequential motor activity, rather than a primary motor disorder. Consonants are usually substituted rather than distorted, as in dysarthria. Patients have special difficulty with polysyllabic words and consonant shifts, as well as in initiating articulation of a word. Errors are inconsistent from one attempt to the next, in contrast to the consistent distortion of phonemes in dysarthria.

The four cardinal features of apraxia of speech are as follows: (1) effortful, groping, or "trial-and-error" attempts at speech, with efforts at self-correction; (2) dysprosody; (3) inconsistencies in articulation errors; and (4) difficulty with initiating utterances. Apraxia of speech is rare in isolation but often contributes to the speech and language deficit of Broca's aphasia. A patient with apraxia of speech, in addition to aphasia, often writes better than speaks, and comprehension is relatively preserved. Patients with apraxia of speech always have damage in the left hemisphere insula, whereas patients without apraxia of speech do not.

Oral or buccolingual apraxia

Buccolingual apraxia is ideomotor apraxia for learned movements of the tongue, lips, and larynx. Oral apraxia can be elicited by asking the patient to lick his or her upper lip, smile, or stick out the tongue.

Aphemia

Aphemia is reserved for a syndrome of near muteness, with normal comprehension, reading, and writing. Aphemia is clearly a motor speech disorder rather than aphasia. Patients are often anarthric, with no speech whatever, and then effortful nonfluent speech emerges. Some patients have persisting dysarthria, with dysphonia and sometimes distortions of articulation that sound similar to foreign accents. In general, aphemia involves lesions near the primary motor cortex and perhaps Broca's area, whereas apraxia of speech may be localized to the insula.

The Foreign Accent Syndrome

The foreign accent syndrome is an acquired form of motor speech disorder related to dysarthria, in which the patient acquires a dysfluency resembling a foreign accent, usually after a unilateral stroke. Lesions often involve the motor cortex of the left hemisphere and may coexist with aphasia.

Acquired Stuttering

An uncommon motor speech disorder following acquired brain lesions is a pattern resembling developmental stuttering, referred to as *acquired* or *cortical stuttering*. Acquired stuttering involves hesitancy in producing initial phonemes, with an associated dysrhythmia of speech. Acquired stuttering overlaps apraxia of speech but may lack the other features. Acquired stuttering is described most often in patients with left hemisphere cortical strokes. Recurrence of childhood stuttering occurs in patients with Parkinson's disease, suggesting involvement of the dopaminergic system.

Opercular Syndrome

The opercular syndrome is a severe form of pseudobulbar palsy in which patients with bilateral lesions of the perisylvian cortex or subcortical connections become completely mute. These patients can follow commands involving the extremities but not of the cranial nerves; for example, they may be unable to open or close their eyes or mouth or smile voluntarily, yet they smile when amused, yawn spontaneously, and even utter cries in response to emotional stimuli. The syndrome is usually seen in adults after multiple strokes but also occurs in children with bilateral malformations of the opercula.

For a more detailed discussion, see Chapter 12 in Neurology in Clinical Practice, 4th edition.

Neurogenic Dysphagia

7

Impaired swallowing, or dysphagia, can originate from disturbances in the mouth, pharynx, or esophagus and can involve mechanical, musculoskeletal, or neurogenic mechanisms. This chapter focuses on neuromuscular and neurogenic causes of dysphagia.

NORMAL SWALLOWING

The process of swallowing can be broken down into three distinct stages or phases: oral, pharyngeal, and esophageal. The oral phase of swallowing comprises the horizontal subsystem and is largely volitional in character, whereas the pharyngeal and esophageal phases comprise the vertical subsystem and are primarily under reflex control. Within the brainstem, swallowing appears to be regulated by central pattern generators that contain the programs directing the sequential movements of the various muscles involved with swallowing.

MECHANICAL DYSPHAGIA

Structural abnormalities from the mouth to the esophagus can interfere with swallowing on a strictly mechanical basis. Such abnormalities include congenital anomalies, tumors, and inflammatory processes of the face and neck.

NEUROMUSCULAR DYSPHAGIA

Several neuromuscular diseases involve the oropharyngeal and esophageal musculature and produce dysphagia as part of a

Table 7.1: Neurogenic dysphagia

Oropharyngeal	Motor neuron diseases
Arnold-Chiari malformation	Amyotrophic lateral sclerosis
Basal ganglia diseases	Multiple sclerosis
Central pontine myelinolysis	Peripheral neuropathic
Cerebral palsy	processes
Drug-related	Charcot-Marie-Tooth
Cyclosporin	disease
Tardive dyskinesia	Guillain-Barré syndrome
Vincristine	(Miller Fisher variant)
Infectious	Spinocerebellar ataxias
Brainstem encephalitis	Stroke
Listeria	Syringobulbia
Epstein-Barr virus	Esophageal
Diphtheria	Achalasia
Poliomyelitis	Autonomic neuropathies
Progressive multifocal	Diabetes mellitus
leukoencephalopathy	Familial dysautonomia
Rabies	Paraneoplastic syndromes
Mass lesions	Basal ganglia disorders
Abscess	Parkinson's disease
Hemorrhage	Chagas' disease
Metastatic tumor	Esophageal motility disorders
Primary tumor	Scleroderma

larger syndrome of weakness. Table 7.1 lists the disorders discussed in several other chapters.

EVALUATION OF DYSPHAGIA

Various diagnostic tests, ranging from simple bedside analysis to sophisticated radiological and neurophysiological procedures, have been developed to evaluate dysphagia. Other specialists perform most of these tests, but neurologists should be aware of when to request services. A barium swallow is the primary test for oral phase and pharyngeal phase dysfunction. Oral phase dysfunction is suspected when the patient has difficulty in initiating swallowing or has repetitive swallowing. Pharyngeal phase dysfunction is suspected when the patient has a retrosternal "hanging up" sensation. The primary test is a modified barium swallow. Complementary tests include pharyngeal videoendoscopy and manometry, electromyography, and video manofluorometry. Esophageal dysfunction is suspected when the patient complains of difficulty with both solids and liquids. The primary tests are videofluoroscopy and endoscopy. Difficulty with solids but not liquids suggests a mechanical obstruction.

For a more detailed discussion, see Chapter 13 in Neurology in Clinical Practice, 4th edition.

Disturbances of Vision

8

VISION LOSS

Type and Severity

Central Visual Field Loss

A defect in the field of vision is called a *scotoma*. Loss of central vision involves the central visual field and quickly becomes symptomatic. Peripheral visual field defects such as homonymous hemianopia may be asymptomatic or referred to the eye with the larger homonymous visual field. In predominantly one-sided involvement of the optic chiasm, a central scotoma may be associated with a contralateral silent temporal hemianopia. The cause of central or centrocecal scotomas is usually a disease of the central retina or the optic nerve. Scotomas caused by macular disease are perceived as a black or gray spot in the visual field. Images may also be distorted so that straight edges or geometric figures appear crooked or distorted (*metamorphopsia*). Retinal disease is always the cause of metamorphopsia. Optic nerve lesions, other than those causing central scotomas, characteristically cause areas of absent vision of which the patient is unaware, often in conjunction with decreased appreciation of color and light brightness. Photopsias (light flashes) may be perceived with vitreoretinal traction, retinal disease (e.g., cancer-associated retinopathy), drugs (e.g., digitalis), during the healing phase of optic neuropathies, and as a migraine aura.

Patterns of Visual Field Loss

Visual field defects are classified as prechiasmal, chiasmal, or retrochiasmal. Unilateral prechiasmal lesions affect the visual field in one eye; chiasmal lesions cause binocular, nonhomonymous field defects; and retrochiasmal lesions cause homonymous field defects with variable degrees of congruity, depending on their location.

Vision Loss of Sudden Onset

The three patterns of sudden loss of vision are transient, nonprogressive, and progressive (Table 8.1).

Unilateral Transient Vision Loss

Amaurosis fugax is a transient monocular blindness (TMB) caused by emboli to the retinal circulation from carotid vessels or from the heart. Typical attacks are sudden in onset, last 5–15 minutes, and are usually associated with scotomas described as a shade or curtain pulled down in front of the eye.

TMB can be caused by retinal artery vasospasm and is called "retinal migraine" only if accompanied by migraine headache. Vasospastic TMB is usually benign and often responds to calcium-channel blockers.

Subacute attacks of angle-closure glaucoma are a consideration in the differential diagnosis of intermittent monocular visual loss, especially if the patient complains of halos around lights. This symptom results from corneal edema related to rapid elevations of intraocular pressure. Eye pain and redness may not be associated. *Vision loss in bright light (hemeralopia or day blindness)* may occur in patients with severe impairment of blood flow, presumably from impaired regeneration of photopigments by ocular ischemia. It suggests an internal carotid artery occlusion. *Cone dystrophy* also causes evanescent visual worsening in bright light.

Temporary loss of vision with elevation of body temperature *(Uhthoff's phenomenon)* is most common in optic neuritis associated with demyelinating disease. A *transient obscuration of vision* is a unilateral or bilateral visual loss lasting only seconds. These occur in patients with chronic swelling of the optic discs. The description is a "gray-out" brought on by postural change or straining. Gaze-evoked transient visual obscurations are typical of orbital tumors but also occur with systemic hypotension, temporal arteritis, or retinal venous stasis. Other causes of recurring, remitting visual loss are cystic lesions, such as sphenoid sinus mucocele, craniopharyngioma, and pituitary tumor.

Bilateral Transient Vision Loss

Other than transient visual obscurations, decreased cerebral perfusion is usually the cause of simultaneous complete or incomplete loss of vision in both eyes. Transient blindness in children may occur as a migraine variant, especially when posttraumatic, and as part of the syndrome of benign occipital

Table 8.1: Causes of vision loss

Causes of progressive vision loss
    Anterior visual pathway inflammation (optic neuritis)
    Sarcoidosis
    Meningitis
    Anterior visual pathway compression
    Tumors
    Aneurysms
    Dysthyroid optic neuropathy
    Hereditary optic neuropathies (Leber's hereditary optic
      neuropathy)
    Optic nerve drusen
    Low-tension glaucoma
    Chronic papilledema
    Toxic and nutritional optic neuropathies
    Drugs (e.g., ethambutol)
    Radiation damage to anterior visual pathways
    Paraneoplastic retinopathy or optic neuropathy
Causes of transient monocular blindness
    Embolic cerebrovascular disease
    Migraine (vasospasm)
    Hypoperfusion (hypotension, hyperviscosity, hypercoagulability)
    Ocular (intermittent angle-closure glaucoma, hyphema,
      optic disc edema, partial retinal vein occlusion)
    Vasculitis (e.g., giant cell arteritis)
    Other (Uhthoff's phenomenon, idiopathic, psychogenic)
Causes of bilateral transient vision loss
    Migraine
    Cerebral hypoperfusion
    Thromboembolism
    Systemic hypotension
    Hyperviscosity
    Vascular compression
    Epilepsy
    Papilledema (transient visual obscurations)
Causes of unilateral sudden vision loss, nonprogressive
    Branch or central retinal artery occlusion
    Anterior ischemic optic neuropathy, arteritic or nonarteritic
    Branch or central retinal vein occlusion
    Traumatic optic neuropathy
    Central serous choroidopathy
    Retinal detachment
    Vitreous hemorrhage
    Functional (psychogenic) vision loss
Causes of bilateral sudden vision loss, nonprogressive
    Occipital lobe infarctions
    Pituitary apoplexy
    Functional (psychogenic) vision loss
    Head trauma

epilepsy. Visual migraine auras are the most common cause of bilateral transient visual disturbances in patients younger than 40 years.

Nonprogressive Unilateral Sudden Vision Loss
Cranial (temporal or giant cell) arteritis is a consideration in people older than 60 years. Retrobulbar optic nerve infarction, also *posterior ischemic optic neuropathy*, may occur with hemodynamic shock. Optic nerve infarction from emboli or related to migraine is exceptionally rare. Branch or central retinal artery occlusions are usually embolic or thrombotic in cause. Altitudinal, quadrantic, or complete unilateral visual field loss may occur with retinal arterial occlusions. Occlusion of the central retinal vein presents as sudden vision loss with a characteristic hemorrhagic retinopathy. It usually occurs in adults with systemic hypertension or diabetes.

Nonprogressive Bilateral Sudden Vision Loss
Sudden, permanent vision loss affecting bilateral vision, if not caused by trauma, is usually the result of an infarct in the visual radiations causing a homonymous hemianopia. The site of infarction is the occipital lobe in patients who are otherwise neurologically asymptomatic. Bilateral occipital lobe infarcts can result in tubular visual fields, checkerboard visual fields, or total cortical blindness. Cortical blindness from bilateral occipito-parietal lobe infarcts, when accompanied by denial of the visual defect and confabulation, is called *Anton's syndrome.*

Vision Loss of Sudden Onset with Progression
Unilateral vision loss that appears suddenly and progressively worsens is often caused by optic nerve demyelination (*optic neuritis*). The usual period for worsening is hours to days but almost never longer than 2 weeks. *Devic's disease* (neuromyelitis optica) is the combination of bilateral optic neuritis and transverse myelitis. A long-standing visual loss, when discovered suddenly, is thought to be sudden in onset. The presentation of *Leber's hereditary optic neuropathy* is acute or subacute. The result is often a permanent loss of central vision, usually in men during early adulthood. Both eyes are affected within 1 year, but rarely simultaneously. Although Leber's hereditary optic neuropathy may cause loss of vision in women, it tends to be less severe than in men.

Gradual Visual Loss

Gradual visual loss is typical of a compressive lesion affecting the prechiasmal or chiasmal visual pathways. Pituitary tumors, aneurysms, craniopharyngiomas, meningiomas, gliomas, and granulomatous disease are the more common causes. Hereditary or degenerative diseases of the optic nerve or retina are considerations in patients younger than 20 years. Considerations at all ages are low-tension glaucoma, chronic papilledema from pseudotumor cerebri, toxic and nutritional amblyopias, several medications (ethambutol, isoniazid, chloramphenicol, diiodohydroxyquin, chloroquine, and phenothiazines), radiation damage to the anterior visual pathways, and a rapidly progressive paraneoplastic retinopathy (cancer-associated retinopathy syndrome). Approximately 75% of patients have some form of visual field loss, which may include arcuate defects, sectoral scotomas, enlargement of the blind spot, and generalized visual field constriction.

ABNORMALITIES OF THE OPTIC NERVE AND RETINA

Optic Neuropathy

The following clinical features suggest optic neuropathy: (1) visual loss in association with a swollen, pale, or anomalous optic disc or (2) a normal disc appearance in the setting of vision loss (visual acuity, color vision, or visual field) combined with an afferent pupillary defect. History and examination often establish the specific etiology. The basis for classification of acquired optic neuropathies depends on whether the optic disc appears normal, swollen, or pale.

Swollen Optic Disc

The clarity of the peripapillary nerve fiber layer is the most important distinguishing feature between acquired disc edema (papilledema) and pseudopapilledema. The most common causes of unilateral optic disc edema are optic neuritis, anterior ischemic optic neuropathy (AION), and orbital compressive lesions. Optic nerve function is usually abnormal in each of these entities. Compressive lesions producing disc edema usually involve the intraorbital portion of the optic nerve. Intracranial compressive lesions rarely produce disc edema, unless they raise intracranial pressure. Graves' ophthalmopathy is a nontumorous cause of compressive disc edema. Less common causes of unilateral optic disc edema include central retinal vein occlusion/obstruction and infiltrative disorders, such as leukemia and lymphoma. Infiltration of the optic nerve can occur secondary to carcinomatous, lymphoreticular, and granulomatous processes.

Bilateral Optic Disc Edema
The term *papilledema* refers specifically to optic disc swelling secondary to increased intracranial pressure. In the acute phase, central visual acuity is generally normal. The most common visual field defects are enlargement of the physiological blind spot, concentric constriction, and inferior nasal field loss. Malignant hypertension, diabetic papillopathy, anemia, hyperviscosity syndromes, pickwickian syndrome, hypotension, and severe blood loss are less common causes of bilateral optic disc swelling.

Optic neuropathies with a completely normal disc appearance are classified as retrobulbar optic neuropathies. The most common causes of unilateral retrobulbar optic neuropathy are optic neuritis (most frequently acute demyelinating optic neuritis) and compressive lesions. Bilateral optic neuropathies in which the optic discs appear normal include nutritional optic neuropathy (including tobacco-alcohol amblyopia), Vitamin B12 or folate deficiencies, toxic optic neuropathy (heavy metals), drug-related optic neuropathy (chloramphenicol, isoniazid, ethambutol, ethchlorvynol, chlorpropamide, and others), and inherited optic neuropathies.

Congenital Optic Disc Anomalies
Congenital optic nerve anomalies include drusen, tilted optic disc, and optic nerve dysplasia.

RETINAL DISORDERS IN NEUROLOGICAL DISEASE

Retinal Arterial Disease

Retinal arterial disease can present as a central or branch retinal artery occlusion or as "amaurosis fugax" (transient monocular visual loss). Carotid artery atherosclerotic disease is the most common cause; cardiac valvular disease is also a consideration. Acute retinal artery occlusion is characterized by retinal whitening (edema) secondary to infarction. After resolution, the retinal appearance typically returns to normal, although the prognosis for visual recovery is generally poor. Retinal emboli are most often located at arteriolar bifurcations. The three major types of retinal emboli are (1) cholesterol (source carotid artery), (2) platelet-fibrin (source cardiac valves), and (3) calcific (source carotid or cardiac).

Vasculitis

In vasculitis, focal areas of retinal infarction develop. These areas, known as *cotton-wool spots*, are usually bilateral and may be extensive. The causes include branch retinal artery occlusions and encephalopathy (Susac's syndrome), ocular ischemic syndrome, and retinal vein occlusion.

Neurological Diseases with Retinal Findings

The cause of retinitis pigmentosa (RP) is a degeneration of the retinal rods and cones. Rods are predominantly affected first, impairing night vision. Visual field loss occurs first in the midperiphery and progresses to severe field constriction. RP usually appears without systemic findings. However, retinal degeneration occurs in Kearns-Sayre syndrome, Laurence-Moon-Bardet-Biedl syndrome, Marie's ataxia, Cockayne's syndrome, Refsum's syndrome, Batten's disease, inherited Vitamin E deficiency, and spinocerebellar ataxia type 7. Inflammatory changes in both the eye and the central nervous system characterize the uveoretinal meningoencephalitis syndromes. The most common, Vogt-Koyanagi-Harada syndrome is characterized by exudative retinal detachments. Retinal findings are common in phakomatoses that affect the nervous system, particularly tuberous sclerosis and von Hippel–Lindau disease.

For a more detailed discussion, see Chapters 14 and 15 in Neurology in Clinical Practice, 4th edition.

Eye Movement and Pupillary Disorders

9

The human fovea is a highly sensitive part of the retina that is capable of resolving angles of less than 100 seconds of arc. The ocular motor system places images of objects of regard on the fovea and maintains foveation if the object or head moves. Each eye has six extraocular muscles, yoked in pairs that move the eyes conjugately (versions) to maintain alignment of the visual axes (Table 9.1).

Five ocular motor subsystems enable the fovea to find and fixate on a target, stabilize an image of the target on each retina, and maintain binocular foveation during head movement, target movement, or both. These systems include (1) the *saccadic system*, which moves the eyes rapidly to fixate on new targets and is the fast component of nystagmus, (2) the *pursuit system*, which enables the eyes to track slow-moving targets to maintain the image stable on the fovea, (3) *vestibular eye movements*, which maintain a stable image on the retina during head movements, (4) the *optokinetic system*, which stabilizes images on the retina in situations such as spinning, and (5) the *vergence system*, which enables the eyes to move disconjugately (converge and diverge) in the horizontal plane to maintain binocular fixation on a target moving toward or away from the subject.

HETEROPHORIAS AND HETEROTROPIAS

Images of the same target must fall on corresponding points of each retina to maintain binocular single vision (fusion). Misalignment of the visual axes because of dysconjugate positioning of the eyes causes diplopia because images of the target fall on noncorresponding (disparate) points of each retina. After a variable period the patient learns to ignore or suppress

Table 9.1: Actions of extraocular muscles

Muscle	Primary	Secondary	Tertiary
Medial rectus	Adduction		
Lateral rectus	Abduction		
Superior rectus	Elevation	Intorsion	Adduction
Inferior rectus	Depression	Extorsion	Adduction
Superior oblique	Intorsion	Depression	Abduction
Inferior oblique	Extorsion	Elevation	Abduction

one image. If suppression occurs before age 9 years and persists, the child fails to develop fully central connections in the afferent visual system. This failure leads to permanently impaired visual acuity (*developmental amblyopia*) in the weaker eye.

When the degree of "misalignment" (the angle of deviation of the visual axes) is constant, the patient has a *comitant* strabismus (*heterotropia*). When the degree of misalignment varies with gaze direction, the patient has a *noncomitant* strabismus (*paralytic or restrictive*). Comitant strabismus is usually a congenital ophthalmological condition, and noncomitant strabismus is usually an acquired neurological condition. The condition of having divergent eyes is called *exotropia* and convergent eyes is *esotropia*; vertical misalignment of the visual axes is called *hypertropia* (determined by the higher eye, irrespective of which eye is paretic). Most people have a latent tendency for ocular misalignment, *heterophoria*, which becomes manifest under conditions of stress, fatigue, or the ingestion of alcohol and sedative medications. When a heterophoria is unmasked, the diplopia is comitant.

DIPLOPIA

The following rules apply when assessing diplopia:

1. *Head tilt* is when the weak extraocular muscle is unable to move the eye, and the head moves the eye. Therefore the head tilts and turns in the direction of action of the weak muscle.
2. The *image from the nonfixing eye is the false image* and displaces in the direction of action of the paretic muscle.
3. The *false image is the most peripheral image* and displaces in the direction of action of the weak muscle.
4. *The images are most widely separated when the patient looks in the direction of the paretic muscle.*

5. *Secondary deviation* (the angle of ocular misalignment when the paretic eye is fixating) is always greater than *primary deviation* (when the good eye is fixating).
6. The cause of *acquired isolated vertical diplopia* is usually superior oblique muscle palsy. The false image always tilts.
7. *Monocular diplopia* is double vision that occurs with one eye covered. The most common cause of monocular diplopia is an optical aberration. Other causes are psychogenic, retinal dysfunction, and disturbances of the cerebral cortex.

SUPRANUCLEAR GAZE DISTURBANCES

The cause of supranuclear gaze palsies is an interruption of the saccadic and pursuit pathways from the cortex to the brainstem eye movement generators; voluntary eye movements are lost and reflex eye movements are spared. *Ocular motor apraxia* is the inability to perform voluntary saccades while spontaneous and reflex eye movements are preserved.

Congenital Ocular Motor Apraxia

Impaired voluntary horizontal pursuit and saccadic movements with preservation of vertical eye movements characterize congenital ocular motor apraxia (COMA). Reflex saccades may be partly retained. By 4–8 months of age, the patient develops a thrusting head movement strategy, often with prominent blinking, to overcome the eye movement deficit. When the patient reaches school age, the apraxia may improve but does not completely resolve. COMA may be associated with hypoplasia of the corpus callosum and midline cerebellum, occipital porencephalic cysts, or bilateral cortical lesions. A similar disorder occurs in children with Pelizaeus-Merzbacher disease, ataxia-telangiectasia (80%), Cockayne's syndrome, and succinic semialdehyde dehydrogenase deficiency.

Spasm of Fixation

Affected patients have difficulty shifting visual attention because of impaired initiation of voluntary saccades when looking at a fixation target but normal initiation of saccades in the absence of a target. Their saccades have a prolonged latency and may be hypometric in the presence of a central visual target; however, blinks or combined eye and head movements may sometimes facilitate normal saccades.

Familial Gaze Palsy

Patients with familial gaze palsy have paralysis of horizontal gaze with impaired optokinetic nystagmus (OKN) and vestibuloocular reflexes (VORs) but intact convergence and vertical eye movements. Inheritance is autosomal recessive. Progressive scoliosis, facial myokymia and twitching, hemifacial atrophy, and situs inversus of the optic discs are sometimes associated.

Acquired Horizontal Gaze Palsy

Acquired horizontal gaze palsy occurs in 20% of patients with acute cerebral hemisphere injuries of any cause. It is a transitory gaze deviation in which the eyes are usually toward the side of the lesion (ipsiversive gaze deviation) because of gaze paresis to the opposite hemiplegic side. After several days the intact hemisphere, which contains neurons for bilateral gaze, takes over, and the gaze palsy resolves.

Wrong-Way Eyes

Conjugate eye deviation to the wrong side, that is, away from the lesion and toward the hemiplegia (*contraversive gaze deviation*), may occur with supratentorial lesions, particularly thalamic hemorrhage, and, rarely, with large perisylvian or lobar hemorrhage.

Periodic Alternating Gaze Deviation

Periodic alternating gaze deviation (PAGD) is a rare cyclic ocular motor disorder in which the direction of gaze alternates every few minutes. Lateral deviation can be sustained for up to 15 minutes; gaze then returns to the midline for 10–20 seconds before changing to the other side. Occasionally, PAGD is associated with pontine vascular disorders, Chiari malformations, Creutzfeldt-Jakob disease, spinocerebellar degeneration, and paraneoplastic brainstem encephalitis.

Ping-Pong Gaze

Ping-pong gaze is a conjugate horizontal rhythmic oscillation that cycles every 4–8 seconds (short-cycle PAGD) and occurs in comatose patients because of bilateral cerebral or upper brainstem damage (disconnection) or because of metabolic dysfunction. The prognosis for recovery is poor except when the cause is toxic or metabolic.

Saccadic Lateropulsion

Saccadic lateropulsion is hypermetric (overshoot) saccades to the side of the lesion and hypometric (undershoot) saccades to the opposite side that occurs with lesions of the lateral medulla. Lateropulsion with a bias away from the side of the lesion (contrapulsion) may occur with lesions involving the region of the superior cerebellar peduncle (outflow tract) and adjacent cerebellum (superior cerebellar artery territory).

Torsional Saccades

Pathological rapid torsional eye deviation during voluntary saccades may occur with large lesions involving the midline cerebellum, deep cerebellar nuclei, and dorsolateral medulla.

Slow Saccades

Saccades of low velocity result from pontine disease in patients with olivopontocerebellar degeneration and other degenerative and metabolic disorders.

Prolonged Saccadic Latency

Prolonged latencies for voluntary saccades occur in patients with acquired immunodeficiency syndrome (AIDS)–dementia complex, and degenerative disorders of the nervous system.

Square Wave Jerks

Square wave jerks (SWJs) are spontaneous, small-amplitude paired saccades that briefly interrupt fixation. They occur in normal elderly people, particularly in darkness without fixation. SWJs are prominent in progressive supranuclear palsy, multiple system atrophy, and cerebellar disease.

INTERNUCLEAR OPHTHALMOPLEGIA

In internuclear ophthalmoplegia, damage to the medial longitudinal fasciculus (MLF) between the third and sixth cranial nerve nuclei impairs transmission of neural impulses to the ipsilateral medial rectus muscle. Adduction of the ipsilateral eye is slow or absent, and abduction of the contralateral eye is normal. Nystagmus of the abducting eye is actually overshoot dysmetria. Stroke and multiple sclerosis are the most common causes.

One-and-a-Half Syndrome

In one-and-a-half syndrome, a lesion in the caudal dorsal pontine tegmentum involving the ipsilateral abducens nucleus or the pontine reticular formation and the ipsilateral MLF causes ipsilateral gaze palsy with an ipsilateral internuclear ophthalmoplegia. Abduction of the contralateral eye is the only horizontal movement left intact. The most common causes are multiple sclerosis and brainstem stroke, followed by metastatic and primary brainstem tumors. Ocular myasthenia may cause a pseudo–one-and-a-half syndrome.

DISORDERS OF VERTICAL GAZE

Disorders of conjugate vertical gaze result from isolated lesions placed discretely in the midbrain pretectal region. Bilateral involvement of the pathways for downgaze or upgaze is caused by diffuse disorders such as progressive supranuclear palsy, Whipple's disease, neurovisceral lipid storage disorders, and complications of AIDS.

A crossed vertical gaze paresis, with supranuclear weakness of elevation of the contralateral eye and weakness of depression of the ipsilateral eye, may occur with a lesion involving the mesodiencephalic junction and medial thalamus.

Tonic Upward Deviation of Gaze

Tonic upward deviation of gaze is a forced upgaze seen in unconscious patients and must be distinguished from oculogyric crises, petit mal seizures, and psychogenic coma.

Benign Paroxysmal Tonic Upward Gaze

Benign paroxysmal tonic upward gaze in young children occurs in association with both downbeat nystagmus on attempted downgaze and ataxia. The duration of deviation is seconds to hours but is usually short and recurrent throughout the day. The cause is unknown. It usually starts in infancy and lasts about 2 years. Tonic upgaze may also occur in normal infants in the first few months.

Tonic Downward Deviation of Gaze

Tonic downward deviation of gaze is a forced downgaze that is associated with impaired consciousness in patients with medial thalamic hemorrhage, acute obstructive hydrocephalus, severe metabolic or hypoxic encephalopathy, or massive subarachnoid hemorrhage. The eyes may also be converged as if looking at the nose. Downward deviation while awake also occurs transiently in otherwise normal infants.

Skew Deviation

Skew deviation is a vertical divergence of the ocular axes caused by a prenuclear lesion in the brainstem or cerebellum that involves the vertical vestibuloocular pathways. A skew is usually comitant; when noncomitant, it mimics a partial third nerve or a fourth nerve palsy. Skew deviations occur most commonly with vascular lesions of the pons or lateral medulla (Wallenberg's syndrome). *Alternating skew deviation*, in which the hypertropia changes sides, results from vascular or demyelinating lesions at the pretectal-mesodiencephalic junction.

Oculogyric Crises

Oculogyric crises are spasmodic conjugate ocular deviations, usually in an upward, sometimes lateral, and occasionally downward direction. Neuroleptic medications, particularly haloperidol, are the usual cause. A typical attack or crisis lasts about 2 hours, during which the eyes are tonically deviated upward repetitively for periods of seconds to minutes.

DISORDERS OF CONVERGENCE

Convergence Paralysis

Convergence paralysis is usually associated with other features of the dorsal midbrain syndrome. Lack of effort is the most common cause of poor convergence, which becomes more difficult with age.

Convergence Insufficiency

Insufficiency is an idiopathic condition that may be psychogenic and usually occurs in women between the ages of 15 and 45 years. It is an imbalance between accommodation and convergence and may cause frank diplopia, although eyestrain, headache, and vague symptoms such as burning eyes are more common.

Spasm of the Near Reflex

Intermittent episodes of convergence, miosis, and accommodation characterize spasm. It may mimic bilateral and occasionally unilateral abducens paresis. The patient may complain of double or blurred vision and is esotropic, particularly at distance. Spasm of the near reflex is usually psychogenic. The differential diagnosis is the same as that for esotropia.

DISORDERS OF DIVERGENCE

Divergence Insufficiency

Sudden-onset esotropia and uncrossed horizontal diplopia at distance in the absence of other neurological symptoms or signs characterize divergence insufficiency. The esotropia may be intermittent or constant, but the patients can fuse at near. The cause of divergence insufficiency is unclear but may result from a break in fusion in a patient with a congenital esophoria, which usually develops later in life.

Divergence Paralysis

Divergence paralysis is difficult to distinguish from divergence insufficiency. It usually occurs with raised intracranial pressure. Horizontal diplopia is present at distance. Patients with bilateral sixth nerve palsies, who recover gradually, may go through a phase during which the esotropia becomes comitant with full ductions, mimicking divergence paralysis.

Cyclic Esotropia

Cyclic esotropia (*circadian, alternate-day*, or *clock mechanism esotropia*) usually begins in childhood, although it can occur in infancy, in later life, or after surgery for intermittent esotropia. The cycles of orthotropia and esotropia may run 24–96 hours.

Ocular Neuromyotonia

Ocular myotonia is a brief episodic myotonic contraction of one or more muscles supplied by the ocular motor nerves, most commonly the third nerve. It usually results in esotropia of the affected eye accompanied by failure of elevation and depression of the globe. Causes include radiation therapy and, less commonly, compressive lesions such as cavernous sinus meningiomas or pituitary adenomas.

NYSTAGMUS

Nystagmus is involuntary biphasic rhythmic ocular oscillations in which one or both phases are slow. The cause is dysfunction of the vestibular end organ, vestibular nerve, brainstem, or cerebellum. The slow phase of jerk nystagmus is responsible for initiating and generating the nystagmus, whereas the fast (saccadic) phase is a corrective movement bringing the fovea back on target.

Nystagmus is categorized as *pendular* or *jerk*. Both can be horizontal or vertical. Jerk nystagmus is named by the direction of the fast phase. Pendular nystagmus is always brainstem or cerebellum in origin, whereas jerk nystagmus can be either central in origin or from peripheral vestibular dysfunction.

Clinical Evaluation

Nystagmus may be congenital or acquired and sporadic or familial.

Nystagmus Syndromes

Congenital Nystagmus
Congenital nystagmus (CN) is usually present from birth but not noticed for several weeks. It may be genetically associated with severe visual impairment. CN is sometimes associated with ocular albinism. Inheritance may be autosomal recessive or X-linked dominant or recessive.

CN is usually horizontal and may be pendular or jerk in primary position. Pendular nystagmus often becomes jerk on lateral gaze. Vision is satisfactory unless retinal disease or optic atrophy is associated. CN damps with convergence, and a null zone exists where nystagmus intensity is minimal. The head frequently oscillates as well. Therapy uses the damping of nystagmus with convergence and the presence of a null zone by changing the direction of gaze with prisms or extraocular muscle surgery to improve head posture and visual acuity.

Spasmus Nutans
Spasmus nutans is a transitory, high-frequency, low-amplitude pendular nystagmus that occurs between the ages of 6 and 12 months and lasts approximately 2 years or longer. Oscillation may occur in any direction and is often dysconjugate, asymmetrical, and variable. It is often associated with head tilt and titubation. Binocular spasmus nutans is benign and

transitory, but monocular spasmus nutans may be associated with tumors of the anterior visual pathways.

Pendular Nystagmus

Pendular nystagmus has a sinusoidal waveform and is usually horizontal. It may be either congenital or acquired. The most common acquired cause is multiple sclerosis, followed by brainstem vascular disease involving the deep cerebellar nuclei or their efferent connections. Lesions of the dorsal pontine tegmentum may also be causative.

Vertical pendular nystagmus closely resembles the vertical ocular oscillation associated with palatal myoclonus (the *oculopalatal syndrome*); lesions of the deep cerebellar nuclei and their connections cause both.

Gaze-Paretic Nystagmus

Gaze-paretic nystagmus is usually symmetrical, with eccentric gaze to either side, but is absent in the primary position. Alcohol or drug intoxication and any lesion that causes a gaze paresis cause it.

Vestibular Nystagmus

Vestibular nystagmus results from damage in the vestibular system from the labyrinth to its central connection. Peripheral vestibular nystagmus (labyrinth and nerve) is usually associated with severe nausea, vomiting, perspiration, and diarrhea (vegetative symptoms). Vegetative symptoms are less severe in central vestibular nystagmus; however, dysconjugate gaze and pyramidal tract signs are often present.

Physiological Nystagmus

End-point nystagmus is a jerk nystagmus seen on extreme lateral or upward gaze. It is symmetrical on right and left gaze.

Upbeat Nystagmus

Upbeat nystagmus is a spontaneous jerk nystagmus with the fast phase upward while the eyes are in primary position. Its amplitude and intensity usually increase on upgaze. Upbeat nystagmus usually suggests structural disease of the brainstem or cerebellar vermis.

Downbeat Nystagmus

Downbeat nystagmus is a spontaneous downward-beating jerk nystagmus present in primary position. Directing the eyes downward and laterally increases the amplitude of the oscillation. It is often associated with structural lesions at the craniocervical junction but also occurs with cerebellar degeneration, metabolic disorders, drug intoxications, magnesium depletion, Wernicke's encephalopathy, brainstem encephalitis, multiple sclerosis, leukodystrophy, and vertebrobasilar ischemia. Downbeat nystagmus may be congenital or, rarely, occur as a transitory ocular oscillation in normal neonates.

Periodic Alternating Nystagmus

Periodic alternating nystagmus (PAN) is a horizontal jerk nystagmus in which the fast phase beats in one direction and then damps or stops for a few seconds before changing direction to the opposite side. It has the same clinical significance as downbeat nystagmus, with which it sometimes coexists. Baclofen successfully treats the acquired form of PAN.

Rebound Nystagmus

Rebound nystagmus is a horizontal gaze–evoked jerk nystagmus in which the direction of the fast phase reverses with sustained lateral gaze. When the eyes return to primary position, the fast phase may beat transiently in the opposite direction. Dysfunction of the cerebellum or the perihypoglossal nuclei in the medulla is causative.

Convergence-Evoked Nystagmus

Convergence-evoked nystagmus is a pendular ocular oscillation induced by voluntary convergence. The movements may be conjugate or dissociated, congenital or acquired, and they occur in patients with multiple sclerosis and Chiari malformations.

Seesaw Nystagmus

In seesaw nystagmus, one eye rises and intorts as the other eye falls and extorts. It occurs with lesions in the region of the mesodiencephalic junction.

Torsional (Rotary) Nystagmus

In torsional nystagmus, the eye oscillates in a pure rotary or cyclorotational plane. It may be present in primary position or with either head positioning or gaze deviation and the cause are usually lesions in the central vestibular connections.

Ictal Nystagmus

Nystagmus often accompanies adversive seizures and beats to the side opposite the seizure focus. Nystagmus as the only motor manifestation of a seizure is unusual.

Lid Nystagmus

Rhythmic jerking movements of the upper eyelids occur (1) synchronous with vertical ocular nystagmus, (2) synchronous with the fast phase of gaze-evoked horizontal nystagmus with the lateral medullary syndrome, and (3) during voluntary convergence with lesions of the rostral medulla.

Episodic Nystagmus
Episodic nystagmus is associated with paroxysmal episodes of vertigo and ataxia, lasting up to 24 hours. The nystagmus may be torsional, vertical, or dissociated. Periodic ataxia occurs with hereditary inborn errors of metabolism, in a familial form without any detectable metabolic defect but with recognized chromosomal abnormalities, and in patients with basilar migraine or multiple sclerosis. Acetazolamide or valproic acid may alleviate or prevent attacks in the familial form.

Treatment

Refraction corrects acuity. With the exception of CN, in which prisms, surgery, and contact lenses are helpful, the treatment of other forms of nystagmus is discouraging. Acquired pendular and downbeat nystagmus sometimes responds to the central muscarinic antagonists benztropine and scopolamine. Clonazepam and baclofen may be useful for acquired PAN, upbeat, and downbeat nystagmus. Gabapentin and trihexyphenidyl have been effective for the pendular nystagmus of multiple sclerosis.

OTHER OCULAR OSCILLATIONS

Voluntary Nystagmus

Voluntary nystagmus is not true nystagmus but ocular flutter under voluntary control. It consists of a series of fast, back-to-back saccadic eye movements, without any interval or slow phase. Occasionally, patients use this ability to feign acquired illness.

Ocular Flutter

Ocular flutter occurs with brainstem or cerebellar disease and consists of horizontal, conjugate, back-to-back saccades that occur spontaneously in intermittent bursts. Attempts at fixation aggravate flutter.

Opsoclonus

Opsoclonus is a spontaneous, chaotic, multivectorial, saccadic eye movement disorder that is virtually always conjugate. It is aggravated by attempts at fixation and may be associated with myoclonic jerks of the limbs and cerebellar ataxia (dancing eyes–dancing feet syndrome). The most common causes are neuroblastoma in children and a paraneoplastic syndrome in adults.

Ocular Dysmetria

Ocular dysmetria occurs with refixation saccades that cause the eyes to overshoot the target. It results from cerebellar dysfunction.

Convergence-Retraction Nystagmus

Convergence-retraction nystagmus is a rapid dysmetric horizontal eye movement induced by attempted upward saccades that occurs in the dorsal midbrain (*Parinaud's*) syndrome.

Ocular Bobbing

Ocular bobbing is a rapid downward movement of both eyes followed by a slow drift back to primary position. The oscillation recurs between 2 and 15 times per minute and occurs in patients, usually comatose, with severe central pontine destruction and horizontal gaze palsies.

Ocular Myoclonus

Ocular myoclonus is a vertical pendular oscillation that is usually associated with similar oscillations of the soft palate (the *oculopalatal syndrome*). It occurs after brainstem infarction, particularly of the pons, involving the central tegmental tract or the dentate nuclei of the cerebellum, with secondary pseudohypertrophy of the inferior olivary nucleus.

PUPILLARY ABNORMALITIES

Anisocoria

Unequal pupils (anisocoria) are the most common sign of disorders affecting the iris or its innervation. The differential diagnosis of anisocoria includes local disease of the eye, parasympathetic defects (affecting the third nerve or pupillary sphincter), sympathetic defects (affecting the iris dilator muscle or its innervation), and simple anisocoria.

Blunt trauma to the eye can damage the pupillary sphincter, causing mydriasis with poor pupillary constriction to both light and near stimuli. Immediately after injury, the pupil may be smaller than normal, but after a few minutes the pupil becomes dilated and poorly reactive. This course of events may simulate uncal herniation.

Syphilis causes several pupillary disorders; the *Argyll Robertson pupil* is the best known, but anisocoria caused by degeneration of iris stroma is the most common. Acute inflammatory disease of the eye (iritis) can cause mild pupillary constriction. The inflamed eye is red, and the patient has photophobia. Ischemia of the iris from angle-closure glaucoma and the ocular ischemic syndrome causes mydriasis and poor pupillary reactivity; other symptoms are poor vision and pain.

Parasympathetic Disturbances

Oculomotor (third) nerve palsy, tonic pupils, and pharmacological mydriasis cause defective parasympathetic innervation. The involved pupil is usually larger but may become smaller after chronic denervation, although it remains poorly reactive. Extraocular palsies accompany pupillary involvement in third nerve palsies. The Holmes-Adie pupillary syndrome (tonic pupils and diminished deep tendon reflexes) is the most common cause of tonic pupils. Other causes include orbital trauma, herpes zoster ophthalmicus, syphilis, temporal arteritis, and peripheral neuropathies. Pharmacological mydriasis usually occurs after accidental or intentional instillation of atropine. Such pupils are larger than the dilated pupils secondary to third nerve palsies.

Sympathetic Disturbances

Sympathetic denervation causes pupillary miosis and ipsilateral ptosis (*Horner's syndrome*).

Simple (Physiological, Essential) Anisocoria

Simple anisocoria occurs in about 20% of the normal population. The difference in pupil size is rarely more than 0.6 mm. The amount of anisocoria may differ in a given individual at different times.

Episodic Anisocoria

Anisocoria may be intermittent. Migraine headaches can cause unilateral mydriasis that may persist for several hours. Unilateral pupillary dilation and other pupillary signs can occur during seizures.

Examination

The pupillary response to light is tested first. If both pupils constrict well, then pupillary diameter is assessed in bright and dim light. If anisocoria is greater in bright light, the iris sphincter on the side of the larger pupil is not working well and the main diagnostic considerations are third nerve palsy and traumatic iridoplegia. If the anisocoria is greater in dim light, the iris dilator muscle on the side of the smaller pupil is working poorly and both Horner's syndrome and simple anisocoria should be considered.

If the pupillary response to light is poor, assess the response to near. A better pupillary constriction to near effort than to light indicates *light-near dissociation*. Poor constriction to both light and near implies a local iris problem, parasympathetic defects, and midbrain disease, but also with aging and anxiety.

The testing of *dilation lag* is used when Horner's syndrome is a consideration. The smaller pupil of Horner's syndrome dilates more slowly in darkness than the normal pupil. The definitive diagnosis of Horner's syndrome requires pharmacological testing.

Assess pupils with a parasympathetic defect for *tonic redilation*, a sign that establishes the diagnosis of tonic pupil. During near effort and convergence, a large, unilateral tonic pupil may constrict, but then with distance refixation it remains constricted for several seconds while the normal fellow eye dilates.

Investigations
Instillation of drugs is often necessary to establish the cause of anisocoria. Cocaine acts by blocking reuptake of norepineph-rine; in a 4–10% solution, cocaine dilates the normal pupil of simple anisocoria but not the sympathetically denervated pupil of Horner's syndrome. Hydroxyamphetamine 1% acts by releasing norepinephrine from the presynaptic terminal and can be used for pharmacological localization of Horner's syndrome. Hydroxyamphetamine dilates normal pupils and those with preganglionic lesions, but not those with postganglionic sympa-thetic lesions. Pilocarpine in a 0.05% solution is too dilute to cause pupillary constriction except in eyes with tonic pupils. Pilocarpine in a 1% solution causes marked pupillary constric-tion in individuals with normal pupils and in those with third nerve palsies but not in those with pharmacological mydriasis.

Examining old photographs with a magnifying glass can help establish the duration of a pupillary abnormality. Any patient with bilateral tonic pupils, poorly reactive or irregular pupils, or pupils with light-near dissociation deserves evaluation for tertiary syphilis.

Other Pupillary Abnormalities

Poorly Reactive Pupils without Anisocoria
Large pupils that are poorly reactive but roughly equal in diameter can occur with hypothalamic and midbrain lesions,

syphilis, botulism, the Miller Fisher variant of the Guillain-Barré syndrome, and autonomic neuropathy. Toxic and pharmacological causes are considerations. Bilateral mydriasis is sometimes congenital. Anxious young adults and teenagers often have large, poorly reactive pupils. Small, poorly reactive pupils, often combined with simple anisocoria, are common in older people. Other acquired causes are syphilis, diabetes, and long-standing Holmes-Adie pupillary syndrome. Patients with glaucoma using pilocarpine drops have small pupils that do not react to light or near stimuli.

Light-Near Dissociation

Light-near dissociation refers to pupils that have marked diminution of constriction to light, with a much better constriction to near stimuli. When the pupils are large, the differential diagnosis includes syphilis, tonic pupils, pretectal lesions, and bilateral afferent pupillary defects (e.g., from bilateral optic atrophy). Small pupils with light-near dissociation can occur in patients with syphilis (Argyll Robertson pupils), long-standing Holmes-Adie pupillary syndrome, and diabetic neuropathy.

Irregular Pupils

Irregular pupils are usually caused by local iris disease. Oval or eccentric pupils (corectopia) may occur with midbrain disease and increased intracranial pressure.

Hippus (Pupillary Unrest)

Shining a light in the eyes of most normal people elicits spontaneous conjugate oscillations in pupillary diameter.

For a more detailed discussion, see Chapters 16 and 17 in Neurology in Clinical Practice, 4th edition.

Dizziness, Vertigo, Hearing Loss, Tinnitus | *10*

Dizziness, vertigo, and disequilibration are common complaints. The patient's history is the best means to establish a diagnosis, as the physical examination and diagnostic test results are often normal. Hearing loss, however, requires audiological testing.

DIZZINESS AND VERTIGO

Symptoms and Signs

Vertigo refers to a hallucination of movement. The sensation of dizziness varies among individuals. The signs that accompany vertigo and dizziness depend primarily on their cause. Patients with an acute peripheral vestibulopathy usually have nystagmus, with the fast phase beating away from the involved ear. Falling during Romberg testing and past-pointing occur toward the side of the involved ear. When dizziness involves lightheadedness from postural hypotension, examination will document the hypotension. Central causes of dizziness are usually associated with other signs of central nervous system dysfunction, such as gaze-evoked nystagmus, facial weakness, other cranial nerve abnormalities, ataxia, hemisensory loss, or even paralysis.

In patients with an acute peripheral vestibular abnormality, the input from one end organ does not match the input from the other end organ. The brain interprets this sensation as movement or vertigo. Many patients with disequilibrium experience anxiety. It is often difficult to tell whether the anxiety is primary or secondary to the disequilibrium; however, vertigo is rarely a cause of anxiety. Establishing a definitive cause for chronic disequilibrium is unusual. However, consider migraine as a cause for recurrent attacks of vertigo.

Differential Diagnosis

The causes of vertigo are (1) peripheral vestibulopathy, (2) central neurological disorders, and (3) systemic conditions. Neurologists consider conditions that affect the vestibular nerve to be peripheral in location because they are extra-axial.

Peripheral Causes of Vertigo

Peripheral causes of vertigo result from dysfunction of vestibular end organs (semicircular canals, utricle, and saccule) (Table 10.1). *Peripheral vestibulopathy* is a preferred term to *vestibular neuronitis*, *labyrinthitis*, and *viral neurolabyrinthitis* because it does not suggest a cause. In the acute phase, many patients present with sudden severe vertigo, nausea, and vomiting without any hearing disturbance or facial weakness. The acute symptoms usually resolve in a few days to 1 week but may recur in weeks or months.

Benign paroxysmal positional vertigo (BPPV) is a symptom complex suggesting benign peripheral (end-organ) disease. Factors that suggest the diagnosis of BPPV include the following: (1) symptoms associated with certain head positions, (2) a brief episode of rotational vertigo, (3) an antecedent episode of severe rotary vertigo, with or without nausea and vomiting and associated with an upper respiratory tract infection, (4) an antecedent history of head trauma, (5) most severe symptoms occurring early in the day, with lessening symptoms as the day progresses, and (6) relative absence of spontaneous symptoms without head movement or position change. The clinical features of BPPV are transitory, rarely lasting more than 40 seconds. They often occur when a certain position is assumed, such as lying down or turning in bed.

Table 10.1: Peripheral causes of vertigo

1. Peripheral vestibulopathy (includes labyrinthitis, vestibular neuronitis, and acute and recurrent peripheral vestibulopathy)
2. Benign positional vertigo (includes benign positional nystagmus and benign paroxysmal vertigo)
3. Posttraumatic vertigo
4. Vestibulotoxic, drug-induced vertigo
5. Ménière's disease
6. Other focal peripheral diseases (includes local bacterial infection, degeneration of hair cells, genetic anomalies of labyrinth, cupulolithiasis, tumor of eighth nerve, otosclerosis, fistula of labyrinth, and, rarely, focal ischemia)

Posttraumatic vertigo that occurs immediately after head injury in the absence of other central nervous system dysfunction implies end-organ damage from fracture of the temporal bone. In posttraumatic vertigo, the symptoms may be those of general peripheral vestibulopathy or benign positional vertigo. The prognosis is usually good, with symptoms gradually resolving within weeks to months. Disabling persistent positional vertigo, unresponsive to medical therapy, does occur.

Drug toxicity from vestibulotoxic drugs usually indicates permanent injury to the peripheral end organ. The aminoglycosides cause such injury. Streptomycin and gentamicin have their greatest effect on the vestibular end organ; kanamycin, tobramycin, and neomycin cause more damage to the auditory end organ. Progressive unsteadiness occurs, particularly with diminished visual input. Vestibular testing documents a progressive bilateral loss of vestibular function.

The characteristic features of Ménière's disease are recurrent attacks of severe vertigo and vomiting, tinnitus, fluctuating but progressive hearing loss, ill-described aural sensations of fullness and pressure in one ear, and spontaneous recovery in hours to days. A sense of disequilibration persists for days afterward. The most consistent pathological finding is an increase in the volume of the endolymphatic fluid and distention of the canals. Most cases are idiopathic.

Other Peripheral Vestibular Conditions
Many other disorders affect the peripheral labyrinth, including acute and chronic otitis media, hereditary degenerative disorders of the end organ, and local tumors. Conditions such as a vertebrobasilar transient ischemic attack (TIA) or focal ischemic stroke of the end organ, particularly in an elderly patient, are often cited as a cause of vertigo. Such isolated involvement is difficult to document, and vertebrobasilar insufficiency is unusual without associated brainstem symptoms and signs.

Central Causes of Vertigo
Normal people experience physiological vertiginous sensations when visual and vestibular inputs are in conflict (such as with motion sickness or watching motion picture automobile chase scenes) or when they are exposed to heights while standing on a ledge. Central pathological causes of vertigo are less common than either peripheral or systemic causes. The main causes are brainstem ischemia and infarction, demyelinating disorders, remote effects of carcinoma, cerebellopontine angle tumors, cranial neuropathies, other intrinsic brainstem disorders, migraine (in children), and spinocerebellar degenerations

Table 10.2: Central neurological causes of vertigo*

---

1. Brainstem ischemia and infarction
2. Demyelinating disease: multiple sclerosis, postinfectious demyelination; remote effect of carcinoma
3. Cerebellopontine angle tumor: acoustic neuroma, meningioma, cholesteatoma, metastatic tumor, etc.
4. Cranial neuropathy: focal involvement of eighth nerve or in association with systemic disorders
5. Intrinsic brainstem lesions (tumor, arteriovenous malformation)
6. Other posterior fossa lesions (primarily other intrinsic or extra-axial masses of the posterior fossa, such as hematoma, metastatic tumor, and cerebellar infarction)
7. Seizure disorders (rare)
8. Heredofamilial disorders (such as spinocerebellar degeneration)

---

*Hearing loss is rare except in the condition listed in No. 3.

(Table 10.2). Brainstem and cerebellar disease often cause pendular nystagmus that results in an illusion of environmental movement characterized by bouncing or jiggling of objects (oscillopsia).

Systemic Causes of Vertigo
Systemic causes of vertigo are conditions that secondarily affect the peripheral vestibular structures, central vestibular structures, or both, to produce vertigo. The main causes are drug ingestion, hypotension, infections, diabetes, hypothyroidism, vasculitis, and systemic conditions such as polycythemia, anemia, dysproteinemia, sarcoidosis, and granulomatous disease.

Other Vestibular Conditions
Many other disorders affect the peripheral labyrinth, including acute and chronic otitis media, hereditary degenerative disorders of the end organ, and local tumors (Table 10.3). Conditions such as a vertebrobasilar TIA or focal ischemic stroke of the end organ, particularly in an elderly patient, are cited as a cause of vertigo but are difficult to document. Vertebrobasilar insufficiency is unusual without associated brainstem symptoms and signs.

Multiple Afferent Sensory Loss
The vestibular system provides (1) spatial orientation at rest or during acceleration, (2) visual fixation during head or body movement (the vestibuloocular reflex [VOR]), and (3) feedback control of muscle tone to maintain posture. The interconnection of these functions is complex. A combination of multiple sensory deficits can produce disorientation or disequilibrium.

Table 10.3: Characteristics of peripheral versus central positional vertigo

Symptom or Sign	Peripheral	Central
Latency (time to onset of vertigo or nystagmus)	0–40 sec (mean 7.8*)	No latency Begins immediately
Duration	<1 min	Symptoms may persist (signs and symptoms of single episode)
Fatigability (habituation) (lessening signs and symptoms with repetition of provocative maneuver)	Yes	No
Nystagmus direction	Direction fixed, torsional, up, upper pole of eyes toward ground	Direction changing, variable
Intensity of signs and symptoms	Severe vertigo, marked nystagmus, nausea	Usually mild vertigo, less intense nystagmus, rare nausea
Reproducibility	Inconsistent	More consistent

*According to Baloh, R. W., Honrubia, V., & Jacobson, K. 1987, "Benign positional vertigo: Clinical and oculographic features in 240 cases," *Neurology* vol. 37, pp. 371–378.

Examination

Every patient should have a screening general physical examination with particular attention to the cardiovascular system and blood pressure on standing when symptoms suggesting presyncope or syncope are present. All patients should have a complete neurological examination. Signs of confusion may suggest overmedication, metabolic encephalopathy, or an acquired dementing process. Focal disturbances in intellectual function, such as a subtle aphasia, may lead to the consideration of a multi-infarction state (multi-infarction dementia) with accompanying brainstem infarctions or of an intracranial mass lesion.

A *directed neuro-otological examination* includes an otoscopic examination of the external auditory canals and the tympanic membranes and a careful search for nystagmus. The ability to maintain fixation on distant objects during head-turn tests the VOR. Further tests include balance during standing, walking, and turning and past-pointing.

Investigations

Screening Tests
The screening tests to evaluate vertigo of unknown cause should include a complete blood cell count, serum glucose and electrolyte measurements, erythrocyte sedimentation rate, thyroid function testing, lipid screens for the presence of hypercholesterolemia or increased triglycerides, and a rheumatological battery. A history of presyncope or syncope is an indication for an electrocardiogram and rhythm strip. Chest palpitations or flutter requires further testing with 24-hour Holter monitoring or with a monitor that can be activated at times of symptoms to record the cardiac rhythm. Tinnitus or hearing loss indicates the need for audiometric testing. Multiple or recurrent cranial neuropathy should prompt magnetic resonance imaging (MRI) of the head.

Vestibular Tests
Vestibular testing may include electronystagmographic testing, specific ocular motor testing, rotational tests, and posturography.

Management of Peripheral Vestibulopathy

Medical Treatment
Therapy is outlined for symptomatic treatment of dizziness presumed to be of peripheral origin (Table 10.4). Although most of the drugs used for dizziness are referred to as *vestibular suppressants*, their mechanism of action is largely unknown. When a definitive diagnosis has been made, therapy must be directed to the underlying disorder. In patients with chronic dizziness, patience is required to relieve anxiety and depression.

Exercise therapy can be extremely beneficial for the treatment of persistent positional vertigo. In the Brandt-Daroff technique, the patient is asked to move rapidly from a seated position to lying on the side. It is more comfortable if the patient rests his or her head on a pillow or other support until the symptoms subside. The patient is to remain in that position for 30 seconds and then return to the upright position and wait until any

Table 10.4: Medical therapy for vertigo

Class	Dose*
Antihistamines	
Meclizine	25–50 mg 3 times/day
Cyclizine	50 mg 1–2 times/day
Dimenhydrinate	50 mg 1–2 times/day
Promethazine	25–50 mg/day
Anticholinergics	
Scopolamine tablets	0.45–0.50 mg 1–2 times/day
Scopolamine transdermal patch	1/day for 3 days
Donnatal[†]	1, 3 times/day
Sympathomimetics	
Ephedrine	25 mg/day
Antiemetics	
Trimethobenzamide	250 mg 1–2 times/day PO
	200-mg suppository
Promethazine	25–50 mg/day
Prochlorperazine	5–10 mg 1–3 times/day PO
	25-mg suppository
Tranquilizers	
Diazepam	5–10 mg 1–3 times/day
Oxazepam	10–60 mg/day
Haloperidol[‡]	0.5–1.0 mg 1–2 times/day
Combination preparations and others (doses as listed above)	
Scopolamine with ephedrine	
Scopolamine with promethazine	
Ephedrine with promethazine	
Diuretics	
Diet	

*Usual adult starting dose; maintenance dose can be increased by a factor of two to three. The most common side effect is drowsiness.
[†]This is a combination preparation, containing a mixture of atropine alkaloids with approximately one-fourth grain (15.0–16.2 mg) phenobarbital.
[‡]Note the very low dose when compared with usual antipsychotic treatment. Nevertheless, the patient should still be observed for dystonias.

recrudescence of symptoms subsides or for a minimum of 30 seconds. The patient is then instructed to move rapidly lateral to the opposite recumbent position, wait for 30 seconds, and then return to the upright position, completing one repetition. Patients are asked to repeat this exercise for 20 repetitions two times a day. Most patients experience significant relief within 1 week. Permanent cure is common despite some recurrences.

Surgical Treatment

Surgical treatment of chronic peripheral vestibular dysfunction is primarily destructive. Labyrinthectomy is recommended for patients with severe Ménière's disease who do not respond to medical therapy and who are having severe recurrent disabling attacks. A medical labyrinthectomy may be performed by the use of the aminoglycosides, which are particularly destructive to the peripheral vestibular hair cells.

Various shunting procedures have been used to treat Ménière's disease and its associated endolymphatic hydrops. Although some patients can benefit, long-term success with such shunting procedures to the mastoid region and to the subarachnoid space has been modest.

Management of Central and Systemic Vestibular Disorders

The management of central vestibular disorders depends on the diagnosis. Medical therapy for peripheral vestibular dysfunction may be useful for central disorders and systemic disorders. Surgical treatment is directed primarily toward removal of the tumors that can affect the peripheral or central vestibular apparatus.

HEARING LOSS AND TINNITUS WITHOUT DIZZINESS OR VERTIGO

Types of Hearing Loss

Hearing loss can result from a lesion anywhere within the auditory system. An abnormality within the outer or middle ear will create a *conductive hearing loss* because of inefficient transmission of sound to the inner ear system. When the loss of hearing is a result of pathology in the cochlea or along the eighth cranial nerve from the inner ear to the brainstem, the loss is referred to as a *sensorineural hearing loss*. Patients may exhibit both conductive and sensorineural loss, which is referred to as a *mixed hearing loss*.

Auditory Neuropathy

Auditory neuropathy (AN) is also known as *auditory dyssynchrony*. A typical presentation of a patient with AN is that of a variable bilateral hearing loss with the following test findings:

1. The presence of otoacoustic emissions indicating normal outer hair cell function

2. The presence of cochlear microphonics on auditory brain-stem responses consistent with functioning outer hair cells
3. Absent or elevated acoustic reflexes

Most children with AN have speech/language delays and require remediation by a speech pathologist. Approximately one third of AN cases are associated with hereditary sensory motor neuropathies or spinocerebellar degenerations.

Examination

Otoscopic examination is essential to determine the patency of the external ear canal and the integrity of the tympanic membrane. If the external canal is occluded by cerumen, simple tests of hearing may be invalidated. A neurologist should be able to recognize an inflamed, bulging, or scarred drum. The office examination of hearing loss includes the *Weber* and *Rinne* tests, in which a tuning fork is used to test air and bone conduction. With a vibrating tuning fork placed on the midline of the skull, the patient is asked to indicate in which ear the sound is heard (Weber's test). In unilateral hearing losses, lateralization to the ear that hears more poorly indicates conductive impairment in that ear. Lateralization to the ear that hears better suggests that the problem in the opposite ear is sensorineural. The Rinne test is a comparison of the patient's hearing sensitivity by bone conduction with that by air conduction. Individuals who hear normally and individuals with sensorineural hearing loss perceive air-conducted sound louder than bone-conducted sound. Individuals with conductive hearing loss have better bone conduction than air conduction. A *mixed hearing loss* consists of a conductive and a sensorineural component in the same ear.

Central Auditory Disorders

Lesions within the central auditory system are difficult to detect or localize. Indeed, many central auditory dysfunctions cannot be demonstrated by conventional audiological measurements. Total removal of one hemisphere of the brain in humans does not result in any major change of auditory sensitivity in either ear.

Tinnitus

Tinnitus is experienced by one third of adults. It may be constant, intermittent, fluctuating, or pulsating and may be perceived as a high- or low-pitched tone, a band of noise, or some combination of such sounds. Most tinnitus sufferers have a concomitant loss of hearing, which may be either conductive or sensorineural. Tinnitus may precede or follow the onset of a loss in hearing, or the two may occur simultaneously.

Subjective Tinnitus
Only the patient hears subjective tinnitus. It may be present in one or both ears or localized within the head. This type of tinnitus can result from a lesion involving the external ear canal, tympanic membrane, ossicles, cochlea, auditory nerve, brainstem, or cortex. The most common cause is cochlear disease.

Objective Tinnitus
Objective tinnitus is less common and perceived not only by the patient but also by the examiner. Objective tinnitus may be vascular (an arteriovenous malformation or fistula) or mechanical in origin. Objective mechanical tinnitus is caused by abnormal muscular contraction of the nasopharynx or middle ear. Objective tinnitus of vascular origin may also be a referred bruit from stenosis in the carotid or vertebrobasilar system.

For a more detailed discussion, see Chapters 17, 18, and 41 in Neurology in Clinical Practice, 4th edition.

Disturbances of Taste and Smell | *11*

The senses of taste and smell rely on chemical stimuli to excite their receptors and are designated the *chemosensory system*. Together they produce the sensation of flavor; dysfunction in one is often perceived as an abnormality in the other.

OLFACTION

Two important nasal chemosensory systems are the free nerve endings of the trigeminal nerve and the sensory receptors of the olfactory system. High concentrations of most odorants stimulate the trigeminal nerve in the walls of the nasal passages and cause a sensation of general nasal irritability. Olfactory receptors respond to chemical stimuli at lower concentrations and with greater selectivity than the trigeminal nerve and are responsible for the discrimination of different odorous substances. In cases of total anosmia, the capacity to distinguish between odors is lost, whereas the response to nasal irritation is generally preserved.

Clinical Evaluation of Smell

When assessing impaired sense of smell, the clinician's main objective is to distinguish intranasal from neurogenic causes. The causes of transitory olfactory loss include viral upper respiratory tract infection, rhinitis, sinusitis, polyps, neoplasms, and abnormalities in mucus secretion. The ability to detect odors may be lost (*anosmia*) or decreased (*hyposmia*), normal smells may be distorted (*parosmia* or *dysosmia*), sensitivity to some or all odorants may be increased (*hyperosmia*), or the ability to discriminate odors may be impaired. Neurogenic olfactory loss produces similar symptoms and is caused by direct olfactory nerve damage (closed-head injury, viral infection, toxic substances) or impairment of normal receptor cell turnover (radiation or antiproliferative drug therapy). Neural olfactory loss can impair discrimination without producing anosmia.

Unilateral loss of smell is not recognized by the patient but when found on examination serves as a useful sign of a neurogenic lesion. Patients complaining of anosmia should be asked about a history of head trauma, recent upper respiratory tract infection, drug use (both prescribed and abused), systemic illness, occupational exposure to toxins, dental procedures and prostheses, smoking and alcohol history, seizure disorder, radiation therapy, and pending litigation (loss of smell is a compensable disorder).

System review should include headache, vision changes, nosebleeds, nasal obstruction, menstrual history, diminished intellectual capacity, and psychiatric disturbances, including mood changes such as depression. Physical examination, in addition to taste and smell testing, should evaluate the ears, nose, mouth, oronasopharynx, and upper cranial nerves. Mental status evaluation for evidence of dementia and depression is important.

Examination of odor discrimination or identification is sufficient to screen for deficits in transport, sensory, and neural olfactory functions. Traditionally, having the patient sniff a familiar substance such as coffee, oil of cloves, or oil of peppermint, held in turn beneath each nostril while the other is occluded, tests olfaction. Suggestion is minimized by having patients close their eyes and by indicating that the bottle may be empty. The patient is asked to identify the odor. Appreciation of an odor, despite the inability to name it, excludes anosmia. Hysterical patients may show unilateral anosmia on the side of an alleged neurological deficit. A malingerer can be detected with ammonia that stimulates the trigeminal nerve, which malingerers deny noticing.

Laboratory Investigation

The extent of the laboratory investigation depends on the history and physical examination. If no obvious cause can be identified, appropriate studies for an underlying systemic illness should include complete blood cell count, routine blood chemistries, serum Vitamin B_{12}, thyroid function tests, glucose concentration, syphilis serology, magnetic resonance imaging (MRI) of the skull and sinuses, and an electroencephalogram. A formal otorhinolaryngological evaluation is essential to exclude local nasal disorders.

Disease Entities

Among the many causes of smell disturbances, except for nasal and paranasal sinus disease, 85% of cases follow upper respiratory tract infections or head trauma or are idiopathic conditions. The high incidence of nasal and parasinus disease causing anosmia and hyposmia underscores the need for a thorough otorhinolaryngological evaluation. Although intracranial causes (excluding head trauma and intracranial surgery) are rarely responsible for loss of smell, they result in the greatest morbidity if not diagnosed.

Olfactory Groove Meningioma

Anosmia may be the first symptom of an olfactory groove meningioma. This treatable condition, if not detected, often enlarges and causes seizures, visual loss, and dementia. Headache is usually present. Cranial MRI establishes the diagnosis.

Head Trauma

Loss of smell may result from damage to the olfactory nerve as it enters the skull at the cribriform plate, damage to the olfactory bulb, and possibly cerebral cortical injury. Shearing forces, fracture of the anterior fossa, and direct contusion are the mechanisms most commonly responsible. The frequency of anosmia and hyposmia after head trauma is 10–20% and is proportional to the severity of the injury. MRI changes are present in 88% of patients, predominantly in the olfactory bulbs and tracts of the inferior frontal lobes. Recovery occurs in up to 40% of patients but is unlikely beyond 1 year after injury.

Aging

Olfactory changes associated with aging include reduced sensitivity, intensity, identification, and discrimination. Age-related deficits can alter food choices and subsequently exacerbate disease states and impair nutritional status and immunity. Use of flavor-enhanced food can help maintain appetite and food enjoyment.

Other Causes

In Parkinson's disease (PD), the degree of olfactory impairment does not correlate with age, disease duration, disease severity, cognitive impairment, and dopaminergic or cholinergic treatment. Hyposmia in asymptomatic relatives of patients with PD suggests subclinical dopamine dysfunction. Olfactory dysfunction occurs in 40% of patients with multiple sclerosis and correlates with the number of demyelinating plaques on MRI involving areas of olfaction in the inferior frontal and temporal lobe regions. An increased sense of smell, *hyperosmia*, is uncommon and may occur with depression and exposure to toxic vapors. *Parosmia*, the distortion of normal smell, may occur with temporal lobe seizures or tumor, olfactory bulb injury, depression, or sinusitis. Approximately 75% of parosmic patients have associated hyposmia or anosmia.

Olfactory hallucinations occur in Alzheimer's disease, depression, schizophrenia, alcohol withdrawal, and uncinate seizures. In seizures, the hallucinations are characteristically unpleasant or foul and rarely appear as isolated epileptic events. Cigarette smoking, several drugs, radiation therapy, and hemodialysis, as well as environmental and industrial toxins, cause disturbances of smell.

TASTE

The gustatory system is responsible for the perception of sweet, salty, bitter, and sour. Disturbances of taste are far less common than disturbances of smell. Patients who complain that food no longer has any taste usually have olfactory dysfunction with normal taste. Disorders of taste are characterized as absence of taste (*ageusia*), diminished sensitivity (*hypogeusia*), increased sensitivity to some or all qualities of taste (*hypergeusia*), distortion of normal taste (*dysgeusia* or *parageusia*), and gustatory hallucinations.

Clinical Evaluation of Taste

Patients presenting with a disturbance of taste should be asked about any associated disorder of smell; any pre-existing medical conditions and their treatment, such as ear infection, ear surgery, Bell's palsy, significant head injury, or tracheal intubation; recent upper respiratory tract illness; dental procedures or prostheses; and a detailed drug history. In addition to a physical examination and testing of taste and smell, special attention should be paid to the oral cavity for evidence of infection, inflammation, degeneration, and masses, as well as atrophy and dryness of tongue, gums, dentition, and surrounding mucous membranes. Specific investigations are ordered when the clinical features suggest a specific cause. If no local cause is suggested, patients with taste abnormalities, particularly unilateral, should have audiological evaluation and imaging studies that include the inner ear.

The sense of taste can be tested with natural stimuli, such as aqueous solutions of sugar, sodium chloride, acetic acid, and quinine. A cotton applicator is used to rub the aqueous solution gently on one quadrant of the protruded tongue. The patient should not talk but should identify the perceived taste by pointing to cards printed with the words *sweet, salt, sour,* and *bitter.* The mouth is rinsed with water between tests.

Disease Entities

The two most common causes of hypogeusia are nasal disorders and a prior respiratory tract infection. Other causes are local disorders involving the tongue, taste buds, or both and damage to neural pathways in the peripheral or central nervous system.

Drugs, Physical Agents, and Aging

Heavy smoking, particularly of pipe tobacco, and pharmaceutical agents, especially antirheumatic drugs, antiproliferative drugs, and drugs with sulfhydryl groups, such as penicillamine and captopril, are common causes of taste dysfunction. Calcium-channel blockers, such as nifedipine and diltiazem, as well as antifungal agents, smokeless tobacco, and sumatriptan nasal spray, may cause abnormalities of taste. Other local causes, in part related to drying of the mouth (xerostomia), include Sjögren's syndrome, radiation therapy, and pandysautonomia; these illustrate the important role saliva plays in taste perception. The taste threshold in the elderly is more than twice as high as that of the general population. Loss of taste may be the initial symptom of primary amyloidosis.

Bell's Palsy

Although Bell's palsy is usually associated with ipsilateral loss of taste over the anterior two thirds of the tongue, the patient usually does not recognize the loss. Recovery of taste within the first 14 days of onset usually predicts complete recovery from paralysis.

Other Causes

Taste disorders after head injury are rare and are almost always caused by disturbance of smell. Impaired taste may occur with jugular foramen tumors and with more diffuse processes, such as idiopathic midline granuloma, high-altitude sickness, and diabetes mellitus.

For a more detailed discussion, see Chapter 20 in Neurology in Clinical Practice, 4th edition.

Cranial and Facial Pain

12

HISTORY

It is usually helpful to begin by asking the patient to describe the pain or by simply asking what kind of help the patient seeks. This approach allows patients to relax and to say what they had planned to say previously. Once the patient has had an opportunity to speak, directed but open-ended questions can be asked.

Types of Headaches

Many individuals, especially those with a long-standing problem, have more than one type of headache. It is valuable to establish this information at the beginning of the interview so that each type of pain can be carefully delineated. In most instances, migraine is one headache and tension headache or rebound headache is the other.

Onset of Headaches

A headache disorder of many years' duration with little change is almost always of benign origin. Migraine headaches often begin in childhood or early adulthood. A headache of recent onset has many possible causes, some benign and others more serious. An increasingly severe headache suggests an expanding intracranial lesion. A new headache in an older patient suggests an intracranial lesion (e.g., subdural hematoma) or giant cell (temporal or cranial) arteritis. Headaches of instantaneous onset suggest an intracranial hemorrhage, usually in the subarachnoid space, but also may be caused by cerebral venous sinus thrombosis, spontaneous cerebrospinal fluid (CSF) leaks, pituitary apoplexy, and severe hypertension. Occasionally, mass lesions produce intermittent acute headaches by interfering with CSF circulation.

Frequency and Periodicity of Episodic Headaches

Migraine may be episodic or chronic. Chronic migraine (formerly referred to as *transformed migraine*) usually occurs in individuals with a history of episodic migraine headaches. Episodic migraine may become chronic with or without medication overuse. *Episodic cluster headaches* typically occur daily for weeks or months and are followed by a long headache-free interval, although chronic cluster headaches may occur daily for years. A related disorder, *chronic paroxysmal hemicrania*, occurs several times per day, often for years. A chronic daily headache lacking migrainous or autonomic features is likely to be a chronic tension-type headache. If there is no regular periodicity, it is useful to inquire about the longest and shortest periods of freedom between headaches. Asking patients to monitor their headache frequency, intensity, and medication use on a "headache calendar" often provides useful information.

Peak and Duration of Headaches

Migraine usually peaks within 1–2 hours of onset and usually lasts 6–36 hours. Cluster headache is typically maximal immediately if the patient awakens with the headache in progress or peaks within a few minutes if it begins during wakefulness. Cluster headaches characteristically last 45–120 minutes but occasionally last a few hours. Headaches similar to cluster headaches but lasting only about 15 minutes several times a day are typical of chronic, or episodic, *paroxysmal hemicrania*. "Ice-pick" head pains (*idiopathic stabbing pain*) are momentary, lasting only seconds. Tension-type headaches commonly build up over hours and may last days to years. These headaches may include some migraine features and were formerly called a *mixed* or *tension-vascular* headache but more appropriately fall under the rubric of chronic migraine. A new sudden, severe headache that is maximal at onset suggests intracranial hemorrhage, cerebral venous sinus thrombosis, or pituitary apoplexy. A chronic, continuous unilateral headache of moderate severity with superimposed attacks of more intense pains that are associated with autonomic features suggests the diagnosis of hemicrania continua, an indomethacin-responsive syndrome. Occipital neuralgia and trigeminal neuralgia manifest as brief shocklike pains, sometimes occurring in a crescendo pattern over a period of seconds to minutes. Occasionally, a duller pain in the same nerve distribution persists longer. Short-lasting unilateral neuralgiform headache with conjunctival injection and tearing (SUNCT) is a rare syndrome manifested by paroxysms of retroorbital pain lasting seconds but with 3–100 episodes per day and the associated autonomic symptoms for which it is named.

Time and Occurrence and Precipitating Factors
Cluster headaches often awaken patients from a sound sleep and have a tendency to occur at the same time each day in a given person. Hypnic headaches typically affect elderly patients, regularly awakening the patient at a particular time of night. Unlike cluster headaches, they are typically diffuse and not associated with autonomic phenomena. Migraine can occur at any time during the day or night but frequently begins in the morning. A headache of recent onset that disturbs sleep or is worse on waking may be caused by increased intracranial pressure (ICP). Tension-type headaches are typically present during much of the day and are often more severe late in the day. Obstructive sleep apnea may be accompanied by the chronic occurrence of headaches on awakening.

Patients with chronic recurrent headaches often can recognize factors that trigger an attack. Migraine headaches may be precipitated by bright light, menstruation, weather changes, caffeine withdrawal, sleeping longer or less than usual, and ingesting substances such as alcohol. Trauma, emotional or physical, may be an important causative factor in the pathogenesis of headache.

If bending, lifting, coughing, or Valsalva maneuver produces a headache, an intracranial lesion, especially involving the posterior fossa, must be considered; however, most exertional and cough headaches are benign. Intermittent headaches that are precipitated by assuming the upright position and are promptly relieved by lying down are characteristic of a CSF leak. If no history exists of a lumbar puncture, head trauma, or neurosurgical procedure, a spontaneous leak may be the cause. Alcohol is often a potent precipitant of cluster headaches.

Headache occurring during sexual activity, especially during or shortly after orgasm, may be of benign origin, especially if a headache has occurred on multiple occasions previously. A single headache in this circumstance, however, may be caused by a subarachnoid hemorrhage.

Lancinating face pain triggered by facial or intraoral stimuli occurs with trigeminal neuralgia. Glossopharyngeal neuralgia is most commonly triggered by chewing, swallowing, and talking, although cutaneous trigger zones in and about the ear are occasionally present.

Location and Evolution
Asking the patient to delineate the location of the pain with a finger is often helpful. Trigeminal neuralgia is confined to one or more branches of the trigeminal nerve. The patient may be able to localize one or more trigger points over the face or in the mouth and then outline the spread of the pain. Pain in the throat may be related to a local process or glossopharyngeal neuralgia. Pain in the lower portion of the face and neck can be produced sometimes by either a cluster or a migraine variant—a so-called *lower half headache.* Carotid dissection commonly presents with neck, face, and head pain ipsilateral to the dissection; this should be considered in any patient with pain of recent onset in these locations.

Migraine is most often unilateral, commonly in the frontotemporal region, but it may be generalized or may evolve from a unilateral location to become generalized. Cluster headaches are virtually always unilateral during an attack and are typically centered in, behind, or about the eye. At different times (different clusters), some patients do experience cluster headaches that have switched sides from a prior cluster.

A typical tension-type headache is generalized, although it may originate across the nuchal muscles only to spread and perhaps predominate in the frontal or occipital region. When pain is localized to an eye, the intraoral region, or the ear, local processes involving these structures must be considered. Otalgia may be caused by a process involving the tonsillar fossa and the posterior tongue. Unilateral facial pain when chronic often does not have an underlying lesion. Occasionally, though, facial pain may be a symptom of nonmetastatic lung cancer.

Quality and Severity

Although it is often difficult for the patient to describe the quality of the pain, this information may be useful. It may be helpful to ask the patient to grade the severity of pain on a scale of 1–10. Migraine often has a pulsating quality that may be superimposed on a more continuous pain. Cluster headache is characteristically severe, boring, and steady and is often described as similar to a "hot poker." SUNCT produces moderately severe pain in the orbital or temporal region and may be described as stabbing or pulsatile. Tension-type headaches are usually described as a feeling of fullness, tightness, or pressure or as being like a cap, band, or vise. Headaches caused by meningeal irritation, whether related to infectious meningitis or a hemorrhage, are typically severe. Trigeminal neuralgia is severe, brief, and stabbing, occurring up to several times per minute; a milder ache may occur between paroxysms of pain. Pain caused by glossopharyngeal neuralgia is similar in character to that of trigeminal neuralgia.

Premonitory Symptoms, Aura, and Accompanying Symptoms

Leading questions may be necessary. Some patients have premonitory symptoms that precede a headache attack by hours. These can include psychological changes, such as depression, euphoria, and irritability, or more somatic symptoms, such as constipation, diarrhea, abnormal hunger, fluid retention, or increased urination. The term *aura* refers to focal cerebral symptoms associated with a migraine attack. These symptoms most commonly last 20–30 minutes and precede the headache. At other times, the aura may continue into the headache phase or arise during the headache phase. Visual symptoms are the most common kind of cerebral dysfunction and may consist of either positive or negative phenomena or a mixture of both. Other hemispheric symptoms, such as weakness, somatosensory disturbances (usually paresthesias), or language dysfunction, may precede the headache. Aura symptoms usually have a gradual onset and spread over minutes. If more than one symptom occurs (e.g., visual and somatosensory), the onsets are usually staggered and not simultaneous. The slow spread is a helpful feature to differentiate these from focal neurological symptoms caused by cerebral ischemia. Symptoms of brainstem origin, such as vertigo, dysarthria, ataxia, quadriparesis, diplopia, and loss of consciousness, accompany basilar migraine. Nausea, vomiting, photophobia, phonophobia, and osmophobia characteristically accompany migraine attacks. In addition, lacrimation, rhinorrhea, and congestion accompany migraine headache in many patients and should not be confused with a headache of sinus origin.

Ipsilateral miosis and ptosis (oculosympathetic paresis or Horner's syndrome), lacrimation, conjunctival injection, and nasal stuffiness frequently accompany cluster headache. Sweating and facial flushing on the side of the pain have been described but are uncommon. Facial swelling, usually periorbital in location, may develop with repeated attacks. Shorter-lived attacks occurring multiple times per day with similar autonomic features suggest a diagnosis of episodic or chronic paroxysmal hemicrania, an indomethacin-responsive syndrome. An oculosympathetic paresis is also a common feature associated with ipsilateral internal carotid artery dissection. In the setting of acute transient or persistent monocular blindness, giant cell arteritis and carotid dissection should be considered.

Temporomandibular joint dysfunction often is characterized by jaw pain precipitated by movement of the jaw, clenching of the teeth, reduction in the range of jaw movement, joint clicking, and tenderness over the joint.

Headache accompanied by fever suggests an infectious cause. Persistent or progressive diffuse or focal central nervous system symptoms, including seizures, suggest a structural cause for a headache. Purulent or bloody nasal discharge suggests an acute sinus cause for the headaches. Likewise, a red eye raises the possibility of an ocular process, such as infection or acute glaucoma. A history of polymyalgia rheumatica, jaw claudication, or tenderness of the scalp and superficial arteries in an elderly person suggests the possibility of giant cell arteritis. Transient visual obscurations, tinnitus, diplopia, and the finding of papilledema may be associated with increased ICP from any cause, particularly idiopathic intracranial hypertension (pseudo-tumor cerebri).

An important principle is that symptoms that accompany a headache can be key in accurate diagnosis.

Aggravating Factors

The worsening of headache as a result of a cough or jolt suggests an intracranial element to the pain, whereas aggravation by torsion of the neck may indicate a musculoskeletal component. Cluster headache sufferers tend to suffer their pain in an agitated state, pacing and moving about, whereas migraineurs prefer to lie still. Precipitation or marked aggravation of headache in the upright position suggests intracranial hypotension.

Mitigating Factors

Rest, especially sleep and avoidance of light, tend to provide relief to the migraineur. Massage or heat may ameliorate the pain associated with a tension-type headache. Local application of pressure over the affected eye or ipsilateral temporal artery, local application of heat, or, rarely, short-lasting intense physical activity may alleviate the pain of cluster headache. Headache caused by intracranial hypotension typically is relieved or markedly benefited by recumbency.

Family History of Headaches

Migraine is often an inherited disorder, and a family history of migraine or "sick headaches" should be sought. Tension-type headaches are also usually familial. Cluster headache is familial in a minority of cases (approximately 7%). Familial hemiplegic migraine is a rare autosomal dominant variant of migraine with aura, wherein the migraine attack includes hemiparesis lasting minutes to weeks.

Prior Evaluation and Medications

The patient should be asked about prior consultations and testing for the headaches. If appropriate, the records and imaging study films can be obtained for review.

Prior Medications

Response to medications should be sought, including those used to treat individual headache attacks and those used prophylactically. The dose, route of delivery, dosage schedule, and duration of treatment should be established. This information also provides an opportunity to determine whether medications such as ergot preparations and analgesics have been overused. It also establishes whether prophylactic medications were optimized. A history of the use of caffeine-containing substances also should be elicited, because they may cause or aggravate headaches.

Disability, Patient Concerns, and Reasons for Seeking Help

The assessment of headache-related disability is important. A baseline determination with follow-up assessments is useful when judging the effects of treatment and can be useful in guiding headache therapy. In addition, disability can be useful in guiding the headache therapy. The Migraine Disability Assessment Scale (MIDAS) is an example of a useful, validated clinical tool.

Headache pain can produce significant fear and anxiety regarding serious disease. The patient should be allowed to articulate any concerns so each aspect can be appropriately addressed by the physician.

Reason for Seeking Help

The reason the patient is seeking help may be irrelevant if the problem is of recent onset. If the problem is chronic, however, it can be useful to inquire why the patient has come for aid at this point.

Other Medical or Neurological Problems

A history of past or current medical and neurological conditions and history of trauma, operations, and medication allergies should be obtained. Additionally, a history of the use of other medications and dietary supplements unrelated to the headaches should be obtained.

EXAMINATION

In the patient with headache, the physical examination often shows no abnormalities. However, findings on examination may yield important clues as to the underlying cause. Even when the results of the examination are normal, both the physician and the patient gain confidence that nothing has been overlooked.

Although, strictly speaking, the history and the examination are separate parts of the evaluation, in practice the examination begins the moment the physician encounters the patient. Careful observation helps determine whether the patient has physical illness, whether he or she appears anxious or depressed, and whether the patient's history is reliable. For instance, with respect to reliability, a patient who is unable to give a reasonably coherent history is suspected of having an abnormal mental status.

It is important to perform a neurological examination, including examination of the mental status, gait, cranial nerves, motor system, and sensory system, as discussed in Chapter 1. A neurovascular examination also should be performed.

The skull and cervical spine should be examined. The skull should be palpated for lumps and local tenderness. There may be tenderness over inflamed sinuses. Thickened, irregular temporal arteries with an associated reduction in pulse suggest giant cell arteritis. Occasionally, other scalp lesions may be present that point to a cause for head pain. In muscle contraction headaches, the scalp muscles may be tender.

A short neck or low hairline suggests basilar invagination or an Arnold-Chiari malformation. In an infant, separation of the sutures suggests increased ICP, most commonly caused by hydrocephalus. Measuring the head circumference is always worthwhile in a child.

The cervical spine also should be tested for tenderness and mobility. Nuchal rigidity on passive neck flexion and Kernig's sign are evidence of meningeal irritation.

Vital signs, especially blood pressure and pulse, always should be assessed. If there is a question of fever, temperature should be measured. The body habitus should be noted. This observation may be particularly relevant in young women with headache possibly related to pseudotumor cerebri who are almost always obese. The general examination also includes auscultation of the heart and lungs, palpation of the abdomen, and examination of the skin.

DIFFERENTIAL DIAGNOSIS

In most cases, the history and examination are all that are needed to make a diagnosis, especially in the patient with a chronic headache. Migraine, tension-type headaches, and cluster headaches usually can be diagnosed with a high degree of certainty, especially if the headaches have been recurrent over a long period and the examination is normal. Then it may be possible to proceed directly to management.

In some situations, however, the diagnosis is uncertain. These situations specifically raise concerns of a serious organic cause for the headaches. Headaches that are progressive are a worrisome indication of a possible intracranial process. A new headache of abrupt onset always raises concern about an intracranial process, especially hemorrhage and sometimes a mass lesion. Headaches that interfere with sleep, although sometimes benign, must be considered to have a potential serious cause. Headaches precipitated by exertion, change of position, cough, sneeze, or strain may be benign, although again they raise the possibility of an intracranial lesion, especially in the posterior fossa. Systemic symptoms, such as weight loss, fever, or those associated with another known systemic disease, such as malignancy or human immunodeficiency virus infection, should be investigated with care. Headaches that are associated with neurological symptoms, except those that are typical for migraine, should raise concern. Unexplained findings on neurological examination and a history of seizures should prompt additional evaluation.

The investigations used to evaluate a patient with headaches can include almost all of the tests used in neurology and neurosurgery, as well as various medical tests. Selection of the appropriate studies depends on the formulation after the history and examination. Indiscriminate use of batteries of tests is unwarranted.

LABORATORY STUDIES

Neuroimaging Tests

Computed Tomographic Scanning and Magnetic Resonance Imaging

Computed tomographic (CT) scanning and magnetic resonance imaging (MRI) are extremely useful tests in the evaluation of patients with headache. Tumors, hematomas, cerebral infarctions, abscesses, hydrocephalus, and many meningeal processes can be identified with CT scanning and MRI. Abnormalities of the skull base, pituitary gland–craniocervical junction, and white matter are better seen with MRI. The cost of an MRI study is severalfold that of a CT scan, but MRI is safer because x-rays are not used to generate the image and the enhancing agent used with MRI (gadolinium) is safer than the iodinated contrast used with CT. CT can detect acute subarachnoid hemorrhage if sufficient bleeding has occurred. If the CT scan is normal and the history is suggestive of recent subarachnoid hemorrhage, a lumbar puncture should be performed. CT scanning can be helpful for evaluating abnormalities of the skull, orbit, sinuses, facial bones, and the cervical spine. Changes associated with intracranial hypotension are best shown with MRI. The cervical spinal cord and exiting nerve roots and the craniocervical junction are much better shown with MRI.

Magnetic resonance angiography (MRA) is a noninvasive method that can demonstrate intracranial and extracranial vascular occlusive disease including large vessel dissection, intracranial arteriovenous malformations, and aneurysms. Intracranial venous sinus thrombosis is best diagnosed with magnetic resonance venography.

Evidence-based guidelines for neuroimaging of patients with nonacute headache found MRI to be more sensitive in finding white matter lesions and developmental venous anomalies than CT.

For acute-onset headache, CT is the optimal imaging study; in patients with subacute and chronic headache, MRI is likely to reveal more, but many of the abnormalities will be incidental.

Plain X-rays of the Skull, Sinuses, and Cervical Spine

Plain x-rays of the skull are unnecessary in the routine evaluation of patients with headache but can be obtained if there has been acute head trauma or if there is an unusual bony abnormality on physical examination. Although plain x-rays of the sinuses can show infection, hemorrhage, or tumor, CT scanning and MRI provide greater definition. The role of the cervical spine in the causation of headaches remains uncertain, but occipitonuchal pain may result from degenerative disc and joint disease of the middle and upper cervical spine. Rheumatoid arthritis can lead to craniocervical junction instability and pain. Tomographic films may be needed to show bony changes in the upper cervical spine and craniocervical junction. Flexion and extension, odontoid, and pillar views of the cervical spine can help to exclude ligamentous damage and fractures in patients with a history of head and neck injury. Congenital abnormalities of the cervical spine, such as the Klippel-Feil syndrome, may be associated with other disorders such as an Arnold-Chiari malformation.

Other Imaging Studies
Panoramic x-ray examination, MRI, or CT of the temporomandibular joints may be helpful in select patients. The presence of temporomandibular joint disease should not be taken as proof that a patient's headaches are related. Dental x-rays are useful if dental-origin pain is suspected.

Cerebral Angiography

Cerebral angiography is rarely needed in the initial investigation of headache. It can be helpful in confirming vascular disease, including arterial dissections, arteriovenous malformations, and intracranial aneurysms, as well as the presence of central nervous system vasculitis.

Radioisotope and Computed Tomographic Studies for Cerebrospinal Fluid Leaks

Isotope cisternography can be helpful in determining the presence and location of a spontaneous, posttraumatic, or postoperative CSF leak. Alternatively, CT scanning of the spine after instillation of contrast into the lumbar spinal fluid can be used to identify the location of CSF leaks.

Cerebrospinal Fluid Tests

CSF examination is used to diagnose or exclude meningitis, encephalitis, subarachnoid hemorrhage, leptomeningeal cancer, and lymphoma and is required to confirm increased or decreased ICP. Measurement of the opening CSF pressure should be performed in all patients.

Electroencephalography

Electroencephalography is not useful in the investigation of headache unless the patient also has a history of seizures, syncope, or episodes of altered awareness.

General Medical Tests

A few blood tests are important in the investigation of headache. Determining the erythrocyte sedimentation rate is essential in the evaluation of giant cell arteritis. Although a normal value does not exclude this condition, it greatly reduces the likelihood. Episodic headaches associated with unusual behavior or impairment of consciousness may suggest an insulinoma. A diagnosis of insulinoma is supported by elevated insulin and C-peptide levels in the face of a low or relatively low fasting glucose level. Levels of carboxyhemoglobin can be measured in patients complaining of early morning headaches during the winter when home heating is used, especially when several members of the same household are affected. Estimation of blood alcohol levels and drug screening may be helpful in certain patients. Sensitive thyroid-stimulating hormone and serum thyroxine levels should be measured in patients with chronic headache because hypothyroidism may present with headaches. Urine concentrations of metanephrines and free catecholamines should be measured if a pheochromocytoma is suspected.

Special Examinations and Consultations

Perimetry is helpful in the delineation of visual field defects. Tonometry is necessary to document elevated intraocular pressure in glaucoma, but unless the eye is red or the cornea is cloudy glaucoma is an unlikely cause of head or even eye pain. These tests are routinely done by ophthalmologists, who also have the equipment and expertise to perform slit-lamp examinations and other specialized examinations.

If pain of dental or temporomandibular joint origin is suspected, a dentist or oral surgeon skilled in the detection and treatment of these disorders should be consulted.

Diagnosis of tumors of the sinuses, nasopharynx, and neck, as well as inflammation of the sinuses, is aided by the expertise of an otorhinolaryngologist.

Temporal artery biopsy is performed to confirm or exclude giant cell arteritis.

In some selected patients (e.g., those with headaches as a manifestation of a chronic pain disorder with or without a history of drug abuse), psychiatric consultation may be helpful for diagnosis and management.

For a more detailed discussion, see Chapter 22 in Neurology in Clinical Practice, 4th edition.

Brainstem Syndromes | *13*

The most effective method of evaluating a brainstem disorder is to organize the differential diagnosis around the objective physical findings. The long tracts of the nervous system traverse the entire brainstem in the longitudinal (rostrocaudal) plane; cranial nerve nuclei and their nerves originate and exit at distinct horizontal levels. The combination of long-tract and cranial nerve signs provides precise localization. Cranial magnetic resonance imaging (MRI) is the main laboratory investigation in the diagnosis of brainstem syndromes.

OCULAR MOTOR SYNDROMES

Combined Vertical Gaze Ophthalmoplegia

Combined vertical gaze ophthalmoplegia is paresis of both upward and downward gaze. Symptoms are relatively non-specific and usually occur when reading, eating from a table, and walking down a flight of stairs. Coma, long-tract signs, and loss of pupillary reflexes are often associated. The diagnosis of combined vertical gaze ophthalmoplegia is appropriate when the ocular findings occur in isolation from long-tract signs. The location of the lesion is the rostral interstitial nucleus of the medial longitudinal fasciculus (MLF), and the usual cause is infarction of the rostral dorsal midbrain.

Upgaze Paresis (Dorsal Midbrain or Parinaud's Syndrome)

The tetrad of findings in the dorsal midbrain syndrome are (1) loss of upgaze, which is usually supranuclear, (2) average-size or large pupils with light-near dissociation or pupillary areflexia, (3) convergence-retraction nystagmus, and (4) lid retraction.

The presence of the full syndrome implies a lesion of the dorsal midbrain (including the posterior commissure), a bilateral lesion of the pretectal region, or a large unilateral tegmental lesion. The most common cause of loss of upgaze is a tumor of the pineal region. The next most common causes are stroke and trauma.

Downgaze Paresis

Isolated downgaze paresis is uncommon. Symptoms include difficulty reading, eating, and walking down stairs. Neurological examination reveals loss of downward pursuit and saccades, occasionally sparing pursuit. The site of the lesion for isolated downgaze paresis is bilateral involvement of the lateral portions of the MLF. The differential diagnosis is ischemic stroke, progressive supranuclear palsy (PSP), and Whipple's disease.

Internuclear Ophthalmoplegia

The characteristic features of internuclear ophthalmoplegia (INO) are paresis of adduction of one eye, with horizontal nystagmus in the contralateral eye when abducted. It is due to a lesion of the MLF ipsilateral to the side of the adduction weakness. The common causes of INO are stroke and multiple sclerosis.

Horizontal Gaze Paresis

Horizontal gaze paresis seldom occurs in isolation. Patients may complain of inability to see or to look to the side. Examination reveals loss of ipsilateral saccades and pursuit but full horizontal eye movements with the oculocephalic maneuver. The location of the lesion for horizontal gaze paresis is the frontopontine tract, mesencephalic reticular formation, pontine reticular formation, and sixth cranial nerve nucleus. Cerebrovascular disease is the likely cause in patients older than 50 years with an acute onset and multiple sclerosis before age 50.

Global Paralysis of Gaze

The common symptoms of global paralysis of gaze are inability to look voluntarily (saccades and pursuit) in any direction. It rarely occurs in isolation. The location of the lesion is the frontopontine tract for saccades and the parietooccipital-pontine tract for pursuit, where they converge at the subthalamic and upper midbrain level. The common causes for these symptoms are Guillain-Barré syndrome, myasthenia gravis, and chronic progressive external ophthalmoplegia.

One-and-a-Half Syndrome

The characteristic features of one-and-a-half syndrome are gaze palsy when looking toward the side of the lesion, together with INO on looking away from the lesion. The common symptoms are diplopia, oscillopsia (the illusion that objects or scenes are oscillating), and blurred vision. Associated findings are skew deviation and gaze-evoked nystagmus on upgaze or lateral gaze, and less commonly on downgaze. The location of the lesion is the peripontine reticular formation (PPRF) or sixth cranial nerve nucleus with extension to involve the internuclear fibers crossing from the contralateral sixth cranial nerve nucleus, which causes the INO. The differential diagnosis is multiple sclerosis, stroke, arteriovenous malformation, or tumor of the lower pons.

SYNDROMES INVOLVING OCULAR MOTOR NUCLEI

Lesions of the third or sixth cranial nerve nuclei are usually associated with long-tract signs and show ocular motility disturbances that are different from lesions of the third or sixth cranial nerve.

Third Cranial Nerve Nucleus

The usual symptoms of nuclear third nerve palsies are diplopia and ptosis. The signs ipsilateral to the lesion are weakness of the inferior and medial recti and of the inferior oblique muscles. Both eyes have limited upgaze because the superior rectus subnucleus is contralateral, and the axons cross within the nuclear complex. Bilateral ptosis and dilated unreactive pupils may be present because the levator subnucleus and Edinger-Westphal nuclei have bilateral representation. Ischemic stroke is the most common cause of nuclear third nerve palsies. Other considerations are hemorrhagic stroke, metastatic tumor, and multiple sclerosis. Disorders that simulate nuclear third nerve palsy are myasthenia gravis, chronic progressive external ophthalmoplegia, and thyroid ophthalmopathy, all of which spare the pupil.

Sixth Cranial Nerve Nucleus

A lesion of the sixth nerve nucleus causes ipsilateral gaze palsy and lateral rectus palsy. The oculocephalic maneuver cannot overcome the gaze palsy because the vestibuloocular reflex synapses are in the nucleus of the sixth nerve. Ipsilateral peripheral seventh nerve palsy is always associated. The differential diagnosis includes stroke, Wernicke's encephalopathy, multiple sclerosis, and a tumor of the pontomedullary junction.

OTHER BRAINSTEM AND ASSOCIATED SYNDROMES

Diencephalic Syndrome (Russell's Syndrome)

The symptoms of diencephalic syndrome are emaciation with increased appetite, euphoria, vomiting, excessive sweating, and an alert appearance with motor hyperactivity. Most cases occur in children younger than 3 years. Laboratory studies may show an elevated serum growth hormone level incompletely suppressed by hyperglycemia. MRI usually demonstrates a hypothalamic mass lesion.

Thalamic Syndrome

The usual features of the thalamic syndrome are pain, numbness, and hemisensory loss. Thalamic pain may be spontaneous or evoked by mild stimulation and often has a disagreeable and lasting quality. Examination shows marked hemianesthesia in which pain and temperature or light touch and vibration sense may be separately impaired. Proprioceptive loss is usually marked, often with astereognosis. Transitory hemiparesis sometimes occurs. The usual cause of thalamic pain is lesions in the ventroposterolateral nucleus of the thalamus. The differential diagnosis is stroke or tumor.

Tectal Deafness

The symptoms of tectal deafness are bilateral deafness, usually sparing pure tones, associated with poor coordination, weakness, or vertigo. The differential diagnosis includes conduction-type hearing loss, cochlear disorders, bilateral eighth cranial nerve lesions, and pure word deafness. The dorsal midbrain syndrome is often associated. The common causes are tumors of the brainstem, cerebellum, or pineal region and trauma or stroke. Tests that reveal central nervous system auditory loss are distorted speech audiometry, dichotic auditory testing, and auditory brainstem-evoked responses. MRI usually establishes the diagnosis.

Foramen Magnum Syndrome

The characteristic features of the foramen magnum syndrome are spastic weakness and sensory loss below the head. The cause is often a benign, completely removable tumor. The initial features are usually neck stiffness and pain that radiates to the shoulder. Other complaints are occipital headache, weakness of the arms or legs, numbness of the hands or arms, clumsiness, and a gait disturbance. Examination usually shows hemiparesis or quad-riparesis and sensory loss. The loss of sensation may affect some modalities more than others and have a "cape" or C2 distribution. Other patterns are a hemisensory loss below the head or restricted involvement of the legs. Pseudoathetosis from loss of joint position sense may be an early sign. Muscle atrophy may occur, often involving the intrinsic muscles of the hands. Neck flexion may induce electric shock–like sensations that radiate down the spine and transmit to the limbs (*Lhermitte's symptom*). These usually occur with lesions of the posterior columns, most commonly multiple sclerosis. Lower cranial nerve palsies are uncommon. The presence of downbeat nystagmus in primary position or lateral gaze strongly suggests a lesion of the craniocervical junction.

Syringobulbia

Syringobulbia is a progressive enlargement of a fluid-filled cavity in the medulla that usually extends into the spinal cord (syringomyelia). The symptoms are those of central medullary and spinal cord dysfunction, including the following: painless burns, hand numbness, neck and arm pain, leg stiffness, and headache, together with oscillopsia, diplopia, or vertigo. Examination reveals signs of lower brainstem dysfunction. Lower motor neuron signs of the ninth through twelfth cranial nerves may be present. Nystagmus, if present, is horizontal, vertical, or rotary. The arms or forequarter may show loss of pain and temperature, with sparing of other sensations. The sensory loss may also be in a hemisensory distribution. Absent or decreased tendon reflexes in the arms are expected. The differential diagnosis is intrinsic central cord and lower brainstem lesion (syrinx, tumor, or trauma) and compressive foramen magnum syndrome caused by a tumor. Less likely causes are multiple sclerosis and spinal arachnoiditis.

BRAINSTEM ISCHEMIC STROKE SYNDROMES

Vertebrobasilar ischemia causes lesions that often have a rostrocaudal or patchy localization. Clinical features may not be explainable in anatomical terms. The ischemic stroke syndromes outlined in this section may occur in isolation, as presented here, or in combination. The combinations can be medial with lateral or often rostrocaudal extension. The main feature of brainstem stroke is the combined involvement of long tracts and cranial nerve nuclei. The cranial nerve palsy is ipsilateral to the lesion and the long-tract signs are contralateral. Another feature is bilateral involvement of the long tracts. This can cause the *locked-in syndrome* or *pseudobulbar palsy*. Blindness occurs with bilateral posterior cerebral artery occlusion and concomitant occipital lobe infarction.

Thalamic Stroke Syndromes

The blood supply to the thalamus is from the posterior cerebral, posterior communicating, basilar communicating, and anterior and posterior choroidal arteries. Table 13.1 lists the thalamic stroke syndromes.

Midbrain Stroke Syndromes

Long-tract signs and third and fourth cranial nerve palsies characterize midbrain ischemia. Supratentorial (anterior circulation) stroke syndromes also may cause midbrain signs when rostrocaudal deterioration occurs. The blood supply of the upper mesencephalon is by perforating branches of the basilar communicating artery supply (P1 segment of the posterior cerebral artery or mesencephalic artery) that connects the basilar artery with the posterior communicating artery. The division of vascular territories is into median and lateral transverse regions. Ipsilateral third cranial nerve palsy associated with contralateral hemiparesis characterizes the medial midbrain syndromes. The lateral syndromes consist of contralateral loss of pain and temperature sensation and ipsilateral Horner's syndrome and loss of facial sensation. Ataxia may occur on either side.

Table 13.1: Ischemic stroke syndromes of the diencephalon

Anterolateral
  Common symptoms
    Contralateral weakness, vision loss
    Confusion
    Disorientation
    Language disturbance
  Signs
    Contralateral
      Hemiparesis
      Hemiataxia
      Hemisensory loss
      Homonymous hemianopia
    Right-sided lesion: visuospatial abnormalities, hemineglect, nonverbal intellect affected
    Left-sided lesion: disorientation, aphasia
  Arterial territory involved: thalamic polar (tuberothalamic) artery
Medial
  Common symptoms
    Disorientation and confusion
    Coma with occlusion of mainstem variant
    Visual blurring
  Signs
    Vertical gaze ophthalmoplegia
    Loss of pupillary reflexes
    Loss of convergence
    Disorientation and confusion, stupor, coma, and various neuropsychiatric disturbances
  Arterial territory involved: posterior thalamosubthalamic paramedian artery (thalamic paramedian or deep interpeduncular profundus artery)
Lateral and posterior internal capsule
  Common symptoms
    Contralateral
      Hemiparesis
      Numbness
    Confusion
  Signs
    Contralateral
      Hemiparesis
      Diminished pain and temperature
      Dysarthria
      Homonymous hemianopia; characteristically with a tongue of visual field spared along the horizontal meridian
      Memory impairment
      With right-sided lesions: visuoperceptual abnormalities
  Arterial territory involved: anterior choroidal artery

Continued

Table 13.1: (continued)

Posterolateral
  Common symptoms
    Contralateral
      Weakness
      Numbness
      Vision loss
      Neglect
      Confusion
  Signs
    Contralateral
      Loss of touch, pain, temperature, and vibration sense (common)
      Hemiparesis in some
      Hemiataxia
      Homonymous hemianopia
      Left hemispatial neglect
      Poor attention span
    Arterial territory involved: geniculothalamic artery

Pontine Stroke Syndromes

Penetrating branches of the basilar artery represent the pontine blood supply. These arteries do not have collateral supply. Lacunar stroke syndromes, which may be clinically indistinguishable from lesions of the internal capsule, are common.

Contralateral hemiparesis, ipsilateral ataxia, internuclear ophthalmoplegia, and conjugate horizontal gaze paresis characterize the *medial syndrome*. The lateral syndrome consists of contralateral hemianesthesia, loss of discriminative sensation, ipsilateral Horner's syndrome, facial hemianesthesia, and ataxia. Caudal pontine lesions cause ipsilateral facial palsy of the lower motor neuron type, sixth nerve paresis, deafness, and vertigo.

Medullary Stroke Syndromes

Four patterns of deficit occur with medial medullary stroke: (1) crossed hypoglossal hemiparesis syndrome, (2) sensorimotor stroke without lingual palsy, (3) pure hemiparesis, and (4) bilateral medial medullary stroke. Ipsilateral paralysis of the tongue and contralateral paralysis of the limbs characterize the medial medullary syndrome. Loss of discriminative sensation is associated when the medial lemniscus is involved. The lateral medullary syndrome (*Wallenberg's syndrome*) is characterized by contralateral loss of pain and temperature sensation and ipsilateral ataxia, Horner's syndrome, ipsilateral sensory loss in the face, dysphagia, hoarseness, diminished gag reflex, and loss of taste. Nystagmus is often present. The critical sign that distinguishes this syndrome from a lateral pontine syndrome is weakness of the ipsilateral palate and vocal cords.

For a more detailed discussion, see Chapter 22 in Neurology in Clinical Practice, 4th edition.

Gait Disorders

14

Many diseases of the motor system produce characteristic disturbances of gait and posture.

HISTORY AND COMMON SYMPTOMS

A detailed account of the walking difficulty and its evolution provides important clues to the underlying diagnosis. The ways to describe walking difficulties are limited. Disturbances almost anywhere in the central or peripheral nervous systems cause tripping and stumbling. The particular circumstances associated with walking difficulty help distinguish weakness from a more global defect of motor control or imbalance. Uneven ground exacerbates most walking difficulties and is not discriminatory.

Weakness

Descriptions of leg weakness vary. Stiffness or heaviness may be the initial symptom of a spastic paraparesis or hemiparesis. A tendency to trip due to catching or scraping the toe on the ground is an initial symptom of spastic equinovarus foot posture or a footdrop. Bilateral symptoms usually indicate a peripheral neuropathy. Difficulty climbing stairs or rising from a seated position suggests proximal muscle weakness, usually from myopathy, whereas weakness of knee extension causes difficulty walking down stairs.

Slowness

Slowness of walking and limb stiffness are common symptoms in extrapyramidal diseases. Associated features are a shuffling gait with small steps and difficulty rising from a chair. Falling backward or forward is an early feature of akinetic-rigid syndromes. Fatigue during walking occurs in muscular weakness of any cause and is usually a symptom of the extra effort required to walk in upper motor neuron syndromes and extrapyramidal disease.

Loss of Balance

The main features of ataxia, midline cerebellar disease, or proprioceptive sensory loss are poor balance, unsteadiness, and a tendency to fall. Patients with cerebellar gait ataxia complain of an inability to walk in a straight line, difficulty turning suddenly, and staggering, whereas those with sensory ataxia complain of increased unsteadiness in the dark. Acute disturbances of balance and equilibrium suggest a vascular insult to the cerebellum, thalamus, or basal ganglia.

Falls

Tripping may be due to footdrop or shallow steps, and proximal muscle weakness may result in the legs giving way. Unsteadiness and poor balance lead to falls in ataxic syndromes. Spontaneous falls or falls following postural adjustments suggest an impairment of postural reflexes. With extreme loss of postural reflexes, patients show marked retropulsion.

Sensory Symptoms and Pain

The distribution of any accompanying sensory complaints provides further information about the site of the lesion producing walking difficulties. It is important to determine whether complaints of leg pain and weakness in patients with difficulty walking share a common cause or whether the pain is of musculoskeletal origin and is exacerbated by walking. The patient may voluntarily engage strategies to minimize pain by avoiding bearing the full weight on the affected limb and by limiting its range of movement (*antalgic gait*).

Incontinence

Loss of the voluntary control of sphincter function in a patient with a spastic gait suggests a spinal cord lesion. Parasagittal cerebral lesions are also a consideration. Impairment of higher mental function may be an important clue to a cerebral cause of paraparesis.

EXAMINATION OF POSTURE AND WALKING

The examination of posture and walking begins with observing the overall pattern of whole-body movement as the patient walks. Normal walking progresses in a smooth and effortless manner, with an upright posture of the trunk, free-swinging motion of the legs, regular and appropriately sized strides, and flowing associated synergistic head, trunk, and arm movements.

Trunk Posture

Flexion of the trunk is a feature of extrapyramidal diseases and cautious gait syndromes, neck extension is characteristic of progressive supranuclear palsy, and an exaggerated lumbar lordosis is secondary to hip-girdle weakness in proximal myopathies and paraspinal muscle spasm. Exaggerated flexion of the trunk and hip when walking occurs in torsion dystonia. Altered truncal postures, particularly in the lumbar region, may be to compensate for a shortening of one lower limb, disease of the hip, knee, or ankle, or in response to leg pain.

Postural Reflexes

Examination of postural reflexes is by gently pulling the upper trunk backward or forward with the patient standing. Impaired postural righting reactions are evident after each displacement by a few short shuffling steps backward (*retropulsion*) or forward (*propulsion*).

Stance

Patients with cerebellar or sensory ataxia, diffuse cerebral vascular disease, and frontal lobe lesions have wide-based gaits.

Initiation of Gait

Difficulty initiating the first step (start hesitation) and episodes of freezing are features of Parkinson's disease and frontal lobe disease. Start hesitation ranges in severity from a few shuffling steps to small shallow steps on the spot without forward progress, to complete immobility with the feet seemingly glued to the floor ("magnetic feet"). Exaggerated upper body movements are an effort to engage the legs in motion.

Stepping

Slowness is characteristic of the akinetic-rigid syndromes but is also seen in ataxic and spastic syndromes. Increasingly rapid small steps (*festination*) are common in Parkinson's disease but are rare in other akinetic-rigid syndromes. Reduced associated trunk movement and arm swing occurs in unilateral upper motor neuron, extrapyramidal, and acute ataxic syndromes. Bilateral loss of synergistic arm movement when walking is an important sign of Parkinson's disease in the early stages, when most symptoms are unilateral.

PHYSICAL SIGNS

Spastic Gait

Spasticity of the arm and leg on one side produces the characteristic clinical picture of a spastic hemiparesis. The arm is adducted, internally rotated at the shoulder, and flexed at the elbow with the forearm pronated, and the wrist and fingers are flexed. The leg, slightly flexed at the hip and extended at the knee, shows plantar flexion and inversion of the foot. Slight lateral flexion of the trunk toward the unaffected side accompanies the swing phase of each step. Hyperextension of the hip on that side allows the slow circumduction of the stiffly extended paretic leg, as it swings forward from the hip, dragging the toe or catching it on the ground beneath. Minimal associated arm swing occurs on the affected side.

Ataxic Gait

The main causes of an ataxic gait are cerebellar disorders, sensory loss, and frontal lobe disorders. Table 14.1 summarizes their features.

Gait in the Elderly

Healthy, neurologically normal elderly people tend to walk at slower speeds than younger people. The slower speed of walking relates to shorter and shallower steps with reduced excursion at lower limb joints. The rhythmicity of stepping is preserved.

Myopathic Weakness and Gait

Weakness of proximal leg and hip-girdle muscles interferes with the stabilization of the pelvis and legs on the trunk during all phases of the gait cycle. Failure to stabilize the pelvis produces exaggerated rotation of the pelvis with each step (waddling or Trendelenburg gait); weakness of hip extension causes slight flexion of the hips and an exaggerated lumbar lordosis.

Table 14.1: Summary of the major clinical features distinguishing different types of gait ataxia

Feature	Cerebellar Ataxia	Sensory Ataxia	Frontal Lobe Ataxia
Trunk posture	Stooped, leans forward	Stooped, upright	Upright
Stance	Wide based	Wide based	Wide based
Postural reflexes	Variable	Intact	Impaired or absent
Initiation of gait	Normal	Normal	Start hesitation
Steps	Staggering, lurching	High stepping	Short, shuffling
Speed	Normal, slow	Normal, slow	Very slow
Heel-toe	Unable	Variable	Unable
Turning corners	Veers away	Minimal effect	Freezing, shuffling
Romberg test	Variable	Increased unsteadiness	Variable
Heel-shin test	Usually abnormal	Variable	Normal
Falls	Uncommon	Yes	Very common

Neurogenic Weakness and Gait

Muscle weakness secondary to a peripheral neuropathy typically affects distal muscles of the legs and results in a steppage gait. The patient lifts the leg and foot high above the ground with each step because of weakness or paralysis of ankle dorsiflexion and a footdrop (steppage gait).

For a more detailed discussion, see Chapter 25 in Neurology in Clinical Practice, 4th edition.

Hemiplegia and Monoplegia

15

Hemiplegia and monoplegia result from focal structural lesions. Imaging studies easily localize the cause.

HEMIPLEGIA

Cerebral lesions are the most common causes of hemiplegia. The lesions may be either cortical or subcortical.

Cortical Lesions

On the cerebral cortex the body is represented as a *homunculus*, with the body draped over the central sulcus, the leg in the interhemispheric fissure, and the face and arm on the lateral aspect of the hemisphere. Function is the basis of cortical organization. Activation of motor neurons causes movement of individual muscles or groups of muscles with a synergistic action. Small lesions of the cortex cause prominent weakness of a limb, but hemiplegia is not expected. Sensory signs usually accompany motor signs. Other signs of cortical dysfunction (e.g., aphasia, hemianopia) depend on the location of the lesion.

Subcortical Lesions

Lesions in the basal ganglia or internal capsule can produce hemiparesis or hemiplegia. The hemiparesis is contralateral and may be without sensory loss (*pure motor stroke*). Depending on the portion of the internal capsule affected, focal weakness of mainly one arm or leg may result, although pure monoplegia is unusual. Thalamic lesions result in sensory loss contralateral to the lesion.

Brainstem Lesions

Brainstem lesions causing hemiplegia are easy to localize because of associated signs of brainstem dysfunction. Motor pathways for the limbs remain crossed until they reach the pyramidal tract decussation in the medulla; a lesion of the pons or midbrain causes contralateral limb weakness. Lesions that affect the medial lemniscus and spinothalamic tract at low medullary levels produce loss of light touch and position sense on the body ipsilateral to and below the lesion and loss of pain and temperature sensation below and contralateral to the lesion. Lesions above the midmedulla produce contralateral disturbance of all sensation. Their distinct features include ipsilateral facial weakness, sensory loss, or both, with contralateral hemiplegia (*crossed neurological signs*). Oculomotor deficits with hemiparesis indicate pontine or midbrain lesions. Horner's syndrome develops ipsilateral to lesions that affect the descending sympathetic tracts in the lateral aspect of the brainstem.

Spinal Cord Lesions

Spinal cord lesions rarely cause hemiplegia but can cause asymmetrical limb weakness that may appear as monoplegia. Tumors affecting nerve roots can compress the spinal cord and cause corticospinal tract signs. Most of the descending corticospinal fibers are ipsilateral to the innervated limbs, so the upper motoneuron deficit is ipsilateral to the lower motoneuron deficit in the arm. High cervical lesions may produce asymmetrical compression of the cord, and although hemiparesis can occur, contralateral involvement is usually present.

Peripheral Lesions

Hemiplegia is unlikely from peripheral lesions, but occasionally tandem lesions affecting a homolateral arm and leg can mimic a central lesion. Important causes include mononeuropathy multiplex and combined cervical and lumbar radiculopathy.

Functional Hemiplegia

Functional weakness includes both conversion reaction and malingering. In conversion reaction, the patient is not conscious of the nature of the hemiplegia. In malingering, the patient makes a conscious effort to fool the examiner. In both conditions, the deficit offers some secondary gain. The following clues are helpful but not compelling in establishing the diagnosis of functional weakness:

1. The hemihypesthesia that accompanies functional hemiplegia often changes from hypesthetic to normal sensation exactly at the midline, whereas in central nervous system disease, sensation changes 1–2 cm before the midline on the abnormal side.
2. *Hoover's sign* is tested while the patient is supine. The examiner places one hand below the normal heel and instructs the patient to raise the weak leg against resistance. The patient with a weak leg pushes the other heel down against the examiner's hand, whereas the patient with functional weakness does not.
3. Functional weakness is not associated with other expected findings, such as tendon reflex changes and pathological reflexes.

MONOPLEGIA

Monoplegia usually signifies a lesion at the level of the spinal cord, root, plexus, or peripheral nerves, but brain lesions are a consideration in the differential diagnosis.

Brain Lesions

Cerebral lesions occasionally produce monoplegia rather than hemiplegia. Focal infarction in the distribution of the anterior division of the middle cerebral artery can affect the arm and the leg, but the face is usually affected. Leg weakness develops with damage to the central medial aspect of the hemisphere. This is most likely with anterior cerebral artery infarction. Usually both legs are involved, giving the appearance of a myelopathy. Brainstem lesions produce hemiparesis or quadriparesis rather than monoparesis because of the proximity of the leg and arm motor axons.

Spinal Cord Lesions

Cord lesions can cause monoplegia in the arm if segmental damage affects mainly the anterior horn cells of one side, with little damage to the contralateral cord or descending tracts. The best example is monomelic amyotrophy. Intradural extramedullary lesions can compress the cord, producing prominent segmental dysfunction, but signs of descending and ascending dysfunction ultimately develop.

Nerve Root Lesions

Nerve root lesions do not cause complete paralysis of all muscles of an arm or leg. Roots serving arm power are C5 through T1. Roots serving leg power are L2 through S1. Loss of relevant tendon reflexes can be present even when no weakness is detectable.

Plexus Lesions

Brachial and lumbar plexopathies produce monoparesis with a distribution that does not conform to a neural or dermatomal distribution. The presence of hyporeflexia rather than hyperreflexia differentiates brachial plexopathy from cerebral lesions and the absence of leg weakness from spinal lesions.

Peripheral Nerve Lesions

Peripheral nerve lesions usually produce monoparesis, with the weakness confined to the individual nerve distribution.

Functional Monoplegia

Most of the discussion of functional hemiplegia applies equally to patients with functional monoplegia. In monoplegia, the affected limb is often an arm, and it is held tightly against the chest.

PITFALLS IN DIAGNOSIS

Intrinsic Weakness of the Small Muscles of the Hand

The ulnar nerve innervates most intrinsic muscles of the hand. An isolated distal ulnar lesion causes profound loss of hand use that is similar to frontocentral cerebral lesions located in the hand region. Median nerve lesions produce impaired hand function because the finger and wrist flexors have greater loss of function than the intrinsic muscles of the hand. Intact function of ulnar- and radial-innervated muscles with the hand stabilized rules out lesions at or above the plexus. Lower brachial plexus lesions cause dysfunction of the intrinsic hand muscles and the long finger flexors. This can be mistaken for central weakness, because the deficit spans peripheral nerve distributions.

Electromyography usually documents the axonal damage after several weeks. A small cerebral cortical lesion can produce disuse of the hand without signs of other deficit. Reflexes are eventually exaggerated. Magnetic resonance imaging is the most sensitive imaging study for a small cerebral lesion.

Radial Neuropathy or Small Cerebral Cortical Infarcts?

Radial neuropathy causes weakness of the wrist extensors, which can result in destabilization of the intrinsic muscles of the hand and long finger flexors. The deficit seems more extensive than expected because opposition from the radial-innervated extensors is required for the median- and ulnar-innervated muscles to function, suggesting a cerebral lesion. Stabilizing the finger flexors and wrist demonstrates intact median and ulnar nerve function and differentiates radial neuropathy from a cerebral lesion.

Leg Weakness: Peroneal Nerve Palsy or Paramedian Cerebral Cortical Lesion?

Peroneal nerve palsy results in weakness of foot dorsiflexion and eversion with relative preservation of other motor functions. Small lesions of the leg region of the homunculus cause similar weakness. However, peroneal palsy does not cause inverter weakness and electromyographic signs of denervation do not develop with cerebral lesions. Cerebral causes of lower leg weakness cause an extensor-plantar response and hyperactivity of the Achilles' tendon reflex, despite clinical evidence of gastrocnemius muscle involvement.

Leg Weakness: Cauda Equina Lesion, Myelopathy, or Paramedian Cerebral Cortical Lesion?

Cauda equina lesions are usually due to acute disc herniations, spondylosis, or tumors in the lumbosacral spinal canal. Compression of the lumbar and sacral nerve roots results in motor and sensory loss. Intermittent claudication of the cauda equina causes severe pain accompanied by neurological dysfunction that is relieved by a few minutes of rest. Standing worsens pain, sensory loss, and weakness. *Spondylotic myelopathy* is compression of the spinal cord by degenerative spondylosis above the cauda equina. Compression produces weakness of the legs and pain near the level of the lesion. Spine pain is not expected. Cauda equina lesions are associated with depressed reflexes, whereas spinal cord and cerebral lesions have hyperactive reflexes and upgoing plantar responses. Sensory loss is more prominent with cauda equina lesions than with higher lesions.

For a more detailed discussion, see Chapter 26 in Neurology in Clinical Practice, 4th edition.

Paraplegia and Spinal Cord Syndromes

16

The localization of spinal cord pathology is by the *level* in the rostrocaudal axis and by *extent* in the transverse plane. These two coordinates are determined by clinically assessing neurological functions served by spinal tracts, anterior horn cells, and nerve roots. The time course during which spinal cord dysfunction evolves is the third factor because it often determines the underlying cause and predicts the prognosis.

SEGMENTAL INNERVATION

Ventral Root Dysfunction

Ventral root dysfunction causes a characteristic pattern of weakness that distinguishes it from peripheral nerve disease. Even though the innervation of each muscle is by multiple roots, ventral root dysfunction may affect one muscle more than others. Such muscles are *segment-pointer muscles* (Table 16.1). Complete lower motor neuron (LMN) paralysis of a muscle or muscle group typically signifies plexus or peripheral nerve disease, rather than a monoradiculopathy. The weakness is often associated with atrophy and fasciculations. The fasciculations may be restricted to the myotomal distribution of the compressed root, occur repetitively in the same fascicle during minimal contraction, and may be absent during complete rest. Muscle tone is either normal or decreased unless pain causes muscle spasm.

Dorsal Root Dysfunction

Dorsal root dysfunction usually causes pain and, to a lesser extent, sensory impairment. The pain may be local or projected in a radicular or nonradicular distribution. The sensory disturbances, reflex changes, and motor abnormalities correspond to the injured nerve root.

Table 16.1: Segment-pointer muscles

Root	Muscle	Primary Function
C3	Diaphragm	Respiration
C4	Diaphragm	Respiration
C5	Deltoid	Arm abduction
C5	Biceps	Forearm flexion
C6	Brachioradialis	Forearm flexion
C7	Triceps	Forearm extension
C8	Intrinsic hand muscles	Finger adduction/abduction
T1	Intrinsic hand muscles	Finger adduction/abduction
L1	Iliopsoas	Hip flexion
L3	Quadriceps femoris	Knee extension
L4	Quadriceps femoris	Knee extension
L4	Tibialis anterior	Foot dorsiflexion
L5	Extensor hallucis longus	Great toe dorsiflexion
S1	Gastrocnemius	Plantar flexion

Source: Modified with permission from Schliack, H. 1969, "Segmental innervation and the clinical aspects of spinal nerve root syndromes," in *Handbook of Clinical Neurology*, vol. 2, eds P. J. Vinken, G. & W. Bruyn, North-Holland Publishing, Amsterdam.

Pain

Local or regional back or neck pain is usually secondary to irritation or damage of innervated structures of the spine. Radicular pain has great localizing value. Irritation of a dorsal root causes pain in the appropriate dermatome. Projected pain arises from one anatomical site and projects to a site some distance from the location of the pathology. When the spine is the source, the projected pain may be either radicular or nonradicular. Projected pain that arises from irritation of posterior nerve roots is of a radicular type, whereas that caused by irritation of other spinal structures is usually of a nonradicular type (*referred pain*). Tables 16.2 and 16.3 list the differential diagnoses of lesions of the cervical and lumbosacral nerve roots.

Dermatomes

The figures on the inside front and back covers illustrate the currently recognized dermatomal map. A few points deserve emphasis: (1) On the trunk, the C4 and T2 dermatomes are contiguous, (2) the thumb, middle finger, and fifth digits are innervated by C6, C7, and C8, respectively, (3) the nipple is at the level of T4, (4) the umbilicus is at the level of T10, and (5) in the posterior axial line of the leg (medial thigh), the lumbar and sacral dermatomes are contiguous.

Table 16.2: Differential diagnosis of lesions of the cervical nerve roots

Roots	C5	C6	C7	C8	T1
Sensory supply	Lateral border upper arm	Lateral forearm including thumb	Over triceps, mid forearm, and middle finger	Medial forearm to include little finger	Axilla down to the olecranon
Sensory loss	As above	As above	Middle fingers	As above	As above
Area of pain	As above, and thumb and index finger	As above, especially thumb and index finger	As above, and medial scapula border	As above	Deep aching in shoulder and axilla to olecranon
Reflex arc	Biceps jerk	Supinator jerk	Triceps jerk	Finger jerk	None
Motor deficit	Deltoid Supraspinatus Infraspinatus Rhomboids	Biceps Brachioradialis Brachialis (pronators and supinators of forearm)	Latissimus dorsi Pectoralis major Triceps Wrist extensors Wrist flexors	Finger flexors Finger extensors Flexor carpi ulnaris (thenar muscles in some patients)	All small hand muscles in some via C8

Continued

Table 16.2: (continued)

Roots	C5	C6	C7	C8	T1
Some causative lesions	Brachial neuritis	Acute disc lesions	Acute disc lesions	Rare in disc lesions or spondylosis	Cervical rib
	Cervical spondylosis	Cervical spondylosis	Cervical spondylosis		Thoracic outlet syndromes Pancoast's tumor
	Upper plexus avulsion				Metastatic carcinoma in deep cervical nodes

Source: Adapted from Patten, J. 1977, *Neurological Differential Diagnosis*, Springer–Verlag, New York.

Table 16.3: Differential diagnosis of lesions of the lumbosacral nerve roots

Roots	L2	L3	L4	L5	S1
Sensory supply	Across upper thigh	Across lower thigh	Across knee to medial malleolus	Side of leg to dorsum and sole of foot	Behind lateral malleolus to lateral foot
Sensory loss	Often none	Often none	Medial leg	Dorsum of foot	Behind lateral malleolus
Area of pain	Across thigh	Across thigh	Down to medial malleolus	Back of thigh, lateral calf, dorsum of foot	Back of thigh, back of calf, lateral foot
Reflex arc	None	Adductor and knee reflex	Knee jerk	None	Ankle jerk
Motor deficit	Hip flexion	Knee extension	Inversion of the foot	Dorsiflexion of toes and foot (latter L4 also)	Plantar flexion and eversion of foot
Some causative lesions		Neurofibroma		Disc prolapse	Disc prolapse
		Meningioma Metastasis Intervertebral disc prolapse (infrequent)		Metastases Neurofibroma Meningioma	Metastases Neurofibroma Meningioma

Source: Adapted from Patten, J. 1977, *Neurological Differential Diagnosis*, Springer–Verlag, New York.

Tendon Reflexes
Tendon reflex abnormalities have precise localizing value. Tendon reflexes that are segmentally hypoactive are sensitive indicators of specific root disturbance and, when hyperactive below a specific spinal level, indicate a myelopathy at or above that level.

Nerve Root versus Peripheral Nerve Lesion
Root lesions rarely cause paralysis of a single muscle or muscle group or autonomic dysfunction, although both can occur with peripheral nerve lesions.

LOCALIZATION OF LESIONS IN THE TRANSVERSE PLANE

Motor Disorders

The findings of LMN dysfunction are weakness associated with atrophy, hypotonia, fasciculations, and depressed tendon reflexes, whereas those findings of corticospinal tract disease are spasticity, hyperreflexia, and an extensor-plantar response. The most important clue suggesting a spinal cord disorder is paraparesis or quadriparesis.

Sensory Disturbances

Subjective sensory complaints generally precede objective sensory signs. Sensory complaints without abnormal sensory signs may be the initial feature of spinal cord disease, but in the absence of sensory complaints the sensory examination is usually normal. The symptoms of dorsal (posterior) column dysfunction are tingling or vibratory paresthesias. The initial feature of spinothalamic tract dysfunction is pain that is poorly characterized and localized.

The lateral spinothalamic tract usually conveys pain sensation, usually measured by pinprick and temperature sensation. These pathways are somatotopically organized so the sacral fibers are most peripheral and the cervical fibers are most central. Because a laterally placed extramedullary lesion compresses the peripheral fibers first and then the more centrally located fibers, a compressive lesion in the rostral spine may give rise to an apparently ascending loss of pain and temperature sensation. These findings underscore the importance of recognizing that a rostral lesion may give rise to a sensory level far below the site of the compression. Therefore image the entire spine when spinal cord compression is suspected.

The posterior columns transmit position and vibration sensation, but both modalities also travel in other pathways. The evaluation of position and vibration sensation impairments in the spinal cord is simple. However, spinal ataxia from posterior column or spinocerebellar tract disturbances may not be self-evident. Both the lateral and the posterior columns convey light touch, and its loss is not an early feature of spinal cord disease.

Autonomic and Respiratory Disturbances

Dysfunction of the spinal cord and cauda equina often causes bladder, bowel, and sexual dysfunction. A high bilateral cervical cord lesion may compromise respiration. Urinary retention and overflow incontinence often follow an acute spinal cord injury. Later, a reflex (*neurogenic* or *spastic*) bladder develops. Slowly evolving upper motor neuron dysfunction results in a reflex bladder without a preceding period of spinal shock and flaccid bladder. Damage in the region of the conus medullaris or the cauda equina produces a decentralized or autonomous flaccid bladder. Voluntary control over bladder function is impaired, the bladder distends, and overflow incontinence occurs. Control over the anal sphincter and the anal reflex is usually lost, and a region of saddle anesthesia may be present. Erectile dysfunction is common in men.

COMMON SPINAL CORD SYNDROMES

Spinal Shock

A complete transverse lesion of the spinal cord results in total loss of motor and sensory functions below the level of the lesion. *Spinal shock* develops after acute injuries. All spinal reflex activity is lost below the level of the lesion, accompanied by motor paralysis and sensory loss.

Incomplete Lesions of the Spinal Cord

Unilateral Transverse Lesion
Hemisection of the spinal cord results in contralateral loss of appreciation of pain and temperature and ipsilateral loss of sensation for position and vibration, as well as upper motor neuron paralysis (the *Brown-Séquard syndrome*). Trauma is the usual cause.

Central Cord Syndrome
Intramedullary lesions cause a dissociated sensory loss in which the decussating fibers at the level mediating sensation of pain and temperature are lost or decreased, whereas the position and vibratory sensibilities remain unimpaired. Central cord lesions may result in a *suspended sensory level* with preservation of sacral sensation, the fibers that are most peripheral in the lateral spinothalamic tracts. The usual causes of acute central cord syndrome include hemorrhage or contusion after trauma, whereas the causes of a slowly evolving central cord syndrome are tumor or syringomyelia.

Anterior Spinal Artery Syndrome
The frequency of spinal cord infarctions has increased because of an increased number of invasive procedures, such as vascular and thoracoabdominal surgery, and improved survival after cardiac arrest and hypotension. The anterior horns and anterolateral tracts are involved. After an initial interval of spinal shock, the clinical syndrome consists of corticospinal tract dysfunction below the level of the infarction; loss of bowel, bladder, and sexual functions; and a sensory disturbance in which posterior column function remains intact while spinothalamic tract function is lost.

Anterior Horn and Pyramidal Tract Syndrome
Disturbances of the anterior horns and pyramidal tracts, along with sparing of the sensory functions and autonomic nervous system, occur in motor neuron disease.

Combined Posterior and Lateral Column Disease
Loss of posterior column and lateral column function causes a spastic ataxic gait. The usual causes are subacute combined degeneration, Friedreich's ataxia, and tabes dorsalis.

CHARACTERISTIC CLINICAL FEATURES OF LESIONS AT DIFFERENT LEVELS

Foramen Magnum

Lesions of the foramen magnum are a challenging diagnostic problem for the clinician. Symptoms are often vague or may be distant from the foramen magnum. A common initial feature is occipital or neck pain, often increased by neck movement that radiates also into the shoulders or the ipsilateral arm. Neurological signs associated with foramen magnum tumors include nystagmus, impaired sensation over the upper face, and sometimes dysarthria, dysphonia, and dysphagia. Spastic weakness is characteristic.

Upper Cervical Spine

Compressive lesions of the upper cervical spine have similar clinical characteristics. Pain in the neck, occipital region, or shoulder is a common initial complaint. Compression of the second cervical root causes scalp pain; compression of the third or fourth roots causes neck or shoulder pain. Neck movement usually provokes the pain. Progressive compression results in unilateral arm weakness that may be upper motor neuron or LMN in type. Weakness then progresses to the ipsilateral leg before affecting the contralateral limbs.

Lower Cervical and Upper Thoracic Spine

The main feature of spinal cord and root compression at the C5 through T1 level is radicular pain. Tendon reflex, motor, and sensory disturbances follow. Table 16.2 summarizes the clinical features associated with dysfunction of these nerve roots.

Thoracic and Lumbar Levels

The thoracic dermatomal landmarks are the nipple (T4), the umbilicus (T10), and the inguinal ligament (L1). A radicular distribution of pain or sensory alterations localizes the abnormality to a specific dermatome.

Conus Medullaris and Cauda Equina

Lesions of the cauda equina and conus medullaris cause local, referred, and radicular pain; sphincter disturbances, loss of buttock and leg sensation; and leg weakness.

DISTINGUISHING INTRAMEDULLARY FROM EXTRAMEDULLARY LESIONS

This distinction is not always possible on clinical grounds, and an imaging study is required. As a rule, extramedullary compression causes ischemia and demyelination in the posterior and lateral column, with relative sparing of the anterior columns.

For a more detailed discussion, see Chapter 27 in Neurology in Clinical Practice, 4th edition.

Proximal, Distal, and Generalized Weakness | *17*

Weakness is decreased muscle strength as measured by the force of a maximal contraction. Fatigue is a failure to maintain an expected contraction. Weak muscles are more easily fatigued than normal muscles, but fatigue may occur in the absence of weakness. Weakness and fatigue may accompany dysfunction at all levels of the neuraxis and systemic diseases.

This chapter emphasizes the types of weakness caused by dysfunction of the motor unit (the motor neuron, peripheral nerve, neuromuscular junction, and muscle). As a rule, neuronopathies cause weakness of the extensors of the arms and the flexors of the legs, together with hyperreflexia and an extensor-plantar response. Neuropathies cause distal weakness, sensory impairment, and areflexia. Disorders of the neuromuscular junction (myasthenias) cause cranial nerve weakness and fatigue. Myopathies cause proximal weakness.

SYMPTOMS OF WEAKNESS

Symptoms of weakness depend more on the muscles involved than on the cause of weakness. Symptoms of ocular muscle weakness are usually ptosis and diplopia but may also include head tilt—either lateral tilt with fourth nerve palsies or backward tilt with ptosis. The initial feature of facial weakness is usually a feeling of stiffness or numbness. Drinking through a straw and blowing up balloons become difficult tasks. Facial expressions change, and the patient may sleep with his or her eyes open. Pharyngeal, palatal, and tongue weakness disturb speech and swallowing. A flaccid palate causes nasal regurgitation, choking spells, and aspiration of liquids. Pseudobulbar palsy causes dysphagia but does not cause nasal regurgitation.

The earliest feature of neck muscle weakness is failure to stabilize the head during sudden stopping and starting. Neck extensor weakness makes the chin fall to the chest during stooping and bending, whereas neck flexor weakness causes difficulty lifting the head off the pillow. Diaphragm muscle weakness causes shortness of breath, especially when lying flat or with exertion. These symptoms first lead to hypoventilation and carbon dioxide retention and then to morning headaches and/or vivid nightmares. Later, hypercapnia results in sedation and a depressed mental state.

Shoulder weakness produces fatigue and impairs tasks that require holding the arms up, such as combing the hair. Hand and forearm weakness are usually first noticed when opening a tightly closed screw-capped jar or when turning a faucet. Weakness of hip muscles causes difficulty arising from the floor or from a deep chair, so the hands push the body up. Descending stairs is difficult with quadriceps weakness, and ascending stairs is difficult with hip extensor weakness. Anterior tibial and ankle evertor weakness first causes repeated ankle sprains followed by footdrop with repeated tripping and a slapping gait. Weakness of both the anterior and the posterior muscles of the lower leg is associated with instability of stance and poor balance.

Weakness of the abdominal muscles makes sit-ups impossible. Focal weakness of the lower abdominal muscles causes a protuberance that mimics an abdominal hernia. Paraspinal muscle weakness prevents a straight posture when sitting or standing as compared with lying on the bed.

EXAMINATION OF THE WEAK PATIENT

The four parts to the examination of patients with muscle weakness are inspection, palpation, muscle strength evaluation, and testing of tendon reflexes. Inspection of facial expression, posture, and functional ability is the most informative part of the examination.

Observation

Patients with severe ptosis throw their head back and elevate the eyebrows in order to see. Facial weakness since childhood gives the face a smooth, unlined appearance. Expression is diminished or altered and drooling is present. Inspection of the tongue may reveal atrophy and fasciculations. When shoulder muscle tone is lost, the point of the shoulder rotates forward so that the backs of the hands face forward and the arms swing loosely in normal walking. Weakness of the serratus anterior muscles and trapezii causes the scapula to rise off the back of the rib cage and protrude (*winging of the scapula*) when the shoulders are abducted. Weakness and wasting of the intrinsic muscles of the hand produce a claw hand. The thumb rotates outward so that it lies in the same plane as the fingers. Slight flexion of the interphalangeal joints is associated with slight extension of the metacarpophalangeal joints. The medial and lateral bellies of the wasted quadriceps muscle fail to appear upon tightening the knee and wasted anterior tibial muscle does not fill the groove on the lateral side of the tibia when the foot is dorsiflexed.

Examination

Inspect all limbs for *fasciculations* and then palpate for consistency. Fibrotic muscle feels rubbery and hard, whereas denervated muscle sometimes separates into strands that roll under the fingers. Muscle may be tender in inflammatory myopathies, but severe muscle tenderness is unusual and suggests hysteria. Percussion of muscle elicits *myotonia*. Assess muscle strength by watching the patient perform the following tasks: blowing up the cheeks, walking on toes and heels, rising from the floor or a low seat, and doing a pushup. The assessment of individual muscle strength, when needed, uses the method and scoring system of the Medical Research Council (Table 17.1).

Abnormal muscle hypertrophy is uncommon when present beyond the expected increase in muscle bulk that accompanies exercise. Generalized muscle hypertrophy occurs in patients with myotonia congenita and paramyotonia congenita, in the rare syndrome of acquired neuromyotonia, and in chronic denervating disorders, especially in the posterior calf muscle in S1 radiculopathies. Focal hypertrophy of calf muscles may occur in Duchenne's and Becker's muscular dystrophy, as well as in the limb-girdle muscular dystrophies, spinal muscular atrophies (SMA), and in some glycogen storage disorders.

Table 17.1: Medical Research Council scale for grading muscle strength

0	No contraction
1	Flicker or trace of contraction
2	Active movement, with gravity eliminated
3	Active movement against gravity
4	Active movement against gravity and resistance
5	Normal power

Fatigue is a common symptom in many neuromuscular disorders and in many medical conditions. However, myasthenia is a probable diagnosis when strength is normal at rest and progressively worsens with use. Test fatigue when suspicious of a neuromuscular transmission disorder by repetitive or sustained contractions.

In disorders of the motor unit, reflexes are either normal, reduced, or absent. Amyotrophic lateral sclerosis is the exception because both upper and lower motor neuron dysfunction coexists. In neurogenic disorders, demyelinating conditions tend to lose reflexes early, whereas axonal neuropathies depress reflexes in proportion to the amount of axonal loss. In myopathies, reflexes tend to diminish in proportion to the amount of muscle weakness. The same is true for postsynaptic neuromuscular transmission disorders. Presynaptic neuromuscular transmission disorders tend to have depressed or absent reflexes at rest that are enhanced with brief periods of exercise.

INVESTIGATING THE WEAK PATIENT

The most useful tests are electrodiagnosis, muscle biopsy, genetic analysis, and measurement of the serum concentration of creatine kinase (CK). In addition, edrophonium chloride testing, exercise testing, nerve biopsy, and biochemical analysis of muscle are useful in specific conditions. The serum CK concentration is normal to moderately increased in neurogenic atrophy and markedly increased in myopathies. Race, sex, age, and activity level influence the normal CK concentration. The normal upper limits (97.5th percentile) are as follows: black men, 520 U/liter; black women and non-black men, 345 U/liter; and non-black women, 145 U/liter. The non-black population includes Hispanics, Asians, and whites.

An experienced clinical neurophysiologist is essential to interpret electrodiagnostic studies. Electrodiagnosis differentiates denervation from myopathy and axonal from demyelinating neuropathies. It localizes abnormalities from the anterior horn cells to the neuromuscular junction and establishes the presence of myotonia and neuromyotonia.

Muscle histology and histochemistry is more useful in myopathic disorders than in neuropathic disorders. It is indispensable for the diagnosis of congenital myopathies, some inflammatory myopathies, and the muscular dystrophies. An important aspect of the muscle biopsy is the analysis of the muscle proteins (e.g., dystrophin, the sarcoglycan complex, and merosin). Proteins may be missing in specific illnesses, and diagnosis is not possible without these analyses. Sampling error is a risk in all muscle biopsies. The muscle chosen should be mildly weak.

Genetic analysis has become a routine part of the clinical investigation of neuromuscular disease and often supplants muscle biopsy and other diagnostic tests. Genetic testing can be used as a diagnostic test in an isolated individual when the gene is well characterized and intragenic probes are available that can determine whether the gene is abnormal. Genetic testing not only allows accurate diagnosis but also is useful for carrier detection and prognosis.

For a more detailed discussion, see Chapter 28 in Neurology in Clinical Practice, 4th edition.

Muscle Pain and Cramps

18

Fourteen percent of the U.S. population between the ages of 25 and 74 years has chronic joint and musculoskeletal pain. The common causes are unaccustomed exercise, trauma, cramps, and systemic infections. Disorders in connective tissue, joints, and bone refer pain to muscle. Depression is approximately twice as common in patients with chronic musculoskeletal pain (18%) than in the general population.

EVALUATION OF MUSCLE DISCOMFORT

History should include the type, localization, and evolution of the pain, drug use, and mood disorders. Measures of strength and endurance are required, but these are difficult to assess in the presence of pain. The sensory examination is important because small-fiber sensory neuropathies commonly cause muscle discomfort. Blood studies may include a complete blood cell count, erythrocyte sedimentation rate, creatine kinase (CK), potassium, calcium, phosphate, and lactate concentrations, thyroid functions, and evaluation for systemic immune disorders. Evaluation of urine myoglobin is required in patients with a high CK concentration and severe myalgia, especially when related to exercise. Electromyography (EMG) is a sensitive test for myopathy and denervation. Nerve conduction evaluation may detect an underlying neuropathy, but small-fiber axonopathies require quantitative sensory testing or skin biopsy with staining of distal nerve fibers. Focal or diffuse muscle abnormalities revealed by magnetic resonance imaging can indicate the best site for muscle biopsy. Muscle biopsy is more likely to be useful when another test is abnormal, such as a high serum lactate or CK concentration or an abnormal EMG. In muscle discomfort syndromes, examination of both muscle and connective tissue

147

increases the yield of diagnostic information. Muscle histochemistry should include, in addition to routine processing, reactions for acid phosphatase, alkaline phosphatase, esterase, mitochondrial enzymes, glycolytic enzymes, and myoadenylate deaminase.

CONDITIONS PRODUCING MUSCLE PAIN

Episodes of pain originating in muscle are commonly associated with exercise, inflammation, and trauma. Exercise can produce muscle pain by several pathways, including exhaustion of fuel supply (with lack of training, vascular insufficiency, or metabolic defects), cramps, or injury to muscle fibers or tendons. When muscle contracts while it is being stretched (eccentric contraction), damage and pain are especially likely. Delayed-onset muscle soreness may be due to several factors, including muscle fiber and connective tissue damage, inflammation, and edema.

Clinical Features of Muscle Pain

General Features of Muscle Pain
Descriptions of muscle discomfort include pain, soreness, aching, fatigue, cramps, or spasms. The perception of pain that originates in muscle is that it arises from deep tissues. The localization of chronic muscle pain is poor and often referred to a deeper location. Autonomic and affective symptoms are often associated. Pain with muscle cramps has an acute onset and short duration. Cramp pain is associated with palpable muscle contraction and immediately relieved by muscle stretching. Localization of pain originating from fascia and periosteum is precise. Cutaneous pain differs from muscle or fascial pain by its distinct localization and sharp, pricking, stabbing, or burning nature. In fibromyalgia syndromes, patients commonly complain that fatigue accompanies their muscle discomfort.

Evaluation of Muscle Discomfort

The basis of classification of disorders underlying muscle discomfort is anatomy, temporal relation to exercise, muscle pathology, and the presence or absence of active muscle contraction during the discomfort. Evaluation of muscle discomfort typically begins with a history, including the type, localization, inducing factors and evolution of the pain, drug use, and mood disorders. The physical examination requires special attention to the localization of weakness. However, accurate assessment of strength may be difficult in the presence of pain.

Muscle Discomfort: Specific Causes

Myopathies may be associated with muscle pain without associated muscle contraction (myalgias). Muscle pain during muscle activity may occur with muscle injury, myopathy, cramps, or long-term tonic contraction. Myopathies that produce muscle pain are usually associated with weakness, a high serum CK concentration, and an abnormal EMG. Only a minority of inflammatory myopathies are associated with pain and muscle tenderness. Myopathies caused by infections, including bacterial, viral, toxoplasmosis, and trichinosis, are usually painful. Metabolic myopathies, including phosphorylase and carnitine palmitoyltransferase II deficiencies, typically produce muscle discomfort or fatigue that arises toward the end or after the completion of exercise and is less prominent at rest. As a rule, disorders of carbohydrate use produce pain and fatigue after short intense exercise, whereas lipid disorders cause muscle discomfort with sustained exercise. Rhabdomyolysis is usually associated with muscle pain and tenderness that can persist for days after the initial event. It may occur with a defined metabolic or toxic myopathy or sporadically, in the setting of unaccustomed exercise, especially with hot weather. Muscular dystrophy and mitochondrial disorders are usually painless, but some patients may experience myalgias and cramps or rhabdomyolysis. Several myopathies defined by specific morphological or physiological changes in muscle commonly have myalgias or exercise-related discomfort as part of their associated clinical syndrome.

Muscle Overuse Syndromes

Cramps are a localized form of muscle contraction and overuse. Pain syndromes associated with cramps include discomfort during a muscle contraction and soreness after the contraction due to muscle injury. Cramps are common in normal people in the gastrocnemius muscle and in patients with denervation. They usually arise during sleep or exercise and are more likely to occur when the muscle contracts in a shortened position. Relief of cramps is attained by stretching the affected muscle. Active stretching, by contracting the antagonist, may be especially effective treatment because it evokes reciprocal inhibition. Cramps that occur frequently in muscles other than the gastrocnemius usually herald an underlying neuromuscular disorder.

The EMG is useful for defining the specific type of cramp. Cramps of muscular origin include electrically active contractions, electrically silent contractures, and myotonic types.

Electrically active muscle cramps due to myopathy are manifest by irregular triphasic action potentials occurring at a rate of 40–60 Hz. Muscle contractures are active muscle contractions in the absence of electrical activity. These electrically silent muscle contractions occur in myophosphorylase deficiency and other glycolytic disorders, Brody's syndrome, rippling muscle disease, and hypothyroidism (myoedema). Exercise provokes prolonged and painful contractures in myophosphorylase deficiency. Myotonic cramps are often not painful. Patients with recessive myotonia congenita often note fatigue.

Neurogenic cramps may arise from peripheral nerves or the central nervous system (CNS). They frequently produce discomfort. The common muscle cramp usually arises from motor nerve terminals. EMG shows irregular triphasic action potentials at 40–150 Hz that increase and then decrease during the course of the cramp. Several drugs may precipitate cramps. The definition of muscle spasms is an intense painful muscle contraction that persists longer than a cramp. There is often palpable tightness and resistance to muscle movement and occasionally a distortion of posture. EMG shows tonic firing of motor unit action potentials. Neurogenic disorders that are associated with cramps, painful muscle spasms, or muscle discomfort include amyotrophic lateral sclerosis, neuromyotonia, spinal stenosis, stiff person syndrome, spasticity, restless legs syndrome, and focal dystonias. Treatment of cramps involves treating the underlying disorder or symptomatic trials of medications. Quinine was effective in treating nocturnal muscle cramps in a double-blind, placebo-controlled trial.

The cause of diffuse muscle contraction syndromes is often a CNS disorder associated with drugs or toxins. These include malignant hyperthermia, neuroleptic malignant syndrome, and toxic disorders related to phencyclidine, amphetamine, tetanus, and strychnine. Diffuse contraction syndromes produce great discomfort when the patient is awake. In the postoperative period, myalgia and fasciculations often occur after the use of succinylcholine (suxamethonium).

Myalgia Syndromes without Chronic Myopathy

Polymyalgia syndromes are pain localized to muscle and other structures without muscle weakness. The pain may produce the appearance of weakness by preventing full effort and is characterized by sudden reductions in the level of effort. Polymyalgic pain is often present at rest and variably affected by movement. Serum CK concentration and EMG are normal.

No major pathological changes occur in muscle unless the discomfort produces disuse and atrophy of type II muscle fibers. Muscle biopsies may show changes associated with systemic immune disorders, including inflammation around blood vessels or in connective tissue. Many polymyalgia syndromes have clear underlying disorders, including systemic immune disease, drug toxicity, and small-fiber polyneuropathies.

Some syndromes associated with muscle discomfort, such as polymyalgia rheumatica, fibromyalgia, and chronic fatigue syndrome, are defined by their clinical features and have no well-defined pathophysiology. Polymyalgia rheumatica usually occurs after age 50 and manifests with pain and stiffness in joints and muscles, weight loss, and low-grade fever. The pain is symmetrical, involves the shoulder, neck, and hip-girdle, and is greatest after inactivity and sleeping. *Polymyalgia rheumatica* can be associated with temporal arteritis. Patients often have an elevated sedimentation rate (>40 mm/hour). Pain improves within a few days after treatment with corticosteroids (prednisone, 20 mg/day). The diagnosis of *fibromyalgia* depends on a history of widespread musculoskeletal pain, most commonly around the neck and shoulders, for 3 months or more, and findings of tender points on the extremities and trunk. Other features are fatigue and disturbed sleep, headache, irritable bowel syndrome, and aggravation of symptoms by exercise, anxiety, or stress. The diagnosis of chronic fatigue syndrome requires symptoms of muscle fatigue for at least 6 months. Myalgias, paresthesias, headache, dizziness, diaphoresis, fainting, and memory loss may also be noted. A low-grade fever, pharyngitis, and enlarged cervical or axillary lymph nodes are sometimes associated. Many patients with chronic fatigue syndrome improve spontaneously over time. Treatment of both fibromyalgia and chronic fatigue syndrome frequently includes the use of tricyclic antidepressants. Among controversial syndromes that include myalgias are myoadenylate deaminase deficiency, adjuvant breast disorders, Gulf War syndrome, and multiple chemical sensitivity.

Pain or discomfort localized to muscle may arise in other structures. For example, hip disease may suggest a painful proximal myopathy with apparent leg weakness. External or internal rotation of the thigh commonly evokes proximal pain, and radiological studies confirm the diagnosis. Disorders of bone and joints, connective tissue, endocrine systems, vascular supply, peripheral nerve and roots, and the CNS may also present with discomfort localized to muscle.

Pain originating from muscle, often acute, may occur in the absence of a chronic myopathy. Muscle ischemia causes a squeezing pain in the affected muscles during exercise. Ischemia produces pain that develops especially rapidly (within minutes) if muscle is forced to contract at the same time and that subsides quickly with rest. Cramps and overuse syndromes are associated with pain during or immediately after muscle use. Delayed-onset muscle soreness occurs 12–48 hours after exercise and lasts for hours to days. It is most commonly precipitated by eccentric contraction or unaccustomed exercise.

For a more detailed discussion, see Chapter 29 in Neurology in Clinical Practice, 4th edition.

The Floppy Infant

19

One of the more common neurological syndromes in the newborn and infant is generalized hypotonia (the *floppy infant*). The differential diagnosis is broad (Table 19.1). Anatomical localization, based on the history and physical examination, narrows the differential diagnosis. A small number of confirmatory tests often provide a specific diagnosis. These may include an imaging study, electrodiagnosis, muscle biopsy, or molecular genetic testing.

CARDINAL FEATURES

Tone

The definition of *tone* is the unconscious and automatic induction of muscle power in response to an applied load. *Resting tone*, assessed by inspection, is present when in an awake alert state at rest. Passive movement of an otherwise immobile muscle induces *static* or *passive tone*. *Postural tone* involves resistance to gravity and maintains a stable posture in space. *Dynamic tone* and *postural tone* are closely related. Tests of dynamic tone require phasic activity such as automatic movements (e.g., walking). Diminished tone in the setting of normal muscle power implies involvement of the central nervous system (CNS). Subdivision of increased tone is, by the characteristics of the resistance, into *spasticity* or *rigidity*.

Power

Muscle power (strength), the maximum force generated, is more easily defined and evaluated than muscle tone. Attention focuses on diminished power because increased muscle power is never pathological. The usual assessment of weakness in infants and children is in relation to developmentally appropriate skills and behaviors because isolated muscle testing may be difficult.

Table 19.1: Important differential diagnoses of the floppy infant (excluding syndromes in which features of cerebral degeneration precede hypotonia or weakness)

Cerebral hypotonia
  Chromosomal disorders
    Trisomy
  Partial chromosome deletion/duplication
    Prader-Willi syndrome*
  Static encephalopathy
    Cerebral malformation
    Perinatal distress
    Postnatal cerebral injury
    Idiopathic disorders
  Single gene disorders
    Zellweger syndrome (peroxisome biosynthesis, multiple)
    Neonatal adrenoleukodystrophy (multiple)
    Oculocerebral renal syndrome (Lowe's) (OCRL, Xq26.1)
    Acid maltase (α2,4-glucosidase deficiency, 17q25.2-q25.3)
    Carbohydrate-deficient glycoprotein syndrome (unknown)
Spinal cord disorders
  Hypoxic-ischemic myelopathy
  Trauma
  Congenital malformation
Motor neuronopathies
  Spinal muscular atrophy (SMA) (SMN, 5q11-13)*
  Congenital cervical SMA (unknown)
  Infantile neuronal degeneration (some have SMA)
  Neurogenic arthrogryposis (some have SMA)
  Vaccine-associated poliomyelitis
  Incontinentia pigmenti (unknown, Xq28)
Polyneuropathies
  Congenital hypomyelinating polyneuropathy
    (myelin P_0 [MPZ], 1q22)
  Dejerine-Sottas syndrome (myelin P_0 [MPZ], 1q22; PMP22,
    1q22)*
  Idiopathic (heritable) motor sensory polyneuropathies
Disorders of neuromuscular transmission
  Congenital (genetic) defect of neuromuscular junction (multiple)
  In utero passive transfer of maternal antijunction antibodies
  Autoimmune myasthenia gravis
  Infantile botulism
Myopathies
  Genetic myopathies
  Central core disease (ryanodine receptor, 19q13.1)
  Congenital fiber-type disproportion myopathies
  X-linked myotubular myopathy (MTM1, Xq28)*

Continued

Table 19.1: (continued)

Autosomal dominant nemaline myopathy (tropomyosin-3, 1q22-q23)
Autosomal recessive nemaline myopathy [Nebulin(?), q21.2-q22]
Congenital myotonic dystrophy (myotonin protein kinase, 19q13.2-q13.3)
Other congenital myopathies (nosologically indistinct)
Infantile myositis
Metabolic myopathies
Acid maltase deficiency (α2,4-glucosidase deficiency, 17q25.2-q25.3)
Cytochrome-*c*-oxidase deficiency (multiple, autosomal, and mitochondrial)
Carnitine dependency with impaired cellular carnitine uptake (unknown)
Multisystem phosphofructokinase deficiency (unknown)
Congenital muscular dystrophies
Fukuyama's (fukutin, 9q31)
Merosin/α_2-laminin deficiency (α_2-laminin, 6q22-q23)
Walker-Warburg (unknown)
Muscle-eye-brain (1p32-p34)

Note: Gene and location, respectively, indicated in parentheses.
*Indicates whether DNA test is practical for diagnosis.

Diminished muscle power is substantial but not conclusive evidence of involvement of the motor unit.

Range of Movement

Joint range can be restricted by muscle fibrosis, ligamentous restrictions, and fibrosis of the joint capsule. *Arthrogryposis* is prenatally acquired restriction of joint range and may be associated with underdevelopment of the joint. A *contracture* is postnatally acquired restriction in joint mobility. Arthrogryposis is caused by several disorders and may affect a single joint or many joints. Involvement of multiple joints is called *arthrogryposis congenita multiplex*. Clubfoot is the most common expression of arthrogryposis. Fetal immobility is believed to cause arthrogryposis, but among the disorders that significantly decrease fetal movement arthrogryposis is frequently associated with some but rarely so in others.

Reflexes

The knee tendon reflexes usually can be elicited shortly after birth. Ankle and biceps reflexes are more inconsistent but are more easily obtained with each succeeding month. In younger infants, the head must be in a midline position because the tonic neck reflex exaggerates tone on the side to which the head is turned. Absent or increased reflexes with normal coordination and power are unlikely to be important. Normal reflexes in the setting of hypotonia or weakness imply localization to the CNS. Motor neuron disorders generally diminish reflex activity in proportion to weakness. Increased ease of reflex elicitation with a normal or diminished response; for example, percussion below the tibial tuberosity provoking reflexive knee extension in a weak limb suggests simultaneous CNS and motor unit involvement. Disorders of the neuromuscular junction usually spare tendon reflexes.

Certain postural responses elicited in infancy may have predictive value. The Moro reflex and tonic neck reflex may be elicited in newborns and infants with cerebral hypotonia even when there is a paucity of spontaneous movement. Their presence shows that the motor unit is intact. The Moro reflex is elicited by startle and is normally present in its full expression up to 6 months. Absence of a Moro reflex is always abnormal and suggests severe central or motor unit dysfunction. Asymmetry of the response also may be either central or peripheral in origin.

The tonic neck reflex is a primitive vestibular reflex that is present from birth to 3 months of age. It must be suppressed before the child can learn to turn over. The tonic neck reflex should be variable, unsustained, and nonobligatory, with other responses easily dominating. An asymmetrical tonic neck response suggests injury to the contralateral hemisphere; a bilateral persistent or obligatory tonic neck response suggests bihemispheric injury.

Endurance

Disorders of the neuromuscular junction are uncommon in infants. Infants do not ordinarily exercise to the point of exhaustion, except possibly while crying vigorously. Thus, neuromuscular junction fatigue is best appreciated in those with difficulty sucking or possibly swallowing. Infants with junctional disorders may show restricted extraocular movement, ptosis, bulbar and facial weakness, and sometimes generalized weakness.

Bulk

Severe loss of muscle bulk follows denervation and is extreme in spinal muscular atrophy. Diminished bulk of muscle may be obscured in infants by abundant subcutaneous fat and sometimes better appreciated by palpation of long bones rather than by inspection. Commensurate decreases in muscle bulk and power occur in severe malnutrition and some poorly characterized developmental myopathies. Although muscle atrophy suggests motor unit disease, it also occurs infrequently with purely central disorders.

Sensation

The sensory examination is difficult to evaluate in infants. It requires considerable time, and small differences in sensibility almost never have diagnostic value. In evaluating the floppy infant, the sensory examination is of greatest value in those with spinal injury or peripheral polyneuropathy, in which sensory and motor fibers are equally affected.

Associated Features

Long-standing immobility in the fetus may produce deformations. In addition to arthrogryposis, hypotonic infants may have a narrow, high-arched palate with mandibular underdevelopment, a short umbilical cord, and demineralization of bones. The hip acetabulum may be shallow and the hips dislocated. If there is difficulty swallowing, polyhydramnios may ensue.

Laboratory Diagnosis

The availability of specific DNA tests for several disorders has greatly improved laboratory diagnosis (see Table 19.1).

Neuroimaging

T1-weighted magnetic resonance imaging (MRI) of the brain is useful for the detection and characterization of occult cerebral malformations. If cerebral malformation is suspected, careful evaluation of skin and eyes may produce clues to the underlying diagnosis. T2-weighted MRI best displays the abnormal white matter signal associated with α_2-laminin deficiency in congenital muscular dystrophy. Spectroscopy studies may show abnormal spectra associated with the mitochondrial encephalomyopathies.

Electrodiagnosis

Nerve conduction studies and electromyography (EMG) are most useful in focusing on a portion of the motor unit for further study. The value of the study is related directly to the skill and experience of the physician performing the test. EMG is usually able to discern myopathic from neuropathic weakness. Specific studies with repetitive stimulation are especially valuable in the diagnosis of the myasthenic syndromes and infantile botulism.

Muscle Biopsy

Muscle biopsy is essential to the diagnosis of congenital myopathies and muscular dystrophies. Histochemical evaluation of quickly frozen muscle tissue is essential to diagnosis. The best anatomical sites for biopsy are those muscles free of myotendinous insertions in which the histochemical fiber types are normally equal in abundance (deltoid, biceps, triceps, and rectus femoris). Careful thought should be given prospectively to the amount of tissue that will be necessary for the potentially relevant histochemical, electron microscopic, enzymatic, or DNA tests.

Nerve Biopsy

Biopsy of the sural nerve is indicated in the setting of unexplained neuropathy when other test results for specific candidate neuropathies are not available or are normal.

Edrophonium Chloride (Tensilon) Test

Edrophonium chloride (Tensilon) is a rapid-acting anticholinesterase that produces a temporary reversal of weakness in patients with many of the myasthenic syndromes. It is most useful when eyelid ptosis or restriction of eye movement is present. In newborns and infants, the total dose is 0.15–0.20 mg/kg; one fourth of this dose is given intravenously each minute until a response is seen or the total dose is given.

For a more detailed discussion, see Chapter 30 in Neurology in Clinical Practice, 4th edition.

Sensory Abnormalities of the Limbs, Trunk, and Face | **20**

SENSORY ABNORMALITIES

Strictly speaking, the term *numbness* means loss of sensation, usually manifest as decreased sensory discrimination and elevated sensory threshold; these are negative symptoms. *Dysesthesia* is an abnormal perception of a sensory stimulus, such as when pressure produces a feeling of tingling or pain. *Paresthesia* is an abnormal spontaneous sensation of similar quality to dysesthesia. Dysesthesias and paresthesias usually occur in peripheral neuropathic processes, such as polyneuropathy or mononeuropathy, but also occur with central conditions such as myelopathy or cerebral sensory tract dysfunction. *Neuropathic pain* can result from damage to the sensory nerves of any cause. *Hyperesthesia* is increased sensory experience with a stimulus. *Hyperpathia* is augmented painful sensation. *Sensory ataxia* is difficulty in coordination of a limb from loss of sensory input, particularly proprioception.

LOCALIZATION OF SENSORY ABNORMALITIES

Table 20.1 presents a general guide to sensory localization and Table 20.2 presents guidelines for diagnoses of the sensory abnormalities.

Peripheral Sensory Lesions

Peripheral nerve and plexus lesions produce sensory loss, which follows the peripheral anatomical distribution. Clues to localization are as follows: Distal sensory loss or pain in more than one limb suggests peripheral neuropathy; sensory loss in a restricted portion of one limb suggests a peripheral nerve or plexus lesion; sensory loss affecting an entire limb is rarely due to a peripheral lesion and suggests a central lesion.

Table 20.1: General guidelines to sensory abnormality localization

Level of Lesion	Features and Location of Sensory Loss
Cortical	Sensory loss in contralateral body, restricted to the portion of the homunculus affected by the lesion. If the entire side is affected (with large lesions), either the face and arm or the leg tends to be affected to a greater extent.
Internal capsule	Sensory symptoms in contralateral body, which usually involved head, arm, and leg to an equal extent. Motor findings commonly present, though not always.
Thalamus	Sensory symptoms in contralateral body including head and may split the midline. Sensory loss without weakness highly suggestive of lesion here.
Spinal transection	Sensory loss at or below a segmental level, which may be slightly different for each side. Motor examination is also key for localization.
Spinal hemisection	Sensory loss ipsilateral for vibration and proprioception (dorsal columns), contralateral for pain and temperature (spinothalamic tract).
Nerve root	Sensory symptoms follow a dermatomal distribution.
Plexus	Sensory symptoms span two or more adjacent root distributions, corresponding to the anatomy of the plexus.
Peripheral nerve	Distribution follows peripheral nerve anatomy or involves nerves symmetrically.

Spinal Sensory Lesions

The following sensory syndromes suggest a spinal lesion: a sensory level, loss of vibration and proprioception ipsilateral to the lesion and loss of pain and temperature sensation contralateral to the lesion (dissociated sensory loss), and sacral sparing.

Cerebral Sensory Lesions

Thalamic lesions. Pure sensory deficit of cerebral origin usually arises from damage to the thalamus. Thalamic pain syndrome is characterized by spontaneous pain localized to the distal arm and leg, exacerbated by contact and stress.

Table 20.2: Guidelines to diagnosis of sensory abnormalities

Abnormality	Features	Lesion	Cause
Distal sensory deficit	Sensory loss with or without pain distal on the legs; arms may also be affected	Peripheral nerve	Peripheral neuropathy
Proximal sensory deficit	Sensory loss on the trunk without limb symptoms	Neuropathy with predominantly proximal involvement	Porphyria, diabetes, other plexopathies
Dermatomal distribution of pain and/or sensory loss	Pain or sensory loss in the distribution of a single nerve root	Nerve root	Radiculopathy due to disc, osteophyte, tumor, herpes zoster
Single-limb sensory deficit	Loss of sensation on one entire limb, which spans neural and dermatomal distribution	Plexus or multiple single nerves	Autoimmune plexitis, hematoma, tumor compression or infiltration
Hemisensory deficit	Loss of sensation on one side of the body, may be associated with pain; face is involved in brain lesions but not with spinal lesions	Thalamus, cerebral cortex or projections, less likely to be brainstem lesion if face involved; spinal cord if face not involved	Infarction, hemorrhage, demyelinating disease, tumor, infection
Crossed sensory deficit: Unilateral facial and contralateral body	Unilateral loss of sensation on the face and contralateral body	Lesion of the uncrossed trigeminal fibers and the crossed spinothalamic fibers	Lateral medullary syndrome

Continued

Table 20.2: (continued)

Abnormality	Features	Lesion	Cause
Crossed sensory deficit: pain/temperature and vibration/ proprioception on opposite sides	Loss of pain and temperature sensation on one side and vibration and proprioception on the other	Spinal cord lesion ipsilateral to the vibration and proprioception deficit and contralateral to the pain and temperature deficit	Disc protrusion, spinal stenosis, intraspinal tumor, transverse myelitis; intraparenchymal lesions are more likely to produce dissociated sensory loss
Dissociated suspended sensory deficit:	Loss of pain and temperature sensation on one or both sides, with normal sensation above and below	Syringomyelia in cervical or thoracic spinal cord	Chiari malformation, hydromyelia, central spinal cord tumor or hemorrhage
Sacral sparing	Preservation of perianal sensation with impaired sensation in the legs and trunk	Lesion of the cord with mainly central involvement, sparing the peripherally located sacral ascending fibers	Cord trauma, intrinsic tumors of the cord

Cortical lesions. Lesions of the postcentral gyrus produce sensory more than motor symptoms. Posterior lesions may spare the primary modalities (pain, temperature, and touch and joint position) but impair higher sensory function (graphesthesia, two-point discrimination, and the perception of double simultaneous stimuli).

For a more detailed discussion, see Chapter 31 in Neurology in Clinical Practice, 4th edition.

Neurological Causes of Bladder, Bowel, and Sexual Dysfunction

21

BLADDER

Anatomy and Physiology

The bladder performs only two functions: storage and emptying. These mutually exclusive activities are controlled by neural programs that exist in centers in the dorsal tegmentum of the pons. Suprapontine influences act to switch from one state to the other. The cortex determines the social and behavioral circumstances under which micturition occurs. Lesions of the superomedial frontal cortex or of the linking pathways usually cause automatic voiding when the bladder is full. Further, the ability to initiate or inhibit voiding consciously is lost. For both normal storage and normal voiding, connections between the pons and the sacral spinal cord must be intact, as must the peripheral innervation, which arises from the most caudal segments of the cord.

During the storage phase, the maintenance of raised intravesical pressure within the bladder outlet is achieved both by sympathetic influences on the smooth muscle of the detrusor in the bladder neck region and by pudendal nerve activation of the striated muscle of the urethral sphincter and the pelvic floor. Inhibition of the parasympathetic outflow prevents detrusor contraction. At the start of voiding, the reciprocal activation/inhibition of the sphincter detrusor reverses. Some seconds after relaxation of the striated muscle of the sphincter, the smooth muscle of the detrusor contracts and the bladder empties.

Physical Examination

Patients with a neurological cause for a urogenital complaint usually have neurological abnormalities of the legs, because the spinal segments that innervate the bladder are caudal to those that innervate the legs. Lesions of the low sacral cord or conus are sometimes an exception, but only the most caudal lesions fail to produce some hyperreflexia in the lower limbs and extensor-plantar responses. Lesions at S1 and S2 usually impair the ankle reflexes, S3 lesions cause foot deformities and fasciculations in the intrinsic foot muscles, and conus lesions cause saddle anesthesia.

After examining the legs, the clinician inspects the lumbosacral spine for signs of underlying congenital malformations such as hypertrichosis, a nevus, sinus, or dimpling in the sacral region. Evidence of extrapyramidal disease, cerebellar ataxia, laryngeal involvement, and postural hypotension suggests multiple system atrophy (MSA). Neuroimaging and neurophysiological testing are unlikely to be informative in patients with urogenital complaints whose neurological examination findings are normal.

Urological Investigations

Patients with urogenital complaints without known neurological disease should first be seen by a urologist to exclude obvious urological disorders such as prostatic hypertrophy. In contrast, a neurologist should see patients who develop genitourinary symptoms as part of an established neurological disease.

Urodynamic Studies
Urodynamic studies examine the function of the lower urinary tract. Included in this term are measurements of urine flow rate, residual volume, cystometry during both filling and voiding, videocystometry, urethral pressure profile measurements, and pelvic floor neurophysiology.

Noninvasive Bladder Investigations
Urinary flowmetry is a valuable noninvasive investigation, particularly when combined with an ultrasound measurement of the postmicturition residual volume. The study provides a graphic printout and an analysis of the time taken to reach maximum flow, maximum and average flow rate, and the voided volume.

Cystometry
Bladder pressure includes measures during both filling and voiding. The essential measurement is the intravesical pressure, but because this also reflects increases in intra-abdominal pressure, the simultaneous rectal pressure recording is subtracted from the measured intravesical pressure to give the true isolated detrusor pressure. Detrusor overactivity is the main abnormality diagnosed through cystometry. The urodynamic finding of

neurogenic detrusor overactivity is indistinguishable from idiopathic detrusor overactivity.

Neurophysiological Investigations

Electromyography
Electromyography (EMG) assesses the extent of relaxation of the urethral sphincter during voiding. Interruption of the neural pathways between the pons and the sacral cord results in loss of coordination of sphincter and detrusor muscle activity (*detrusor-sphincter dyssynergia*), a disorder that arises because of spinal cord disease. A highly abnormal result in a patient with mild parkinsonism establishes a diagnosis of probable MSA.

Other Neurophysiological Investigations of the Pelvic Floor
Other neurophysiological means of assessment rest largely on measurements of conduction velocity or latency and therefore correlate less well with function.

Management of Bladder Disorders

Detrusor Overactivity
Detrusor overactivity is the main cause of incontinence in patients with neurogenic bladder disorders. Spontaneous increases in bladder pressure develop that cannot be suppressed. These occur at volumes less than normal capacity, so frequency is associated. Anticholinergic medications are the mainstay of treatment for detrusor overactivity. The first-line medications in this group are oxybutynin and tolterodine. The starting dose for oxybutynin is 2.5 mg twice daily (up to a maximum of 20 mg daily in divided doses), and for tolterodine 2 mg twice daily; newer once-daily formulations are available for both medications. The main side effect is dry mouth, and less commonly blurred vision, drowsiness, and constipation occur.

Injection of botulinum-A toxin into the detrusor smooth muscle treats bladder overactivity. The effect is thought to last 6–12 months. Desmopressin spray, first introduced to treat diabetes insipidus and widely used for children with nocturnal enuresis, reduces nocturnal frequency in neurogenic bladder. One or two nasal puffs of desmopressin from a metered-dose spray administered on retiring reduce urine output for the following 6–8 hours. An oral preparation is also available.

Incomplete Bladder Emptying or Urinary Retention
The use of *intermittent catheterization* greatly facilitates the management of neurogenic bladder. Incomplete emptying

exacerbates detrusor hyperreflexia, and an overactive bladder constantly stimulated by a residual volume responds by contracting and producing symptoms of urgency and frequency. A significant residual volume is 100 ml. Because the principle of intermittent catheterization is to reduce the postmicturition residual volume, advise at least twice-daily catheterization for most patients. If urge incontinence is the main problem and the bladder empties completely, some men are able to wear an external device attached around the penis to manage bladder disorders. The simplest and least obtrusive is placement of a self-sealing latex condom sheath each night or kept in place for up to 3 days. An external appliance for women is not available.

When the patient is no longer able to perform self-catheterization, or when urge incontinence and frequency are unmanageable, an in-dwelling Foley catheter becomes necessary. In patients with spinal cord disease, this point may be reached when the patient is no longer bearing weight and is confined to a chair. A preferred alternative to an in-dwelling urethral catheter is a suprapubic catheter.

The implantation of a nerve root stimulator is a consideration for patients with a complete spinal cord transection in whom the caudal section of the cord and its roots are intact. An external switching device activates the stimulating electrodes, placed around the S2-S4 roots. Stimulating individual roots or combinations of roots achieves micturition, defecation, and erection.

A surgical procedure to rectify a disorder causing incontinence in an otherwise fit and healthy individual is often highly successful, and even after spinal cord injury a surgical option may be the best solution for long-term bladder management. However, this does not apply to patients with progressive neurological disease causing incontinence.

BOWEL

Anatomy and Physiology

Lower bowel function exists mostly in the storage mode. A combination of the acute anorectal angle, caused by puborectalis contraction, and internal anal sphincter tone, determined by sympathetic activity, maintains continence. In neurological health, contraction of the external anal sphincter and pelvic floor delays defecation when necessary.

The process of defecation involves a series of neurologically controlled actions that begin in response to the conscious sensation of a full rectum. Raising the intra-abdominal pressure and straining down, causing descent of the pelvic floor, starts defecation. The internal anal sphincter pressure falls, due to the rectoanal inhibitory reflex, and the pubococcygeus and striated external sphincter muscles relax.

Management of Fecal Incontinence

Pelvic floor incompetence can occur from cauda equina lesions or pudendal nerve injury. Referral to a colorectal surgeon is necessary for consideration of a sphincter or postanal repair. Healthy nonsphincter striated muscle, such as the gracilis, transposed around the anal canal creates an anosphincter. Advise patients with partial spinal cord disease who complain of constipation or occasional fecal incontinence to use suppositories and attempt to empty the bowel at a predictable and convenient time.

SEXUAL FUNCTION

Anatomy and Physiology

Excitement, plateau, and resolution are the normal sexual responses in men and women. Erection results from increased blood flow into the corpus cavernosum because of relaxation of the smooth muscle in the cavernosal arteries and a reduction in venous return. The major peripheral innervation determining erection is the parasympathetic, which arises from S2-S4 segments and travels to the genital region in the pelvic nerves. Psychogenic erection requires cortical activation of erectogenic pathways via the spinal cord. Men with low spinal cord lesions preserve responsiveness. Reflex erections occur as the result of cutaneous genital stimulation. In women, the main parasympathetic innervation is from the pelvic nerves, the sympathetic innervation from the hypogastric nerves, and bilateral somatic innervation from the pudendal nerves.

Sexual Dysfunction

Sexual dysfunction is more common in both men and women with epilepsy. Sexual apathy is the most common dysfunction in patients with temporal lobe epilepsy. The deficit results from specific temporal lobe involvement.

Male Erectile Dysfunction

The introduction of orally active erectogenic agents (Viagra) transformed the treatment of male erectile dysfunction (MED). Penile erection is achieved with appropriate stimulation 1 hour after ingestion. Adverse effects are unusual and mild. Viagra is effective in men with diabetes-induced MED, spinal cord injury, and multiple sclerosis. Other agents becoming available differ in terms of speed of onset and duration of effect.

Ejaculatory Failure

Ejaculatory failure commonly accompanies erectile failure of neurogenic origin in men with spinal cord disease, whereas in diabetics, preservation of ejaculation function is better than erectile function. Much less can be done for ejaculatory failure than MED.

Sexual Dysfunction in Women

Knowledge is sparse concerning sexual dysfunction of women with neurological disease. Women with spinal cord disease, such as multiple sclerosis, encounter difficulties with intercourse because of poor bladder control, lower limb spasticity, and loss of sensation. Loss of perineal sensation is a major problem for women with cauda equina lesions and may be a persisting cause of dissatisfaction, even after establishing adequate means of managing bladder and bowel dysfunction.

For a more detailed discussion, see Chapters 32 and 42, in Neurology in Clinical Practice, 4th edition.

Arm and Neck Pain

22

Pain may arise from portions of the nervous system or non-neural structures of the neck and arm. Nerve root irritation frequently generates neck muscle spasm. Such spasms fall into the "neurological" category.

HISTORY

Neurological Causes of Pain

Muscle Spasm
Posterior cervical muscle spasm causes local pain aggravated by neck movement. Palpable spasm and tenderness of the neck and shoulder muscles supports the diagnosis. Pain radiation is upward to the occipital region and then over the top to the bifrontal area. Pain is constant and described as aching, bursting, or a tight band or pressure on top of the head. Abnormalities of the facet joints of the cervical spine, the vertebrae, and the intervertebral discs cause similar pain. Muscle spasm restricts neck mobility. Neck movements assess muscle spasm. Normally in flexion the chin can touch the sternum, and in rotation the chin should be able to approximate the point of the shoulder.

Central Pain
Central dysfunction affecting sensory tracts in the spinal cord may generate pain or paresthesias in the arm or down the trunk and lower limbs. Pathological processes in the cervical cord cause an electric-like sensation that spreads to the arms, down the spine, and even into the legs with neck flexion (*Lhermitte's sign*). Sharp superficial burning or itching pain suggests dysfunction in the spinothalamic system, whereas deep, aching, boring pain with paresthesia suggests dysfunction in the posterior columns.

171

Nerve Root Pain

Nerve root pain radiates down the limb in dermatomal distribution. Neck movement, coughing, or sneezing aggravates arm pain.

Plexus Pain

Pain in the arm can result from damage to the brachial plexus or individual nerves in the arm. Infiltrative or inflammatory lesions of the brachial plexus produce severe brachialgia radiating down the arm and spreading to the shoulder region. Radiation to the ulnar two fingers suggests origin in the lower brachial plexus, and radiation to the upper arm, forearm, and thumb suggests an upper brachial plexopathy. Patients with a thoracic outlet syndrome complain of brachialgia and numbness or tingling in the upper limb or hand when working with objects above the head.

Nerve Pain

Ulnar nerve entrapment produces numbness or pain radiating down the medial aspect of the arm to the little and ring fingers. Median nerve entrapment in the carpal tunnel produces tingling in the thumb, index, and middle fingers.

Non-neurological Causes of Pain

Pain arising in muscles is deep, aching, and boring. Patients with fibromyalgia may have pain in the neck, shoulders, and arms and trigger spots that are tender even to light pressure. Movement of the joint initiates and aggravates pain originating in the joints and tendons. Pain on shoulder joint movement is unlikely to be neuropathic.

EXAMINATION

The physical examination localizes a neurological deficit to the spinal cord, nerve roots, or peripheral nerves. Evaluation for non-neurological pathology is important because orthopedic and rheumatological problems often simulate or complicate neurological presentations. Detailed knowledge of motor and sensory neuroanatomy is required for accurate localization.

Motor Signs

The examination begins with inspection, paying special attention to atrophy of muscles of the shoulders, arms, and the small muscles of the hands. Fasciculations are often caused by anterior horn cell disease, but patients with cervical spondylosis and radiculopathy fasciculate as well. A good confirmatory sign of cervical radiculopathy is *Spurling sign*. With the patient's head inclined toward the painful side, apply pressure from the crown. This may produce sharp pain radiating down the arm and forearm. Although the specificity for radiculopathy is in the range of 93%, sensitivity is only about 30%.

Test muscles in the cervical and upper thoracic myotomes individually. When unilateral weakness is present, the contralateral side can act as a control. A standard measure of strength is necessary for accurate evaluation when bilateral weakness is present. If the examiner can overcome the action of a patient's muscle by resisting or opposing its action using an equivalent equipotent muscle (fingers test fingers, whole arm tests biceps), then that muscle in the patient is by definition weak. Grade the amount of weakness present using the 5-point Medical Research Council (MRC) grading scale. Grade 5 represents normal strength. Grade 4 represents "weakness" somewhere between normal strength and the ability to move the limb only against gravity (grade 3). Grade 4 covers such a large range that expansion is required (mild, moderate, or severe). Movement of the joint with the effect of gravity eliminated is graded 2. Grade 1 is just a flicker of contraction.

The distribution of weakness helps to localize the problem to the nerve root, peripheral nerve, muscle, or even the upper motor neuron. It is useful to use a simplified schema of anatomical localization in the evaluation of weakness caused by nerve root lesions because overlap of myotomes complicates the analysis.

Examination of the legs is required even when the complaints are limited to the arms. Sensory or motor dysfunction in the legs, when combined with the presence of radicular signs in the arms, indicates a spinal cord lesion.

Sensory Signs

The testing of sensation is in a standardized manner starting with pinprick appreciation at the back of the head (C2). Next, test the cervical dermatomes and proceed stepwise down the shoulder, over the deltoid down the lateral aspect of the arm to the lateral fingers, and then proceed to the medial fingers and up the medial aspect of the arm. Repeat the procedure with a wisp of cotton and test tubes filled with cold and warm water to test temperature sensation. Vibration sense testing is restricted to the fingers. Testing position sense in the distal phalanx of a finger requires immobilizing the proximal joint and supporting the distal phalanx on its medial and lateral sides. Then move the terminal phalanx up and down, and the patient reports movement and its direction. Loss of position sense in the fingers usually indicates a high cervical cord lesion. Light tapping over an accessible plexus or peripheral nerve may elicit distal tingling in the distribution of the plexus or nerve (Tinel's sign). This may be positive over the brachial plexus in the supraclavicular fossa, the ulnar nerve at the elbow, or the median nerve at the wrist.

Tendon Reflexes

Examination of the tendon reflexes helps localize segmental nerve root levels affected. An absent or decreased biceps reflex localizes the root level to C5, and an absent triceps reflex localizes the level to C6 or C7. In patients with cervical spondylosis who have both a radiculopathy and an associated myelopathy, the reflexes may be preserved or even increased despite the radiculopathy. The most common disc prolapse at C5-C6 may result in a radiculopathy and myelopathy at that level. The clinical features are absent or decreased biceps and brachioradialis reflexes, an increased triceps reflex, and spread of the brachioradialis reflex to the finger flexors to produce a finger jerk. Hoffmann's reflex may be present.

Nonneurological Signs

Passive abduction and internal and external rotation at the shoulder should not cause pain. The complaint of pain on movement or at a point in the abductor arc indicates local shoulder joint disease. The usual cause is shoulder tendonitis or pericapsulitis. The tendons anteriorly and at the lateral point of the shoulder may be tender to pressure. Bursitis is suggested when pain is more diffuse and tenderness localizes anterior to the shoulder joint. Tenderness over the medial or lateral epicondyle at the elbow indicates local inflammation, and pain on active or passive wrist or finger joint movement suggests tendonitis or arthritis.

For a more detailed discussion, see Chapter 33, in Neurology in Clinical Practice, 4th edition.

Low Back and Leg Pain

23

Low back pain is a common cause of neurological consultation. Leg pain may accompany low back pain or occur independently. The differential diagnosis of low back and leg pain includes neural, bony, and non-neurological causes. Most low back pain is secondary to radiculopathy, or mechanical factors, urolithiasis, tumors, and other intra-abdominal processes are considerations. The differential diagnosis of low back pain alone is different from back and leg pain. The causes of *low back pain without leg involvement* include ligamentous strain, facet pain, muscle strain, bony destruction, and inflammation. The combination of *low back plus leg pain* suggests a radiculopathy or plexopathy. *Leg pain without low back pain* suggests sciatic neuropathy, femoral neuropathy, peroneal neuropathy, meralgia paresthetica, and peripheral neuropathies. The important abdominal causes of low back pain are urolithiasis, ovarian cysts and carcinoma, endometriosis, and cystitis.

HISTORY AND EXAMINATION

History focuses on mode of onset, character, distribution, associated motor and sensory symptoms, bladder or bowel control, exacerbating and remitting factors, and predisposing factors such as cancers and osteoporosis. An acute onset of low back pain that radiates down the leg suggests a lumbosacral radiculopathy. Onset with exertion suggests a herniated disc. Progressive development of symptoms suggests an expanding lesion such as a tumor or a gradually expanding disc extrusion. Symptoms are usually more prominent than signs of neurological dysfunction.

The neurological examination helps determine whether abnormal neurological signs accompany the symptoms. Test all of the following muscle groups: hip flexors, extensors, adductors, and abductors; knee extensors and flexors; and the ankle and foot muscles. Sensory examination includes the femoral, peroneal, tibial, and lateral femoral cutaneous nerves, as well as the lumbar and sacral roots. Testing of the Achilles' and patella reflexes and the plantar response is essential.

Exacerbation of pain may occur by stretching damaged nerves. Straight-leg-raising testing augments pain in a lumbosacral radiculopathy. Hip extension exacerbates pain of upper lumbar radiculopathy or damage to the upper parts of the lumbar plexus.

DIFFERENTIAL DIAGNOSIS

Tables 23.1 and 23.2 provide a differential diagnosis of low back and leg pain. Some basic guidelines for differential diagnosis are as follows:

- Pain confined to the low back is generally a result of low back pathology.
- Pain confined to the leg is usually a result of leg pathology.
- Pain in both the low back and the leg is usually a result of lumbar radiculopathy or less commonly lumbosacral plexopathy.

Table 23.1: Classification of low back and leg pain

Type	Examples
Mechanical pain	Facet pain
	Bony destruction
	Sacroiliac (SI) joint inflammation
	Osteomyelitis
	Lumbar spondylosis
Neuropathic pain	Polyneuropathy
	Radiculopathy from disc disease, zoster, diabetes
	Mononeuropathy, including sciatic, femoral, lateral femoral cutaneous, peroneal neuropathies
	Plexopathy from cancer, abscess, hematoma, autoimmune processes
Non-neurological pain	Urolithiasis
	Retroperitoneal mass
	Ovarian cyst or carcinoma

Table 23.2: Differential diagnosis of low back and leg pain

Disorder	Clinical Features	Diagnosis
Radiculopathy	Back pain radiating into the leg in a dermatomal distribution; sensory loss or motor loss is in a root distribution; increased pain with coughing or straining	Suspected when neuropathic pain radiates from the back down into the leg in a single nerve distribution; disc or mass can be seen on MRI or CT; zoster and diabetes can cause radiculopathy without studies being abnormal
Plexopathy	Back and leg pain that has a neuropathic character, dysesthesias, burning, or electric; back pain can develop when the cause is a mass lesion in the region of the plexus	Suspected when patient has leg pain in more than one peripheral nerve distribution; MRI of the plexus or CT of the abdomen/pelvis can show mass or hematoma
Spinal stenosis	Pain in the low back, buttocks, and legs, especially with standing, walking, and lumbar spine extension	MRI or CT scan shows obliteration of the subarachnoid space

CT = computed tomography; MRI = magnetic resonance imaging.

- Clinical findings confined to one nerve root distribution are usually due to intervertebral disc disease or lumbosacral spondylosis.
- Involvement of several nerve distributions is usually a result of plexus or cauda equina lesions.
- Bilateral lesions suggest proximal damage affecting the roots of the cauda equina.
- Impaired bladder control indicates either a cauda equina lesion or a bilateral sacral plexopathy.
- Multiple lesions may complicate neurological localization.
- Non-neurological disorders cause low back pain.

EVALUATION

Magnetic Resonance Imaging

Magnetic resonance imaging (MRI) assesses the morphology of the lumbosacral spine, the lumbosacral plexus, and the peripheral nerves in the pelvis and legs. MRI of the lumbosacral spine has the highest yield when the patient has back pain associated with radicular distribution of pain. Contrast enhancement is required to visualize intraspinal pathology.

Nerve Conduction Study and Electromyography

Nerve conduction study (NCS) and electromyography (EMG) are important for neurological localization. Electrical studies are useful for localization by determining the denervated muscles and the localization of the nerve lesion. Mechanical low back pain is not associated with EMG or NCS abnormalities.

Radiographs

Bone radiographs are useful after acute bony trauma and isolated low back pain. Potential findings are degenerative joint disease, vertebral body collapse, bony erosion, subluxation, or other fracture.

Bone Scan

Bone scan is important when neoplastic bone involvement is considered.

For a more detailed discussion, see Chapter 34 in Neurology in Clinical Practice, 4th edition.

Neurological Complications of Systemic Disease

24

CARDIAC DISORDERS AND THE NERVOUS SYSTEM

Congenital Heart Disease

The possible neurological complications of congenital heart disease (CHD) in children include cerebral hypoxia, neurological abnormalities secondary to the cardiac anomaly, associated cerebral malformations, and complications of diagnostic and therapeutic interventions. Patients with acyanotic CHD have left-to-right shunts (atrial septal defects, ventricular septal defects, and patent ductus arteriosus). The neurological complications are secondary to emboli or bacterial abscess. Congenital stenosis of the great vessels does not cause cyanosis. Aortic stenosis is occasionally responsible for decreased cardiac output with secondary cardiac arrhythmia, cerebral hypoxia, and seizures. Pulmonary stenosis rarely causes neurological complications. Coarctation of the aorta may be associated with cerebral aneurysms.

Tetralogy of Fallot, transposition of the great vessels, truncus arteriosus, tricuspid atresia, and complete anomalous pulmonary venous return cause cyanotic CHD. Blood flow to the heart and brain does not first traverse the pulmonary vascular bed. This can result in cerebritis, brain abscess, or stroke. The clinical features of cerebral embolization are sudden alteration of consciousness, dysphasia/aphasia, seizures, and hemiparesis. Transthoracic echocardiography demonstrates cardiac vegetations and magnetic resonance imaging (MRI) shows cerebral ischemia. Antibiotics are the mainstay of treatment.

Most children with CHD have normal intellectual development. Delay in the surgical repair of cyanotic CHD increases the incidence of developmental delay. Reasons for developmental delay include brain malformations, chronic hypoxia, cerebral infarction, and seizure disorders.

Cardiogenic Embolism

Cardiogenic emboli are most prevalent in patients with mitral stenosis, intramural thrombi, prosthetic cardiac valves, atrial myxoma, infective endocarditis, sick sinus syndrome, and atrial fibrillation. Cardiac emboli are a consideration in young people with either valvular heart disease or mitral valve prolapse. Emboli are more likely when atrial fibrillation is associated with valvular heart disease.

Diagnosis
Transesophageal echocardiography is the preferred technique to evaluate atrial disease and to demonstrate a patent foramen ovale. Transthoracic echocardiography is preferred to visualize the ventricular apex, mitral or aortic valvular disease, and left ventricular thrombus. Transesophageal echocardiography is appropriate to investigate adults younger than 45 years with suspected cardiogenic emboli and older people without signs of cardiac disease, but transthoracic echocardiography is generally adequate in children and adults with clinical evidence of cardiac disease.

Management
Long-term oral warfarin is the treatment for atrial fibrillation unless specific contraindications exist or the atrial fibrillation is an isolated finding in people younger than 60 years without other evidence of cardiovascular disease. Aspirin (325 mg/day) is used when warfarin is contraindicated. Warfarin is usually started 3 weeks before elective cardioversion in people with atrial fibrillation of more than 2 days' duration and continued until normal rhythm is maintained for 4 weeks.

Reduced Cerebral Perfusion

Brain function is critically dependent on the cerebral circulation. The brain receives about 15% of the total cardiac output.

Syncope
Transitory reduction in cerebral perfusion causes syncope. Visual disturbances, paresthesias, and lightheadedness sometimes precede syncope. Syncope is always associated with loss of muscle tone and pallor. Tonic posturing and irregular jerking movements, which are easily mistaken for seizures, may follow. Cardiac causes of syncope include obstructed outflow, arrhythmias, sick sinus syndrome, and paroxysmal tachycardia. Benign syncope occurs in 15% of children and is probably a familial trait. The *prolonged QT interval syndrome* is an autosomal dominant trait that causes syncope in patients between 2 and

6 years of age. Measuring the QT interval on a standard electrocardiogram or a rhythm strip confirms the diagnosis. Additional causes of syncope are central and peripheral dysautonomias, postural hypotension, and endocrine and metabolic disorders.

Cardiac Arrest

Ventricular fibrillation or asystole causes circulatory failure that, depending on its duration, can cause irreversible anoxic-ischemic brain damage. The prognosis generally depends on age, the duration of the arrest before starting cardiopulmonary resuscitation, and the interval before starting defibrillating procedures. Circulatory arrest caused by ventricular fibrillation has a better prognosis than asystole.

In the mature brain, gray matter is generally more sensitive to ischemia than white matter, and the cerebral cortex is more sensitive than the brainstem. Cerebral or spinal regions lying between the territories supplied by the major arteries (watershed areas) are especially vulnerable to ischemic injury. An arrest of less than 5 minutes causes temporary loss of consciousness and impaired cognitive function. A sometimes fatal demyelinating encephalopathy may follow recovery 7 to 10 days later. The main features are progressive intellectual decline, seizures, visual agnosia, cortical blindness, amnestic syndromes, and personality changes. Prolonged cardiac arrest causes widespread and irreversible brain damage characterized by prolonged coma or a persistent vegetative state.

Neurological Complications of Diagnostic and Surgical Intervention

Injury to the endothelial lining of the vessel is an inherent risk of introducing catheters, balloons, or other devices into the vascular system. The main risk is the possibility of thrombus formation and the subsequent dispersion of emboli to the brain and other organs. The emboli more often involve the posterior than the anterior circulation.

The successful repair of complex congenital heart disorders at an earlier age has increased survival but also increased morbidity. The occurrence of seizures varies from 5% to 25% in the early postoperative period. The incidence of stroke, during and after surgery, is 25%. Altered intravascular endothelial surfaces and prosthetic devices facilitate thrombus formation and embolization by decreasing blood flow. This increased risk of stroke necessitates the use postoperative anticoagulation. Choreoathetosis may follow hypothermic heart surgery. Movement disorders occur in 1% or less of children following such surgery. The abnormal movements persist for several months and are part of a generalized encephalopathy.

Early complications of cardiac transplantation are organ rejection with consequent cardiac failure and side effects of immunosuppressive drugs. Infections are the most important late complications. The infecting organisms include *Aspergillus, Toxoplasma, Cryptococcus, Candida, Nocardia,* and viruses.

Cognitive changes after cardiac bypass surgery are detectable in 53% of patients at discharge and 42% after 5 years. Compression or traction injuries to the brachial plexus, especially the lower trunk, as well as phrenic and recurrent laryngeal nerves, may occur during cardiac surgery. Stroke occurs in approximately 5% of patients undergoing coronary artery bypass surgery.

DISEASES OF THE AORTA

Spinal cord ischemia is the main consequence of aortic disease. In general, aortic pathology that causes cord ischemia is above the origin of the renal arteries. Spinal cord ischemia from aortic disease usually causes a complete transverse myelopathy or an anterior spinal artery syndrome. The causes of neurogenic claudication are ischemia of the nerve roots or cauda equina, intermittent cord ischemia from spinal vascular malformations, or aortic disease. Pain, weakness, or a sensory disturbance develops in one or both legs while walking and is relieved by rest.

Aortic Aneurysm

Marfan's syndrome is associated with an unusually high incidence of dissecting aneurysm of the ascending aorta. The neurological features are acute cerebral or cord deficits from ischemia. Acute chest pain is often associated.

Thoracic aortic aneurysms suggest tertiary syphilis. Cerebral emboli are a complication of thoracic aortic aneurysms. Atherosclerosis is the usual cause of abdominal aortic aneurysms. These aneurysms may compress the femoral or obturator nerves. Occlusive disease of the terminal aorta may cause an ischemic neuropathy of one leg, characterized by pain and loss of sensation in the feet.

Aortitis

The causes of aortitis include syphilis, Takayasu's disease, irradiation, transient emboligenic aortoarteritis, and connective tissue diseases. Ischemia or aneurysm causes the neurological complications of aortitis. Corticosteroids are the treatment of choice.

Coarctation of the Aorta

Congenital coarctation of the aorta is a narrowing of the thoracic aorta just after the origin of the left subclavian artery. Acquired coarctation may follow irradiation during infancy. A narrowed segment, atypically located for congenital coarctation and unrelated to prior irradiation, suggests Takayasu's disease. Headache occurs in more than 25% of patients with coarctation. Complications include subarachnoid hemorrhage from cerebral aneurysm, episodic loss of consciousness, and ischemia of the lower spinal cord. Surgical repair of the underlying coarctation is required.

Subclavian Steal Syndrome

Occlusion of either the innominate or the left subclavian artery before the origin of the vertebral artery reverses the direction of blood flow in the vertebral artery on the affected side. The syndrome is usually asymptomatic but may cause ischemia in the posterior cerebral circulation during exercise of the relevant arm. Neurological features are weakness, vertigo, visual complaints, and syncope. A diminished or absent pulse and a reduced systolic pressure compared with the opposite arm is typical. Reconstructive surgery is sometimes helpful but unnecessary in most patients.

Complications of Aortic Surgery

Spinal cord infarction is the most serious neurological complication of aortic surgery. Cerebrospinal fluid (CSF) drainage and distal aortic perfusion may be important adjuncts to corrective surgery, significantly reducing the incidence of paraplegia and paraparesis. Other complications include neuropathy, radiculopathy, postsympathectomy neuralgia, and disturbances of penile erection or ejaculation.

CONNECTIVE TISSUE DISEASES AND VASCULITIDES

In connective tissue diseases and vasculitides, the causes of neurological complications are ischemia from vasculitis, other organ failure, or immunosuppressive therapy. The common direct central nervous system (CNS) features are cognitive or behavioral changes and focal neurological deficits. Peripheral neuropathies are common and take the form of mononeuritis multiplex, distal axonal polyneuropathy, compression neuropathy, sensory neuronopathy, trigeminal sensory neuropathy, acute or chronic demyelinating polyneuropathy, or plexopathy.

Behçet's Disease

The combination of uveitis and oral and genital ulcers defines Behçet's disease. Aseptic meningitis or meningoencephalitis occurs in 20% of patients. The causes of focal or multifocal deficits are ischemic disease of the brain or spinal cord. Cerebral venous sinus thrombosis may occur. The CSF shows a mild pleocytosis, and the protein concentration may be increased. Peripheral nerve involvement is rare. Treatment is with corticosteroids. Heparin is the treatment of cerebral venous sinus thrombosis.

Giant Cell Arteritis

Headache is the most common initial complaint of patients with giant cell arteritis, but some also complain of masticatory claudication. The temporal and other scalp arteries are often erythematous, tender, and nodular. A more serious initial symptom is acute transitory or permanent blindness, affecting one or both eyes, caused by ischemic optic neuropathy. Peripheral neuropathies occur in up to 15% of patients. One half of patients have an elevated erythrocyte sedimentation rate (ESR), and polymyalgia rheumatica is often associated. High-dose corticosteroids are initiated immediately upon diagnosis. The clinical response and ESR are used to monitor the clinical response. Despite the use of a tapered corticosteroid dose, treatment is required for 18–24 months.

Polyarteritis Nodosa

Peripheral neuropathy occurs in up to 60% of patients. It usually begins as a painful mononeuropathy multiplex that in polyarteritis becomes more confluent and resembles a polyneuropathy. CNS involvement occurs later in the course. Common features are headache, cognitive decline, acute confusion, and affective or psychotic disorders. Ischemic or compressive myelopathies from extradural hematomas are rare complications. An infantile form of polyarteritis is probably the same or similar to Kawasaki disease.

The 6-month survival rate of patients with untreated polyarteritis nodosa is only 35%. Weight loss, fever, cutaneous abnormalities, and arthralgia are common. Hypertension and renal, cardiac, pulmonary, or gastrointestinal involvement may occur. Laboratory studies show multiorgan and immunological abnormalities. Nerve or muscle biopsy often shows the necrotizing vasculitis, and angiography shows segmental narrowing or aneurysmal distention, especially in the renal, mesenteric, or hepatic vessels. Treatment is with corticosteroids, sometimes combined with cyclophosphamide.

Rheumatoid Arthritis

Rheumatoid arthritis is the most common of the connective tissue diseases. Systemic vasculitis occurs in up to 25% of adult patients, but the CNS is rarely affected. Involvement of the cervical spine or atlantoaxial dislocation may cause myelopathy, headache, hydrocephalus, or compression of the vertebral arteries, brainstem, and cranial nerves. Hyperextension of the neck may cause subluxation. A distal sensory or sensorimotor polyneuropathy is common. Mononeuropathy multiplex and entrapment or compression neuropathies also occur. Several antirheumatic agents have adverse effects on the neuromuscular system. Gold causes peripheral neuropathy in up to 1% of patients. Chloroquine can cause neuropathy, myopathy, or both, and D-penicillamine causes disturbances of taste, an inflammatory myopathy, and a reversible form of myasthenia gravis.

Juvenile Rheumatoid Arthritis

The characteristics of juvenile rheumatoid arthritis (JRA) include chronic inflammation of one or more joints in children younger than 16 years in whom other causes for the arthritis are excluded. All of the different features of JRA are attributable to complex autoimmune disease. No identifiable infectious agent causes JRA. About 10% of children with JRA have a *systemic form* characterized by recurrent fevers, a faint evanescent skin rash, irritability, malaise, and anorexia. Some have severe joint pain and myalgia before joint involvement. Pericarditis and myocarditis are common and life threatening. Laboratory studies (in systemic JRA) show anemia and thrombocytosis. Children with systemic JRA are typically seronegative for rheumatoid factor (RF) and antinuclear antibodies (ANAs). An acute encephalopathy with increased intracranial pressure may be associated. Electroencephalographic (EEG) study results are abnormal even in the absence of clinical seizures.

Other types of JRA include a *pauciarticular* form in which one or several joints are affected and a *polyarticular* form in which five or more joints are involved. Focal neurological findings are uncommon and can be secondary to soft tissue involvement. Sensorimotor polyneuropathies are uncommon. Serum creatine kinase concentrations are elevated in one third of children, but proximal weakness or histological evidence of myositis is uncommon. Decreased mobility of the neck, secondary to fusion of the cervical vertebrae, can occur in both the systemic or the polyarticular form of JRA. Torticollis may be the presenting feature. Cervical myelopathy from atlantoaxial dislocation is a rare event in children. The management of JRA is usually with aspirin or nonsteroidal anti-inflammatory agents. Some require corticosteroids, intravenous immune globulin (IVIG), immunosuppressive agents, or parenteral gold salts. Physical and occupational therapy lessen the discomfort of joint or muscle stiffness.

Systemic Lupus Erythematosus

Most patients with systemic lupus erythematosus (SLE) have neurological complications, often during the first year. The mechanism is unknown. Neither the presence of antineuronal and antiastrocyte antibodies nor the deposition of antibody in the choroid plexus correlates with CNS involvement. The most common neurological manifestations are episodic affective or psychotic disorders and seizures. Disturbances of consciousness sometimes occur, especially in patients with systemic infections. Focal neurological deficits may result from stroke. Dyskinesias, especially chorea, occur in some patients with SLE. Peripheral nervous system (PNS) involvement occurs less often. The characteristic features are usually a distal sensory or sensorimotor polyneuropathy. Corticosteroids, immunosuppressive agents, and plasmapheresis are beneficial when necrotizing vasculitis causes neuropathy.

Sjögren's Syndrome

The main features of Sjögren's syndrome are xerostomia and xerophthalmia. Women are more often affected than men. Definitive diagnosis requires a positive result of the rose bengal dye test for keratoconjunctivitis, evidence of diminished salivary gland flow, abnormalities on biopsy of a minor salivary gland, and an abnormal test result for RF or ANAs. Neurological complications are uncommon and include psychiatric disturbances, migrainous episodes, aseptic meningitis, meningoencephalitis, an acute or chronic myelopathy, and polyneuropathy. Cranial MRI may show hyperintense small subcortical lesions.

Wegener's Granulomatosis

Neurological involvement occurs in up to 50% of patients with Wegener's granulomatosis. Peripheral involvement is usually a mononeuropathy multiplex or a symmetrical polyneuropathy. Vasculitis or extension of granulomas from the upper respiratory tract causes neurological complications. The clinical syndromes are basal meningitis, temporal lobe dysfunction, cranial neuropathies, cerebral infarction, or venous sinus obstruction.

RESPIRATORY DISEASES

Ventilation requires the integrity of the CNS and PNS to support its coordinated motor activity.

Hypoxia

The neurological manifestations of hypoxia depend on its rate of onset, duration, and severity. Hypercapnia is always concurrent with hypoxia, and the features of each are difficult to distinguish. The characteristic encephalopathy caused by chronic pulmonary insufficiency includes headache, disorientation, confusion, and depressed cognitive function. Examination may show postural tremor, myoclonus, asterixis, brisk tendon reflexes, and papilledema.

High-altitude sickness occurs at heights of more than 10,000 feet. The features are headache, lassitude, anorexia, nausea, difficulty concentrating, and sleep disturbances. At higher altitudes, consciousness may be disturbed and coma may occur. Cerebral edema is the cause of increased intracranial pressure and causes papilledema, retinal hemorrhages, cranial neuropathies, focal or multifocal motor and sensory deficits, and behavioral disturbances. Corticosteroids relieve the syndrome.

Hypocapnia

The hypocapnia that results from hyperventilation causes cerebral vasoconstriction, a shift of the oxyhemoglobin dissociation curve so peripheral availability of oxygen is reduced, and an alteration in the ionic balance of calcium. The clinical features are lightheadedness, paresthesias, visual disturbances, headache, unsteadiness, tremor, nausea, palpitations, muscle cramps, carpopedal spasms, and loss of consciousness.

Sarcoidosis

Sarcoidosis is a primary granulomatous disorder of the respiratory system. Cranial neuropathies from chronic basal meningitis are the main neurological complication. Facial palsies, sometimes bilateral, are common. The optic nerve may be swollen or atrophied. The causes of visual changes are increased intracranial pressure, direct involvement of the optic nerves or their meningeal covering, or uveitis. Unilateral or bilateral recurrent laryngeal, trigeminal, or auditory nerve involvement also may occur.

Disturbances of the hypothalamic region are associated with diabetes insipidus, abnormal thermoregulation, amenorrhea, impotence, hypoglycemia, disturbed sleep, obesity, personality changes, and hypopituitarism. Other neurological features depend on intracranial or intraspinal meningeal or parenchymal involvement. An enlarging granuloma may mimic a cerebral tumor. Peripheral neuropathy and myopathy from granulomatous involvement may occur.

Management

Neurosarcoidosis often remits spontaneously, but progressive neurological disease occurs in about 30% of patients. The diagnosis relies on histological confirmation and is difficult in the absence of cutaneous or pulmonary involvement. Corticosteroids are the recommended treatment.

Systemic Inflammatory Response Syndrome

Neurological complications may occur when infection and trauma have induced a systemic inflammatory response affecting the microcirculation to multiple organs. For example, patients with sepsis and multiorgan failure sometimes develop an axonal neuropathy (*critical illness neuropathy*) that comes to attention when ventilatory support is withdrawn. Corticosteroids and neuromuscular blocking drugs may induce a myopathy, especially in patients with obstructive airways diseases. Its highest prevalence is among asthmatics who require ventilatory support in addition to corticosteroids and who have also received vecuronium.

HEMATOLOGICAL DISORDERS

Anemias

Anemia often causes nonspecific behavioral symptoms such as lassitude, lightheadedness, inattentiveness, irritability, headache, and unsteadiness. Severe anemia may rarely cause focal neurological deficits in patients with pre-existing cerebral atherosclerotic disease.

Megaloblastic Anemia

Vitamin B12 deficiency causes myelopathy, encephalopathy, optic neuropathy, peripheral neuropathy, or some combination of these disorders. The neurological complications do not necessarily correlate with the presence or severity of associated megaloblastic anemia. Folic acid masks the anemia without preventing the neurological complications. Treatment with intramuscular injections of Vitamin B12 reverses the neurological disorder.

Sickle Cell Disease

Children with sickle cell disease are unusually susceptible to infections with *Streptococcus pneumoniae*, *Haemophilus influenzae*, and *Mycoplasma pneumoniae*. CNS infection provokes stroke, the most common neurological complication of sickle cell disease. Chronic symptoms of silent stroke include recurring headache, seizures, abnormalities of speech and language, and learning disabilities. The baseline prevalence of silent infarcts is 22% among children aged 6 to 19 years. Transcranial Doppler ultrasonography is a useful screening technique to demonstrate vascular narrowing. Partial-exchange transfusions are beneficial in terminating an occlusive crisis in children. Sufficient packed red blood cells are given to reduce the hemoglobin S to no more than 30% to 35%. Higher levels are associated with a significant risk of recurrent stroke.

Thalassemias

Extramedullary hematopoiesis occurs in the liver, spleen, and lymph nodes of patients with severe forms of β-thalassemia but may also occur in the spinal epidural space and cause a compressive myelopathy. Treatment includes local irradiation, surgical decompression, corticosteroids, and repeated blood transfusions.

Proliferative Hematological Disorders

Leukemias

The causes of neurological complications from leukemia are leukemic infiltration of the nervous system, hemorrhage, infection, electrolyte disturbances, hyperviscosity, and complications of treatment. Localized leukemic deposits are more likely to affect the brain than the spinal cord; peripheral nerve involvement is rare.

Plasma Cell Dyscrasias

Classification of the plasma cell dyscrasias is by the protein synthesized. Multiple myeloma is the most common plasma cell dyscrasia. It is associated with a monoclonal immunoglobulin G (IgG) or immunoglobulin A (IgA) paraprotein in the serum or urine. The clinical features are pain, fracture, and destruction of bone. The POEMS syndrome consists of *p*olyneuropathy, *o*rganomegaly, *e*ndocrinopathy, *M* protein, and *s*kin changes in patients with plasma cell dyscrasia.

Waldenström's Macroglobulinemia

Waldenström's macroglobulinemia is a plasma cell dyscrasia associated with immunoglobulin M (IgM) gammopathy. Neurological complications are common. A progressive sensorimotor polyneuropathy is secondary to the binding of monoclonal IgM to peripheral nerves or from lymphocytic infiltration of the nerves.

Monoclonal Gammopathy of Undetermined Significance

Many patients with a monoclonal gammopathy have no evidence of serious underlying pathology, but some eventually develop a malignant plasma cell dyscrasia. Chronic inflammatory demyelinating polyradiculoneuropathy is the characteristic polyneuropathy associated with monoclonal gammopathy of undetermined significance.

Amyloidosis

Amyloidosis may occur as a familial disorder with dominant inheritance. The main neurological complication is a small fiber sensory neuropathy, with marked impairment of pain and temperature appreciation and lesser involvement of other sensory modalities.

Cryoglobulinemia

Cryoglobulins are proteins that precipitate in the cold and dissolve when heated. They are classified as (1) monoclonal IgM, IgG, IgA, or light chains (type 1), (2) mixed but with one monoclonal immunoglobulin (type 2), or (3) polyclonal without any monoclonal protein (type 3).

Lymphoma

The causes of neurological complications of lymphoma are direct spread of tumor, compression of the nervous system by extrinsic tumor, or paraneoplastic syndromes.

Polycythemia

The thrombotic and hemorrhagic complications of polycythemia affect the nervous system by occlusion of small or large arteries, or venous channels may cause cerebral infarcts that are sometimes recurrent and fatal.

Hemorrhagic Diseases

Hemophilia
Intracranial hemorrhage is the major cause of death in hemophilia. Hemorrhages may be epidural, subdural, subarachnoid, or intracerebral and may occur spontaneously or after trivial head injury. Peripheral neuropathies are secondary to compression of individual nerves by intramuscular or retroperitoneal hematomas.

Thrombocytopenia
Thrombocytopenia, the reduced production or increased breakdown of platelets, may lead to hemorrhage. Thrombotic thrombocytopenic purpura is a disorder of uncertain cause that often has a fatal outcome. Treatment options are plasma exchange or infusion, splenectomy, and administration of corticosteroids or antiplatelet agents.

Antiphospholipid Antibody Syndromes
Antiphospholipid antibodies (the lupus anticoagulant and anticardiolipin antibodies) are detectable in several disorders, but especially in SLE and Sneddon's syndrome. The presence of antiphospholipid antibodies increases the risk of thrombotic disease.

Liver Disease

Patients with acute hepatic failure often develop severe cerebral edema.

Portal Systemic Encephalopathy
Chronic liver disease causes a portal systemic encephalopathy. The encephalopathy may have an insidious onset. A flapping tremor (*asterixis*) may be the only other neurological sign. EEG abnormalities correlate with the severity of encephalopathy.

Chronic Nonwilsonian Hepatocerebral Degeneration
Some patients with chronic liver disease develop a permanent neurological deficit, even in the absence of prior portal systemic encephalopathy. The neurological features are similar to those of Wilson's disease: intention tremor, ataxia, dysarthria, and choreoathetosis.

Gastrointestinal Diseases

Nutritional deficiency is the usual cause of neurological complications from gastrointestinal disorders.

Gastric Surgery
Neurological complications occur in 10–15% of patients after gastric resection. Impaired Vitamin B12 absorption because of the loss of gastric intrinsic factor may be responsible in part for neuropathy or myelopathy. Gastric plication has been associated with encephalopathy, myelopathy, polyneuropathy, Wernicke's syndrome, and a nutritional amblyopia.

Small Bowel Disease
Neuropathy and myelopathy are associated with the malabsorption syndromes caused either by small bowel disease, biliary atresia, or blind loop syndrome or with previous extensive gastrointestinal resection. The findings may include pigmentary retinal degeneration, external ophthalmoplegia, dysarthria, peripheral neuropathy, and pyramidal and cerebral signs in the limbs.

Whipple's Disease
Whipple's disease is a multisystem disorder believed to be caused by infection with the bacillus *Trophermyma whippleii*. The characteristic features are steatorrhea, abdominal pain, weight loss, arthritis, and lymphadenopathy. Neurological involvement is rare but may occur in the absence of gastrointestinal symptoms. The most common neurological feature is dementia.

Renal Failure

Uremic encephalopathy resembles other metabolic encephalopathies. A length-dependent, symmetrical sensorimotor polyneuropathy is a common complication of uremia. Uremic optic neuropathy causes a rapidly progressive vision loss that responds to hemodialysis and corticosteroid treatment.

Neurological Complications of Dialysis
Shift of water into the brain is the probable cause of the dialysis disequilibrium syndrome. Headache, irritability, agitation, somnolence, seizures, muscle cramps, and nausea during or after hemodialysis or peritoneal dialysis are the characteristic features. Patients undergoing dialysis for longer than 1 year may develop a fatal encephalopathy called *dialysis dementia*. Dialysis dementia has become less common since the removal of aluminum from dialysates. Deferoxamine, a chelating agent that binds aluminum, is the drug often prescribed for patients with dialysis dementia. The optimal duration of treatment is unclear.

For a more detailed discussion, see Chapters 54A and 54B in Neurology in Clinical Practice, 4th edition.

Trauma of the Nervous System | 25

CRANIOCEREBRAL TRAUMA

Traumatic brain injury (TBI) is the leading cause of morbidity and mortality in the United States for people aged 1–45 years. An estimated 1.6 million people sustain a TBI each year. Approximately 270,000 require hospitalization, 52,000 die of their injuries, and 80,000 have severe neurological disabilities. Another 760,000 are treated and released from emergency departments or clinics, and approximately 400,000 people with mild or moderate TBI do not even seek medical attention. The leading causes of TBI are motor vehicle crashes (MVCs), violence, and falls. Adolescents, teenagers, and the elderly are most at risk. Falls are the leading cause of head injury in people 65 years and older, whereas the leading cause of head injury in younger people is MVCs. At all ages, the risk of TBI in males is twice that in females. In the United States an estimated 5.3 million people are living with a permanent TBI-related disability, the direct and indirect costs estimated to exceed $4 billion a year. TBI-related death rates have been falling in the United States, with one study documenting a 22% decline from 1979 to 1992. A significant reduction in MVC-related TBI is primarily responsible. At the same time, however, some large cities are seeing a rise in gunshot wounds to the head, and deaths from this cause often exceed MVC-related fatalities.

Pathophysiology

The main categories of intracranial lesions are focal or diffuse, although both may occur in the same patient. Focal hematomas may be epidural, subdural, or intracerebral hematomas and frequently represent surgical emergencies. Diffuse lesions are concussions or diffuse axonal injury (DAI). In general, the greater the velocity of the force and head movement, the greater the likelihood of diffuse parenchymal sequelae and the less the likelihood of focal injuries or hematomas.

Axonal Injury
DAI is probably the most important factor in determining outcome in blunt head injury and is the most common cause of coma in the absence of an intracranial mass lesion. The characteristics of DAI are widely distributed axonal swellings of the cerebral white matter, corpus callosum, and upper brainstem, as well as hemorrhagic lesions of the corpus callosum and one or both dorsolateral quadrants of the rostral brainstem.

Acute Subdural Hematoma
Acute subdural hematoma (SDH) is the most common focal intracerebral lesion. SDH occurs in approximately 30% of patients with severe head injury. It has the highest morbidity and mortality of all traumatic focal lesions because of underlying parenchymal injury and intracranial hypertension. Morbidity and mortality depend on three factors: (1) the size of the volume change, (2) the rate of the volume change, and (3) the initial intracranial compliance.

Epidural Hematoma
Epidural hematoma is less common than SDH but has a better overall outcome, provided it is detected and evacuated quickly. The cause of the hematoma is a skull fracture that ruptures the meningeal arteries, usually middle meningeal. Less underlying parenchymal brain injury is associated.

Contusion and Intracerebral Hematoma
Contusions and intracerebral hematomas represent a continuum. Contusions are bruises of the brain characterized by extravasation of blood from small lacerated vessels, whereas intracerebral hemorrhages are large blood clots in the brain parenchyma.

Subarachnoid Hemorrhage
Subarachnoid hemorrhage (SAH), or bleeding into the subarachnoid space, is common in TBI. Isolated SAH does not require surgical intervention, although one must be alert for cerebral vasospasm, raised intracranial pressure (ICP), and hydrocephalus.

Secondary Injury

Posttraumatic ischemia activates a cascade of metabolic events leading to the excessive generation of oxygen-free radicals, excitatory amino acids, cytokines, and other inflammatory agents. TBI also increases extracellular potassium levels, which result in an imbalance of intracellular and extracellular K^+, disruption of the $Na-K^+$-ATPase cell membrane regulatory mechanisms, and subsequent cell swelling. Severe TBI reduces extracellular magnesium levels, thereby impairing normal glycolysis, cellular respiration, oxidative phosphorylation, and the biosyntheses of DNA, RNA, and protein.

Management of Traumatic Brain Injury

The acutely traumatized brain is vulnerable to further injury from systemic hypotension, cerebral hypoperfusion, hypercarbia, hypoxemia, and elevated ICP. Prevention of these complications is essential for limiting secondary brain injury. The initial prehospital evaluation of trauma patients always begins with evaluation of and securing a patent airway, as well as restoration of normal breathing and circulation. Rapid fluid resuscitation and restoration of a normal blood pressure is critical. A systolic blood pressure of less than 90 mm Hg is associated with a doubling of the mortality rate following severe TBI. The immediate concern after TBI is a determination of the need for craniotomy to evacuate an intracranial mass lesion such as a hematoma or contusion. Head computed tomography (CT) scanning identifies posttraumatic intracranial lesions, brain swelling, patency of the basal cisterns, and other characteristics that guide subsequent treatment.

Physical Therapy and Rehabilitation

The increased number of survivors of TBI has increased the demand for high-quality, well-organized TBI rehabilitation programs. The primary goal of these programs is to reintegrate patients with TBI back into their communities by either restoring normal or near-normal functional capacities or teaching alternative strategies to help them function at a high level despite their disability.

Prognosis

Several clinical and radiological characteristics have proven useful for outcome prediction when used in concert. The best outcome predictors are age, initial Glasgow Coma Scale (GCS) score (particularly the motor component), pupil size, and reaction to light, ICP, and the nature and extent of intracranial injuries (see Table 2.3). Age is perhaps the most important factor limiting good outcomes following TBI. The likelihood of death, persistent vegetative state, or severe disability is 92% for those older than 60 years, 86% for those older than 56 years, and

50% for younger patients. The second most important predictor of outcome is the initial postresuscitation GCS score. Good outcomes occur in only 4% of those with an initial GCS score of 3, 6% if the initial GCS score is 4, and 12% if the initial GCS score is 5.

Penetrating Head Trauma

The most common cause of penetrating head injury is gunshot wounds. Although the incidence of TBI caused by MVCs is declining, the incidence of gunshot wounds to the head is increasing. The number of firearms-related deaths surpasses MVCs as the single largest cause of death related to TBI. Gunshot wounds to the head usually cause massive destruction of brain tissue, severe brain swelling, and death. The initial assessment and resuscitation of patients with penetrating head injuries is the same as that for those with closed head injuries. Most patients with gunshot wounds to the head die before or shortly after admission to the hospital.

SPINAL CORD TRAUMA

Half of spinal cord injuries (SCIs) occur in the cervical region, with the rest evenly distributed in the thoracic, lumbar, and sacral regions. Thoracic spine injuries have the highest rate of complete recovery and cervical spine injuries have the poorest rate of recovery. Early diagnosis, early stabilization of spinal fractures, aggressive management of comorbid disease, and multidisciplinary rehabilitation have resulted in increased survival and quality of life for these patients. Approximately 15% of patients with SCI worsen neurologically immediately after admission to the hospital. Missed or poorly managed spinal injuries are often the cause.

Grading of Spinal Cord Injury

The currently adopted standard is the American Spinal Injury Association/International Medical Society of Paraplegia (ASIA/ IMSOP) scale in conjunction with the Medical Research Council muscle grading system.

Level of Spinal Cord Injury

The term *spinal cord level* establishes the functional level of injury in patients with SCI. The ASIA/IMSOP scales form the

Table 25.1: ASIA/IMSOP impairment scale

Grade A	Complete	No motor or sensory function preserved in the sacral segments S4-S5.
Grade B	Incomplete	Sensory but not motor function is preserved below the neurological level and extends through the sacral segments S4-S5.
Grade C	Incomplete	Motor function is preserved below the neurological level, and the majority of key muscles below the neurological level have a muscle grade less than 3.
Grade D	Incomplete	Motor function is preserved below the neurological level, and the majority of key muscles below the neurological level have a muscle grade greater than or equal to 3.
Grade E	Normal	Motor and sensory functions are normal.

Modified and reprinted with permission from the American Spinal Injury Society (ASIA) and International Medical Society of Paraplegia (IMSOP).

basis for the strictest definition of SCI level (Table 25.1). A determination is made of sensory and motor levels for both sides of the body, along with zones of partial preservation. The definition of spinal cord level is the caudal-most segment of the spinal cord demonstrating normal function. In practice, it is more common to report the level at which normal motor and sensory function exists on both sides of the body or to report the level at which the grade of motor function is 3 of 5 or better. Because the spinal cord is shorter than the spinal column, a significant disparity often exists between the spinal cord and skeletal levels of injury.

Complete SCIs are those injuries that meet the criteria for the ASIA/IMSOP scale grade A injury. Because a zone of partial preservation often exists below the lowest level considered normal, the definition includes those patients with complete absence of normal motor and sensory function starting four levels below the caudal-most normal level. Patients with incomplete injuries compose grades B, C, and D.

Spectrum of Disease

SCI represents a spectrum of diseases, not all of which are permanent. Disorders such as "stingers" and transient paraplegia are at one end of the spectrum. These represent self-limited injury to the spinal cord and nerve roots. Disorders such as the progressive myelopathy associated with severe cervical spinal stenosis and chronic progressive conditions with an insidious onset and a reversible course are the middle of the spectrum. Disorders with immediate irreversible paralysis, such as spinal cord transection and vascular injury, are at the other end of the spectrum. SCI most often occurs in the setting of pre-existing pathology, even in young adults.

PERIPHERAL NERVE TRAUMA

Traumatic injury to the peripheral nervous system (PNS) is a relatively common and underrecognized source of significant physical disability. Possible mechanisms of peripheral nerve damage are laceration, compression, crush, or stretch. Most injuries arise from MVCs, but they are also common in sports, in the operating room, from drug injections, and from gunshot wounds. As many as 5% of all admissions to a level I trauma center have a peripheral nerve, nerve root, or plexus injury. Upper extremity nerve and plexus injuries are more common than lower extremity injuries. The radial, ulnar, and median nerves are most often affected. In the lower limb, the sciatic nerve and peroneal nerves are most often affected.

Classification of Nerve Trauma

Neurapraxia
The cause of neurapraxia is a mild compression or stretch injuries, which produce a physiological block in conduction rather than axonal loss. Large fibers are usually affected, and recovery occurs over hours to days.

Axonotmesis
Axonotmesis is a condition in which the axon has lost continuity but its endoneurial nerve sheath is intact. The entire distal nerve degenerates, as do the first few proximal internodes. Because the nerve sheath is intact, the axon regenerates down its proper course and functional recovery is expected.

Neurotmesis
Neurotmesis is the most severe injury. Disruption occurs to the endoneurial, perineurial, and frequently epineurial parts of the nerve, as well as the axon. Regrowth is unusual. Surgical repair is required for recovery.

Mechanisms of Nerve Injury

Laceration
Most laceration injuries are neurotmetic and require surgical repair. Delayed repair causes the nerve to retract, and secondary grafting is required. Functional recovery is reduced.

Compression
Most compressive injuries occur after prolonged immobilization (Table 25.2). The injury is usually neurapraxic, axonotmetic, or both. Spontaneous recovery is the rule.

Stretch
Stretch is the most common mechanism of serious nerve injuries. All grades of injury may occur. Sensation impairment without motor impairment is possible, but the reverse is unusual.

Stretch Avulsion
Most avulsion injuries occur at the nerve rootlet level. This may be suspected by an associated Brown-Séquard's syndrome, Horner's syndrome, phrenic palsy, severe paraspinal denervation, or other indications of very proximal nerve root injury.

High-Velocity Missile Injury
High-velocity missiles generate shockwave pressures on impact. Abrupt stretching and deformity may occur to structures adjacent to and distant from the missile path. Laceration and stretch injuries occur to the nerves. Surgery is required for nerve and vascular repair.

Time Course of Spontaneous Nerve Recovery

Recovery time depends on the level of injury in relation to muscles innervated, the specific nerve, or plexal element involved, and the severity of injury. The time needed for recovery increases by 2 weeks when an axon is discontinuous and 4 weeks with sutured axonotmetic injuries. In general, the regenerative rate is faster in the proximal limb than in the distal limb. The overall growth rate for recovery of motor function is 1 mm per day (1 inch per month). No clinical recovery 8 weeks after nerve injury usually indicates a severe injury. The functional potential of motor recovery decreases with time because of changes in the muscle. Sensory recovery may occur over several years.

Evaluation of Nerve Trauma

Clinical and Electrodiagnostic Examination
The most important aspect of the history is the time interval that has elapsed between sustaining the injury and presenting for

Table 25.2: Some examples of predominantly compressive nerve injuries

Nerve and Site of Injury	Clinical Picture	Pathophysiology
Radial nerve at spiral groove of humerus; compression	Saturday Night Palsy; wrist and finger drop with sparing of triceps function	Demyelinating conduction block Generally recovers over 6–8 weeks
Common peroneal nerve at fibular head; compression	Acute footdrop: weakness of ankle dorsiflexion, foot eversion, great toe extension; sensory loss on dorsum of ankle and foot	Demyelinating conduction block Generally recovers over 6–8 weeks
Upper trunk of brachial plexus between clavicle and first rib; compression and/or traction	Classic postoperative brachial plexopathy Paralysis of shoulder abduction and elevation Paresthesiae into lateral forearm	Predominantly demyelinating conduction block; lesser component of axon loss Usually recovers over 3 months; can be delayed recovery up to 1 year
Infraclavicular brachial plexus by pseudoaneurysm or hematoma secondary to transaxillary arteriography; compression	Median neuropathy, Combined median and ulnar neuropathy, Combined median, ulnar, axillary, musculocutaneous neuropathies	Predominantly demyelinating conduction block if decompressed within first few hours Axon loss if not repaired
Ulnar nerve at olecranon groove or within cubital tunnel; compression	Paresthesiae, pain in medial hand, and weakness of intrinsic hand muscles	Varies between demyelinating conduction block and axon loss; combined conduction block and axon loss

evaluation. Significant motor recovery is unlikely 4 years after injury. The mechanism of the injury is also important, and intraoperative transection of a nerve by a scalpel portends a better prognosis than a laceration from a chain saw. The elderly and those with diabetes or renal failure are less likely to enjoy a good functional outcome after nerve injury. A good outcome is likely if the target organ is 3 inches from the injury site on the nerve, but not with greater distances. Electrodiagnostic examination, especially assessment of sensory nerve action potentials and compound muscle action potentials, provides information about the site of the injury, its underlying pathophysiology, and the rate of recovery of the injury. The timing of this test is vital and is of both practical and prognostic importance. In the case of a severe axon-loss injury, electrodiagnostic study results will be entirely normal for the first 2 days. The optimal time for study is after 2 weeks. Repeated examinations assess for electrophysiological recovery or worsening.

Neuroradiological Assessment

MRI neurography is an exciting advance. This modality can differentiate axonotmesis and neurotmesis lesions and detect neuroma formation at nerve repair sites. Using specialized phased array coils, one may even be able to identify which fascicles within a nerve trunk are injured and which are spared.

Surgical Repair of Nerve Trauma

A specialized intraoperative technique called *nerve action potential recording* enables the surgeon to locate abnormal sites of nerve conduction due to axon loss and/or neurapraxia and to define the healthy margins of the nerve. Obvious cases of neurapraxia do not require surgical intervention because an excellent spontaneous recovery is expected. In cases of axonotmesis, which account for approximately 70% of all serious nerve injuries, spontaneous recovery is not expected and surgical intervention is required. The extent and timing of surgery depends on the severity of the injury. Most nerve injuries occur in closed wounds and are difficult to judge. Failure of recovery progress for 2–3 months in the case of a suspected focal lesion and 4–5 months for a suspected lengthy lesion usually indicates a more severe injury that requires surgical inspection.

For a more detailed discussion, see Chapters 56A, 56B, 56C, and 56D in Neurology in Clinical Practice, 4th edition.

Vascular Diseases of the Nervous System | 26

ISCHEMIC CEREBROVASCULAR DISEASE

At least 500,000 Americans experience a new or recurrent stroke annually. Stroke remains the third leading cause of death and the leading cause of disability in adults. Table 26.1 lists modifiable and unmodifiable risk factors for ischemic stroke. The incidence of stroke increases with advancing age. Men develop ischemic strokes at higher rates than women up to the age of 75 years. Heredity seems to play a minor role in the pathogenesis of cerebral infarction. At least 25% of the adult population has arterial hypertension (systolic blood pressure > 140 mm Hg or diastolic blood pressure > 90 mm Hg). Arterial hypertension is a predisposing factor for ischemic stroke by aggravating atherosclerosis and accelerating heart disease, increasing the relative risk of stroke threefold to fourfold. Ischemic stroke results from thromboembolism. The emboli arise from intracranial or extracranial arteries, emboli of cardiac origin, hypercoagulable states, occlusion of small penetrating arteries of the brain, or nonatherosclerotic vasculopathies. Specific therapy determines the long-term prognosis.

Cholesterol-lowering agents reduce the total mortality rate.

Threatened Ischemic Stroke

Approximately 80% of ischemic strokes occur in the carotid or anterior circulation, and 20% occur in the vertebrobasilar or posterior circulation. A *transient ischemic attack* (TIA) is a prognostic indicator of stroke. One third of patients with untreated TIA have a stroke within 5 years of the TIA and half of these in 1 year. Myocardial infarction is the main cause of mortality after TIA. Asymptomatic carotid disease is a greater risk factor for heart attack than for stroke. Lowering cholesterol reduces the incidence of both stroke and TIA. Chronic

Table 26.1: Risk factors for ischemic stroke

Nonmodifiable	Modifiable
Age	Arterial hypertension
Gender	Transient ischemic attacks
Race/ethnicity	Prior stroke
Family history	Asymptomatic carotid bruit/stenosis
Genetics	Cardiac disease
	Aortic arch atheromatosis
	Diabetes mellitus
	Dyslipidemia
	Cigarette smoking
	Alcohol consumption
	Increased fibrinogen
	Elevated homocysteine
	Low serum folate
	Elevated anticardiolipin antibodies
	Oral contraceptives
	Obesity

nonvalvular atrial fibrillation increases the risk of stroke fivefold to sixfold. Cigarette smoking is an independent risk factor for ischemic stroke in men and women of all ages and a leading risk factor of carotid atherosclerosis in men. Although moderate alcohol consumption reduces the risk of ischemic stroke, high alcohol consumption increases the risk of stroke.

Clinical Syndromes of Cerebral Ischemia

Transient Ischemic Attacks

A TIA is a focal neurological deficit of sudden onset caused by ischemia of the brain, retina, or cochlea, lasting less than 24 hours, and followed by complete recovery. Most TIAs last only 5–20 minutes. Small infarctions are the usual cause of episodes lasting longer than 1 hour. Table 26.2 summarizes the clinical syndromes of the carotid and vertebrobasilar arteries. TIAs occur before 25–50% of atherothrombotic infarcts, 11–30% of cardioembolic infarcts, and in 11–14% of lacunar infarcts.

Subclavian Steal Syndrome

A high-grade subclavian artery stenosis or occlusion proximal to the origin of the vertebral artery causes reversal of flow in the vertebral artery. Symptoms of brainstem ischemia are precipitated by actively exercising the ipsilateral arm. Brainstem

Table 26.2: Recognition of carotid and vertebrobasilar transient ischemic attacks

Symptoms suspicious for carotid transient ischemic attacks
   Transient ipsilateral monocular blindness (amaurosis fugax)
   Contralateral body weakness or clumsiness
   Contralateral body sensory loss or paresthesias
   Aphasia with dominant hemisphere involvement
   Various degrees of contralateral homonymous visual field defects
   Dysarthria (not in isolation)
Symptoms suspicious for vertebrobasilar transient ischemic attacks
   Usually bilateral weakness or clumsiness, but may be unilateral
     or shifting
   Bilateral, shifting or crossed (ipsilateral face and contralateral
     body) sensory loss or paresthesias
   Bilateral or contralateral homonymous visual field defects or
     binocular vision loss
   Two or more of the following symptoms: vertigo, diplopia,
     dysphagia, dysarthria, and ataxia
Symptoms not acceptable as evidence of transient ischemic attack
   Syncope, dizziness, confusion, urinary or fecal incontinence,
     and generalized weakness
   Isolated occurrence of vertigo, diplopia, dysphagia, ataxia,
     tinnitus, amnesia, drop attacks, or dysarthria

infarction is an uncommon complication of the subclavian steal syndrome.

Carotid Artery System Syndromes
Amaurosis fugax is a sudden onset of transitory monocular blindness (a fog, haze, curtain, shade, blur, cloud, or mist). Vision loss is sudden, often brief, and painless. The duration is usually 1–5 minutes and rarely lasts more than 30 minutes. Anterior cerebral artery (ACA) territory infarctions account for fewer than 3% of cerebral infarcts. Contralateral weakness involving the leg more than the arm is characteristic.

Vertebrobasilar System Syndromes
Ischemia in the posterior system causes vertigo, ataxia, nystagmus, dysmetria, and cranial nerve dysfunction.

Diagnosis and Treatment of Threatened Ischemic Stroke

An ischemic stroke develops when there is interrupted cerebral blood flow to an area of the brain. Ischemic strokes account for approximately 80–85% of all strokes. Ischemic strokes may result from (1) large artery atherosclerotic disease resulting in stenosis or occlusion, (2) small vessel or penetrating artery disease (lacunes), (3) cardiogenic or artery-to-artery embolism, (4) nonatherosclerotic vasculopathies, (5) hypercoagulable disorders, or (6) infarcts of undetermined causes.

Although most arterial disorders leading to stroke are caused by atherosclerosis, several nonatherosclerotic vasculopathies are responsible for ischemic strokes. These uncommon conditions, more common in children than adults, represent 5% of all ischemic strokes. Hypercoagulable disorders are associated with an increased risk of cerebrovascular events, particularly those of an ischemic nature and may account for a considerable number of cryptogenic strokes. These disorders account for 1% of all strokes and for 2–7% of ischemic strokes in young patients. Secondary hypercoagulable states include malignancies, the postpartum period, oral contraceptives, and smoking.

Preventing Stroke Recurrence: Medical Therapy
General measures in preventing stroke recurrence include control of associated risk factors and the use of antithrombotic agents (platelet antiaggregants and anticoagulants). A large proportion of strokes should be preventable by controlling blood pressure, treating atrial fibrillation, and stopping cigarette smoking. Oral anticoagulation with warfarin is indicated for primary and secondary prevention of stroke in patients with nonvalvular atrial fibrillation.

Treatment of Acute Ischemic Stroke
Modern therapy for acute ischemic stroke is being approached in four ways. First are general measures aimed at prevention and treatment of complications. Second are those reperfusion strategies directed at arterial recanalization. Third are cytoprotective strategies aimed at cellular and metabolic targets. The fourth approach aims at the inhibition of the inflammatory processes associated with cerebral ischemia. Eventually, combined therapy is used for the treatment of acute ischemic stroke. If patients meet appropriate criteria, thrombolytic therapy may be administered. Thrombolytic therapy is able to recanalize acute intracranial occlusions, and a strong correlation exists between arterial recanalization and neurological improvement in acute cerebral ischemia.

INTRACEREBRAL HEMORRHAGE

Intracerebral hemorrhage (ICH) accounts for approximately 10% of strokes. Genetic factors, such as the possession of the 2 and 4 alleles of the apolipoprotein E, play an important role in the occurrence of certain forms of ICH, such as lobar hemorrhages.

Mechanisms of Intracerebral Hemorrhage

Hypertension
The main cause of ICH is hypertension. Hypertension is the dominant risk factor in all forms of ICH, with the exception of lobar hemorrhages. Bleeding into an underlying brain tumor is the cause in fewer than 10% of cases.

Bleeding Disorders, Anticoagulants, and Fibrinolytic Treatment
Abnormalities of coagulation rarely cause ICH. Treatment with oral anticoagulants increases the risk 8-fold to 11-fold. Potential risk factors for intracranial bleeding in anticoagulated patients include advanced age, hypertension, preceding cerebral infarction, head trauma, and excessive prolongation of the prothrombin time.

Cerebral Amyloid Angiopathy
Cerebral amyloid angiopathy is a selective deposition of amyloid in cerebral vessels that weakens the wall. The frequency increases steadily with age and rarely occurs before the age of 55 years.

Sympathomimetic Agents
Amphetamines cause ICH after intravenous, oral, or intranasal use. The hemorrhages occur within minutes to a few hours after drug use. Most are located in the subcortical white matter of the cerebral hemispheres.

Hemorrhagic Infarction
The cause of hemorrhagic infarction is arterial or venous occlusion rather than vascular rupture. These occur in the setting of cerebral embolism or cerebral infarction secondary to venous occlusion.

Clinical Features of Intracerebral Hemorrhage

The location of the hematoma determines the symptoms. The initial focal neurological deficit progressively worsens during the first hours as the hematoma enlarges. A concomitant deterioration in the level of consciousness suggests increased intracranial pressure (ICP). Seizures at onset are rare, except with lobar ICH, in which it occurs in 28% of patients. Computed tomography (CT) is a sensitive test that shows fresh blood in the brain parenchyma, features of local mass effect, and ventricular extension of blood. Magnetic resonance imaging (MRI) adds precision in determining the timing of the hemorrhage.

Management of Intracerebral Hemorrhage

The two main issues in the treatment of ICH are as follows: (1) the type and intensity of medical interventions required to improve prognosis and (2) the choice between medical and surgical therapy. Most treatments include lowering ICP or preventing its increase. General measures include control of hypertension and treatment of seizures. Pharmacological correction of severe hypertension is mandatory in the acute phase. The aim is maintenance of normal cerebral perfusion pressure levels (50–70 mm Hg) and a mean arterial pressure of less than 130 mm Hg. Intravenous labetalol is the antihypertensive agent of choice. Seizures, a feature of lobar rather than deep ganglionic ICH, occur at onset. Patients who did not have early seizures are not at great risk of late epilepsy, and the routine prophylactic use of anticonvulsants is not justified.

Choice between Medical and Surgical Therapy in Intracerebral Hemorrhage

The current treatment of ICH in most patients is medical. Surgical therapy is an option when progressive deterioration in the level of consciousness occurs in patients with putaminal and lobar hemorrhage, as well as in many instances of cerebellar hemorrhage. CT criteria for early selection of candidates for surgical therapy are large hematomas (diameter ≥3 cm), presence of hydrocephalus, and obliteration of the quadrigeminal cistern. With cerebellar hemorrhage, early signs of pontine tegmental compression and development of obtundation and extensor-plantar responses are indications for emergency surgical therapy.

INTRACRANIAL ANEURYSMS AND SUBARACHNOID HEMORRHAGE

Clinical Syndromes

The main features of a major aneurysmal rupture include a sudden explosive headache, decreased level of consciousness, photophobia, meningismus, nausea, and vomiting. The prognosis is better if treatment occurs before these develop. Therefore, recognizing the signs and symptoms associated with aneurysmal expansion or a minor hemorrhage is important. Sentinel headaches occur in approximately one half of patients before rupture. Other associated symptoms may include nausea, neck pain, lethargy, and photophobia. The presumed cause of these symptoms is a noncatastrophic leak associated with blood in the cerebrospinal fluid (CSF). Hemorrhage into the wall of an aneurysm produces *thunderclap headache*, which is not associated with red blood cells in the CSF. Other premonitory features may include diplopia, visual field deficits, or facial pain.

Physical Findings

The size and location of the aneurysm determines the physical findings in patients with unruptured aneurysms. Symptoms associated with aneurysms of the anterior communicating artery are visual field defects, endocrine dysfunction, or localized frontal headache. Aneurysms of the internal carotid artery cause oculomotor paresis, visual field deficits, impaired visual acuity, endocrine dysfunction, and localized facial pain. Large aneurysms of the internal carotid artery cause a cavernous sinus syndrome. Aphasia and focal arm weakness occur with middle cerebral artery aneurysms. An unruptured internal carotid artery aneurysm, arising at or near the origin of the posterior communicating artery, causes third nerve dysfunction. Because the pupilloconstrictor fibers lay superficially, external pressure usually causes a dilated pupil. Ischemic nerve lesions, such as diabetes, usually spare the pupil. Aneurysmal rupture can result in hemorrhage into the subarachnoid space alone or in combination with subdural hematoma, intracerebral hematoma, or intraventricular hemorrhage. The immediate physical findings can vary from slight meningismus and headache to profound neurological deficits with coma.

Because treatment and prognosis depend on the clinical status of the patient, a grading scale based on the neurological presentation of the patient is routine. The two systems most commonly used are the Hunt and Hess classification and the World Federation of Neurological Surgeons' grading scale (Table 26.3).

Laboratory Studies

The laboratory evaluation of patients suspected of having a ruptured or an unruptured intracranial aneurysm uses a combination of CT, MRI, magnetic resonance angiography (MRA), lumbar puncture, and angiography. CT delineates the amount and location of blood in the subarachnoid space. CT may not detect small amounts of subarachnoid blood. A lumbar puncture should follow a normal CT scan in a patient with the appropriate history of subarachnoid hemorrhage (SAH). If the CT shows blood, a lumbar puncture is unnecessary. If either CT or lumbar puncture is positive, immediately obtain four-vessel

Table 26.3: Hunt and Hess and World Federation of Neurological Surgeons' scales

Hunt and Hess
  Grade 0: Asymptomatic
  Grade I: Slight headache, no neurological deficit
  Grade II: Severe headache but no neurological deficit other than perhaps a cranial nerve palsy
  Grade III: Drowsiness and mild deficit
  Grade IV: Stupor, moderate to severe hemiparesis, and possible early rigidity and vegetative disturbances
  Grade V: Deep coma, decerebrate rigidity, and moribund appearance
World Federation of Neurological Surgeons' scale
  Grade I: GCS 15; motor deficit absent
  Grade II: GCS 13 or 14; motor deficit absent
  Grade III: GCS 13 or 14; motor deficit present
  Grade IV: GCS 7–12; motor deficit absent or present
  Grade V: GCS 3–6; motor deficit absent or present

GCS = Glasgow Coma Scale.

angiography because multiple aneurysms occur in approximately 20% of patients.

Treatment and Prognosis

The management of patients in good condition with uncomplicated aneurysms is operative intervention to secure the aneurysm. The benefits of early surgery are prevention of rebleeding, improved management of vasospasm, and a shorter hospital course with potentially fewer complications. Delayed ischemic deterioration is a major cause of morbidity and mortality after SAH. The major branches of the circle of Willis exposed to blood develop vasospasm, which lasts for 1–2 weeks or longer. Ischemic complications occur in 30% of patients who have had an SAH. CT predicts the occurrence of vasospasm because it shows the amount of blood in the subarachnoid space.

Standard medical therapy for the prevention and treatment of vasospasm includes a regimen of volume expansion, augmentation of cardiac index with dobutamine, and induced systemic hypertension. Angioplasty with a silicone balloon to treat vasospasm is indispensable in the comprehensive management of SAH and provides functional improvement in patients who would otherwise suffer from ischemic neurological deterioration. Six months after discharge from hospital following SAH, 58% of patients have good recovery, 9% are moderately disabled, 5% are severely disabled, 2% survive in a vegetative state, and 26% are dead.

Central Nervous System Complications

Hydrocephalus caused by SAH can be immediate or delayed. Acute dilatation occurs in 20% of patients. Delayed ventricular dilatation usually occurs after the tenth day in 23% of patients. Approximately 3% to 5% of patients with SAH have seizures during their hospitalization. Epilepsy develops, usually in the first 18 months, in 15% of patients who suffer an SAH.

The basis of management of patients with SAH for prevention and treatment of cerebral vasospasm is optimization of volume status and cardiac output. In addition, nimodipine is effective for the prevention of delayed ischemia deficits. Magnesium sulfate may prevent or reverse vasospasm. Endovascular treatment, such as angioplasty with a silicone balloon to treat vasospasm, is indispensable in the comprehensive management of patients with SAH and can provide dramatic improvement in the function.

Unruptured Aneurysms

The International Study of Unruptured Intracranial Aneurysms (ISUIA) examined the issue of treatment for unruptured aneurysms. The risk of rupture of an aneurysm smaller than 10 mm was 0.05% per year. The risk of rupture increases to 0.5% per year in patients with a history of SAH. Aneurysms larger than 10 mm had an approximately 1% per year risk of rupture, with or without a history of SAH. Current data on unruptured aneurysms do not support the use of or the size of the lesion as the sole criterion on which to base treatment decisions. Elective aneurysm surgery is cost-effective if the surgical morbidity and mortality remain at low levels, patient life expectancy is at least 13 years, and knowledge of the aneurysm decreases the quality of life.

Subarachnoid Hemorrhage in Pregnancy

SAH, the third most common nonobstetrical cause of maternal death, accounts for approximately one half of all intracranial bleeding in pregnancy and carries a grave prognosis. The management of pregnant women with incidentally discovered aneurysms is not well defined, and individualized treatment is required. Once SAH occurs, neurosurgical consideration should take precedence over obstetrical concerns. The time of aneurysm rupture in normal pregnancies is as follows: 8% ruptured in the first 3 months, 22% in the next 3 months, 59% between the seventh and tenth month, 3% during labor, and 8% in the puerperium.

ARTERIOVENOUS MALFORMATIONS

Arteriovenous malformations (AVMs) are developmental abnormalities of blood vessels in which primitive direct communication between otherwise normal arterial and venous channels is preserved. The most devastating consequences of these lesions occur because of intracranial hemorrhage. Seizures are the most common feature preceding hemorrhage. Other vascular malformations that come to clinical attention are venous angiomas, cavernous malformations, and capillary telangiectasia.

Clinical Features

The features of an AVM that bring patients to medical attention are (1) intracranial hemorrhage, (2) seizures, (3) focal neurological deficits, (4) impairment of higher cortical function, (5) headache, and (6) bruit. Some are discovered incidentally, when neuroimaging is done for other reasons. The presence and character of a neurological deficit can localize the site of hemorrhage. Intracranial hemorrhage from an AVM does not have a pattern of early rebleeding and is rarely associated with vasospasm. An unruptured AVM carries a 4% yearly risk of hemorrhage. The mortality rate from the first hemorrhage varies between 6% and 14%. Once an AVM has bled, the likelihood of recurrent hemorrhage is approximately 6% for the first year and 2–4% for the subsequent years.

Laboratory Studies

Although MRI and MRA provide information for both the diagnosis and the therapy for AVMs, only arteriography defines the predominant afferent and efferent vessels and determines how the AVM affects the blood supply to the surrounding brain. An AVM may receive arterial input from any of the major cerebral arteries.

Venous angiomas are vascular malformations composed entirely of venous structures. Often, they are incidental findings on MRI. Unlike angiography, MRI visualizes *cavernous malformations* because the afferent vessels are small and thrombosed and the flow in the vessels is low. *Capillary angiomas* or *telangiectasias* are small solitary groups of abnormally dilatated capillaries. They rarely give rise to spontaneous hemorrhage and are usually a postmortem finding. *Cryptic malformation* is a term used to describe a small malformation that is undetectable by angiography but demonstrable by pathological examination to be responsible for intracranial hemorrhage.

Treatment

The overall course of patients harboring an AVM is not benign. In addition to the effects of a major hemorrhage, neuronal damage from repeated minor hemorrhages or ischemia of adjacent brain from cerebral steal can result in progressive neurological deterioration. The yearly mortality is 1–2%. A surgical option is a consideration in all patients.

The decision to pursue treatment requires a comparison of the natural history of AVM and the risks of therapy for each individual. A hemorrhage from a small accessible AVM located in a noncritical area of the brain warrants intervention, whereas a large lesion with a complex blood supply located in a critical area that has never bled generates considerably more controversy. The management of large lesions, previously classified "unresectable," is by a regimen of preoperative embolization and staged resection. Radiosurgery has become an important tool for the treatment of some AVMs. The risks and benefits of the therapeutic options for patients with AVMs are better appreciated by direct comparison (Table 26.4).

SPINAL CORD VASCULAR DISEASE

Clinical Presentation and Course

Weakness, numbness, pain, and urinary complaints are common presenting symptoms of spinal cord ischemia. The weakness may progress gradually or be maximal at onset. Because of the vulnerability of the thoracic cord to flow-related ischemia, paraparesis is more common than quadriparesis. Numbness, accompanied by paresthesias, often parallels the weakness and occasionally precedes it. Back pain in a radicular distribution is common. Visceral referred pain can mistakenly suggest an intraabdominal process. Urinary dysfunction is typical, usually in the form of retention, but bladder and bowel incontinence may develop after the initial spinal shock resolves.

Table 26.4: Comparison of treatment modalities

Treatment Modality	Advantages	Disadvantages
Microsurgical excision	Immediate elimination of risk of hemorrhage	Risk of immediate new neurological deficit
Endovascular embolization	Immediate reduction in size of AVM; immediate closure of intranidal aneurysms; no general anesthesia; short hospitalization	Rarely achieves total and permanent obliteration of AVM; risk of immediate new neurological deficit from hemorrhage or ischemia
Stereotactic radiosurgery	Noninvasive treatment; short hospitalization	Latency of 13 yr with risk of hemorrhage until complete obliteration of AVM; risk of delayed neurological deficit from radiation damage

AVM = arteriovenous malformation.

Source: Adapted with permission from Steinberg, G. K. & Marks, M. P. 1997, "Intracranial arteriovenous malformation: Therapeutic options," in *Cerebrovascular Disease,* eds H. H. Batjer, L. R. Caplan, L. Friberg, Lippincott–Raven, Philadelphia.

Examination initially reveals flaccid paresis with diminished superficial (abdominal, cremasteric) and tendon reflexes below the level of ischemia. Spasticity and hyperreflexia, accompanied by extensor-plantar responses, usually evolve with ischemia above the lumbar segments. The rare posterior spinal artery syndrome is notable for preservation of strength and reflexes. Sensory loss is nearly universal in spinal cord ischemia. The cutaneous distribution of sensory loss and the modalities involved predict the lesion location.

The course of spinal ischemic syndromes is variable. TIAs of the cord may occur, with weakness and numbness lasting 15 minutes. Infarction of the spinal cord causes paresis within minutes of the initial symptoms or precipitating event. Pain is often persistent and is a major contributor to long-term disability in spinal cord vascular syndromes. Return of function depends on the degree of parenchymal damage. Unless significant motor recovery occurs in the first 24 hours, the likelihood of major improvement is low.

Investigations

MRI is the imaging procedure of choice. The pattern of signal changes and their time course are similar to those for cerebral infarction.

Treatment

The medical management of spinal cord ischemia is generally supportive and focused on reducing risk for recurrence. This includes maintenance of adequate blood pressure, early bed rest, and reversal of proximate causes such as hypovolemia or arrhythmias.

SPINAL VASCULAR MALFORMATIONS

Spinal vascular malformations consist of normal-sized to enlarged arteries and enlarged tortuous veins without an intervening capillary network. A commonly accepted classification system categorizes spinal vascular malformations into four types:

1. *Type I*: dural arteriovenous fistula (AVF); subtypes IA (single feeding artery) and IB (multiple feeding arteries)
2. *Type II*: intramedullary glomus-type AVM
3. *Type III*: intramedullary juvenile-type AVM is more extensive than a glomus-type AVM and often has an

extramedullary component and sometimes an extradural component

4. *Type IV*: intradural, extramedullary (perimedullary) AVF: subtypes IVA, IVB, and IVC correspond to lesions with progressively increased arteriovenous shunting manifested as increased number, size, and tortuosity of feeding arteries

Clinical Presentation and Course

The onset can be acute or insidious, and the course may include remissions and relapses. The most common complaints at onset are pain, weakness, and sensory symptoms. The predilection of spinal vascular malformations for the lower thoracic and lumbar regions results in complaints referable to those levels. The onset of symptoms is often associated with trauma, exercise, pregnancy, or menstruation. The interval between symptom onset and accurate diagnosis may be years. Severe locomotor disability develops in approximately 20% by 6 months after onset of symptoms and in 50% by 3 years. Once leg weakness or gait difficulties start, they tend to progress rapidly.

Investigations

MRI, with contrast-enhanced three-dimensional MRA, is the diagnostic procedure of choice in the initial evaluation of suspected spinal vascular malformations. MRI can discriminate extramedullary from intramedullary lesions, document thrombosis of the malformation following ligation or embolization of the feeding vessels, and demonstrate changes in the spinal cord (e.g., edema and hemorrhage) distinct from, yet caused by, the vascular malformation.

Treatment

The treatment of spinal vascular malformations is by surgical resection and/or angiographically directed embolization of the malformation. A sequential approach of embolization, followed by definitive surgical therapy, is common.

CENTRAL NERVOUS SYSTEM VASCULITIS

Isolated Vasculitis of the Central Nervous System

Clinical Features

The usual picture is one of progressive, cumulative, and multifocal neurological dysfunction. When isolated central nervous system (CNS) angiitis presents as a stroke, it is usually because of ICH, which occurs in approximately 15% of patients. The disease rarely causes cerebral infarcts or TIAs in the absence of clinical or laboratory evidence of a widespread CNS inflammatory disorder, such as a CSF pleocytosis. Nonfocal symptoms such as headache and confusion are the most common presenting features. Aside from confusion, the most common sign at presentation is hemiparesis. Ataxia of limbs or gait, focal cortical dysfunction including aphasia, and seizures are also common.

Laboratory Findings
General laboratory investigations are usually unremarkable. Sedimentation rate may be elevated, but usually not to the degree seen in temporal arteritis. The laboratory is of use only in eliminating systemic vasculitis, neoplasm, infection, or other diagnoses. Cerebral angiography is entirely normal in many pathologically documented cases, and the arteriographic changes of vasculitis, when seen, are not specific. The typical findings are widespread segmental changes in the contour and caliber of vessels. MRI lacks specificity.

Therapy
High-dose prednisone plus cyclophosphamide is the treatment of choice. Prednisone fails to control progression in most patients.

Central Nervous System Vasculitis Associated with Systemic Disorders

Cutaneous Herpes Zoster Infection
CNS vasculitis associated with herpes zoster usually presents as a severe hemispheric stroke in the weeks or months after an ipsilateral ophthalmic division infection in an elderly patient. Angiography shows ipsilateral segmental stenoses of proximal middle and anterior cerebral arteries. The efficacy of acyclovir and corticosteroids is unknown.

Intravenous Drug Abuse
The usual clinical feature is SAH or ICH following the use of intravenous or even oral methamphetamine. Whether the "vasculitis" reported in the angiograms of these patients is a true inflammatory process or a vasculopathy induced by an unusual reaction to the drug, hypertension, or other factors is unknown.

Lymphoma
Rare patients with systemic lymphoma, nearly always Hodgkin's disease, have an isolated CNS vasculitis in the absence of parenchymal or meningeal involvement by lymphoma.

For a more detailed discussion, see Chapters 57 and 57E in Neurology in Clinical Practice, 4th edition.

Cancer and the Nervous System | *27*

The number of newly diagnosed primary brain tumors continues to increase annually, with an estimated 39,455 patients diagnosed in 2002.

EPIDEMIOLOGY

Primary brain tumors are a diverse group of neoplasms arising from different cells of the central nervous system (CNS). Light microscopy is used to classify these tumors according to predominant cell type and to grade them for malignancy based on the presence or absence of standard pathological features. Gliomas are the most common brain tumors and may arise from astrocytes (astrocytomas), oligodendrocytes (oligodendrogliomas), or ependymal cells (ependymomas). Astrocytomas account for approximately 80% of all malignant brain tumors.

A slight male predominance exists in the incidence of malignant brain tumors. However, when all brain and CNS tumor types are examined, the disparity between the sexes is less apparent. The increasing incidence rate for brain tumors is confined mainly to the elderly population with no clear ethnic, gender, or geographical differences. Genetic syndromes account for approximately 1–5% of brain tumors.

PATHOLOGY AND MOLECULAR GENETICS OF NERVOUS SYSTEM TUMORS

Nervous system tumors, like other human neoplasms, are clonal proliferations that develop as a result of changes in key growth-regulatory genes. Such genes fall into several classes: (1) growth-promoting oncogenes, which are abnormally activated in tumors, (2) growth-checking tumor suppressor genes, which are inactivated in tumors, (3) cell death genes, which are impaired in tumors, and (4) DNA repair genes, which are improperly regulated in tumors. In combination, these genetic changes result in a powerful growth advantage that enables the cells to proliferate, evolve, and disseminate. Table 27.1 lists the common CNS tumors by location, age, and imaging characteristics.

CLINICAL FEATURES AND COMPLICATIONS OF BRAIN TUMORS

Primary and metastatic brain tumors may present with acute changes in neurological function, such as seizures or confusion, or with gradual and progressive changes in motor or sensory function, personality, or cognition. Headache is probably the most common initial symptom.

Clinical Features

Headache
Headaches are caused either by increased intracranial pressure (ICP) or by direct impingement or traction of pain-sensitive structures. Supratentorial tumors impinging on cranial nerve–innervated structures cause frontal headache, whereas posterior fossa tumors cause cervical pain from irritation of structures innervated by cranial nerves IX and X. About 20% of patients with brain tumors have headache at presentation and 60% develop headache later in the course. Increased severity in the morning with a tendency to improve by afternoon or evening is typical. A good response to simple analgesics is common and triptans may be effective.

Seizures
The incidence of seizures in brain tumor is 35%. Seizures often precede brain tumor diagnosis. Seizures may be focal at onset, reflecting the brain tumor location, or be secondarily generalized. Viscerosensory auras are common auras of temporal lobe onset. Frontal lobe seizures cause dizziness, a rising epigastric sensation, and fear, whereas occipital tumors cause visual auras.

Cognitive Dysfunction
Cognitive dysfunction is probably the most common problem in patients with brain tumors. Tumor location determines the specific clinical features. Frontal lobe tumors cause executive dysfunction. Left hemispheric tumors cause language

Table 27.1: Common CNS tumor diagnoses by location, age, and imaging characteristics

Location	Child/Young Adult	Older Adult
Cerebral/supratentorial	Ganglioglioma (TL, cyst-MEN) DNT (TL, intracortical nodules) PNET (solid, E) AT/RT (infant)	Grade II–III glioma (NE) GBM (ring E, butterfly) Metastases (gray–white junctions, E) Lymphoma (periventricular, E)
Cerebellar/infratentorial	Pilocytic astrocytoma (cyst-MEN) Medulloblastoma (vermis, E) Ependymoma (fourth v., E) Choroid plexus papilloma (fourth v.) AT/RT (infant)	Metastases (multiple, E) Hemangioblastoma (cyst-MEN) Choroid plexus papilloma (fourth v.)
Brainstem	"Brainstem glioma" (pons) Pilocytic astrocytoma (dorsal brainstem)	Gliomatosis cerebri (multifocal)
Spinal cord (intra-axial)	Ependymoma Pilocytic astrocytoma (cystic)	Ependymoma Diffuse astrocytoma (ill-defined) Paraganglioma (filum terminale)
Extra-axial/dural	Secondary lymphoma/leukemia	Meningioma Metastases Secondary lymphoma/leukemia
Intrasellar	Pituitary adenoma Craniopharyngioma Rathke's cleft cyst	Pituitary adenoma Rathke's cleft cyst

Continued

Table 27.1: (continued)

Location	Child/Young Adult	Older Adult
Suprasellar/hypothalamic/ optic pathway/third v.	Germinoma/germ cell tumor Craniopharyngioma Pilocytic Astrocytoma	Colloid cyst (third v.)
Pineal	Germinoma/germ cell tumor Pineocytoma Pineoblastoma Pineal cyst	Pineocytoma Pineal cyst
Thalamus	Pilocytic Astrocytoma AA/GBM	AA/GBM Lymphoma
Cerebellopontine angle	Vestibular schwannoma (NF2)	Vestibular schwannoma Meningioma
Lateral ventricle	Central neurocytoma SEGA (tuberous sclerosis) Choroid plexus papilloma Choroid plexus carcinoma (infant)	Central neurocytoma SEGA (tuberous sclerosis) Choroid plexus papilloma Subependymoma
Nerve root/paraspinal	Neurofibroma (NF1) MPNST (NF1)	Schwannoma Meningioma Secondary lymphoma Neurofibroma (NF1) MPNST

AA = anaplastic astrocytoma; AT/RT = atypical teratoid/rhabdoid tumor; DNT = dysembryoplastic neuroepithelial tumor; E, enhancing; GBM = glioblastoma; MPNST = malignant peripheral nerve sheath tumor; NE, nonenhancing; NF1 = neurofibromatosis type 1; NF2 = neurofibromatosis type 2; PNET = primitive neuroectodermal tumor; SEGA = subependymal giant cell astrocytoma; V, ventricle.

dysfunction and right hemisphere tumors cause problems with visual perception and scanning.

Nausea and Vomiting
Nausea and vomiting may result from increased ICP. Tumors of the posterior fossa have a direct effect on the emetic centers. The vomiting is then repetitive and intractable.

Endocrine Dysfunction
Hypothyroidism, decreased libido, and other symptoms of endocrine dysfunction may follow treatment of brain tumors or may be an initial feature. Tumors of the hypothalamic–pituitary axis may cause gonadotrophin and growth hormone deficiency, as well as hypopituitarism.

Visual Symptoms
Contralateral flashing lights may be due to seizures from an occipital lobe tumor, whereas loss of vision on one side may indicate a tumor in the parietal or temporal lobe. Diplopia usually indicates increased ICP. Transitory episodes of altered consciousness and visual disturbances caused by transitory elevations of ICP (plateau waves) are treatable with acetazolamide.

Investigations

Imaging
Magnetic resonance imaging (MRI) is the investigation of choice. Computed tomography (CT) is useful in excluding hemorrhage into an intracranial mass and in estimating mass effect. MRI provides better definition of brain tumor size, edema, mass effect, and midline shift, as well as evidence of herniation. It is also sensitive for leptomeningeal disease.

Evaluation for Primary Tumors in Suspected Metastases
Contrast CT scans of the neck, chest, abdomen, and pelvis are used to look for the primary cancer. Positron emission tomography (PET) increases the sensitivity for detection of primary tumors such as lung cancer and melanoma.

Brain Tumor–related Complications

Seizures
Surgical removal of the tumor improves seizure control. Both conventional and stereotactic radiation therapy (RT) may result in better seizure control. Seizure frequency may worsen during RT. Antiepileptic drugs may be subdivided into "conventional"

versus "new" and enzyme inducing versus non–enzyme inducing. The newer generation of antiepileptic drugs, such as gabapentin and levetiracetam, are preferred because they are not metabolized by the liver and have less potential for drug interactions.

Cerebral Edema

Both primary brain tumors and metastases usually induce vasogenic cerebral edema. This may result in headache, altered mental status, and neurological deterioration. When brain tumors cause obstructive hydrocephalus, increases in intraventricular pressure may result in transependymal spread of fluid into the periventricular interstitial space, or interstitial edema. Patients with vasogenic edema usually require hospitalization. Intravenous mannitol is often used to reduce ICP. The benefit of mannitol lasts on average 24–48 hours before a rebound increase in pressure occurs. Corticosteroids are the mainstay of treatment for vasogenic cerebral edema. The effect of corticosteroids is sustained, but long-term use is associated with several side effects. Very high doses of dexamethasone (30–36 mg daily in divided doses) are initiated, and the dose is tapered once clinical improvement is noted.

Venous Thrombosis

Deep venous thrombosis occurs in 36% of patients with malignant glioma. The initial feature is unilateral foot, calf, or thigh pain and/or swelling. Superficial venous distention, increased temperature, and erythema may be present. Corticosteroids may blunt symptoms, and local swelling and erythema at the site of thrombosis may be minimal. Anxiety may be the only initial manifestation of pulmonary thromboembolic disease. Venous Doppler studies of the leg are required when venous thrombosis is suspected. Ventilation-perfusion scans or CT angiograms should be ordered when Doppler study results are positive or when symptoms suggest pulmonary embolism. The most important aspect of management of this problem is prevention. Immediate anticoagulation with low-molecular-weight or fractionated heparin is indicated once deep venous thrombosis is confirmed. Oral anticoagulation is continued for at least 6 months. When pulmonary embolism occurs, treatment is continued indefinitely.

BRAIN TUMORS IN CHILDREN

Primary brain tumors are the most common solid tumors of childhood, representing 20% of all childhood cancers in the

United States. They are second only to leukemia in frequency among all childhood cancers. Approximately 85% of primary brain tumors in children 2–12 years of age are located in the posterior fossa. Most primary brain tumors are located in the supratentorial compartment in children younger than 2 years and older than 12 years. Seventy percent of primary brain tumors are gliomas and only 5% of CNS tumors arise from the spinal cord. No geographical or ethnic predominance exists.

The presentation usually involves changes in personality, nausea, vomiting, and morning headaches. Neurological deficits may not become evident until a month or two after the onset of symptoms. An accurate pathological diagnosis is critical for the management. Certain neoplasms have a benign course and good prognosis after gross total resection, despite a malignant appearance on MRI and pathology. Because of the potentially severe side effects of adjuvant radiation and chemotherapy, these modalities should be reserved for truly malignant tumors that carry a poor prognosis. The prognosis and management of pediatric brain tumors is determined by such factors as histopathology, extent of resection, age of the patient, and the presence or absence of metastases. Chemotherapy is assuming an increasingly important role in the management of many types of malignant tumors in children. In many cases, chemotherapy may improve survival and reduce the chances of neurotoxicity by delaying the need for RT in young children.

METASTATIC DISEASE

Brain Metastases

Parenchymal brain metastases are the most common direct neurological complication of systemic cancer. The incidence of brain metastases varies with the tumor type. Overall, lung cancer accounts for 40–50% of all patients with brain metastases, and breast cancer 15–20%. Melanoma, renal cell carcinoma, and gastrointestinal tract tumors each account for an additional 5–10% of cases. The frequency of metastases in various locations reflects the relative proportion of cerebral blood flow. Eighty percent arise in the supratentorial compartment. Pelvic and gastrointestinal tract primary tumors are more likely to metastasize to the posterior fossa than the supratentorial region. Brain metastases are the initial manifestation of an underlying primary tumor in 10–30% of cases.

Pathophysiology and Pathology
Parenchymal brain metastases generally arise from hematogenous spread, typically through the arterial circulation. Tumor emboli, like all emboli, tend to lodge at the gray–white junction because the caliber of blood vessels narrows at this site. The histopathology of brain metastases usually closely resembles that of the underlying systemic tumor. Metastases from certain primary tumors (melanoma, choriocarcinoma, and renal cell carcinoma) have a tendency for intratumoral hemorrhage.

Clinical Presentations
Symptoms of brain metastases may arise 20 years after discovery of the primary tumor or may antedate discovery of the underlying systemic cancer. The presenting features are usually progressive over days to weeks, although occasional patients present with seizures or intratumoral hemorrhage. Half of all patients complain of headache, and one third have mental status changes. Headache in the absence of other symptoms is more likely to be due to multiple metastases than a single metastasis. Seizures are present at diagnosis in 18% of patients with brain metastases. Mental status changes and hemiparesis are each present in about 60% of patients. Despite the frequent occurrence of increased ICP, papilledema is detected in only 10% of patients.

Neuroradiology
Non–contrast-enhanced MRI is as sensitive as contrast-enhanced CT scan for detection of brain metastases. Metastases larger than 1 cm in diameter almost always produce an abnormality on T2-weighted images, whereas those smaller than 0.5 cm rarely do.

Management
Corticosteroids improve symptoms associated with brain metastases in two thirds of patients. Their use improves median survival in otherwise untreated patients from 1 to 2 months. Seizures are the initial feature in 10–20% of patients with brain metastases and respond to anticonvulsant drugs. However, the prophylactic use of anticonvulsant drugs in patients who have not had a seizure is not warranted.

The goals of RT are to alleviate neurological deficits attributable to tumor and to shrink the tumor(s) and prolong survival. Three fourths of patients undergoing RT experience symptom palliation, and two thirds maintain improvement. Whole-brain RT is tolerated well. Patients should expect temporary alopecia and fatigue. Headache and nausea occasionally occur but are generally alleviated with corticosteroids and antiemetics. However, up to 30% of long-term survivors develop cognitive impairment by 1 year. Surgical intervention in patients with accessible single brain metastases has become the standard of care. Metastases from highly radioresistant tumors like melanoma and renal cell carcinoma, which respond very poorly to fractionated radiotherapy, respond virtually as well to stereotactic radiosurgery.

Spinal Cord Metastases

Epidural spinal cord compression (ESCC) refers to compression of the spinal cord or cauda equina from a neoplastic lesion outside the spinal dura. Breast, lung, and prostate cancer each account for about 20%, whereas renal cell carcinoma, non-Hodgkin's lymphoma, and multiple myeloma typically account for 5–10% each. Ewing's sarcoma and neuroblastoma are particularly common causes in children.

Clinical Presentations

Back pain is usually the first symptom of ESCC. The pain usually precedes the development of neurological symptoms by approximately 2 months. Motor involvement is present in 80% of patients. Once weakness is present, progression is often rapid, and diagnostic workup and therapy must proceed expeditiously. Pretreatment neurological function is a major predictor of posttreatment outcome. Currently, about 50% of patients with ESCC are ambulatory, 35% are paraparetic, and 15% are paraplegic at diagnosis. Weakness is typically bilateral and symmetrical; the iliopsoas muscles may be disproportionately affected. Sensory loss is detectable in about three fourths of patients at diagnosis. Bowel and bladder dysfunction are evident in most patients with ESCC.

Neuroradiology of Epidural Spinal Cord Compression

The availability of MRI has revolutionized the definitive diagnosis of ESCC. MRI produces excellent images of the spinal cord, thecal sac, and bony spine, demonstrating metastases in each of these areas when they are present.

Definitive Therapy

Corticosteroids are routinely used in patients with ESCC. Radiotherapy is the treatment of choice for most patients with ESCC. In general, almost all patients who are ambulatory at the onset of radiotherapy will remain ambulatory at its conclusion. Among patients who are paraparetic and unable to walk, one third will regain ambulation. Only 2–6% of patients regain the ability to walk when treatment is delayed until after the patient is paraplegic. Median survival following ESCC is approximately 6 months but is better in patients who remain ambulatory. Locally recurrent ESCC occurs in one half of 2-year survivors. Chemotherapy is a rational means of treating ESCC when the causative tumor is chemosensitive. Most common solid tumor causes of ESCC are not chemosensitive.

Intramedullary Spinal Cord Metastasis
Metastases are capable of spreading to the substance of the spinal cord, either by hematogenous spread or secondary to leptomeningeal invasion and subsequent centripetal growth. Most patients with this complication have either concomitant or prior brain metastases. Treatment generally consists of corticosteroids and fractionated radiotherapy, which usually stabilize neurological function for several months.

Leptomeningeal Metastases

Involvement of the leptomeninges by tumor is an increasingly common problem in patients with cancer and leads to significant morbidity and mortality. Factors that have contributed to the increased incidence are a greater awareness of the condition among oncologists, improved diagnostic tests, and longer survival among patients with systemic malignancies. Longer survival of patients with systemic cancers results in a higher incidence of CNS metastases.

Tumor cells usually reach the leptomeninges by direct extension from pre-existing tumor in the brain parenchyma or epidural space or by hematogenous spread.

Clinical Features
Leptomeningeal metastases (LM) is usually a late complication of systemic cancer, occurring 6 months to 3 years after the diagnosis of the primary tumor. It usually occurs in the setting of active disease outside the nervous system, although as systemic therapy improves increasing numbers of patients are developing LM as the sole site of relapsed disease. In 5% of patients, meningeal involvement is the initial presentation of a neoplasm. Cerebral symptoms occur in up to 50% of patients. Thirty percent of patients have cranial nerve symptoms and 50% will have cranial nerve signs. Approximately 60% of patients have spinal symptoms, especially in the lumbosacral region, as a result of involvement of nerve roots. The most common symptoms are pain, weakness, and paresthesias.

Diagnosis
Examination of the cerebral spinal fluid (CSF) is the most important test for the diagnosis of LM. The finding of malignant cells in the CSF is the definitive diagnosis. The opening pressure

is elevated in half of patients, the CSF protein is elevated in most, and low CSF glucose (hypoglycorrhachia) is present in 30%. MRI is the most sensitive neuroimaging test for detecting LM.

Treatment

The goal of therapy is to improve or stabilize the patient's neurological status and prolong survival. The specific treatment depends on the tumor type, site of leptomeningeal tumor, and the clinical condition of the patient. Without treatment, the median survival of patients with LM is 4–6 weeks. The patients who benefit most from treatment are those with minimal neurological deficits, good performance status, and slowly progressive systemic disease with little or no systemic metastases. RT is limited to symptomatic areas and sites of bulky disease. The administration of chemotherapy for LM is directly into the CSF, using an intraventricular cannula with a subcutaneous reservoir under the scalp (Ommaya or Rickham reservoirs). Only a limited number of chemotherapeutic agents are available for intrathecal administration. Methotrexate is the most widely used drug.

Prognosis

Without treatment, patients with LM usually survive only 1–2 months, with occasional long-term survival. With treatment, the median survival increases to 3–6 months.

Skull Metastases

Skull metastases occur in 15–25% of all patients with cancer, usually in the setting of bony metastases elsewhere in the body. At least half are asymptomatic. Skull metastases usually arise from hematogenous spread via either the arterial circulation or Batson's plexus. The most common primary tumors that metastasize to the skull base and calvaria are breast, lung, and prostate, followed by renal, thyroid, and melanoma. Calvarial metastases are often asymptomatic. Contrast-enhanced MRI is the most useful diagnostic test. Asymptomatic metastases often require no specific therapy. Symptomatic lesions respond well to RT. The prognosis of skull metastases depends on systemic tumor control and local factors, including invasion of venous sinus or dura, leptomeninges, and brain parenchyma. In general, better outcomes are associated with starting treatment less than 1 month after diagnosis.

Dural Metastases

Dural metastases occur in up to 20% of patients in autopsy studies, but symptomatic lesions are much less common. The most common tumors giving rise to dural metastases are non–small cell lung, prostate, and breast cancer. Dural metastases cause symptoms by compressing or invading the underlying brain, by obstructing adjacent venous sinuses, or by producing subdural fluid collections and hematomas. MRI usually establishes the diagnosis. Patients usually respond to treatment with RT. The prognosis for patients with dural metastases is slightly better than for parenchymal metastases (median survival of 24 weeks versus 18 weeks).

Plexus Metastases

Brachial Plexopathy
Invasion of the brachial plexus is by local spread of tumor from lung or breast carcinoma or axillary lymph nodes. Rarely, tumor may reach the brachial plexus by hematogenous or lymphatic spread. The lower trunk of the brachial plexus is usually involved. Most patients experience constant severe pain radiating from the shoulder down the medial aspect of the arm into the fourth and fifth digits. Numbness and paresthesias may be associated. CT or MRI of the brachial plexus usually establishes the diagnosis. The treatment is RT. Approximately half of patients experience improvement in pain, but neither strength nor sensory symptoms improve.

Lumbosacral Plexopathy
Lumbosacral plexopathy usually results from direct extension of tumor or from metastases to local lymph nodes or bone. The most common tumors associated with lumbosacral plexopathy are colorectal cancer, lymphoma, cervical carcinoma, and sarcomas. The initial features are pain, numbness, paresthesias, weakness, and edema of the leg. Impotence and incontinence may occur. Examination findings may include weakness, sensory loss, reflex asymmetry, leg edema, and rarely a pelvic mass on rectal examination. Bilateral lumbosacral plexopathies occur in 25% of patients; the usual cause is metastatic breast cancer. Treatment of neoplastic lumbosacral plexopathy involves RT and, occasionally, surgery.

Peripheral Nerve Metastases

Very rarely, mononeuropathies, mononeuropathy multiplex, and even a symmetrical polyneuropathy may result from direct nerve infiltration by tumor. Lymphomas and leukemias, particularly chronic lymphocytic leukemia, have been associated with peripheral neuropathy due to malignant infiltration of nerve.

PARANEOPLASTIC DISORDERS

Paraneoplastic neurological syndromes (PNS) are a heterogeneous group of disorders caused by cancers not located in the CNS. Their mechanism is other than metastases or any of the other complications of cancer or its treatment. Paraneoplastic disorders may affect any part of the nervous system (Table 27.2) and their frequency varies according to the type of syndrome and cancer. In general, they are difficult to diagnose and treat. The onset of symptoms may occur before the presence of systemic cancer is known, making diagnosis all the more difficult. The onset of neurological features is often acute or subacute, followed by stabilization within a few weeks. This time course suggests that by the time of diagnosis, the pathological damage is already irreversible. For all PNS, treatment of the tumor is the

Table 27.2: Paraneoplastic neurological syndromes

Syndromes affecting the central nervous system
    Cerebellar degeneration
    Encephalomyelitis
    Opsoclonus-myoclonus
    Stiff-person syndrome
    Necrotizing myelopathy
    Motor neuron syndromes (amyotrophic lateral sclerosis, subacute motor neuronopathy, upper motor neuron dysfunction)
Syndromes affecting the visual system
    Retinopathy
    Optic neuritis
    Uveitis (usually in association with encephalomyelitis)
Syndromes affecting the peripheral nervous system
    Sensory neuronopathy
    Vasculitis of the nerve and muscle
    Subacute or chronic sensorimotor peripheral neuropathy
    Sensorimotor neuropathies associated with plasma cell dyscrasias and B-cell lymphoma
    Autonomic neuropathy
    Brachial neuritis
    Acute polyradiculoneuropathy (Guillain-Barré syndrome)
    Peripheral nerve hyperexcitability
Syndromes affecting the neuromuscular junction and muscle
    Lambert-Eaton myasthenic syndrome
    Myasthenia gravis
    Dermatomyositis
    Acute necrotizing myopathy
    Carcinoid myopathy
    Cachectic myopathy

Table 27.3: Paraneoplastic antineuronal antibodies, associated syndromes, and cancers

Antibody	Syndrome	Associated Cancers
Anti-Hu	Focal encephalitis, PEM, PCD, PSN, autonomic dysfunction	SCLC, other
Anti-Yo	PCD	Gynecological, breast
Anti-Ri	PCD, opsoclonus-myoclonus	Breast, gynecological, SCLC
Anti-Tr	PCD	Hodgkin's lymphoma
Anti-CV2/CRMP5	PEM, PCD, peripheral neuropathy	SCLC, other
Anti-Ma proteins*	Limbic, brainstem encephalitis, PCD	Germ cell tumors of testis, other solid tumors
Anti-amphiphysin	Stiff-person syndrome, PEM	Breast
Anti-VGCC†	LEMS	SCLC
Anti-AChR†	MG	Thymoma
Anti-VGKC†	PNH	Thymoma, others
Anti-recoverin‡	Retinopathy	SCLC
Anti-bipolar cells of the retina	Retinopathy	Melanoma

*Patients with antibodies to Ma2 are usually men with testicular cancer. Patients with additional antibodies to other Ma proteins are men or women with a variety of solid tumors.

†These antibodies can occur with or without a cancer association.

‡Other antibodies reported in a few or isolated cases include antibodies to tubby-like protein and the photoreceptor-specific nuclear receptor.

most effective step in controlling or at least stabilizing the neurological disorder.

Pathogenesis

Most paraneoplastic disorders are immune mediated. The expression of neuronal proteins by a tumor provokes an immune response against both the tumor and the nervous system. This hypothesis is supported by the frequent detection in the serum and CSF of antibodies reacting with antigens expressed by the tumor and nervous system (onconeuronal antigens) (Table 27.3). Most antibodies associated with PNS of the CNS are considered highly specific for the presence of cancer. In contrast, antibodies associated with some paraneoplastic disorders of the neuromuscular junction and peripheral nerves (i.e., Lambert-Eaton syndrome) may occur with or without cancer.

General Diagnostic Approach

The specificity of paraneoplastic antineuronal antibodies for some types of cancer makes them useful diagnostic tools (see Table 27.3). In approximately 60% of patients, the neurological symptoms precede the tumor diagnosis. Therefore in the right clinical context the detection of a paraneoplastic antibody in the serum or CSF focuses the search for the neoplasm. Clinical experience suggests that finding high titers of paraneoplastic antibodies in the CSF is confirmatory evidence of the paraneoplastic disease.

For a more detailed discussion, see Chapters 58A, 58B, 58C, 58E, 58F, 58G, and 58H in Neurology in Clinical Practice, 4th edition.

Infections of the Nervous System | 28

BACTERIAL INFECTIONS

Bacterial Meningitis

Bacterial meningitis is an inflammatory response to bacterial infection of the pia arachnoid and cerebrospinal fluid (CSF) of the subarachnoid space. Acute bacterial meningitis occurs throughout the world. In the United States, the incidence of bacterial meningitis is between 3 and 5 per 100,000 people per year. Worldwide, three main pathogens *Haemophilus influenzae*, *Streptococcus pneumoniae*, and *Neisseria meningitidis* account for 75–80% of cases after the neonatal period. *Escherichia coli* and other enteric bacilli, *Listeria monocytogenes*, and group A streptococci are major pathogens in neonatal meningitis.

Clinical Features
Headache, fever, and neck stiffness, often with signs of cerebral dysfunction, make up the clinical presentation of adults with bacterial meningitis. Nausea, vomiting, myalgia, and photophobia are also common. Confusion, delirium, and a declining level of consciousness are the main cerebral symptoms. Seizures occur in approximately 40% of patients. Focal neurological deficits, seizure activity, and encephalopathy may arise from cortical and subcortical ischemia and/or infarction, from increased intracranial pressure (ICP), or from development of subdural empyema. The typical features are typically absent in neonates; high-pitched crying, refusal to feed, irritability, and listlessness may be the only clinical clues.

Diagnosis
The patient with suspected bacterial meningitis requires blood cultures and urgent lumbar puncture (LP). Cranial computed tomography (CT) before LP is indicated when focal findings or clinical evidence of raised ICP is present. CSF examination reveals elevated pressure (200–500 mm H_2O) and protein

(100–500 mg/dl), decreased glucose, and marked pleocytosis (100–10,000 white blood cells [WBCs]/µl) with 60% or greater polymorphonuclear leukocytes.

Treatment
Antibiotic selection depends on the clinical setting in conjunction with allergies, local resistance patterns, and CSF results. Table 28.1 outlines initial empirical therapy. Ampicillin or penicillin G and a third-generation cephalosporin are typical first-line agents. Table 28.2 summarizes current antimicrobial recommendations for bacterial meningitis caused by specific bacterial pathogens. Optimal duration of therapy for bacterial meningitis is not established. The available evidence on adjunctive dexamethasone therapy confirms benefit for *H. influenzae* type b meningitis in reducing audiological sequelae and suggests benefit in reducing audiological and neurological sequelae in pneumococcal meningitis in children.

Brain Abscess

Pathogenesis
A brain abscess consists of suppurative necrosis of the brain parenchyma. Brain abscesses usually develop by spread from a contiguous infected cranial site, such as ear, sinus, or teeth. Hematogenous spread from a remote source is often in the setting of congenital heart disease with right-to-left shunt or pulmonary disorders such as lung abscess, bronchiectasis, or arteriovenous fistula. Metastatic or bloodborne abscesses are usually found at the gray–white matter junction, in the distribution of the middle cerebral artery, and are often multiple.

Clinical Features
Patients with brain abscess present with clinical features of an expanding mass lesion, progressive headache, altered mentation, seizures, or focal deficit. One half develop nausea and vomiting and only one half have fever. Acute worsening of headache and nuchal pain, together with an increase in temperature, can signify rupture of the abscess into the subarachnoid space, a serious event.

Diagnosis
Neuroimaging studies reveal one or more ring-enhancing masses with slight surrounding edema. The ring of enhancement may be thicker near the cortex and thinner near the ventricle. An early lesion in the cerebritis stage appears as a nonenhancing, focal, low-density area on CT or hypointensity on magnetic resonance imaging (MRI) scans. Peripheral leukocytosis may be mild or

Text continued on p. 243.

Table 28.1: Empiric antibiotic therapy of bacterial meningitis

Age of Patient	Likely Organism	Antimicrobial Therapy*	Adverse Effects
0–12 weeks	Group B Streptococcus E. coli L. monocytogenes	Third-generation cephalosporin + ampicillin (+ dexamethasone first 2 days in >4-week-old infant)	Vomiting, diarrhea, maculopapular rash, eosinophilia, biliary pseudolithiasis
3 months–50 years	S. pneumoniae N. meningitidis H. influenzae	Third-generation cephalosporin + vancomycin (± ampicillin)	Nausea, vomiting, diarrhea, maculopapular rash, eosinophilia, biliary pseudolithiasis, leukopenia, "red man"† syndrome
>50 years	S. pneumoniae L. monocytogenes Gram-negative bacilli	Third-generation cephalosporin + vancomycin + ampicillin	Nausea, vomiting, diarrhea, maculopapular rash, eosinophilia, biliary pseudolithiasis, transient increase in liver enzymes, leukopenia, "red man" syndrome
Base of skull fracture	Staphylococci Gram-negative bacilli S. pneumoniae	Third-generation cephalosporin + vancomycin	Nausea, vomiting, diarrhea, eosinophilia, biliary pseudolithiasis, leukopenia, "red man" syndrome

Continued

Table 28.1: (continued)

Age of Patient	Likely Organism	Antimicrobial Therapy*	Adverse Effects
Head trauma, neurosurgery, CSF shunt	Staphylococci Gram-negative bacilli S. pneumoniae	Vancomycin + ceftazidime	Nausea, vomiting, diarrhea, transient increase in liver enzymes, leukopenia, "red man" syndrome
Immunocompromised state	L. monocytogenes Gram-negative bacilli S. pneumoniae H. influenzae	Vancomycin + ampicillin + ceftazidime	Nausea, vomiting, diarrhea, maculopapular rash, eosinophilia, biliary pseudolithiasis, transient increase in liver enzymes, leukopenia, "red man" syndrome

*For all age groups from 3 months onward, an alternative treatment is meropenem + vancomycin. In case of severe penicillin allergy, consider vancomycin + chloramphenicol for meningococcus and trimethoprim/sulfamethoxazole for listeria. A higher failure rate has been reported with chloramphenicol or regimen without vancomycin in meningitis with drug-resistant pneumococcus.

†"Red man" syndrome ranges from mild flushing of upper body and erythema, reported in up to 70%, which may rarely extend to pruritic rash, high fever, and exfoliative dermatitis. Caused by hypersensitivity reaction to vancomycin and related antibiotics.

Table 28.2: Antibiotic treatment for bacterial meningitis*

Antibiotic	Bactericidal/ Bacteristatic	Therapeutic to Toxic Ratio	Cerebrospinal Fluid Penetration	Organism	Intravenous Dose (Adult)	Remarks
Penicillins						
Penicillin G	Cell wall damaged; bactericidal	Wide, except in renal failure and the elderly	3+	N. meningitidis, some S. pneumoniae, group B Streptococcus	24 million U/day (q4h)	Some S. pneumoniae and N. meningitidis may be resistant
Ampicillin	Bactericidal	Wide	3+	As for penicillin G + some H. influenzae, L. monocytogenes, 60–70% E. coli	12 g/day (q4h)	Inactivated by β-lactamase†
Extended- spectrum penicillins	Bactericidal	Wide	3+	As for ampicillin + P. aeruginosa, K. pneumoniae, indole positive Proteus, Serratia	Carbenicillin, 18–30 g/day (q4h); ticarcillin, 12–20 g/day (q4h); azlocillin, piperacillin, and mezlocillin, 10–15 g/day (q4h)	Used in combination with an aminoglycoside; β-lactamase sensitive†
Antistaphy- lococcal penicillins	Bactericidal	Wide	2+	S. aureus, S. epidermidis	Methicillin, nafcillin, and oxacillin, 8–12 g/day (q4h)	Except methicillin- resistant strains
Vancomycin	Bactericidal	Narrow	3+	S. aureus including methicillin-resistant strains, S. epidermidis, penicillin-resistant pneumococci, enterococci, diphtheroids, and F. meningosepticum	3 g/day (q6h)	Ototoxic, nephrotoxic effects additive with aminoglycoside; can be used in penicillin allergy

Continued

Table 28.2: (continued)

Antibiotic	Bactericidal/ Bacteristatic	Therapeutic to Toxic Ratio	Cerebrospinal Fluid Penetration	Organism	Intravenous Dose (Adult)	Remarks
Third-generation cephalosporins	Bactericidal	Wide	3+	Broad-spectrum; some gram-positive and especially gram-negative E. coli, Klebsiella, Proteus, Serratia, N. meningitidis, H. influenzae (including β-lactamase-secreting strains)	Cefotaxime, 8–12 g/day (q4h); Ceftriaxone, 4 g/day (q12h); Ceftazidime, 8 g/day (q6h)	Inactive against enterococci, many penicillin-resistant pneumococci, L. monocytogenes, Clostridium difficile†; Ceftazidime, not cefotaxime/ceftriaxone, active against Pseudomonas
Chloramphenicol	Bacteristatic; bactericidal in therapeutic concentrations against Haemophilus, S. pneumoniae, and meningococcus	Narrow; peak serum levels should be maintained between 15 and 25 mg/liter	4+	H. influenzae, S. pneumoniae, N. meningitidis	4 g/day (q6h) PO administration> IV provided no vomiting	H. influenzae resistance occurs; drug superseded by third-generation cephalosporins in developed countries§
Aminoglycosides	Bactericidal but not uniformly so because of acidic pH and low CSF levels	Narrow	1+; consider intrathecal or intraventricular administration	Gram-negative enteric organisms, P. aeruginosa	Netilmicin, tobramycin, and gentamicin, 200 mg/day (q8h) Kanamycin, amikacin, 1 g/day (q8h)	Dose-related vestibular, hearing, and renal toxicity‖

Trimethoprim-sulfamethoxazole	Bacteriostatic or bactericidal	Narrow	4+	Broad-spectrum *S. pneumoniae, H. influenzae,* meningococcus, gram-negatives, *Staphylococcus, L. monocytogenes, Nocardia*	Trimethoprim, 1.2 g/day sulfamethoxazole, 6 g/day (q12h) (trimethoprim 15 mg/kg/day PO q12h)	Not widely used (cause of kernicterus in newborns)
Metronidazole	Bactericidal	Narrow	4+	Anaerobes	1.5 g/day (q8h)	With large doses, prolonged therapy causes seizures, peripheral neuropathy
Rifampin	Bactericidal	Narrow	4+	Prophylaxis for meningococcus and *H. influenzae;* given with vancomycin for resistant *Staphylococcus* and *F. meningosepticum*	600 mg/day PO	Avoid widespread use in areas where tuberculosis is endemic, as it produces resistant strains
Fluoroquinolones	Bactericidal	Narrow	Ciprofloxacin 1+; Ofloxacin 2+; Pefloxacin 3+	Gram-negative including *P. aeruginosa* and *Staphylococcus;* use selectively for multidrug-resistant gram negative bacteria and *M. tuberculosis;* prophylaxis for meningococcus	Ciprofloxacin, 1.5 g/day (q12h) Pefloxacin and ofloxacin, 800 mg/day (q12h)	Not in prepubertal children or pregnant women; neuropsychiatric side effects; lowers seizure threshold; raises theophylline level

Continued

Table 28.2: (continued)

Antibiotic	Bactericidal/ Bacteriostatic	Therapeutic to Toxic Ratio	Cerebrospinal Fluid Penetration	Organism	Intravenous Dose (Adult)	Remarks
Unique β-lactams	Bactericidal	Narrow	2+, 3+	Broad-spectrum most gram-positive and gram-negative nosocomial *Fonterobacter* and *Acinetobacter*, polymicrobial bacteremia	Imipenem, 2 g/day (6qh)	Except methicillin-resistant *S. aureus*, enterococcus; not often used in meningitis¶ if alternative exists

4+ = excellent; 3+ = very good; 2+ = good; 1+ = poor; CSF = cerebrospinal fluid.

*Readers should check the product information sheet included in the package of each drug and follow those instructions.

†β-Lactamase inhibitors (e.g., clavulanate or sulbactam) may be used with ampicillin, amoxicillin, or ticarcillin to inhibit β-lactamases. They are not always effective.

‡Ceftriaxone can be administered once a day if necessary. It is eliminated by kidneys and liver, and impaired function of either organ does not lead to excess drug accumulation. Ceftazidime is especially effective against *Pseudomonas* species. As single agents, ceftriaxone and cefotaxime are the most frequently used in childhood meningitis. Avoid ceftriaxone in babies younger than 3 months because it displaces bilirubin.

§Avoid in newborns ("gray baby syndrome"). Serum levels should be monitored. Levels >40 mg/L are toxic. Levels >25 mg/L can give dose-related reversible marrow suppression. Idiosyncratic irreversible marrow aplasia (1:30,000 patients) is the most feared complication.

¶Also causes neuromuscular blockade—caution in myasthenia gravis, respiratory failure, and postoperatively when curare has been used.

‖CNS toxicity includes seizures (2–8% of patients).

absent and is not a reliable diagnostic aid. The risk of herniation or precipitating rupture precludes the use of LP.

Treatment
Successful treatment of brain abscess requires antibiotics in all patients and surgery in many. Current recommendations for empirical therapy, based on location of abscess and inferred source of infection, are metronidazole with either penicillin or a third-generation cephalosporin for frontal abscesses; penicillin, metronidazole, and ceftazidime for temporal or cerebellar abscesses; nafcillin, metronidazole, and cefotaxime for multiple (metastatic) abscesses; nafcillin and cefotaxime for penetrating wounds; and vancomycin and ceftazidime for postoperative abscesses. Intravenous treatment must continue for 6–8 weeks followed by oral therapy for 2–3 months. Surgical excision may shorten the course of intravenous therapy by 1 or 2 weeks. Adjunctive medical therapy for medical or surgical cases includes corticosteroids for mass effect, hyperosmolar agents for worsening cerebral edema and raised ICP, and prophylactic or symptomatic anticonvulsants.

Subdural Empyema

Subdural empyema is a collection of pus between the dura and arachnoid. It is usually a consequence of ear or sinus infection.

Clinical Features
The typical features are headache, fever, stiff neck, seizures, focal neurological symptoms and signs, and rapid deterioration. Consider the diagnosis in patients with meningeal signs and deficits indicating extensive unilateral hemispheric dysfunction or in patients with sinusitis who develop meningeal signs. Children younger than 5 years may develop subdural empyemas after *H. influenzae* or gram-negative bacterial meningitis. The clinical features are irritability, poor feeding, and increasing head circumference.

Diagnosis
Subdural empyema and bacterial brain abscess share many aspects of diagnosis and management. Bacterial pathogens for both disorders are similar, although subdural empyemas are less often mixed. Neuroimaging studies help establish the diagnosis but may underestimate the size of the empyema. In infants, subdural taps establish the diagnosis.

Treatment
Combined medical and surgical management should proceed emergently. Untreated subdural empyemas are uniformly fatal.

Burr holes work well for early cases, but pus may reaccumulate. Craniotomy is required in posterior fossa cases or if cranial osteomyelitis coexists. Overall, mortality is 14–18%.

Cranial Epidural Abscess

Cranial epidural abscess, an infection in the space between the dura and skull, begins as cranial osteomyelitis complicating ear, sinus, or orbital infection, as well as nasopharyngeal malignancy. Diagnosis, urgent management, and prognosis are similar to those for subdural empyema.

SEPTIC VENOUS SINUS THROMBOSIS

Septic thrombosis of cerebral veins or venous sinuses may complicate meningitis or epidural or subdural abscesses, or it may develop during the intracranial spread of infection from extracranial veins. Once established, infection and clot spread through the venous system, aided by the absence of valves in intracranial veins. Specific presenting features vary with the site involved and include headache, altered mentation, seizures, cranial neuropathies, fluctuating focal deficits, non–arterial-distribution strokes, and increased ICP. CT scan or MRI demonstrates the primary infection or clot within the sinus. Treatment against the primary infection is required.

Spinal Epidural Abscess

Infection develops in the epidural space by direct extension of vertebral osteomyelitis or soft tissue infections (retroperitoneal, mediastinal, perinephric, psoas, or paraspinal abscess), following penetrating trauma or decubitus ulcers, or by hematogenous spread from skin or parenteral drug use. Localized back pain and radicular pain are common early symptoms, frequently over-shadowed by rapid evolution of paraparesis or quadriparesis. Once diagnosed by MRI or myelography, urgent surgical decompression and antibiotic therapy are required.

MYCOBACTERIAL DISEASES

Tuberculosis

Although tuberculosis (TB) commonly involves the lungs, it can produce disease in nearly every organ system. Neurological disease such as tuberculous meningitis, tuberculoma, or tuber-culous involvement of the spine with myelopathy complicates

1% of TB infections. Human immunodeficiency virus (HIV) infection has been associated with increasing numbers of new cases and with a higher risk of extrapulmonary TB.

Pathogenesis

Neurological TB may develop during primary infection or reactivate because of immunosuppression. Tubercle bacilli spread hematogenously from the lung or other organs, form tubercles in the brain parenchyma, and at a later stage rupture into the subarachnoid or ventricular space.

Clinical Syndromes

TUBERCULOSIS MENINGITIS Untreated TB meningitis (TBM) is always fatal. TBM typically follows a subacute course with low-grade fever, headache, and intermittent nausea and vomiting, followed by more severe headache and fever, neck stiffness, drowsiness, and cranial nerve palsies. The characteristic features of more intense disease are meningismus, seizures, focal neurological deficits, and signs of increased ICP. Identifying tubercle bacilli on CSF acid-fast bacilli (AFB) smear or culture establishes the diagnosis. CSF culture results are positive for *M. tuberculosis* in 45–70% of patients but may take 6–8 weeks to become positive. A presumptive diagnosis based on clinical criteria is sufficient to start empirical anti-TB therapy. CSF examination demonstrates normal or elevated opening pressure, elevated protein (80–400 mg/dl), low glucose (<40 mg/dl), and pleocytosis (averaging 200–400 WBCs/µl) with lymphocytic predominance. Polymerase chain reaction (PCR) techniques have sensitivities of 70–75% and are now routinely available for the diagnosis of TBM, with reported sensitivities of 70–75%.

TUBERCULOMAS Tuberculomas, the parenchymal form of TB, occur as single or multiple brain or spinal cord lesions and present with signs and symptoms of space-occupying lesions. On CT or MRI scan, the lesions may be of low or high intensity, with ring enhancement. Multiple small (1–2 mm) lesions characterize miliary disease. In regions where TB is prevalent, histological confirmation is not required to initiate anti-TB therapy.

SPINAL TUBERCULOSIS The midthorax is the most common site of spinal involvement. Back pain is the chief complaint and examination shows paraspinal muscle spasm or angling of the spine caused by collapse of a vertebra (gibbus). MRI is the best imaging technique. A recommended regimen for initial treatment is with isoniazid (INH) 10 mg/kg per day, rifampin (RIF) 10 mg/kg per day, pyrazinamide 35 mg/kg per day, and ethambutol 25 mg/kg per day or streptomycin (SM) 10 mg/kg per day. After

2 months, if clinical improvement is satisfactory, further treatment uses a simplified protocol of two drugs, INH and RIF, for an additional 10 months. In areas with high prevalence of drug-resistant disease and HIV infection, treatment begins with five to seven drugs until drug susceptibility is established.

Concurrent use of oral pyridoxine (25–50 mg/day) with INH prevents neuropathy. Monthly hearing evaluations are necessary and SM discontinued at first sign of vestibular toxicity. Regular measures of liver enzyme concentrations are required because of potential INH, RIF, and pyrazinamide hepatotoxicity. Continue treatment despite elevated liver enzyme concentrations in the absence of clinical signs of liver toxicity. The following are indications for the use of corticosteroid therapy: (1) increased ICP, (2) complicated meningitis with hydrocephalus, vasculitis, or arachnoiditis, (3) very high CSF protein with impending spinal block, (4) tuberculoma with surrounding edema, (5) ocular lesions, (6) replacement therapy for adrenal insufficiency, and (7) severely debilitated patients with drug-sensitive strains.

During treatment, CSF is re-examined to monitor treatment efficacy. Repeated neuroimaging studies 2–3 months after the start of treatment and again at 3–6 month intervals verify improvement. Tuberculoma requires 2 years of treatment. Chemotherapy alone is effective treatment for most spinal TB without cord involvement.

Complications
Complications of untreated, late, or incompletely treated central nervous system (CNS) TB include progressive hydrocephalus, which may require shunting, blindness caused by damage to the optic nerves and chiasm in the suprasellar cistern, the syndrome of inappropriate secretion of antidiuretic hormone, tuberculoma-associated edema, vasculitis, stroke, arachnoiditis, spinal cord atrophy, and syringomyelia.

Prevention
Vaccination is by intracutaneous injection of bacille Calmette-Guérin (BCG) vaccine. Variation in protection varies from 6–77% but appears to prevent meningitis in children in developed countries.

Leprosy (Hansen's Disease)

Leprosy, caused by *Mycobacterium leprae*, mainly infects the peripheral nerve and skin. It is the most common cause of crippling hand disease in the world and a common cause of blindness. The spread of leprosy is by the respiratory route or by skin-to-skin contact. Not completely excluded is transmission by insects.

Clinical Features

The unique clinical features of leprosy result from the peripheral nerve tropism of *M. leprae* and its preference for temperatures of 7° to 10°C lower than core body temperature. The long incubation period varies from 6 months to 40 years and is a consequence of its very slow growth, doubling only once every 11–13 days. Patients with good resistance develop *tuberculoid leprosy* (TL), with multifocal, often asymmetrical, lesions of nerve and sometimes skin. Early signs include hypopigmented anesthetic skin patches, areas of cutaneous sensory loss without skin patches, and multifocal or diffuse skin infiltration. Sensory impairment proceeds in a predictable sequence, with loss of temperature sensation first, followed by pain, and then touch, with sparing of proprioception and vibration. Diminished sweating is associated.

Patients with impaired cell-mediated immunity develop *lepromatous leprosy* (LL) characterized by widespread symmetrical areas of anesthesia and anhidrosis. In addition, skin lesions (macules, papules, nodules, or extensive skin infiltration) occur with either normal sensation or diminished sensation in anesthetic areas. Unlike TL, the lesions and anesthetic areas are not in the same place. In leprous neuritis, deep reflexes are usually intact until a later stage. The sensory loss spreads to the cool areas of the face and affects the nose. Painless corneal ulceration results from loss of corneal sensation and weakness of eye closure. Hair is lost over all the skin lesions. Hypertrophy and infiltration of the facial skin and forehead lead to leonine facies. Borderline (dimorphous) leprosy, an intermediate form with features of both TL and LL, includes the polyneuritic form of leprosy.

Diagnosis

Consider the diagnosis of leprosy in patients with transient, recurrent, or persistent numbness or paresthesias or when a chronic, asymptomatic, atypical skin rash does not respond to standard treatments. Radial nerve sensory conduction study is one of the more sensitive indicators of disease. Demonstrating *M. leprae* in skin, nasal mucous membrane, or biopsy establishes the diagnosis. Nerve biopsy is performed in purely neural cases or when a skin biopsy has not been diagnostic.

Treatment

Therapy consists of starting two or more drugs as soon as the diagnosis is made and classification as multibacillary or paucibacillary is determined. Multibacillary leprosy is treated with RIF 600 mg once a month, dapsone (a folate antagonist) 100 mg daily, and clofazimine 50 mg daily plus 300 mg once a month for a minimum of 2 years and typically 5 years. Paucibacillary leprosy is treated with RIF 600 mg once a month and dapsone 100 mg daily for 6 months. Additional drugs include the thioamides, fluoroquinolones, minocycline, and clarithromycin. Hemolytic reaction to dapsone is a concern in patients with glucose-6-phosphate dehydrogenase deficiency.

Prevention
Chemoprophylaxis of household contacts is not routine, although children in contact with a lepromatous patient should receive monthly RIF for 6 months. BCG or vaccines derived from killed or chemically modified *M. leprae* and research strains have a variable protective effect.

SPIROCHETAL DISEASES

Spirochetes belonging to the genera *Treponema*, *Borrelia*, and *Leptospira* are important human pathogens. Except for the endemic treponemal diseases, all produce multiphasic or relapsing diseases with multifocal neurological involvement. Suboptimal diagnostic methods, incomplete treatment, and potential relapses despite therapy hamper diagnosis and management.

Syphilis

The spread of syphilis, a chronic multisystem disease caused by the spirochete *T. pallidum*, is venereal or vertical (i.e., mother to child). The characteristic of venereal acquired disease is episodes of active disease separated by periods of latency, with neurological involvement in secondary and later stages. Symptomatic neurosyphilis develops in 4–9% of patients with untreated syphilis. Meningovascular syphilis occurs in 2–3%, general paresis in 2–5%, and tabes dorsalis in 1–5%.

Clinical Features
One or more primary skin lesions, called *chancres*, characterize *primary syphilis*. These develop at the site of inoculation an average of 20 days after exposure. Dark-field microscopy demonstrates spirochetes in the lesions. Neurological disease is not a feature of primary syphilis. *Secondary syphilis* occurs 2–12 weeks after contact. Disseminated infection manifests clinically by constitutional symptoms such as fever, malaise, generalized

lymphadenopathy, rash, and neurologically as syphilitic meningitis or cranial neuropathies, including hearing loss and ocular changes. Approximately 30% of patients with secondary syphilis develop CSF changes indicating meningeal infection, but only 1–2% of patients are symptomatic. CSF shows lymphocytic pleocytosis, elevated protein, and low-to-normal glucose. After the second stage resolves, the patient enters a latent asymptomatic period, with disease apparent only by serology.

One third of untreated patients develop late syphilis (tertiary syphilis), a slowly progressive inflammatory disease that includes gummatous (granulomatous), cardiovascular, and neurological forms. Early neurological manifestations of tertiary neurosyphilis include pure meningeal or meningovascular disease, with a 5- to 10-year latency from primary infection, and parenchymal forms, which occur 10–30 years after initial infection. General paresis refers to parenchymal cerebral involvement, and tabes dorsalis to syphilitic myeloneuropathy. Syphilitic gumma, granulomas that present as space-occupying lesions in brain or cord, may occur at any stage of disseminated disease. All neurological complications of syphilis occur in HIV disease, which accelerates the onset and progression of neurosyphilis.

Syphilitic meningitis typically occurs earlier than other forms of neurosyphilis and is often asymptomatic. General paresis, the encephalitic form of neurosyphilis, typically presents as progressive dementia beginning 15–20 years after original infection (range, 3–30 years). Tabes dorsalis, the spinal form of syphilis, develops approximately 15–20 years after the original infection (range, 5–50 years). At birth, congenitally infected infants may show signs of serous nasal discharge (snuffles), rash, condylomata, hepatosplenomegaly, or osteochondritis. If left untreated, the classic stigmata of Hutchinson's teeth, saddle nose, interstitial keratitis, saber shins, mental retardation, hearing loss, and hydrocephalus develop.

Diagnosis

Diagnosis uses treponemal and nontreponemal serological tests. Treponemal tests include fluorescent treponemal antibody absorption, microhemagglutination assay, fluorescent treponemal antibody absorption double staining, hemagglutination treponemal test for syphilis, and *T. pallidum* immobilization. Treponemal test results become positive 3–4 weeks after inoculation and usually remain positive for life. Nontreponemal or reagin tests detect antibodies to membrane lipids of *T. pallidum*, using antigens such as cardiolipin, lecithin, or cholesterol, and include the Veneral Disease Research

Laboratories (VDRL) test and rapid plasma reagin test. Results become positive 5–6 weeks after exposure and usually become negative in the year following adequate treatment.

The Centers for Disease Control and Prevention (CDC) recommends CSF examination for all patients with syphilis who have neurological or ophthalmic symptoms and signs or active tertiary disease (aortitis, gumma, and iritis) or have failed therapy. In addition, the CDC advises that HIV-infected patients with late latent syphilis or latent syphilis of unknown duration undergo LP before treatment.

Treatment
Optimal treatment of neurosyphilis is aqueous penicillin G at doses of 18–24 million units per day intravenously (3–4 million units every 4 hours) for 10–14 days. In penicillin-allergic patients, alternatives include oral doxycycline 200 mg twice daily for 4 weeks or skin testing to confirm allergy and consideration of desensitization.

After therapy, follow-up is required in patients with documented neurosyphilis. Clinical symptoms or signs of syphilis should prompt consideration of re-treatment, as should a fourfold increase of serum titers or failure of titers greater than 1–32 to decrease at least fourfold by 12–24 months. If pleocytosis was present, repeat LP every 6 months until cell count normalizes. Re-treatment is required if CSF cell count does not decrease after 6 months or normalize after 2 years.

Lyme Disease (Borreliosis)

Borrelia burgdorferi is the organism responsible for Lyme disease. Transmission is by the hard-shelled deer ticks: *Ixodes dammini* in the eastern United States, *Ixodes pacificus* in the western United States, and *Ixodes ricinus* in Europe.

Clinical Features
The spectrum of Lyme-related neurological disease is uncertain. Best agreement exists for the early neurological syndromes, which include lymphocytic meningitis, cranial neuropathy (commonly unilateral or bilateral Bell's palsy), and painful radiculoneuritis. Optic neuritis, mononeuritis multiplex, and Guillain-Barré syndrome are uncommon manifestations. Neurological complications of more advanced Lyme disease include encephalomyelitis, with predominant white matter involvement and peripheral neuropathy. Lymphocytic meningitis is usually acute but may cause chronic or relapsing meningitis and communicating hydrocephalus. Radiculoneuritis, beginning

as a painful limb disorder, may continue with exacerbations and remissions for up to 6 months. Encephalopathy with memory or cognitive abnormalities, confusional states, accelerated dementia, and normal CSF study results may occur.

Dermatological manifestations include erythema chronicum migrans and acrodermatitis chronicum atrophicans. Other extraneural features include *Borrelia* lymphocytoma, occurring 6–12 months after infection, recurrent monoarthritis or polyarthritis, and second- or third-degree cardiac conduction block.

Diagnosis

The best clinical marker is the erythema chronicum migrans rash. The presence of consistent clinical features together with CSF pleocytosis, serum anti–*B. burgdorferi* antibodies, and evidence of intrathecal antibody production establish the diagnosis. Serological testing by enzyme-linked immunosorbent assay (ELISA) is an initial screen, followed by Western blot confirmation. Culture of organisms and PCR testing of CSF are also available.

Treatment

Parenteral antibiotics treat infections that have crossed the blood-brain barrier. Ceftriaxone (2 g once daily intravenously) or penicillin (3–4 million units intravenously every 3–4 hours) for 2–4 weeks are first-line drugs. Tetracycline and chloramphenicol are alternatives in penicillin- or cephalosporin-allergic patients. CSF examination toward the end of the 2- to 4-week treatment course and again 6 months after the conclusion of therapy assesses the need for continuing treatment.

OTHER SELECT ORGANISMS

Rocky Mountain Spotted Fever

Rocky Mountain spotted fever, a tickborne infection caused by *Rickettsia rickettsii*, is the most virulent of the spotted fevers. Delayed treatment is associated with 20% fatalities. The illness begins with fever, headache, myalgia, and gastrointestinal symptoms 2–14 days after the tick bite. The rash appears first around the wrist and ankles from days 3–5 of the illness and spreads to the soles of the feet and forearms. Petechial and ecchymotic rashes, indicating microcirculatory injury, may foreshadow gangrene of the digits or rhabdomyolysis. Other complications include renal failure and pulmonary edema. CNS manifestations accompany severe cases. Meningitis or meningoencephalitis with microinfarcts causes focal neurological deficits, transient deafness, depressed consciousness, or coma. CSF examination reveals elevated protein and lymphocytic or polymorphonuclear pleocytosis in approximately 30% of patients, with low glucose in fewer than 10%.

Demonstration of *R. rickettsii* is by direct immunofluorescence or immunoperoxidase staining of skin biopsy in patients with rash. Treatment is with oral or intravenous tetracycline (25–50 mg/kg per day) or chloramphenicol (50–75 mg/kg per day) in four divided doses or oral doxycycline 100 mg twice a day for 7 days and continued for 2 days once the patient has become afebrile.

Cat-Scratch Disease

Bartonella henselae is the organism responsible for cat-scratch disease, a slowly progressive regional adenitis associated with aseptic meningitis in immunocompetent individuals and encephalitis, myelitis, or radiculoneuritis in HIV-infected patients. ELISA tests and PCR amplification from infected tissues are available. Treatment of encephalitis is with intravenous gentamicin.

Campylobacteriosis

Campylobacter, among the most common bacterial infections of humans worldwide, causes both acute enteric and systemic illnesses. Sources of infection include raw milk, water, and poultry. *Campylobacter jejuni* has been identified as the most common antecedent pathogen for the Guillain-Barré syndrome, accounting for an estimated 20–40% of all cases. The onset of Guillain-Barré syndrome is usually 2–3 weeks after the diarrheal illness and follows an estimated 1 per 1000–2000 *Campylobacter* infections. The isolation of *Campylobacter* infection from stool or blood establishes the diagnosis. Erythromycin, 250 mg orally four times daily for 5–7 days, is effective treatment.

Botulism

Botulinum toxin blocks acetylcholine release at peripheral synapses, leading to the paralytic and autonomic clinical features of botulism. Common early symptoms of botulism are diplopia, ptosis, dysarthria, and dysphagia. Extraocular and bulbar muscle weakness progress rapidly to the limbs, typically symmetrically, and to respiratory muscles. Alertness and cognition are normal, unless hypoxemia or hypercarbia supervene because of respiratory failure. Reflexes are depressed or absent, and sensation is normal. Impaired cholinergic transmission also involves autonomic synapses, as indicated by dilated poorly reactive pupils, dry mouth, paralytic ileus, and occasionally bradycardia.

Preservation of alertness and lack of sensory or upper motor neuron signs distinguish botulism from acute brainstem disorders. The descending paralysis of botulism closely resembles the Guillain-Barré syndrome, except sensation is normal, tendon reflexes are better preserved, and the CSF content is normal. In a patient with a compatible clinical syndrome, the diagnosis of botulism is confirmed by toxin assay or by culturing *C. botulinum*.

Once taken up by neurons, botulinum toxin is invulnerable to antibody inactivation and irreversibly blocks exocytosis. In adults, trivalent (types A, B, and E) equine antitoxin is given if initial testing reveals no hypersensitivity reaction. In infants, supportive care, including mechanical ventilation in many patients, is the mainstay of therapy. Treatment of infant botulism usually does not include antitoxin administration or antibiotics.

VIRAL INFECTIONS

The most common viruses causing nervous system disease in the United States are listed in Table 28.3. In Europe and the United States, the most common causal agents of aseptic encephalitis and meningitis are enteroviruses (coxsackie and echoviruses), arboviruses, and herpes simplex virus (HSV). Worldwide, there are more than 50,000 encephalitis deaths from rabies each year, and in Asia at least 35,000 cases and 10,000 deaths from Japanese encephalitis (JE). In the United States, nearly 4000 cases of West Nile virus encephalitis, with 250 deaths, occurred in 2002. The treatment, prophylaxis, and immunotherapy of specific viral infections are summarized in Table 28.4.

Herpesviruses

Herpesviruses are ubiquitous viruses that cause acute infection but share the biological capacity of latency, the ability to remain quiescent for periods in the host and later reactivate.

Herpes Simplex Viruses Type 1 and 2 (HSV-1, HSV-2)
Herpes Simplex Encephalitis
HSV-1 encephalitis accounts for 10% of encephalitis cases in the United States. Mortality in untreated cases is 70%. One third of infections are primary infections, and the rest are reactivation

Text continued on p. 259.

Table 28.3: Primary causes of viral nervous system infection in North America

Agent		Meningitis	Encephalitis	Postinfectious ADEM	Myelitis
Nonpolio enteroviruses	Echovirus	***	*		*
	Coxsackievirus	***	*		*
Arboviruses (U.S. & Canada)					
Togaviruses Flavivirus	St. Louis encephalitis virus (SLE)	*	**		
	West Nile virus	*	**		*
	Powassan		***		*
Alphavirus	Eastern equine (EEE)	*	**		
	Western equine (WEE)	**	**		
	Venezuelan equine (VEE)	**	*		
Reoviridae: orbivirus	Colorado tick fever	*	**		
Bunyavirus	California (La Crosse)	*	*		
	Jamestown Canyon	*	*		
	Snowshoe hare				

Herpesviruses				
HSV-1	*		**	**
HSV-2	**		**	**
VZV	**	*	**	**
CMV	*		**	*
EBV	*	*	**	*
HHV-6	*		**	*
HHV-7			*	
HHV-8				
Herpes B virus	*		*	
Lymphocytic choriomeningitis virus (LCMV)	**	*	***	**
Mumps virus	*		*	**
HIV	*		*	**
Rabies virus	*	*	*	
Measles virus	*	**	**	
Rubella virus	*	*	*	
Poliovirus (now eradicated from Western hemisphere)	**	*	*	*
Adenovirus			*	*
Vaccinia	*			
Influenza		*		*
Parainfluenza		*	*	*
Rotavirus		*		*
Parvovirus B-19		*	*	*

Table 28.4: Treatment and prophylaxis of viral infections

Antiviral Class	Antiviral Agent	Dose	Indications	Toxicity or Cautions
Nucleoside analogs	Acyclovir	10 mg/kg/dose (IV) q8h × 14–21 days	HSV encephalitis in adults	Renal impairment
		20 mg/kg/dose (IV) q8h × 21 days	Neonatal HSV encephalitis	
		500 mg/m²/dose (IV) q8h × 21 days (equivalent to 10–12 mg/kg/dose in adults and up to 20 mg/kg/dose in infants)	VZV encephalitis in normal or immunocompromised pt	
		15 mg/kg/dose (IV) q8h × 10–14 days	Herpes B virus	
		800 mg (PO) 5X/day × 7 days	Dermatomal zoster or primary VZV in immunocompromised pt	Low solubility
	Famciclovir	200 mg (PO) tid × 7 days	Dermatomal zoster or primary VZV in immunocompromised pt	Headache, nausea

Valacyclovir	1 g (PO) qid × 7 days	Dermatomal zoster or primary VZV in immunocompromised pt	Thrombotic thrombocytic purpura/hemolytic uremic syndrome in HIV patients
Ganciclovir	5 mg/kg (IV) q12h × 14–21 days	CMV, Herpes B virus	Bone marrow suppression
Valganciclovir	900 mg (PO) bid × 21 days (induction), then 900 mg (PO) qd (maintenance)	CMV Retinitis	Bone marrow suppression
Ribavirin	2 g (IV) × 1, then 1 g (IV) q6h × 4 days, then 0.5 g (IV) q8h × 6 days	Lassa fever	Hemolytic anemia
Cytarabine	20–35 mg/kg/day × 7 days	Measles virus PML	Bone marrow suppression
Trifluridine	2 mg/kg (IV) × 5 days × 4 wks 1% ophthalmic solution	Herpetic keratoconjunctivitis Acyclovir-resistant HSV/VZV	
Foscarnet	90 mg/kg (IV) q12h × 14–21 days	Ganciclovir-resistant CMV	Hypocalcemia, renal impairment
Pyrophosphate analogue			

Continued

Table 28.4: (continued)

Antiviral Class	Antiviral Agent	Dose	Indications	Toxicity or Cautions
Other	Amantadine	100 mg (PO) bid × 5 days	Influenza A	CNS + anticholinergic-like side effects
	Rimantidine	100 mg (PO) bid × 5 days	Influenza A	Less CNS side effects
	Oseltamivir	75 mg (PO) bid × 5 days	Influenza A and B	
	Zanamivir	10 mg (PO) bid × 5 days	Influenza A and B	
	Interferon-α	3 million U/day (SC)	PML, acyclovir-resistant VZV, hepatitis C	Flulike side effects
Cytokine		10^5–10^6 U/m^2 body surface (intrathecal)	SSPE	
Supplements	Vitamin A	400,000 IU (IM)	Acute measles in vitamin A deficiency	

CNS, central nervous system; CMV, human cytomegalovirus; HSV, herpes simplex virus; PML, progressive multifocal leukoencephalopathy; SSPE, subacute sclerosing panencephalitis; VZV, varicella zoster virus.

and centripetal spread of virus latent in the trigeminal ganglia. Half of the population has antibodies to HSV-1 by age 15 years, and 90% by adulthood.

Fever and headache are consistent features. The onset may be abrupt, with focal or generalized seizures, or more protracted, with behavioral changes, an amnestic syndrome, aphasia, or other focal signs. The CSF shows increased pressure, with lymphocytic pleocytosis, elevated protein concentration, and normal or low glucose. PCR techniques detect HSV DNA in the CSF. MRI shows areas of high signal intensity on T2-weighted images in frontotemporal regions. Therapy with acyclovir at 10 mg/kg every 8 hours for 10–14 days is used without brain biopsy. Treatment with acyclovir reduces mortality from 70% to 20%. One third of patients recover from the infection with little to no permanent neurological impairment.

Neonatal Herpes Simplex Virus Type 2; Human Herpesvirus Type 1

Half of all infants with neonatal HSV-2 infections have CNS disease. It presents as either disseminated disease with signs of brain involvement at age 1 week or as encephalitis at 2 weeks of age. Skin vesicles suggest the diagnosis; CSF PCR tests provide confirmation. The presence of vesicular skin or mucosal lesions in an infant of this age, even in the absence of fever or systemic symptoms, warrants immediate evaluation. Intravenous acyclovir, at 20 mg/kg every 8 hours, is empirical treatment of neonates with possible HSV disease while awaiting results of CSF HSV PCR. Treatment of infants with isolated skin, eye, and mouth disease is 14 days, and for those with sepsis or evidence of CNS infection it is 21 days.

Varicella Zoster Virus; Human Herpesvirus Type 1

Primary infection with varicella zoster virus (VZV) causes chickenpox. A self-limited cerebellar ataxia often follows natural childhood infections and immunization. Primary VZV may produce encephalitis in immunocompromised patients who require treatment with intravenous acyclovir within 24–72 hours after onset of the rash. Reactivation of endogenous latent virus produces *herpes zoster*, or *shingles*. The virus reactivates in response to waning cell-mediated immunity to VZV. Herpes zoster typically begins with pain and paresthesias in one or two adjacent spinal or cranial dermatomes. A pruritic vesicular eruption in the same area follows the pain in 3–4 days. The eruption lasts 10 days to 2 weeks. Involvement of the first division of the trigeminal ganglion produces *ophthalmic zoster* and of the geniculate ganglion (*otic zoster*) produces facial paresis plus tympanic membrane and external auditory canal rash. Herpes zoster is usually the first clinical presentation of underlying HIV infection. Antiviral treatment of acute VZV encephalitis and myelitis is intravenous acyclovir, at the high dose of 20 mg/kg (or 500 mg/m^2) every 8 hours. Postherpetic neuralgia is less likely to occur after acyclovir treatment. A short course of corticosteroids, tapered over 3 weeks, may be helpful for both pain and optic neuritis. VZV can also cause both granulomatous arteritis leading to stroke and/or multifocal infarcts and small vessel vasculopathy (leukoencephalitis).

Human Cytomegalovirus; Human Herpesvirus Type 4
Cytomegalovirus (CMV) infection is the most common congenital infection of humans. Up to 10% of infants born to mothers with primary CMV infection are symptomatic at birth. Ten percent of symptomatic infants die and 80% of survivors suffer severe neurological morbidity. Infection by passage through the birth canal or following breast-feeding in the perinatal period accounts for additional cases. Persistent high levels of viral replication in the eye, brain, and retina of the maturing fetus produce encephalitis, ependymitis, and retinitis, a pattern similar to that seen in patients with opportunistic CMV infection in the setting of HIV infection. CT scans characteristically show periventricular calcifications. Diagnosis of congenital CMV infection depends on the detection of virus by culture in urine, saliva, or CSF during the first 3 weeks of life.

Epstein-Barr Virus; Human Herpesvirus Type 5
Primary infection occurs as infectious mononucleosis. Nervous system disease occurs in fewer than 1% of cases as aseptic meningitis, encephalitis, cerebellitis, transverse myelitis, optic neuritis, cranial neuropathies, the Guillain-Barré syndrome, and small fiber sensory or autonomic neuropathy syndromes. Serum heterophile antibodies, serum and CSF Epstein-Barr virus (EBV)–specific antibodies, or EBV DNA in CSF are each diagnostic. CSF PCR for EBV is positive during the acute phase of illness in children with infectious mononucleosis and neurological complications such as transverse myelitis, meningoencephalitis, and aseptic meningitis.

Human Herpesvirus Type 6
Human herpesvirus (HHV) type 6 is a prevalent T-lymphotropic virus causing a spectrum of diseases ranging from inapparent infection to disseminated fatal disease. Exanthem subitum (or roseola) of infants or lymphadenopathy syndromes are the most common presentations of primary infection. Primary infection may result in meningoencephalitis in immunocompetent children.

Poliovirus and Other Nonpolio Enteroviruses

The enterovirus family comprises more than 70 serotypes within the Picornaviridae family. The subgroups are the polioviruses, coxsackieviruses A and B, echoviruses, and the newer sequentially numbered enteroviruses. The most common forms of infection by any of the enteroviruses are subclinical or mild febrile illness. Collectively, the enteroviruses are the leading causes of viral meningitis for which a pathogen is identifiable. However, severe neurological syndromes, including encephalitis and acute anterior poliomyelitis, are associated with several of these agents. Poliovirus, one of the most virulent members of the enterovirus group, is the agent of acute anterior poliomyelitis (infantile paralysis). Clinically apparent infection with poliovirus results in aseptic meningitis (8% of cases) or paralytic illness (1% of all cases). Headache, fever, signs of meningeal irritation, drowsiness, and seizures follow a 7- to 14-day incubation period. Asymmetrical flaccid weakness of limbs, diaphragm, or cranial nerve–innervated muscles develops within days and progresses on average for 3–5 days. Cerebellitis, transverse myelitis, and facial paresis also occur. Serology, virus isolation, or PCR amplification of poliovirus RNA from CSF confirms the diagnosis.

Nonpolio Enteroviruses

The nonpolio enteroviruses cause a spectrum of CNS and peripheral nervous system (PNS) disease, including aseptic meningitis, encephalitis, acute anterior poliomyelitis, acute cerebellar ataxia, peripheral and optic neuropathy, cranial polyneuritis, and epidemic myalgia. In neonates, encephalitis is generally part of an overwhelming sepsis-like illness, with up to 10% mortality. Congenital CNS defects are associated with infection acquired *in utero*. Infection of hypogammaglobulinemic patients commonly leads to progressive meningoencephalitis. Certain strains have also been associated with an acute motor neuron disease in association with epidemic hemorrhagic conjunctivitis.

Arboviruses

The term *arbovirus* ("*ar*thropod-*bo*rne *virus*") is a general term for viruses transmitted to humans by mosquito and tick (arthropod) vectors. Arboviruses exist in nature in complex cycles involving birds and mammals, which serve as reservoirs of disease. When transmitted to humans, arboviruses can cause fever, headache, meningitis, and encephalitis. Considered together, arboviruses represent the leading cause of encephalitis worldwide. The salient features of arboviral infections occurring in the United States are summarized in Table 28.5.

Rabies

Rabies is an almost global human encephalitic disease with nearly 100% mortality. Reservoirs of infection are nonimmunized dogs, wild carnivores (skunks, foxes, raccoons, wolves, jackals, wild dogs, merkats, and the mongoose), and bats. Human rabies cases are attributable to an animal bite. The incubation period is usually from 1 to 2 months but may vary from 1 week to several years. An acute neurological phase culminating in coma follows a prodrome of headache, fever, paresthesias, and pain at the inoculation site. Up to 80% of patients exhibit hydrophobia or aerophobia: spasms of pharyngeal and nuchal muscles lasting from 1–5 minutes. Attacks increase in frequency and are accompanied by agitation, hallucinations, autonomic hyperactivity, and seizures. Body temperature may reach 105° to 107°F. Paralytic myelitic rabies accounts for 20% of cases. The clinical features are paresthesias, weakness, and flaccid paralysis in the bitten extremity progressing to quadriplegia. Paralytic rabies is most often associated with bat rabies virus strains.

Intracerebral inoculation of mice with patient saliva and examination of skin from the face or neck within the hairline (nuchal biopsy) and corneal smears for the presence of rabies antigen by immunofluorescence are the most rapid methods of antemortem diagnosis. The presence of neutralizing antibodies in the serum and CSF of an unimmunized patient is diagnostic but is not a highly sensitive method. Active disease produces high titers (>1:5000), which may be helpful for diagnosing acute rabies in previously immunized individuals. High titers also distinguish acute rabies from postvaccination encephalomyelitis associated with vaccines derived from animal neural tissue. PCR protocols for detection of viral sequences in brain specimens are established. Preexposure prophylaxis is available to veterinarians, animal handlers, laboratory workers, or travelers to endemic areas.

Childhood Xanthems

Measles
Despite the availability of an effective vaccine, measles, a highly contagious respiratory-borne disease, is still an important cause of childhood mortality and blindness in developing countries, as well as in sporadic outbreaks in industrialized nations. Measles

Table 28.5: Details of North American arboviruses

Agent	Geographical Distribution	Reservoir	Vector	Season	Group Affected	Mortality	Neurological Sequelae
Eastern equine	Atlantic and Gulf coasts, Great Lakes region	Birds	Mosquito	June–Aug	Children	50–70%	80% (esp. young)
Western equine	Western U.S. and Canada	Birds and small mammals	Mosquito	June–Sept	Infants, adults >50 years	Adults: 3–5% Infants: 10–20%	Adults: 5% Infants: 50%
Venezuelan equine	Texas and Florida	Horses, small animals	Mosquito	Rainy season May–Sept	Adults	<1%	Rare
St. Louis	Throughout U.S., but greatest prevalence in Texas, Florida, and Ohio-Mississippi River Valley	Birds	Mosquito	June–Aug	Adults >50 years	2–20%	25–50% mild <10% severe
California (La Crosse)	Midwest and Northeast U.S., Southern Canada	Chipmunk, squirrel, small mammals	Mosquito	June–Sept	Children	<1%	Rare
West Nile virus	Throughout U.S.	Birds	Mosquito	June–October	All ages, adults >50 with severe disease	Evolving data 5%	Evolving data
Powassan	North Central U.S., Eastern Canada	Squirrel, porcupine, groundhog	Tick	Spring/Summer		Rare	35%
Colorado tick fever	U.S. and Canadian Rocky Mountains	Chipmunk, squirrel, rodent	Tick	March–Sept	Children and adults	<1%	Rare

causes four major CNS syndromes: acute encephalitis, postviral encephalomyelitis, measles inclusion body encephalitis, and subacute sclerosing panencephalitis (SSPE).

Rubella

Rubella is usually a mild illness with maculopapular rash, fever, and lymphadenopathy. Gestational rubella, especially infection acquired during the first trimester, causes the congenital rubella syndrome. Sequelae in survivors include mental retardation, sensorineural hearing loss, motor and posture abnormalities, cataracts, pigmentary retinopathy, and congenital heart disease. Late-onset rubella encephalitis, *progressive rubella panencephalitis*, may follow congenital rubella or natural childhood rubella.

Mumps

Mumps virus causes a mild childhood illness with parotitis but has the capacity for widespread invasion of visceral organs, the vestibular labyrinths, and the CNS. The frequency of mumps meningitis and encephalitis varies in different epidemics from less than 1% to 70%. Vaccination with live attenuated virus at 12–15 months of age and an additional booster dose at 4–6 years of age achieves mumps prevention. Recent studies evaluating the use of the current measles-mumps-rubella vaccine (containing Jeryl-Lynn strain) have not documented any association between vaccination and encephalitis, aseptic meningitis, or autism.

Arenaviruses

Arenaviruses are rodent-borne viruses. Human infection occurs from contact with infected rodent excreta. The arenaviruses of neurological consequence are lymphocytic choriomeningitis virus (LCMV), Lassa fever, and Argentine hemorrhagic fever viruses.

Hemorrhagic Fever Viruses

Dengue (Flavivirus)

In terms of size of epidemics and severity of disease, dengue fever and dengue hemorrhagic fever are the most important arthropod-borne viral diseases of humans. Dengue virus cycles between humans and mosquitoes. Dengue fever begins, after a 2- to 7-day incubation period, as a sudden febrile illness with headache, myalgias, arthralgias, prostration, abdominal discomfort, and rash. Neurological complications including encephalopathy, encephalitis, and mononeuritis multiplex involving cranial and peripheral nerves, and Guillain-Barré and Reye's syndromes.

Filoviruses

Ebola and Marburg viruses are the two known members of the Filoviridae. Outbreaks of Ebola virus occur in Africa. Both viruses lead to fulminating hemorrhagic fever with severe shock and high mortality. Headache and meningismus are the initial features. Hemorrhage, hypotension, hepatic failure, and disseminated intravascular coagulopathy follow. Muscle necrosis caused by disseminated intravascular coagulopathy and intramuscular hemorrhage follows early myositis or muscle pain.

Papovaviruses and Progressive Multifocal Leukoencephalopathy

Progressive multifocal leukoencephalopathy (PML), a subacute demyelinating disease of the CNS, is a result of infection of oligodendrocytes by an opportunistic papovavirus. JC virus causes all documented cases. Although the JC virus is not associated with illness when contracted in early childhood, JC virus persists in the host and reactivates when cell-mediated immunity is impaired. Onset is subacute, with features of multifocal asymmetrical white matter involvement. The disease progresses to dementia as the number of lesions increases. CSF cell counts and protein levels are usually normal. MRI shows focal or multifocal lesions of subcortical white matter. PCR amplification detects JC virus DNA in CSF. No specific therapy is available

Retroviruses: HIV, HTLV-I, HTLV-II

Human Immunodeficiency Virus

HIV infection is associated with several neurological manifestations, either as part of the primary disease process or as neurological complications of secondary opportunistic infections occurring in the immunodeficient state. Aseptic meningitis may occur at the time of HIV infection as a component of the acute retroviral syndrome. HIV-associated dementia, neurocognitive defects, vacuolar myelopathy, and encephalitis are all progressive complications of HIV disease. Table 28.6 lists the major HIV-associated CNS disorders classified by neuroanatomical localization. HIV infections are associated with amyotrophic lateral sclerosis (ALS)–like syndromes. These differ from classic ALS by younger age at onset, progression over weeks, presentation as monomelic syndromes, and improvement or stabilization with highly active antiretroviral therapy.

Table 28.6: Major HIV-associated CNS disorders classified by neuroanatomical localization

Meninges
Aseptic HIV meningitis
Cryptococcal meningitis
Tuberculous meningitis
Syphilitic meningitis
Listeria monocytogenes meningitis
Lymphomatous meningitis (metastatic)
Brain
Predominantly nonfocal
HIV-associated dementia (HAD)
HIV-associated minor cognitive motor dysfunction (MCMD)
Toxoplasmic encephalitis
Cytomegalovirus (CMV) encephalitis
Aspergillus encephalitis
Herpes encephalitis
Metabolic encephalopathy (alone or concomitantly)
Predominantly focal
Cerebral toxoplasmosis
Primary CNS lymphoma (PCNSL)
Progressive multifocal leukoencephalopathy (PML)
Cryptococcoma
Tuberculoma
Varicella-zoster virus (VZV) encephalitis
Stroke
Spinal cord
Vacuolar myelopathy (VM)
Cytomegalovirus (CMV) myeloradiculopathy
VZV myelitis
Spinal epidural or intradural lymphoma (metastatic)
HTLV-1-associated myelopathy

Human T-Lymphotropic Viruses Types 1 and 2
Human T-lymphotropic virus type 1 (HTLV-1) is endemic in southern Japan, Taiwan, Okinawa, the Caribbean basin (including northeast South America), central and west Africa, southern India, and the Seychelles. In the United States and western Europe, the incidence of HTLV infection is higher among intravenous drug users and homosexuals. Most seropositive individuals are asymptomatic; fewer than 1% of infected patients develop spastic paraparesis. Spread of HTLV-1, as with other retroviruses, is by sexual, parenteral, or vertical transmission. Neurological findings include spastic paraparesis, impotence, urinary and fecal incontinence, and generalized

hyperreflexia, except in cases of concomitant sensory neuropathy. Inflammatory myositis, cerebellar ataxia, nystagmus, vertigo, deafness, optic neuritis, adult T-cell leukemia, uveitis, inflammatory arthropathy, and lymphocytic alveolitis may be present. Serological testing uses an ELISA, followed by Western blot confirmation. Treatment is against the inflammatory components of disease.

Influenza

Influenza virus is associated with myositis, Reye's syndrome, acute encephalopathy/encephalitis, and postinfluenzal encephalitis 2–3 weeks after recovery. The acute encephalopathy/encephalitis that has been reported to occur within 1–3 days of onset of respiratory symptoms (associated with both influenza A and influenza B) has a high rate of mortality and morbidity. The postencephalitis syndrome, accompanied by inflammatory spinal fluid, is transitory, with full recovery in most cases. The treatment and prevention of influenza A is with oral amantadine or rimantadine.

FUNGAL INFECTIONS

More than 20,000 fungal species are identified and form an integral part of our ecosystem. More than 250 fungal species are pathogenic. From the common candidal infections to the deadly mucormycosis, fungal infections influence all levels of clinical practice. Most pathological fungi exist in yeast and filamentous states, depending on growth conditions and temperature. In the yeast state, they are unicellular, round to elongated, and reproduce by budding or fission. In the filamentous or mold state, they grow by extension of their tips forming tubular structures called *hyphae*, which often have septae that divide them into many segments. Spores are the reproductive elements of the hyphae. Spores develop into yeast when infecting humans or animals but remain in the filamentous form when grown *in vitro*.

Fungi have varying predilection for involvement of the CNS. In general, fungi found in the meninges and the CSF are in the yeast phase (e.g., *Cryptococcus*), whereas those causing brain parenchymal infection are in the filamentous stage (e.g., *Aspergillus*). CNS fungal diseases are often misdiagnosed or undiagnosed during life. Although many therapeutic options have developed to treat superficial fungal infections, invasive and deep CNS fungal infections are often tenacious to therapy.

Epidemiology and Current Trends

The incidence of CNS fungal infections varies greatly with the geographical location. For example, histoplasmosis is common in areas infested with bats, and cryptococcosis and histoplasmosis are common in patients exposed to birds. Histoplasmosis is commonly seen in central United States (Ohio River Valley) and in restricted areas of the tropics. *Haemophilus duboisii* is frequently found in west Africa. Coccidioidomycosis is mainly found in southwestern United States (San Joaquin Valley) and in Central America, where it resides in the soil. Blastomycosis is endemic in the Ohio and Mississippi basins in the United States. Other fungi such as *Cryptococcus, Aspergillus,* Zygomycetes (*Mucor*), and *Candida* species are more universally distributed. With respect to clinically recognized fungal CNS illnesses, *Cryptococcus* and *Candida* infections are the most common, followed by *Coccidioides, Aspergillus*, and the Zygomycetes. Fortunately, other fungi involve the CNS rarely. *Candida* and the Zygomycetes rarely invade the deep viscera or CNS in the normal host and are therefore considered opportunistic in nature in immunocompromised hosts.

Fungal disease of the CNS has become increasingly common as a consequence of the AIDS epidemic and the use of aggressive immunosuppressive regimens for cancer and for solid organ and bone marrow transplantations. A study from the San Francisco Bay area found that more than 75% of patients who had invasive mycoses had serious underlying medical conditions that affected their immune systems. Only 9% were thought to be healthy at the time of the systemic fungal infection. The authors reported an overall incidence of invasive mycotic infections at 178 per million per year in 1992/1993, but the rate climbed to 5000 per million per year in individuals who were infected with HIV. The study found that the rates of invasive fungal infections per million per year for individual fungi were highest for *Candida* and *Cryptococcus* (73% and 66%, respectively). In another study from Australia, the two most common strains of *Cryptococcus* had different epidemiological features. *Cryptococcus neoformans* variant *neoformans* primarily caused meningitis in immunosuppressed patients, whereas *C. neoformans* variant *gattii* infected healthy hosts. The reason for this difference is unclear. No specific epidemiological data are available from the developing countries.

Pathogenesis

Fungi produce disease by direct invasion, by allergic phenomenon, or by liberating toxins; for example, ergotism resulting from rye ergot, which thrives on cereals, especially ground-nuts, and trichothecene mycotoxins, which are misused in aerosol form as "yellow rain" in biological warfare to produce an illness characterized by weakness, ataxia, hypothermia, and shock.

Fungi are generally not invasive unless there are predisposing factors. They gain entry into the body mainly by inhalation of spores. This causes a localized lung infection, which may be asymptomatic or produce mild respiratory symptoms and is usually successfully terminated by a functional immune system. Failing this, the infection reaches the bloodstream and produces fungemia. If the fungemia overcomes the host's reticuloendo-thelial, cellular, and humoral defense systems and penetrates the blood-brain or blood-CSF barrier, it reaches the brain paren-chyma or the meninges. Fortunately, in the healthy individual, this seldom happens. In-dwelling arterial or venous catheters can also be infected (*Candida*), forming a direct source for fungemia. Less common routes of infection are the skin (sporo-trichosis), the mouth, the gastrointestinal tract (*Candida*), and the nasal sinuses (*Aspergillus* and Zygomycetes). Finally, direct inoculation of fungi into skull fractures or during neurosurgical procedures that place in-dwelling devices such as intraventricular shunts also predisposes to CNS infection. Certain conditions predispose a patient to infection with a particular fungus (Table 28.7).

Central Nervous System Fungal Syndromes

Myriad clinical presentations of the CNS fungal infections occur. Meningitis, meningoencephalitis, cerebral abscess, CNS granu-loma, rhinocerebral necrotic mass, and base of skull lesions are the common modes of presentation. Cerebrovascular accidents and epidural fungal abscess are rare. The manner in which fungal CNS disease manifests is largely determined by the growth characteristics of the particular fungal species during systemic invasion. Fungi that are true yeast when invasive (e.g., *Cryptococcus*) most often present as chronic meningitis. Fungi that are pseudohyphae (e.g., *Candida*) often present with encephalitis as a consequence of multiple intraparenchymal microabscesses. Those that are true hyphae (e.g., *Aspergillus*) can present as strokelike illness because of their propensity to invade blood vessels. Clinicians must be aware that these presentations are not mutually exclusive and that it is not uncommon for the various forms of clinical illness to coexist.

Table 28.7: Therapy for CNS fungal infections

| | | Clinicopathological Features | | | |
| | | Meningitis | Abscess | Infarct | |
Organism	Predisposing Cause				Therapy in Immunocompetent Host	Immunosuppressed Host Without AIDS
C. neoformans	Inherited immunodeficiency (CGD, SCID, etc.), HIV/AIDS, cytotoxic agents, corticosteroids	++++	+	+	AMP B, 0.5–1 mg/kg/day, plus FLU 100 mg/kg/day (in four divided doses) for 6–10 wks or this combination for 2 wks followed by FLUCO 400 mg/day for 10 wks. Consolidation with FLUCO 6 mo–1 yr.	AMP B, 0.7–1 mg/kg/day, plus FLU 100 mg/kg/day (in four divided doses) for 2 wks followed by a minimum FLUCO 400 mg/day for 10 wks. Then reduce it to 200 mg/day for life. An alternative regimen AMP B 0.5–1 mg/kg/day plus FLU 100 mg/kg/day for 6–10 wks followed by FLUCO maintenance. In case of intolerance to AMP B, FLUCO 400–800 mg/day with FLU 100–150 mg/kg/day for 6 wks can be used. Followed by FLUCO.

C. immitis	Inherited immunodeficiency (CGD, SCID, etc.), HIV/AIDS, cytotoxic agents, corticosteroids	+++	+	+	FLUCO 400–800 mg/day for 1–4 yrs or IV 0.25 to 1.5 mg/kg/day with or without IT AMP B dose 3 times/wk for many wks then gradual tapering to biweekly and then monthly, a cumulative dose of 35–100 mg in conjunction with IV AMP B 0.5 mg/kg/day up to a total cumulative dose of 0.5–2.0 g for 1 yr.	AMP B 0.5 mg/kg/day up to a total cumulative dose of 0.5–1.0 g for 1 yr, followed by FLUCO, 200–400 mg/day for life.
H. capsulatum	Inherited immunodeficiency (CGD, SCID, etc.), HIV/AIDS, cytotoxic agents, corticosteroids	++++	+	+	AMP B 0.7–1.0 mg/kg/day. Maintenance ITRA, 400 mg/day for 4–12 wks for 6 mo.	AMP B, 1.5 to 2 g total, followed by ITRA, 400 mg/day for 6 mo or for life.
C. albicans	Inherited immunodeficiency (CGD, SCID, etc.), HIV/AIDS, cytotoxic agents, corticosteroids, cancer, trauma, indwelling catheters, prematurity, alcoholism, intravenous drug abuse, malnutrition, pregnancy	++	++	(Microabscesses)	AMP B, 0.5–1 mg/kg/day, with FLU, 100 mg/kg/day (in 4 divided doses) for 4–6 wks.	AMP B, 0.5–1 mg/kg/day, with FLU, 100 mg/day (in four divided doses) for 4–6 wks or longer.
Z. rhizopus	Diabetic ketoacidosis, intravenous drug abuse, iron chelation therapy	+	+++	++++	AMP B, 1–1.5 mg/kg/day up to a total dose of 3 g. Surgical debridement.	AMP B, 1.5 mg/kg/day up to a total dose of 3 g. Prophylaxis life long.

Continued

Table 28.7: (continued)

Organism	Predisposing Cause	Clinicopathological Features			Therapy in Immunocompetent Host	Immunosuppressed Host Without AIDS
		Meningitis	Abscess	Infarct		
A. fumigatus	Inherited immunodeficiency (CGD, SCID, etc.), HIV/AIDS, cytotoxic agents, corticosteroids	+	+++	++++	AMP B, 0.7–1.5 mg/kg/day, up to a total dose of 3 g, followed by ITRA, 400–800 mg/day for extended period.	AMP B, 1.5 mg/kg/day, up to a total dose of 3 g followed by ITRA, 400–800 mg/day for life.
B. dermatitidis	—	++++	+	+	AMP B, 2–3 g total until stable, followed by ITRA, 400 mg/day for 6 mo.	AMP B, 2–3 g total until stable, followed by ITRA, 400 mg/day for 6–12 mo or life.

AMP B, Amphotericin B; CGD, chronic granulomatous disease; FLU, Flucytosine; FLUCO, Fluconazole; IT, intrathecal; ITRA, Itraconazole; IV, intravenous; mo, months; SCID, severe combined immunodeficiency; wks, weeks; yr, year.

Individual Fungal Pathogens

The True Yeasts

CRYPTOCOCCUS *Cryptococcus* is by far the most common cause of fungal meningitis and meningocerebral syndromes. Cryptococcosis is a systemic infection caused by the encapsulated yeast fungus, *C. neoformans*, which has a ubiquitous distribution in soil and pigeon excreta. Infection occurs by inhalation. Occasionally a mild pulmonary infection may occur at the time of invasion. Meningitis is the most common neurological presentation, although multiple small cryptococcomas or a single large granulomatous lesion and abscess may also occur, presenting with symptoms of a mass lesion, seizures, or focal neurological deficits. Cystic lesions or hydrocephalus may develop in patients who survive. Rarely, chronic infection presents with a dementia-like syndrome. The progression of the disease depends on the degree of immunosuppression. A papular or ulcerative skin lesion, lytic bone lesions, prostatitis, and pulmonary and renal involvement occur in disseminated systemic cryptococcosis.

HISTOPLASMA Inhalation of infectious spores found in soil containing bird excreta causes histoplasmosis. The primary infection may be subclinical and many cases are diagnosed by chest radiography done for another reason. Acute pulmonary histoplasmosis may result in an influenza-like illness that may be accompanied by erythematous skin eruptions. The disease, often mistaken for miliary TB, presents as an acute or chronic febrile illness with diffuse pulmonary infiltrate, abnormal liver function, mucosal ulceration, and less often with neurological involvement (10–20%) in the form of a basilar meningitis, focal cerebritis, or CNS granuloma. Headache, fever, and neck stiffness are seen in about half of the cases. Manifest disease may occur even after leaving an endemic zone, indicating the importance of taking a travel history. Diffuse disease is seen in immunocompromised hosts and at the extremes of age. Approximately 50% of patients who have a CNS infection develop subacute meningitis, whereas 40% have cerebral abscess. The meningitis usually occurs in the setting of disseminated infection but may occur by itself.

BLASTOMYCES Blastomycosis is a systemic disease caused by *Blastomyces dermatitidis*, which proliferates as a saprophyte in soil, and it typically infects healthy individuals. Inhalation of the mycelial form results in the disease. Both systemic and cutaneous forms of blastomycosis may follow pulmonary infection. Neurological involvement occurs in 6–35% of individuals with disseminated blastomycosis and is characterized by intracranial or spinal abscesses or meningitis. Meningitis is often accompanied by rapid deterioration. Infection of vertebrae may lead to osteolytic lesions, which are often painless and may spread to the contiguous soft tissue. For some reason, blastomycosis is not significantly more common in HIV or AIDS and it is not identified as an AIDS-defining infection.

COCCIDIOIDES　Inhalation of airborne spores of *Coccidioides immitis* found in soil results in coccidioidomycosis. Although most cases are self-limiting, chronic pulmonary, skin, or disseminated disease occurs in approximately 1% of patients. The male gender, extremes of age, non-Caucasian race, pregnancy, and immunosuppressed state are known to predispose to disseminated coccidioidomycosis. Lytic skull and vertebral lesions are seen in approximately one third of patients with disseminated disease. The vertebral arch is most frequently involved initially. Involvement of the vertebral body and disc space classically seen in TB is uncommon. Meningitis may be the presenting feature and usually occurs within 6 months of symptomatic or asymptomatic primary infection. Nonspecific signs and symptoms of headache, fever, malaise, and weakness are common, but seizures, cranial nerve palsies, and focal neurological deficits may also occur. The meningitis, if present, is more intense than cryptococcal meningitis. Prominent basilar meningitis frequently leads to the development of obstructive hydrocephalus and meningeal vasculitis may cause occlusions of arteries, leading to cerebral infarcts. If untreated, more than 50% of patients with coccidioidal meningitis die within 8 months.

PARACOCCIDIOIDES　Paracoccidioidomycosis is endemic in Central and South America, particularly Brazil, where it resides in soil and chiefly affects laborers in rural areas. Pulmonary infection is usually self-limiting. Dissemination occurs in immunosuppressed patients. Progressive pulmonary disease and extrapulmonary involvement of skin, lymph nodes, and the CNS are common clinical manifestations. Cerebral and cerebellar masses are also seen.

The Pseudohyphae
CANDIDA　The *Candida* species are normal commensals of the human respiratory, gastrointestinal, and genitourinary tracts. Although *Candida* is the fourth most common organism isolated from blood, CNS infection is uncommon in healthy hosts. In the immunodeficient host, it causes nosocomial and disseminated infection. *Candida albicans* is the most important pathogenic species causing neurological involvement. Patients with malignancies, debilitation, those receiving corticosteroids or

broad-spectrum antibiotics, transplant recipients, critically ill neonates, and postoperative neurosurgery patients are predisposed to *Candida* infection. Involvement of multiple organs, including the brain parenchyma, meninges, and eye, is often seen in disseminated disease. Intracranial abscesses, small vessel thromboses, and microinfarcts occur in areas of vasculitis and tend to have a predilection for the middle cerebral artery. Hemorrhage may occur because of mycotic aneurysms. Coexistence of ophthalmological and dermatological infection provides a helpful clue to the diagnosis. Patients with endophthalmitis often report blurred vision, eye pain, or scotoma. White cotton-like exudates are seen in the retina on funduscopic examination.

The True Hyphae

ASPERGILLUS *Aspergillus* has a predilection for growing on stored grain and decaying vegetation. It mainly affects the paranasal sinuses and causes a hypersensitivity pneumonitis. CNS disease results from direct extension and invasion or embolization. Dissemination from a primary pulmonary focus occurs in immunosuppressed patients, particularly transplant recipients. The posterior circulation is particularly vulnerable resulting in vertebrobasilar strokes. A strokelike syndrome occurs from direct vessel wall invasion, resulting in vasculitis or from rapidly progressing parenchymal granuloma or brain abscess. *Aspergillus* sinusitis may infiltrate intracranially causing a rhinocerebral syndrome. Pulmonary infection may invade the thoracic vertebrae and then the epidural space, causing spinal cord compression. Meningitis is generally rare but may occur after transsphenoidal surgery and in intravenous drug abusers.

Zygomycetes (Mucormycosis)

The Zygomycetes belong to a group of saprophytic fungi growing on decaying vegetation or food of high sugar content. Infection is usually sporadic with a worldwide distribution. Diabetes and acidosis are the most common predisposing conditions; however, malignancies, high-dose corticosteroids, renal transplantation, and iron chelation therapy in hemochromatosis also predispose individuals to this infection. Mucormycosis causes pulmonary and cutaneous manifestations. Rhino-orbitocerebral invasion and cerebral mucormycosis occur after head or orbital trauma. *Mucor* invades through vascular channels, producing occlusive ischemic lesions in single or several anatomically related sites. Within the CNS, zygomycosis causes an acute necrotizing tissue reaction and thrombosis of neighboring vessels. Cavernous sinus and internal carotid artery thromboses are common. A black regional discharge, such as from the nose, indicates necrosis of the underlying tissue and should suggest the diagnosis of mucormycosis. Ocular manifestations occur because of ischemia and present with loss of vision, optic nerve pallor, corneal ulcer, ocular gangrene, choroidal infarction, and central retinal or ophthalmic artery occlusion.

Other Fungal Pathogens
Sporotrichosis is caused by infection by *Sporothrix schenckii*. Cutaneous sporotrichosis presents as single or multiple chronic ulcers, spreading along regional lymphatics. Disseminated infection affects the CNS (meningitis), joints, and lungs. *Pseudallescheria boydii* is another uncommon opportunistic pathogen. It characteristically presents as neutrophilic meningitis or multiple brain abscesses. Factors predisposing to CNS infection by *P. boydii* include immunosuppression or aspiration of contaminated water (near drowning).

Diagnosis

Fungal infections of CNS may challenge physician's diagnostic skills. To diagnose them early, physicians must have a high index of suspicion in any case presenting as chronic meningitis. The chronic nature of fungal infections often results in patients being anemic with elevated total leucocyte counts and erythrocyte sedimentation rate. Renal involvement results in the presence of red blood cells (RBCs), WBCs, casts and protein in urine. Urinary sediment may demonstrate fungal hyphae or yeasts depending on the load of infection. Culture of urine in fungal media often shows growth, especially in cryptococcosis. Chest x-ray may be useful in cases of concomitant lung infection. Patients with chest x-ray films showing infiltrates or abscess should undergo sputum cultures and bronchoscopy and, if needed, a biopsy. Complaints of localized bone pain should always be subjected to bone scan, as the lesion can be biopsied or aspirated. Joint radiographs are helpful if fungal arthritis is present.

Neuroimaging in the form of contrast-enhanced MRI or CT scans of the brain is important in identifying the involvement of neuraxis. MRI is superior to CT in its higher sensitivity and resolution. Meningeal enhancement, especially in the basal cisterns, is commonly seen and suggests the presence of subacute or chronic meningitis. Infections such as cryptococcal meningitis may have multiple small cerebral abscesses caused by fungal invasion of the Virchow-Robin spaces around the meningeal vessels penetrating the brain parenchyma. Hydrocephalus resulting from blockage of CSF flow at the level of the basal cisterns or at the outflow pathways from the fourth ventricle by arachnoiditis may also be observed. If the fungus directly invades the brain, neuroimaging often demonstrates an enhancing localized cerebral mass with variable surrounding edema. Large space-occupying abscesses or granulomas are associated generally with *Aspergillus, Mucor, Candida, Blastomyces,* and *Pseudallescheria.* Bland or occasionally hemorrhagic cerebral infarcts may be seen if meningitis causes vasculitis with thrombosis of arteries or veins. In suspected rhinocerebral syndromes, sinus and orbit imaging must be reviewed. Mucosal thickening, air-fluid levels, or erosion of bone in the walls of the sinus or orbit suggests rhinocerebral infection.

LP and analysis of the CSF are the most crucial tests in establishing the diagnosis of fungal meningitis. The cerebrospinal pressure is often elevated. The fluid is usually clear and colorless unless either the WBC count or the protein concentration is significantly elevated because of other associated infection in an immunocompromised host. The leucocyte count may range from 50 to 1000 cells/mm^3 with a lymphocytic predominance. A neutrophilic predominance should raise the suspicion of aspergillosis, mucormycosis, or *Pseudallescheria* infection. An eosinophilic pleocytosis suggests coccidioidal infections. CSF glucose levels are usually, but not always, decreased and range from 10 to 39 mg/dl. Very low glucose levels (<10 mg/dl) are unusual and suggest the possibility of coexisting bacterial infection. CSF protein levels are elevated and range from 50 to 1000 mg/dl. A suspicion of a subarachnoid block must arise if the protein level is very high. Gram's stain of CSF is unhelpful unless concomitant bacterial infection exists. Rarely hyphae of *Aspergillus* and coccidioides may be seen on microscopic examination of the CSF sediment. India ink examination is useful for *Cryptococcus.* An identifiable capsule and budding yeasts may be seen. A negative control of India ink should be examined to exclude the possibility of contamination of the ink with the fungus. CSF test for cryptococcal antigen latex particle agglutination is more sensitive than the India ink preparation. Other tests are still being developed for fungi; for example, PCR to detect fungal nucleic acid in fluids. Fungal culture growth, except in cryptococcal infection, is time consuming and does not always isolate the organism. Coccidioidomycosis, histoplasmosis, and blastomycosis yield a growth in only 50% of cases. The yield is even lower for other fungi. The sensitivity and specificity of CSF smear and culture increase with repeated examinations of large volumes of CSF, centrifuging the CSF, and subjecting the sediment to culture. The isolation of fungus is important as drug sensitivity patterns can be determined. However, one must also be aware of the possibility of contamination, especially in the case of *Candida* and *Aspergillus*.

Serological tests can be performed on blood and CSF. CSF serological tests may be difficult to interpret. In the early stage, the presence of low titers could indicate active infection, immunosuppressed state, or a past infection that is inactive. A high antibody titer suggests an active systemic infection.

If biopsy of a lesion is obtained, it should be subjected to culture in addition to the histopathological investigations. Often a biopsy is the only way to identify infection caused by *Mucor* and *Aspergillus*. Attempts to harvest fungi from other involved sites, such as skin, lung, lymph node, joint, paranasal, or bone marrow, enhance the rate of detection by 10–35%.

Therapy of Fungal Infections

Antifungal Agents

Amphotericin B is the treatment of choice for most fungal infections of the CNS (see Table 28.7). This agent is a polyene compound that binds to the ergosterol component of fungal cell membranes. It acts by increasing the permeability of the cell membrane, resulting in the leakage of intracellular contents and lysis of the cells. The serum half-life of amphotericin B is approximately 12–24 hours, with peak serum levels lasting 6–8 hours. Excretion is chiefly in the urine. Depending on achievable concentrations, it is either fungistatic or fungicidal. It has no effect on other classes of pathogens.

Limitations of amphotericin B include its poor penetration of the blood-brain barrier, making it difficult to achieve effective fungicidal levels in brain. The drug also has renal toxicity (up to 80%) and it causes electrolyte wasting (K^+ and Mg^{2+}), normochromic-normocytic anemia and a flulike allergic reaction after intravenous use. CNS toxicity limits its intrathecal use. Occasionally, life-threatening reactions like anaphylaxis, acute hepatic failure, seizures, ventricular fibrillation, and cardiac arrest may occur. Premedication with diphenhydramine, hydrocortisone, and ibuprofen for the fever and chills, antiemetics for nausea, and oral potassium supplement to guard against hypokalemia reduces adverse effects. Renal toxicity of amphotericin B is related to its peak serum concentrations and the cumulative dose. Patients should be monitored by frequent urinalyses for detection of RBC or WBC casts, serum creatinine levels, and creatinine clearance. Inability to use this drug orally limits its use in therapy. Idiosyncratic reactions may force cessation of medication. Amphotericin B should be avoided in patients who are hypersensitive to the drug, unless it is the only possible therapy in the face of a life-threatening fungal disorder. In spite of all these limitations, it is the initial choice in induction therapy for most CNS infections, particularly those that are life threatening. New lipid formulations of amphotericin B (vide infra) have been developed to overcome the toxicity, and they, although expensive, are as effective as the original drug.

Flucytosine, which was initially developed as an antineoplastic agent, is commonly given as an adjunct to amphotericin B to patients with invasive infections by *Cryptococcus*, *Candida*, and *Aspergillus*. The drug interferes with the metabolism of fungal nucleic acid and disrupts its genetic code. It is rapidly absorbed from the alimentary tract, has minimal protein binding, and is excreted unchanged in urine. CSF concentrations reach 75% of serum. The serum half-life is 3–5 hours. When given alone, flucytosine has few side effects, which include rash, eosinophilia, diarrhea, and hepatic dysfunction; however, in combination with amphotericin B, bone marrow suppression is the major side effect. Blood levels exceeding 100 µg/ml are associated with increased incidence of these complications. Existing renal failure calls for adjustment of dosage. A twice-weekly leukocyte count and platelet count are mandatory in these cases. Flucytosine blood level estimations are done in reference mycology laboratories and are important in patients with azotemia. Blood levels for flucytosine should be drawn 2 hours after the last flucytosine dose and just before the next dose once or twice a week and should be between 50 and 100 µg/ml.

Fluconazole and itraconazole are synthetic broad-spectrum antifungal agents that belong to the triazole (azoles) class. They act by inhibition of the synthesis of ergosterol and cause accumulation of substituted sterols, which interfere with the permeability of the fungal cell membrane. Fungal cell membranes are far more sensitive to these agents than mammalian ones. Azole antifungals are generally considered to be fungistatic rather than fungicidal. The advantage of these drugs is that they are less toxic, can be administered orally, and have good blood-brain barrier penetration. The disadvantage is a lower cure rate. The cure rate is low for cryptococcosis and still lower for aspergillosis with azoles alone. *In vitro* and animal studies have suggested that concomitant administration of amphotericin B and azole drugs may show antagonistic effects. The use of azoles is hence limited for maintenance therapy to prevent recurrences of coccidioidal, cryptococcal, and histoplasma meningitis.

Itraconazole has properties similar to fluconazole except for its poor penetration of the blood-brain barrier. Adverse effects of azoles are uncommon but include nausea, abdominal pain, headache, dizziness, rash, reversible alopecia, pedal edema, and transiently increased liver enzymes. Physicians must watch for drug interactions of antifungal azoles with other drugs to prevent side effects or lack of effectiveness of the primary medication.

Newer Agents

Lipid amphotericin preparations (liposomal amphotericin B, amphotericin B cholesteryl, and amphotericin B lipid complex) have the advantage of lower toxicity and infusion-related side effects. The half-life of these preparations varies and the larger particles are mostly cleared by the reticuloendothelial system faster. The disadvantages of lipid formulation are higher cost and lower CNS permeability compared to the original drug. The CSF/plasma concentration at steady state for amphotericin B is typically less than 25%, and lower for lipid formulations. Doses of lipid formulations range from 3 to 5 mg/kg per day. There seems to be no major difference in the overall efficacy between the two preparations. A favorable initial response of amphotericin B may permit a switch to a less toxic antifungal preparation after a period. Voriconazole, a new triazole derivative, has broad-spectrum antifungal activity and is especially useful for aspergillosis and candidiasis. Doses vary from 50 to 200 mg per day. SCH59562 is another triazole with apparently greater potency than voriconazole and is under investigation. Agents that boost the immune system, which is often deranged in patients with fungal infections, may help treat invasive fungal infection. Cytokines and γ-interferon are being tried in CNS fungal infections and continue to remain experimental at this stage.

Surgery

Surgical procedure may be critical for CNS fungal treatment, especially in cases of invasive rhinocerebral fungal disease. Surgical biopsy may also be essential for establishing the diagnosis. Among the procedures of therapeutic relevance are exenteration of infected facial, nasal, and intracranial tissues in cases of mucormycosis and aspergillosis, extirpation or drainage of fungal cerebral abscess, repair of rare mycotic aneurysm, and surgical drainage of hydrocephalus complicating fungal meningitis. Hydrocephalus can occur in any fungal meningitis and is seen in as many as 15% of cases of cryptococcal meningitis. Acute hydrocephalus may require emergent ventricular drainage and chronic hydrocephalus a ventriculoperitoneal shunt. Ventricular shunt in the face of active fungal meningitis may produce ventriculitis. In cryptococcal meningitis with communicating hydrocephalus, daily LP may also alleviate symptoms. However, LP is contraindicated in patients with intracranial mass lesions, such as fungal abscess and intracranial shifts on imaging studies. With elevated ICP, LP should be performed cautiously, especially in patients with low-lying cerebellar tonsils, to avoid tonsillar herniation. The latter has even been observed following LP in the absence of focal mass brain lesion.

Treatment of Specific Infections

Cryptococcal Central Nervous System Infection

Practice guidelines by the Infectious Diseases Society of the United States of America have suggested therapy beginning with amphotericin B in the dose of 0.5–1.0 mg/kg per day plus flucytosine at 100 mg/kg per day for 6–10 weeks in immunocompetent hosts with CNS cryptococcal disease. An alternative regimen is to use this combination for 2 weeks followed by fluconazole at 400 mg per day for 10 weeks or more, especially if the patient develops amphotericin B toxicity. The consolidation therapy with fluconazole may be continued for 6 months to 1 year depending on the clinical and CSF response. In patients with HIV infection, induction with amphotericin B (0.7–1.0 mg/kg per day) plus flucytosine (100 mg/kg per day) for 2 weeks followed by fluconazole (400 mg/day) is recommended. The fluconazole dose can later be reduced to 200 mg/day but generally has to be continued for life in patients with HIV or AIDS. An alternative regimen consists of amphotericin B in dosage of 0.5 to 1.0 mg/kg per day plus flucytosine at 100 mg/kg per day for 6–10 weeks followed by fluconazole maintenance therapy. If the patient does not tolerate amphotericin B, fluconazole (400–800 mg/day) with flucytosine (100–150 mg/kg per day) for 6 weeks can be used. Renal function must be monitored and serum flucytosine blood levels be kept between 50 and 100 μg/ml. Neutropenia requires that the treatment be halted. Repeated LP evaluation at 2 weeks of therapy to obtain CSF for antigen titers and fungal culture is needed to ensure the response to treatment. Relapse rates may be as high as 50%. An important predictor of final outcome in patients with HIV is the CSF culture sterility after 14 days after the initiation of treatment. Patients likely to have poor response are those with a high cryptococcal antigen level, low CD4 count, and low serum albumin level. Mass lesions larger than 3 cm may require surgery. Prophylaxis with fluconazole in AIDS is important, because about 5% to 10% of patients develop cryptococcal meningitis, especially when their CD4 count falls to less than 100 cells/mm.

Coccidioidal Central Nervous System Infection

Prolonged treatment is usually required for coccidioidal CNS infections. Recent reports suggest that long-term oral fluconazole is as effective as amphotericin B and is now the treatment of choice. Its use in the dosage of 400 mg/day orally for 4 years has been shown to result in improvement in 75% cases. Occasionally higher doses of 600–800 mg/day may be required. Signs of improvement may come only 4–8 months after beginning the treatment. Intrathecal administration of amphotericin B in a dose of 0.25–1.5 mg three times a week for several weeks with a gradual tapering to biweekly and then monthly to a total cumulative dose of 35–100 mg may be given in difficult-to-control infections. Intrathecal drug is given in conjunction with intravenous amphotericin B (0.5 mg/kg per day, up to a total cumulative dose of 3 g). The duration of treatment may need to be extended up to 1 year. As many as 78% of patients may relapse on discontinuing the therapy. This is especially so in immunocompromised patients. Hence, lifelong maintenance with fluconazole (200 mg per day) may be required.

Histoplasmal Central Nervous System Infection

Intravenous amphotericin B (0.7–1.0 mg/kg per day, for a total cumulative dose of at least 30 mg/kg or 1.5 to 2.0 g) is used in most cases. Intrathecal amphotericin B in a dose of 0.25–1.0 mg on alternate days can be given if there is no contraindication. Four to 12 weeks of induction therapy is required. Maintenance therapy is required because many patients show relapse following induction therapy alone.

Central Nervous System Mucormycosis

Mucormycosis generally occurs in the rhino-orbitocerebral form in patients with diabetic ketoacidosis or other associated illnesses (see Table 28.7). Surgical debridement is required, diabetes should be controlled, and in patients with hemochromatosis, desferrioxamine should be discontinued. Amphotericin B should be administered in rapidly increasing doses to 1.0–1.5 mg/kg per day, with an anticipated dose of 2.5–3.0 g. Hyperbaric oxygenation has been suggested by some investigators. The prognosis is generally poor.

Therapy of other major CNS fungal diseases is summarized in Table 28.7. Cure rates for cryptococcal meningitis are about 75%, coccidioidal meningitis 50%, *Histoplasma* meningitis 40%, and for aspergillosis and Zygomycetes approximately 25%. Outcome in immunosuppressed patients is less favorable and many of these patients die as a result of concomitant infections. Short- and long-term complications in CNS fungal infections are as high as 40–75% and these include hydrocephalus, infarction, cranial nerve palsies, seizures, and dementia.

PARASITIC INFECTIONS

Parasites are a group of organisms that thrive on or in the body of other organisms, deriving protection and nutrition from them. Whereas protozoa are microscopic single-celled organisms, helminths are macroscopic multicellular organisms ranging from a few millimeters to several meters in size. Changes in social, technical, political, behavioral, and economic factors have resulted in a dramatic increase in the incidence of some human parasitic infections. At least 10% of the world population is infected by *Entamoeba histolytica*, a common gut pathogen. It is estimated that one third of the world population harbors helminthic infestations. *Plasmodium falciparum* is the species responsible for 40–60% of the 200 million annual cases of malaria and 95% of malarial deaths, and thus it remains one of the top infectious disease killers in the world. Of the 1–2 million annual deaths caused by malaria, most are the result of cerebral malaria. Parasitic infections are not restricted to tropical regions. Migrations of individuals across the continents and increasing travel have enabled them to spread all over the globe. Emergence of the pandemic of AIDS has caused an exponential increase in the number of individuals affected by certain parasites. Apart from an absolute increase in the incidence, altered immunity of patients with AIDS has resulted in atypical presentation of these diseases. Parasites that are well tolerated by the human body do not elicit an inflammatory response. On the other hand, parasites that are not well tolerated develop an intense inflammatory reaction around the larvae or the adult worms, resulting in a multitude of symptoms.

Protozoan infections are responsible for acute meningitis or meningoencephalitis (*Naegleria*, African trypanosomiasis), encephalopathy (*Plasmodium* species), chronic meningitis (*Acanthamoeba*, *Toxoplasma*), space-occupying lesions of the brain (*Toxoplasma*, *E. histolytica*), neuropathy (Chagas' disease, filariasis), myositis (*Trichinella*, cysticercosis), and chorioretinitis (*Toxoplasma*). Helminths cause nervous system involvement because of their size, mobility, and challenge to the host immune response. Helminths can cause meningoencephalitis (*Taenia solium*, *Trichinella*, *Angiostrongylus*, *Gnathostoma*, *Toxocara*,

Strongyloides, Schistosoma, etc.), encephalopathy (*Trichinella, Loa loa*), cerebral mass lesions (*Taenia, Echinococcus, Gnathostoma, Schistosoma*), and ocular involvement (*Taenia, Angiostrongylus, Gnathostoma, Loa loa, Toxocara*) (Table 28.8). Invasion through the foramina of skull and vertebral column and of tissues surrounding nerves can cause features of nerve or nerve root compression or compressive myelopathy (*Schistosoma*). Ectoparasites do not invade the tissues of the host but release toxins that may affect the nervous system.

It would hardly be possible within the confines of this chapter to discuss with any degree of completeness the innumerable rare parasitic infections that affect the CNS. Rather we will introduce some general clinical approach to parasitic CNS infections, and deal in greater detail with important or relatively common parasitic CNS diseases. A summary of parasitic CNS infections in given in Table 28.8.

Clinical Approach to Parasitic Central Nervous System Infection

Because of the diversity of parasitic organisms that may infect the human CNS, a number of factors are important in the assessment of a possible parasitic etiology for a patient's complaints. These factors include issues related to the patient's work, travel and recreational history, immune status, and presenting neurological and other systemic symptoms. The specific laboratory tests required, ranging from standard blood biochemical assays to imaging of the brain and CSF analysis, are dictated by the nature of the patient's illness.

Geographical, Travel, and Other Exposure History
The cornerstone for the diagnosis of parasitic infections is a thorough history of the patient's illness. Epidemiological aspects of the illness are particularly important because the risk of acquiring many parasites is closely related to occupation, recreation, or travel to areas of high endemicity. A history of travel to, residence or work in, or immigration from areas of the world in which various parasites occur offers a clue to the possible parasitic etiology of a patient's disease. Some parasitic infections may become manifest early after a traveler's return to home; most important among them in terms of mortality is malaria. For patients with a history of recent travel, the onset of gastrointestinal symptoms only after return suggests protozoan diseases. Diseases that may become manifest some years after an individual leaves an endemic region include schistosomiasis, some forms of filariasis, strongyloidiasis, echinococcosis, and

Table 28.8: Parasitic infections of the central nervous system

Parasite	Range	Neurological Manifestations	Treatment of Choice	Alternative Regimen
Protozoans				
Plasmodium falciparum	Africa, South America, Southeast Asia, Pacific Islands, Haiti	E, Sz	Guided by local resistance pattern (see text) Oral: Chloroquine phosphate 600 mg base (1 g), then 300 mg base (500 mg) at 6, 24, and 48 h (if resistance, quinine sulfate plus pyrimethamine-sulfadiazine, or plus tetracycline, or plus clindamycin) Parenteral: Quinine dihydrochloride 20 mg/kg loading (maximum 600 mg) over 1/2 hr followed by 10 mg/kg every 8 hour IM or PO for 7 days	Oral: Mefloquine 750 mg followed by 500 mg 6–8 h later, or halofantrine 500 mg/q6h for 3 days, repeated after 1 week
Naegleria fowleri	Southern United States, Australia, Europe	ME	Amphotericin B 1 mg/kg/day IV for uncertain duration	—
Acanthamoeba spp.	Europe	ME, E, O	Amphotericin B 1 mg/kg/day IV plus vitampin for uncertain duration	—
Entamoeba histolytica	Tropics worldwide	M	Metronidazole 750 mg IV q8h for 10 days followed by iodoquinol 650 mg tid for 20 days	Tinidazole 600 mg bid or 800 mg tid for 5 days followed by iodoquinol 650 mg tid for 20 days
Trypanosoma brucei rhodesiense	Africa	ME	Melarsoprol 2–3.6 mg/kg/day IV for 3 days, after 1 week 3.6 mg/kg/day IV for 3 days, repeated after 10–21 days; or eflornithine 100 mg/kg qid for 14 days, then 300 mg/kg/day for 3–4 weeks	Tryparsamide 30 mg/kg (max 2 g) IV up to total 12 injections, may be repeated after 1 month, plus suramin 10 mg/kg IV q5d to total of 12 injections, sometimes repeated after 1 month

Continued

Table 28.8: (continued)

Parasite	Range	Neurological Manifestations	Treatment of Choice	Alternative Regimen
Trypanosoma brucei gambiense	Africa	ME	Melarsoprol 2–3.6 mg/kg/day IV for 3 days, after 1 week 3.6 mg/kg/day IV for 3 days, repeated after 10–21 days; or eflornithine 100 mg/kg qid for 14 days, then 300 mg/kg/day for 3–4 weeks	—
Trypanosoma cruzi	Central and South America	ME, M, St	Nifurtimox 8–10 mg/kg/day in 4 doses for 120 days	Benznidazole 5–7 mg/kg/day for 30–120 days
Toxoplasma gondii	Worldwide	ME, Sz, M, O	Pyrimethamine 25–100 mg/day plus sulfadiazine 1–1.5 g qid plus folinic acid 10 mg/day for 3–4 weeks	Clindamycin 1.8–2.4 g/day in divided dosage plus pyrimethamine 25–100 mg/day plus folinic acid 10 mg/day for 3–4 weeks or spiramycin 3–4 g/day in pregnancy, continue until delivery
Helminths				
Cestodes				
Taenia solium (cysticercosis)	Worldwide	ME, Sz, M, Sp, O	Albendazole 15 mg/kg/day in 2 doses for 8–28 days, or praziquantel 50 mg/kd/day in 3 doses for 14 days or repeated as necessary, with concurrent glucocorticoids for CNS disease	Surgery
Echinococcus gramulosus	Worldwide	Sz, M, Sp, O	Surgical excision if possible and albendazole 400 mg once; or albendazole 15 mg/kg/day for 40 days, repeated after 2 weeks	—

Echinococcus multilocularis	Arctic	Sz, M	Surgical excision	—
Taenia multiceps (Coenurosis)	Worldwide	M, O	Surgical excision	—
Spirometra spp. (Sparganosis)	Worldwide, mainly Asia, Africa	ME, Sz, M, St	Surgical excision	—
Diphyllobothrium latum	Worldwide	E, Sp, O, N (vitamin B_{12} deficiency)	Praziquantel 10 mg/kg 1 dose, vitamin B_{12}	—
Hymenolepis nana	Worldwide	E, Sz	Praziquantel 25 mg/kg 1 dose	—
Nematodes				
Trichinella spp.	Worldwide	ME, E, Sz, St	Glucocorticoids (for severe symptoms) plus mebendazole 200–400 mg tid for 3 days, then 400–500 mg tid for 10 days	—
Angiostrongylus cantonensis	Asia, Africa, Pacific, Caribbean	ME, Sz, O	Supportive therapy and glucocorticoids as needed	—
Gnathostoma spinigerum	Asia, Israel	ME, Sz, M, St, Sp, O	Surgical removal plus albendazole 400–800 mg/day for 21 days	—
Onchocerca volvulus	Africa, Central and South America, Yemen		Ivermectin 150 µg/kg/day once, repeated every 3–12 months	—
Loa loa	Africa	E, O	Diethylcarbamazine, day 1: 50 mg, day 2: 50 mg tid, day 3: 100 mg tid, days 4–21: 9 mg/kg/day in 3 doses	—
Toxocara spp.	Worldwide	ME, Sz, O	Thiabendazole 25 mg/kg bid for 5 days, supportive therapy and glucocorticoids	Diethylcarbamazine 2 mg/kg tid for 7–15 days, or mebendazole 100–200 mg bid for 5 days, or albendazole 400 mg bid for 3–5 days

Continued

Table 28.8: (continued)

Parasite	Range	Neurological Manifestations	Treatment of Choice	Alternative Regimen
Baylisascaris procyonis	Worldwide	ME, Sz	Thiabendazole 25 mg/kg bid for 5 days, supportive therapy and glucocorticoids	Mebendazole 100–200 mg bid for 5 days, or albendazole 400 mg bid for 3–5 days
Strongyloides stercoralis	Worldwide	ME, St	Thiabendazole 25 mg/kg bid for 3–7 days or longer if host is immunosuppressed	Ivermectin 200 µg/kg/day for 1–2 days, or albendazole 400 mg bid for 3 days
Ascaris lumbricoides	Worldwide	Sz	Mebendazole 100 mg bid for 3 days, or piperazine 75 mg/kg (max 3.5 g) for 2 days	Pyrental pamoate 11 mg/kg (max 1 g) or albendazole 400 mg once
Wuchereria bancrofti	Coastal areas in tropics and subtropics	N	Diethyl carbamazine 6 mg/kg/day in 3 divided doses for 12 days	Surgical resection

ME, meningoencephalitis; E, encephalitis; Sz, seizures; St, stroke; Sp, spinal cord; N, nerve.

cysticercosis. Consumption of contaminated or undercooked food may be associated with trichinosis, cysticercosis, toxocariasis, or eosinophilic meningitis (*Angiostrongylus cantonensis*). Other relevant exposure history includes blood transfusion (malaria, filariasis, Chagas' disease) and wading or swimming in a freshwater lake or pond (*Naegleria* meningitis, schistosomiasis). Residence in an institutional setting, where fecal-oral hygiene may be lacking, raises the possibility of exposure to gut parasites, such as *Entamoeba* and *Strongyloides*.

Immune Status

In patients infected with HIV, especially those with low $CD4^+$ T-cell counts, specific protozoan diseases, such as toxoplasmosis or trypanosomiasis, may develop opportunistically. Patients who are asplenic are at risk not only for overwhelming infections from encapsulated bacteria, but also for fulminant intraerythrocytic protozoa, including malaria. In patients developing symptoms of enterocolitis while receiving corticosteroids, the possibility of exacerbation of unsuspected strongyloidiasis or amoebic colitis should be considered.

Laboratory Investigations

Most protozoa and helminths are excreted from the body in the feces. Stool samples therefore should be collected and examined for ova and parasites in appropriate clinical settings. Because of cyclic shedding of most parasites in the feces, a minimum of three samples collected on alternate days should be examined. Microscopic examination of feces is not complete until direct wet mounts have been evaluated.

Eosinophilia in blood may offer a hematological clue to the presence of parasites. Protozoan infections restricted to the CNS, however, do not cause eosinophilia. Thus eosinophilia in the face of CNS parasitic infection mandates a consideration of the multicellular helminthic parasites that characteristically elicit this abnormality. Helminth-elicited eosinophilia, however, may be suppressed by glucocorticoid therapy or by intercurrent bacterial or viral infections. The magnitude of eosinophilia generally correlates with the extent of tissue invasion by the helminths. Marked eosinophilia (>2500 eosinophils/µl) develops during early tissue migration of nematodes. Eosinophilia is also marked in the early stages of trematode infections, including schistosomiasis (Katayama's fever), paragonimiasis, and fascioliasis, during the stage of muscle invasion (trichinosis), during tissue migration of adult worms (loiasis and gnathostomiasis), and with heavy infections in visceral larva migrans. Eosinophilia persisting for more than a year may be indicative of strongyloidiasis, visceral larva migrans, filarial infection, trematode infections, or cysticercosis. Leakage of fluid from echinococcus cysts can cause intermittent eosinophilia. Eosinophilia may be the only clue to the presence of helminthic infection, and it should prompt an evaluation for such infection.

Laboratory procedures may detect parasites in body fluids. The most common parasites detected in Giemsa-stained blood smears are the *Plasmodium* species, microfilariae, and African trypanosomes. The diagnosis of malaria and the critical distinction between the various *Plasmodium* species is made by the microscopic examination of stained thick and thin blood films.

The value of serum antibody assays is generally limited in parasitic CNS infections. The detection of serum antibody to *Plasmodium* is primarily an epidemiological tool and is of limited use for establishing the diagnosis of malaria in an individual patient. Filarial antigens cross-react with those from other nematodes, and antibody assay cannot distinguish between past and current infections. Despite these specific limitations, the restricted geographical distribution of many of the tropical parasites increases the usefulness of antibody detection as a means of establishing diagnosis in travelers from industrialized countries who have returned from the tropics. The presence of a specific IgM antibody in CSF indicates active CNS disease, such as in CNS toxoplasmosis. PCR for the detection of *Plasmodium* DNA is now available.

Imaging Studies
Contrast-enhanced MRI or CT studies of the brain and spinal cord can identify meningeal enhancement (parasitic meningitis), parameningeal infections (including parasitic granulomas), or intraparenchymal lesions (cysticercosis, echinococcosis). Imaging studies are also useful to localize areas of meningeal or parenchymal disease prior to meningeal or brain biopsy or lesion resection.

Cerebrospinal Fluid Analysis
Once the clinical syndrome is recognized as a potential manifestation of parasitic CNS infection, LP and CSF analysis are essential. However, if the possibility of raised ICP exists, a brain imaging study should be performed before LP. In patients with communicating hydrocephalus caused by impaired absorption of CSF, LP is generally safe and may lead to temporary improvement. However, if ICP is elevated because of a mass lesion or a block in ventricular CSF outflow (obstructive hydrocephalus), then LP carries the potential risk of brain

herniation and death. Acute obstructive hydrocephalus usually requires direct ventricular drainage of CSF.

The CSF pressure should be measured and samples sent for cell count and differential, measurement of glucose and protein, microbial stain, and other investigations. When eosinophils predominate or are present in limited numbers in a primary mononuclear cell response in the CSF, parasitic disease must be considered (*A. cantonensis, Gnathostoma spinigerum, T. canis, T. gondii*, cysticercosis, schistosomiasis, and echinococcal disease). Centrifugation of CSF and wet mount preparation with Giemsa stain may reveal parasites in African trypanosomiasis and *Naegleria fowleri*. IgM antibodies against *T. gondii* in blood or CSF suggest recent infection. Other specific CSF tests should be ordered as indicated on the basis of the clinical picture.

Meningeal or Brain Biopsy

A diagnostic brain biopsy should be considered in patients who are severely disabled, who need chronic ventricular decompression, or whose illness is progressing rapidly. Targeting regions that enhance with contrast on MRI or CT scan can increase the diagnostic yield of biopsy. Single symptomatic lesions (*Cysticercus, Echinococcus*) can be resected for both diagnosis and treatment. The activities of surgeon, pathologist, microbiologist, and cytologist should be coordinated so an adequate sample is obtained and appropriate histological and molecular studies, including PCR, are performed.

Protozoan Infection of the Central Nervous System

Cerebral Malaria

Malaria caused by organisms in the genus *Plasmodium* is one of the oldest and most dreaded protozoan diseases, affecting more than 500 million people each year throughout the world. The endemic zones for malaria, sub-Saharan Africa, Asia, and Central and South America, account for most cases. In hyperendemic areas most children acquire infection with *Plasmodium* before they reach 5 years of age. Infants younger than 6 months enjoy immunity inherited from their mothers. World Health Organization defines cerebral malaria as unexplained unconsciousness lasting 30 minutes or more in a patient with asexual forms of *P. falciparum* in the peripheral blood smear. It occurs in about 0.5–1.0% of infections with *P. falciparum*. Although many cases are caused by *P. falciparum*, a few case reports of cerebral malaria caused by *Plasmodium vivax* are recorded.

Natural transmission of all species of *Plasmodium* occurs by the female *Anopheles* mosquito. Accidental transmission occurs through blood transfusion, laboratory accidents, experimental infection, and zoonotic infection. The female *Anopheles* mosquitoes inject the sporozoites form of *Plasmodium* into the host body during a blood meal. Sporozoites undergo successive developmental stages of trophozoites, schizont, and merozoites that are liberated into the circulation by rupture of erythrocytes, thus ending the asexual cycle.

PATHOGENESIS Pathogenesis of cerebral malaria is ill understood. Evidence based on animal models suggests that the fundamental process in cerebral malaria is the increased cytoadherence caused by formation of knobs on parasitized RBCs (pRBCs) containing schizonts. Other endothelial factors such as leucocyte differentiation molecule (LD36), intercellular adhesion molecule-1 (ICAM-1), and thrombospondin, an extracellular matrix protein, may help in the process of cytoadherence. Additionally, an immune-mediated proinflammatory response caused by tumor necrosis factor-α (TNF-α), interleukin-1 (IL-1), and other cytokines may aggravate cytoadhesion, leading to cerebral microvascular occlusion, cerebral anoxia, and ischemic cerebral damage. Activation of nitric oxide synthetase and the complement cascade induced by prostaglandins and glyco-phosphatidylinositol, leading to inflammation, may also be contributory. Hypoglycemia and acidosis, common complications of cerebral malaria, produce or worsen encephalopathy and neurological deficit.

PATHOLOGY Pathological description in cerebral malaria is necessarily based on severe cases, which are eventually fatal. Grossly, the brain is heavy and the meningeal vessels are congested, giving a pink hue to brain. Microscopically engorged blood vessels containing pRBCs with asexual forms of parasite can be seen. Petechial hemorrhages showing engorged blood vessel in the center and a surrounding ring of extravasated RBCs are called *ring hemorrhages* and are a characteristic finding in cerebral malaria. "Durks nodules" are granulomas consisting of central demyelinated core with inflammatory cells in the ring hemorrhage. Immunohistochemical staining shows amyloid precursor protein in ring hemorrhages indicative of axonal damage.

CLINICAL FEATURES The incubation period depends to a large extent on the immune status, species of *Plasmodium*, dose of inoculation and pretreatment with prophylactic drugs. In *P. falciparum* the mean incubation period is 12 days but may be 6–12 hours in children and if a massive dose is inoculated. The prodrome consisting of lassitude, myalgia, headache, and chills usually precedes the acute attack. High-grade fever (104° to 105°F), shaking chills, and rigors with diaphoresis announce the presence of malaria. Rarely, patients may have hypothermia from shock and endotoxemia. The periodicity of fever in *P. falciparum* malaria is once every third day, but it may not be obvious because of multiple exposures and several cycles of parasitemia. Being a systemic disease, malaria may cause such symptoms as nausea, vomiting, abdominal pain, cough, tachycardia, arthralgia, myalgia, and weakness. Most patients have enlarged liver and spleen with chest rales and muscle tenderness.

Cerebral symptoms start with seizures (generalized or partial), acute-onset delirium, or coma. In children, seizures are more common (70%) as compared to adults (20%), and one third of patients may present with status epilepticus. Other CNS manifestations include headache, meningismus, focal neurological deficits (aphasia, ataxia, hemiplegia, chorea, and tremor), neuro-ophthalmological signs (conjugate gaze disturbance, oculomotor palsies, ocular bobbing, and nystagmus), retinal hemorrhages (up to 15%), and rarely papilledema (<1%). In endemic areas, the presence of febrile encephalopathy with nearly normal CSF findings warrants a diagnosis of cerebral malaria. Systemic effects of severe malaria often complicate the clinical picture and adversely affect the prognosis. The systemic effects include severe anemia, renal complications with oliguria/anuria and azotemia, jaundice, pulmonary edema, adult respiratory distress syndrome, resistant hypoglycemia, secondary infections, and septicemia.

Cerebral malaria carries a mortality of 20–50%, being higher in children. Important prognostic factors are level of consciousness at the time of presentation and the presence of complications. Additionally, recurrent seizures, absent corneal reflex, decerebrate rigidity, retinal hemorrhage, age younger than 3 years, high degree of parasitemia, peripheral schizothemia, RBC mass less than 20%, peripheral leucocytosis, lactic acidosis, elevated CSF lactate, elevated serum transferases, and low antithrombin III levels are associated with a poor prognosis. Although complete recovery occurs in most who survive, sequelae are reported in 10–18%, being higher in children. Ataxia, hemiparesis, memory disturbance, neuropsychological deficits, visual field defects, vertigo, cognitive impairment, behavioral abnormalities, and psychosis are common sequelae, which are mostly reversible in 4–8 weeks. A postmalaria neurological syndrome characterized by acute-onset confusion, seizures, ataxia, myoclonus, tremor, and aphasia is described in patients successfully treated for cerebral malaria in the absence of parasitemia. The pathogenesis of this syndrome is not understood, but immunological mechanism seems to be involved, because the condition is responsive to corticosteroids.

DIAGNOSIS Diagnosis and species identification requires examination of thick and thin smears of peripheral blood stained with Giemsa or Field's stain for the presence of ring-shaped trophozoites. Cerebral malaria usually occurs when more than 10% of peripheral RBCs are parasitized. Absence of trophozoites in the peripheral smear may occur because of sequestration of pRBCs in the cerebral circulation or earlier treatment with antimalarial drugs, as it is a common practice in endemic areas to treat all fevers with antimalarial drugs. If the initial smear is negative, two or three smears 6–8 hours later should be repeated (at least three smears should be declared negative before excluding the diagnosis of malaria).

CSF examination is necessary to exclude other causes of febrile encephalopathies (meningitis, encephalitis, enteric encephalopathy, yellow fever, viral hemorrhagic fever, relapsing fever, leptospirosis, and heat stroke). In cerebral malaria, the CSF is largely normal. However, mild lymphocytic pleocytosis (10–50 cells/μl), and mildly elevated protein (up to 200 mg/dl) may be seen. Neuroimaging with CT and MRI in cerebral malaria is usually normal or it shows edema or cortical or subcortical infarcts in the watershed zones in a small number of cases (15–20%). Recently, a dipstick antigen capture assay for malarial antigen PfHRP2 has shown 75–96% sensitivity and 87–100% specificity. However, its cost prohibits its use where it is maximally needed. Immunochromatographic tests and PCR for malarial parasites in the CSF and blood are also available. Electroencephalograms (EEGs) show a number of abnormalities such as diffuse slowing of background, burst suppression, or spikes and wave discharges but is nonspecific for diagnostic purpose. Cerebral malaria may occur with negative blood smears. A high index of suspicion in endemic areas is the key to successful treatment in a case of high fever, rigors, encephalopathy, seizures, anemia, jaundice, diarrhea, hemorrhages, renal failure, and respiratory distress. In such cases with a history of malaria exposure, treatment with antimalarial drugs should be initiated even before evidence of parasitemia becomes available.

TREATMENT Mortality in cerebral malaria is 20–50% and virtually 100% if untreated for 48 hours. In endemic areas, if cerebral malaria is suspected, treatment should be started without waiting for laboratory confirmation.

In most tropical and endemic countries, the parasite has developed resistance to chloroquine because of its widespread use. Quinine dihydrochloride is the drug of choice. Because of alteration in the pharmacokinetics of quinine related to the volume of distribution and renal clearance in severe malaria, an intravenous loading dose of 20 mg of quinine dihydrochloride in dextrose or saline per kilogram over 30 minutes is advocated to achieve rapid therapeutic concentration in severe cases. The loading dose can be omitted if the patient has already received quinine. Maintenance dose is 10 mg/kg infused over 2–8 hours. The maximum daily dose is 1800 mg. This dose can be used for all age-groups. Therapeutic minimal parasiticidal concentration after oral treatment is achieved in about 4 hours. Once patients regain consciousness, oral treatment with quinine at 10 mg/kg every 8 hours can be started. Total duration of treatment is 7 days. Alternatively, 600 mg of quinine can be given orally thrice a day in an adult. In patients who do not tolerate quinine because of severe vomiting, hypersensitivity or hypoglycemia, quinidine gluconate in doses of 10 mg/kg base can be infused intravenously over 1 hour under cardiac monitoring, followed by continuous intravenous infusion at the rate of 0.02 mg/kg per hour for 7–10 days or longer. Concurrently or immediately following quinine dihydrochloride, tetracycline (250 mg every 6 hours) or pyrimethamine (25 mg)-sulfadiazine (500 mg) every 8 hours should also be administered. In multidrug-resistant malaria artemisia derivatives (derived from traditional Chinese medicine *ginghaosu*), artemether and artesunate, are used. The dose of artemether is 3.2 mg/kg intramuscularly as a loading dose followed by 1.6 mg/kg intramuscularly every day for 4 days plus mefloquine 750 mg orally on the last day of treatment; or artesunate 2 mg/kg intravenous loading dose, followed by 1 mg/kg intravenously at 4 hours and 24 hours, then daily for 6 days. In children, mefloquine solution given by nasogastric tube in a single dose of 25 mg/kg has been found to be as effective as intravenous quinine.

Treatment of Complications Hypoglycemia, resulting from consumption of glucose by parasites, malabsorption, and increased pancreatic secretion of insulin induced by quinine, may be severe in young children and pregnant women and is an important prognostic factor. It should be suspected in patients who show deterioration despite adequate treatment and is treated by infusion of 50% dextrose. Anemia can be severe, with hematocrit levels falling by 8–10% in 48 hours in severe parasitemia. Blood transfusion should be given to keep the hemoglobin at 7 g/dl. In children, exchange transfusion is safe because it also clears the parasite load and does not alter hemodynamics. Raised ICP is also common in children and requires ICP monitoring. Use of corticosteroids has been reported to be associated with increased risk of seizures and gastrointestinal hemorrhages in patients with cerebral malaria. However, there is insufficient evidence to contraindicate the use of corticosteroids in cerebral malaria. Other complications such as renal failure, lactic acidosis, disseminated intravascular coagulation, shock, gastrointestinal hemorrhage, pulmonary edema, and gram-negative septicemia need to be managed as they appear. Adjuvant therapy with Vitamin A, immunoglobulins, monoclonal antibodies, and others has been used without change in morbidity or mortality.

PREVENTION Area-specific guidelines for malaria control can be obtained from the regional World Health Organization centers. Chemoprophylaxis with adequate drugs can be used for prevention of transmission of the disease. It should be given to all individuals traveling to malaria-endemic zones. Vector control is difficult because of resistance of mosquitoes to various insecticides. Recently, the entire genome of *P. falciparum* and *Anopheles* mosquito has been decoded, and this may help in finding ways to better control malaria.

African Trypanosomiasis
African trypanosomiasis or sleeping sickness (*malaise du sommeil*) is caused by *Trypanosoma brucei gambiense* (Gambian trypanosomiasis) or *Trypanosoma brucei rhodesiense* (Rhodesian trypanosomiasis).

African trypanosomiasis occurs in a wide belt of the African continent between latitude of 10 degrees north to 25 degrees south. Gambian trypanosomiasis is more widely distributed in western and central Africa, whereas Rhodesian trypanosomiasis is limited to east and southeast Africa. The official incidence of about 20,000–50,000 cases per year is probably an underestimation, as a large number of cases are not reported because of unavailability of medical facilities. In the wild, reservoir hosts are pigs and dogs for *T. brucei gambiense* and antelope, wild hogs and cattle for *T. brucei rhodesiense*. It is spread by tsetse fly of the genus *Glossina*. Humans contract the disease by the bite of tsetse fly when they go hunting, searching for water and food in areas where the infected reservoirs and vector abound. About 25–50 million people in sub-Saharan Africa live in the endemic zone, wherein more than 200 hyperendemic zones are recognized. Other causes of spread include laboratory accident, blood transfusion, transplacental spread, and perhaps by bites of other insect vectors.

PATHOGENESIS AND PATHOLOGY The pathogenesis of CNS trypanosomiasis is poorly understood. Inoculation of the parasite by the tsetse fly is followed by formation of a nodule caused by an inflammatory response and parasitic replication (stage 1). Recurrent bouts of parasitemia follow thereafter resulting in the hemolymphatic stage (stage 2). The parasites gain access to the brain and meninges through the choroid plexus and Virchow-Robin spaces (stage 3). African trypanosomes are densely coated with a glycoprotein called the *variant surface glycoprotein*, which keeps on changing its antigenic character with each new population of trypanosomes. This may result in letting the trypanosome escape immunological control even after the mounting of IgM antibodies against a large number of antigenic subtypes. Mechanism of damage to the host tissue is unknown.

The characteristic pathological finding of CNS trypanosomiasis is meningoencephalitis, with infiltration of perivascular and Virchow-Robin spaces by dense lymphocytic and plasmacytic inflammatory infiltrate, accompanied by glial proliferation. The meninges are covered by a milky white exudate, especially in the region of vertex where the meninges are adherent to each other and the skull. The choroid plexus shows inflammation, round cell infiltration, and edema. The brain is swollen with cerebral vascular congestion. Perivascular demyelination of the subcortical white matter is seen in most cases. Hemorrhagic leukoencephalopathy with fibrinoid necrosis of parenchymal vasculature may also occur.

CLINICAL FEATURES Characteristically the disease can be recognized as occurring in stages. The first stage is characterized by formation of a chancre at the site of the fly bite, the second stage is the hemolymphatic stage, and the third stage is the systemic stage with involvement of the CNS. A firm tender nodule (chancre), 2–5 cm, develops in 20–50% of patients 10–14 days after the bite of the tsetse fly. This may ulcerate with enlargement of regional lymph nodes, lasting for 1–2 weeks. This is followed within 1–5 weeks by the hemolymphatic stage characterized by high-grade intermittent fever, sweating, nausea, vomiting, general malaise, arthralgia, and generalized lymphadenopathy, often coinciding with bouts of parasitemia. Other symptoms are headache, dizziness, tachycardia, debility, amenorrhea, and sterility as parasitemia worsens. During this stage, each bout of parasitemia is associated with the liberation of successive generation of parasites with slightly different surface antigens. Treatment, if commenced at this stage, is associated with good prognosis. The hemolymphatic stage can lead to the systemic stage with CNS involvement or several cycles of hemolymphatic stage may occur before the CNS is involved. The pace of disease is rapid in Rhodesian trypanosomiasis, whereas it is more chronic and indolent in Gambian disease, with easy identification of different clinical stages.

The systemic stage is also associated with liberation of new generation of parasites lasting 1–6 days at several week intervals. The systemic stage is characterized by serous effusions, pancarditis, deep hyperesthetic pain out of proportion to injury (Kerandel's sign), and lymphadenopathy, particularly of the posterior cervical lymph nodes (Winterbottom's sign) in the Gambian form. CNS involvement is indicated by the presence of psychological and behavioral changes. Initial symptoms of lethargy, apathy, indifference, euphoria, or depression give way to insomnia (10%), daytime hypersomnolence, disturbance of circadian rhythm, chorea, rigidity, tremors, ataxia, and hemiplegia. Less commonly, seizures, cranial neuropathies, and altered mentation occur. Eventually patients develop increasing drowsiness and finally coma. Untreated patients with *T. rhodesiense* infection generally die 6–9 months after the onset of the disease.

DIAGNOSIS Diagnosis is made by demonstration of parasites in the peripheral blood, lymph node aspirate, bone marrow, or CSF. Examination of wet peripheral smear of blood stained with Giemsa stain can demonstrate motile parasites. Repeated examination is necessary because parasitemia is intermittent. Using thick smear, microhematocrit centrifugation, anion exchange, or buffy coat preparation can increase the chances of parasite detection. CNS involvement is confirmed by demonstration of the motile trypanosome in the CSF, although it occurs in only 17% of severe cases of sleeping sickness. CSF examination shows lymphocytic pleocytosis and elevated protein, IgM levels, oligoclonal bands, and morular or Mott cells, which are modified plasma cells containing large eosinophilic inclusions. Although these cells are not pathognomonic of trypanosomiasis, their presence in large numbers is fairly characteristic of the disease. Neuroimaging with CT scan shows meningeal, choroidal, or parenchymal enhancement but is not specific. EEG shows diffuse nonspecific generalized slowing of background activity, especially in the later stages.

The elevation of IgM in both serum and CSF can be used as a screening test in endemic regions. Serological techniques such as indirect hemagglutination and immunofluorescence to detect trypanosomal antigen are reported to be sensitive but high antigenic variability of these parasites poses a major diagnostic problem. ELISAs and immunofluorescent antibody tests allow detection of antibodies in the CSF. Animal inoculation technique, although sensitive, is time consuming, expensive, and impractical in field conditions. The disease should be differentiated from febrile disorders with lymphadenopathy, headache, sleep disorders, malaria, infectious mononucleosis, arboviral encephalitides, leukemia, lymphoma, TB, syphilis, brucellosis, relapsing fever, toxoplasmosis, and onchocerciasis.

TREATMENT Before initiating therapy, confirmation of the diagnosis is essential because most of the drugs used for the treatment of trypanosomiasis are highly toxic. *T. brucei gambiense* in the hemolymphatic stage is treated with intramuscular pentamidine at 3 mg/kg per day for 10 days. For *T. brucei rhodesiense* in the hemolymphatic stage, intravenous suramin in the dose of 20 mg/kg per day with a maximum of 1 g/day is given on days 1, 3, 7, 14, and 21. A suramin test dose of 200–300 mg is essential, because a severe idiosyncratic reaction presenting with shock is not uncommon. Suramin is nephrotoxic; hence, it cannot be given to patients with pre-existing renal disease. Prolonged use of suramin results in an axonal sensorimotor neuropathy. Both suramin and pentamidine do not cross the blood-brain barrier and therefore are not effective in the meningoencephalitic stage of the disease.

For meningoencephalitic trypanosomiasis eflornithine (difluoromethyl ornithine [DFMO]), a polyamine synthetase inhibitor, has shown promise but is expensive. A 14-day course of DFMO in the dose 100 mg/kg intravenously every 6 hours for primary meningoencephalitic trypanosomiasis and a 7-day course for treating relapses are recommended. Because the response of *T. brucei gambiense* to DFMO is variable, organic arsenicals continue to be the mainstay in the treatment of Gambian trypanosomiasis.

Melarsoprol (an organic arsenical) is given intravenously three to four times per day, 200–500 mg (maximum 3.6 mg/kg) per injection. The treatment is given for 3 days and three such treatment cycles are given with an interval of 7 days in between two cycles. Arsenical encephalopathy is a dreaded complication, occurring in about 15–20% patients. It is characterized by recurrent seizures, cognitive impairment, and progressive coma, occurring between the first and fifteenth day of treatment. It is fatal in about 10% of patients. A high CSF pleocytosis and simultaneous use of thiabendazole increase the risk of arsenical encephalopathy. Premedication with corticosteroids, nutritional supplementation for malnourished patients, and prophylactic anticonvulsants are recommended before commencing melarsoprol therapy. MRI may assist to distinguish arsenical encephalopathy from relapse. Focal bilateral high-signal areas in white matter on T2-weighted MRI indicate recurrence of infection or incomplete treatment.

Continuous surveillance for 2–3 years is essential because relapses are common. Relapses are indicated by headache, fever, worsening neurological signs, seizures, and worsening of CSF profile. Relapses in *T. brucei gambiense* infection are treated with eflornithine and in *T. brucei rhodesiense* with melarsoprol. Eradication of infection is achieved in about 90% of cerebral cases. However, sequelae in the form of insomnia, irritability, and poor impulse control may occur.

PREVENTION Preventive measures include eradication of the tsetse fly, use of protective clothes, reservoir control, regular medical surveillance, and treatment of early cases in endemic areas.

American Trypanosomiasis
Existing as an acute or chronic disease, American trypanosomiasis or Chagas' disease is caused by the hemoflagellate protozoa, *Trypanosoma cruzi*. The disease occurs in Central and South America. Chagas' disease causes cardiac and gastrointestinal tract autonomic de-efferentation years after primary infection. Although rare, CNS involvement should suggest concurrent HIV infection.

Chagas' disease is a zoonotic disease, transmitted by the reduvid bug of the genus *Triatoma*. The trypanosome inhabits the gut of the bug. The bug bites at night and defecates at the time of biting. The infection is transmitted by rubbing the fecal matter containing the metacyclic stage of the parasite into the tiny skin puncture, other abrasions of the skin, or by rubbing the eyes or other mucosal surface with infected fingers. The infection can also be transmitted transplacentally, by blood transfusion, or from organ transplant.

CLINICAL FEATURES Acute Chagas' disease, mostly in children, is a flulike illness occurring about 1 week after inoculation, with fever, lymphadenitis, malaise, hepatosplenomegaly, facial edema, tachycardia, and rarely meningoencephalitis. The portal of entry may show nodular or ulcerative swelling (chagoma) in about 25% of cases. In 50% of cases, the primary site is the outer canthus of the eye, with unilateral palpebral edema, and periauricular lymph node enlargement (Romaña's sign). Early myocarditis, meningoencephalitis, or reactivated Chagas' disease suggests concurrent HIV infection. CNS involvement manifests as seizures, tremors, rigidity, paralysis, and altered mentation. Death in the acute stage is caused by acute myocarditis, congestive cardiac failure, or meningoencephalitis.

Chronic Chagas' disease develops years or decades after initial infection, with clinical features suggesting involvement of heart, gastrointestinal tract, and nervous systems. Cardiac involvement is most common in chronic disease with congestive cardiomyopathy, syncopal attacks, and systemic and CNS embolization from mural thrombi of a left ventricular apical aneurysm. Destruction of autonomic ganglion in the heart results in postural hypotension, dizziness, and rhythm disturbance, whereas similar involvement of the gastrointestinal tract results in megacolon and megaesophagus. CNS involvement in chronic Chagas' disease is caused by embolization of cerebral vessels from intramural cardiac thrombi or from formation of mass lesions with seizures, hemiparesis, cerebellar ataxia, or other focal deficit.

Transplacental transmission of *T. cruzi* results in congenital Chagas' disease with premature birth and developmental delay in the survivors.

DIAGNOSIS   In the acute stage, the diagnosis can be established in about 90% of patients by the presence of parasites in thick or thin smears of peripheral blood or buffy coat during febrile episodes. Aspiration of spleen, liver, lymph nodes, and bone marrow may show the parasites in macrophages. Serological tests include hemagglutination, immunofluorescence, and complement fixation tests, which become positive after about 1 month and remain so for life. Chronic Chagas' disease is diagnosed serologically. False-positive serology can occur in syphilis, leishmaniasis, malaria, leprosy, or collagen vascular disease.

TREATMENT   Treatment for Chagas' disease is unsatisfactory because it only reduces the duration of symptoms and mortality. As soon as infection with *T. cruzi* is suspected, treatment should be started without waiting for laboratory confirmation. In acute Chagas' disease, nifurtimox in a dose of 8–10 mg/kg for adults, 12.5–15.0 mg/kg for adolescents, and 15–20 mg/kg for children (1–10 years of age) is recommended in four divided doses for

90–120 days. Adverse effects include abdominal pain, anorexia, nausea, vomiting, weight loss, and neurological side effects (restlessness, disorientation, insomnia, neuritis, and seizures). Alternatively, benzimidazole, at 5 mg/kg per day orally for 60 days, may be used. Side effects include peripheral neuropathy, granulocytopenia, and rash.

PREVENTION Vector control by spraying insecticides, improving housing, and screening of donated blood may check transmission of the parasite. Mosquito nets, insect repellents, and the use of protective clothing provide additional protection. Tourists traveling to endemic areas should avoid sleeping in dilapidated houses. Laboratory workers should wear gloves and eye protection.

Amoebic Infections of the Central Nervous System

Protozoan free-living amoebae are widely distributed in nature and are particularly found in moist soils and in warm freshwater. Amoebic infections of the brain are extremely rare, but they have a very high mortality. Two clinicopathological syndromes are recognized: primary amoebic meningoencephalitis (PAM) and granulomatous amoebic encephalitis (GAE). Amoebae from the genera *Naegleria* cause PAM, and those from the genera *Acanthamoeba* cause GAE. *Naegleria fowleri* exists in three forms: trophozoites, flagellates, and cysts. The trophozoite and flagellate forms are highly motile and transform into cystic form under nutritionally deprived conditions. The parasite excysts when the conditions become favorable through the pores in the cyst wall. The most potent stimulus for the excystment is the presence of molecular carbon dioxide in the environment. *Acanthamoeba* lacks the flagellate stage, and the trophozoites are larger than *Naegleria*. The cysts are stellate and have a small opening at one end from which the excystment occurs. *Leptomyxida*, another free-living amoeba, has been identified as a cerebral pathogen and the genus *Balamuthia mandrillaris* is a rare cause of GAE.

N. fowleri has been isolated from puddles, pools, mud, rivers, and sewage disposals. They have also been isolated from air conditioners and thermal effluents from factories. Children acquire PAM as they swim or play in water contaminated by these free-living amoebae. The disease has a male-to-female ratio of 2:1 for *Naegleria* and 5:1 for *Acanthamoeba*. PAM is more common in children. Granulomatous amoebic meningitis can be seen at any age. *Acanthamoeba* causes GAE in immunocompromised hosts, such as patients with AIDS, those on long-term antibiotics or corticosteroids, and transplant recipients on immunosuppression. CNS invasion is generally through the nasopharynx or respiratory tract. The incubation period of the disease is not known but is probably long.

Pathogenesis and Pathology
The parasites enter the brain by passing through the cribriform plate along the fila of the olfactory nerve to enter the frontal lobes and cause a necrotizing inflammation with extensive destruction. *Acanthamoeba* can also invade the CNS through this route, through the bloodstream, or through a primary corneal infection acquired by using contact lenses stored in contaminated saline solution. A large number of proteolytic enzymes are produced by the amoebae, which destroy the tissues around the area of invasion.

The meninges in PAM are hyperemic with diffuse superficial hemorrhages and are ensheathed in purulent basal exudates, most intense around the olfactory bulbs. There is extensive necrotizing destruction of the cerebral parenchyma, more so in frontal and temporal lobes. Histopathology reveals polymorphonuclear inflammatory infiltrate with interspersed trophozoites in and around the subarachnoid space. The inflammatory infiltrate is devoid of cysts and flagellate forms. Extracerebral tissues are usually spared, but pulmonary and myocardial infiltration has been reported. GAE is characterized by formation of small necrotic abscesses.

Clinical Features
PAM presents with acute onset of fever, headache, vomiting, and photophobia with altered mentation. In the acute phase, the disease closely resembles acute pyogenic meningitis; however, seizures and focal neurological deficits are more common in PAM. Patients may complain of anosmia or cacosmia because the olfactory bulbs are involved early in the course of the disease. Rapid deterioration occurs, as patients do not respond to antibiotics, which are often given for suspected bacterial meningitis. The common preterminal event is raised ICP and consequent cerebral herniation.

GAE has a slow and insidious course suggestive of an intracranial space-occupying lesion and rarely as insidiously progressive meningoencephalitis. The lesions in GAE are most commonly localized in the posterior fossa. The patients gradually deteriorate and eventually die after 2–3 weeks. *Acanthamoeba* keratitis has been reported in patients who use soft contact lenses kept in contaminated saline solutions. Rarely the corneal infection spreads intracranially. *Balamuthia* meningitis affects the cortex more frequently, especially the temporal lobes.

Diagnosis
CSF examination reveals polymorphonuclear leukocytosis, with hypoglycorrhachia, and increased protein, but the Gram's stain and the culture are negative. Rarely, their typical "sluglike" movements in a wet drop preparation of fresh CSF can identify the actively motile trophozoites. The CSF picture of patients with GAE is suggestive of granulomatous infection, with moderately raised protein, a near-normal or slightly low CSF glucose, lymphocytic CSF pleocytosis, and absence of motile trophozoites.

Most patients with PAM have normal CT and MRI scans of the brain. In GAE, cerebral lesions resembling space-occupying lesions are seen. PAM needs to be differentiated from acute bacterial meningitis or brain abscess rupturing into the subarachnoid space. The differential diagnosis of GAE is chronic meningitis of fungal or tuberculous origin, brain abscess, neoplastic lesions, and encephalitis. A similar clinical syndrome may occur in CNS vasculitis. PAM and GAE are so rare and with so high mortality that these are usually diagnosed postmortem, unless diagnosed and treated very early.

Treatment
Diagnosis is usually delayed in amoebic CNS infections, and the therapeutic response to available drugs is poor. Many drugs, including amphotericin B, misonidazole, rifampin, trimethoprim, phenothiazines, and quinghousu, have been tried. *Acanthamoeba* is more resistant to treatment than *Naegleria*. Because there are no established guidelines for treatment because of the rarity of the disease, treatment is individualized. The best response has been observed with a combination of chemotherapeutic agents, which includes amphotericin B given by intrathecal and intravenous routes, in maximal possible doses.

Cerebral Amoebiasis
E. histolytica, the most common intestinal parasite colonizing the large bowel in humans, causes local ulceration of the wall of the colon and presents as amoebic dysentery. It is endemic in Southeast Asia, India, and South America. Humans are the primary host and are infected by consuming water and food contaminated with feces. The amoebae enter the bloodstream and colonize in distant organs, causing "metastatic abscesses." The liver is affected in about 10% of patients, resulting in amoebic liver abscess. Cerebral involvement is seen in about

0.1% of all patients. Cerebral abscess is almost always associated with hepatic abscess.

PATHOGENESIS AND PATHOLOGY   The abscesses are located at the gray–white matter junction in the cerebrum or cerebellum. Proteolytic enzymes of the amoebae cause tissue destruction locally with granulomatous inflammatory infiltrate. The brain appears edematous, with patchy meningeal exudates. The cut surface reveals a necrotic and hemorrhagic center surrounded by poorly differentiated rim with perifocal edema. The rim consists of dense inflammatory infiltrate comprising of mononuclear cells and RBCs. Amoebae or tissue cysts can be identified in the tissue sections.

CLINICAL FEATURES   The disease affects predominantly young adults, with a male-to-female ratio of 10:1. Clinical features are not specific. Intestinal complaints usually predominate initially. Febrile encephalopathy and focal neurological signs should raise the possibility of this disease. Cerebral abscesses have been reported in patients without clinical amoebic colitis. An invasive amoebiasis is usually evident in other organs such as the liver and lungs. Focal neurological signs, fever, lethargy, seizures, and varying degrees of altered mental status are common symptoms.

DIAGNOSIS   Isolated cerebral abscesses are rare. Imaging of liver and brain are helpful. CT scans show single or multiple abscesses, particularly in the frontal lobes or basal ganglia, which appear as low attenuating ring-enhancing lesions with marked perifocal edema. T1-weighted MRI scans show the abscess as a central hypointensity surrounded by an isointense rim, enhancing on gadolinium. On T2-weighted images, they are hyperintense with a hypointense rim. Antiamoebic antibodies are detected in most patients.

TREATMENT   Medical therapy consists of metronidazole at 1 g, followed by 500 mg every 6 hours intravenously or 750 mg intravenously three times a day for 10 days, followed by iodoquinol at 650 mg three times a day for 20 days. In children the dose of metronidazole is 30–50 mg/kg per day in divided doses. Emetine in a dose of 1 mg/kg per day to a maximum of 60 mg/day can also be used. Chloroquine has also been tried in a dosage of 600 mg/day for 2 days followed by 300 mg/day for 2–3 weeks. The result of medical treatment is universally poor. Combining surgical resection of the abscess with antiamoebic therapy may improve survival. The results of all forms of treatment are poor and the mortality is 90%.

Toxoplasmosis

Toxoplasmosis is caused by *Toxoplasma gondii*, an intracellular protozoa, first described by Janku in 1923 in the retina of a child. Common manifestations of toxoplasmosis are chorioretinitis and meningoencephalitis. After the pandemic of HIV/AIDS beginning in the 1980s, toxoplasmosis has acquired the dubious distinction of being the most common cause of cerebral mass lesion in patients with AIDS.

The only definitive hosts for *T. gondii* are domestic cats, which get infected by eating infected rodents or oocysts passed in the feces of cats that harbor the parasite in their intestines. The tissue cysts of the parasite in these animals infect the intestinal epithelial cells and develop into merozoites. The sexual cycle starts when some of the merozoites develop into gametocytes, which fuse and form diploid oocysts, which are excreted in the feces. Under favorable conditions, that is, warm and humid climate, sporogony occurs in the oocysts. Sporulated oocysts are infective, and if ingested by rodents, cats, or other small animals, they release large numbers of sporozoites in the small intestine. Sporozoites penetrate the gut wall, replicate, and spread hematogenously to most mammalian tissues. Once in a cell, sporozoites undergo fission until the host cell ruptures and liberates sporozoites that infect the surrounding cells. Over time, tissue cysts are formed containing many parasites, which are now called *bradyzoites* as they divide slowly. The tissue cysts are immunologically inert and remain so for years, failing to elicit an inflammatory response. Reactivation of tissue cysts occurs if cell-mediated immunity wanes, as occurs in patients with cancer, organ transplant recipients, patients on chronic corticosteroids, and those with AIDS. Most human infections are acquired by ingesting oocysts contaminating food, hands, or soil or tissue cysts contained in raw or undercooked meat. Transplacental transmission is also common. Rarely, organ transplantation and blood transfusion may be the route of entry of the parasite.

PATHOGENESIS AND PATHOLOGY   The toxoplasma gains entry into the host macrophages and occupies a "parasitophorous vacuole." Whereas activated macrophages destroy the parasite with clearance of parasitemia, resting macrophages allow intracellular replication of the parasite. The mechanism by which toxoplasma survive the tissue macrophages is not known. Because the disease is mild and not fatal in the immunocompetent host, pathological reports are scant. The lesions are found in eyes, brain, and other organs. In the brain, they are present in both gray and white matter and appear as moth-eaten, necrotic honeycombed areas, infiltrated with inflammatory cells, particularly in the perivascular area with pyknotic nuclei. In congenital toxoplasmosis, the lesions are most intense in the cortex, the basal ganglion, and the periventricular area. Calcification within the areas of necrosis is common. Hydrocephalus occurs as a result of obstruction of the aqueduct of Sylvius or foramen of Monro by active ependymitis or deposition of necrotic debris in the ventricles. Periventricular and periaqueductal vasculitis and necrosis are almost pathognomonic of congenital toxoplasmosis.

CLINICAL FEATURES Primary infection in an immunocompetent host is usually asymptomatic. Acute infection is associated with fever and lymphadenitis in 10–20% of patients, 1–2 weeks after ingestion of cysts. A maculopapular rash similar to infectious mononucleosis occurs in a few patients. Rarely, immunocompetent hosts develop disseminated toxoplasmosis with CNS involvement. Meningoencephalitis, seizures, drowsiness, confusion, and coma are often the presenting symptoms. The CSF in CNS toxoplasmosis shows lymphocytic pleocytosis, mildly elevated protein level, and normal sugar concentration. Acute chorioretinitis may precede or follow CNS toxoplasmosis.

Congenital toxoplasmosis is transmitted transplacentally when a woman acquires *Toxoplasma* infection during pregnancy. The infant may be born with bilateral chorioretinitis (blindness and strabismus), CNS involvement (e.g., epilepsy, psychomotor retardation, microcephaly, periventricular calcification, hydrocephalus, and pituitary insufficiency), or systemic effects (e.g., jaundice, hepatosplenomegaly, anemia, low birth weight, lymphadenitis, and pneumonitis).

Ocular toxoplasmosis occurs during primary infection when it is usually unilateral, during congenital infection when it is usually bilateral, and during reactivation of previous infection in an adult. *Toxoplasma* chorioretinitis usually involves the posterior pole near the macula. Pain in the eye, photophobia, and diminution of vision occur in the acute stage. Focal yellow-white patches of necrotizing retinitis along with retinal edema and exudates give way to darkly pigmented scars after healing. Uveitis, scotoma, defect in central vision, photophobia, glaucoma, cataract, microphthalmia, and strabismus may be associated. Papilledema may occur because of CNS involvement.

DIAGNOSIS Serodiagnostic tests for toxoplasmosis are available. Antitoxoplasma IgG antibody detection done by Sabin-Feldman dye test is useful in *Toxoplasma* encephalitis up to 8 weeks as the titers decline slowly after that. Titers above 1:1024 are indicative of acute infection. The test is 93% sensitive but lacks specificity. IgM antibody detection by double-sandwich ELISA is sensitive and indicates infection in the past 2–3 months. Acute congenital toxoplasmosis is diagnosed by finding high or rising IgG titers or positive IgM titers. Negative IgG in an immunocompetent host with chorioretinitis almost excludes toxoplasmosis. CSF examination in a patient with encephalitis shows monocytic pleocytosis, raised protein level, and DNA sequences of *T. gondii*, which can be detected by PCR. Plain x-ray films of the skull may show characteristic spotty intracranial calcifications, which are localized in the periventricular area on CT scan. In the acute stage, *Toxoplasma* abscesses are seen as multiple round, nodular, or ring-enhancing lesions with intense edema in the immunocompetent hosts. MRI is more sensitive than CT in detecting these lesions. Differential diagnoses of such lesions on neuroimaging are tuberculomas, lymphoma, metastases, and pyogenic abscesses. Tissue diagnosis by biopsy of the intracranial lesion is the gold standard but is seldom indicated. It is indicated only if the condition worsens after initiation of therapy, if there is a solitary large lesion on MRI, or if a patient develops these lesions while on prophylaxis of *Pneumocystis carinii* pneumonia. Differential diagnosis of neonatal toxoplasmosis includes human CMV, herpes, rubella, syphilis, or *E. coli* meningitis, sepsis, and erythroblastosis fetalis.

TREATMENT A combination of pyrimethamine (a dihydrofolate reductase inhibitor) in a loading dose of 200 mg followed by 50–75 mg/day (or 1 mg/kg per day up to maximum of 100 mg/day) in three divided doses and sulfadiazine (a dihydrofolate synthetase inhibitor) 4–6 g/day (or 100 mg/kg per day, up to maximum 8 g/day) for 3–4 weeks is recommended. Immunocompromised hosts require lifelong prophylaxis. Supplement of folinic acid (10 mg/day) prevents hematological complications. The drug is effective against tachyzoites (in active macrophages) but ineffective on the cystic stage. Alternatively, clindamycin (600 mg orally or parenterally every 6 hours) is recommended. It has poor CSF penetration, and side effects include neutropenia, rash, pseudomembranous enterocolitis, myositis, and elevated creatine kinase levels. Another drug atovaquone, a hydroxynaphthoquinone derivative, in doses of 750 mg four times a day has shown promise. Patients who cannot tolerate standard therapy may be treated with azithromycin, roxithromycin, or clarithromycin.

Immunologically competent adults and children with only lymphadenopathy do not require specific therapy unless the symptoms are severe. Ocular toxoplasmosis should be treated with pyrimethamine plus either sulfonamide or clindamycin for 1 month. Congenital toxoplasmosis is treated with pyrimethamine (0.5–1.0 mg/kg) and sulfadiazine (100 mg/kg) orally for 1 year. Additionally, spiramycin (100 mg/kg) plus prednisolone (1 mg/kg per day) has shown good results. The choice of antiparasitic agent for its safety and efficacy profile for congenital toxoplasmosis remains unsettled.

PREVENTION Prevention requires clean habits while handling pet cats and dogs. Stray dogs and cats should be avoided and meat should be properly cooked and stored at −20°C. Immunocompromised hosts, especially those with AIDS, require lifelong prophylaxis with 25–50 mg of pyrimethamine and 1–2 g of sulfadiazine per day after recovery from toxoplasmic encephalitis. Patients intolerant to sulfadiazine should receive clindamycin (1200 mg/day in three divided doses).

Helminthic Infections of the Central Nervous System

Twenty species of the helminths affect the CNS in humans. Of these, cysticercosis and echinococcosis are by far the most common.

Cestodes

CYSTICERCOSIS Cysticercosis is invasion of tissues by the larval stage of pork tapeworm, *Taenia solium*. Neurocysticercosis (NCC), invasion of the nervous system by larvae, is an important public health problem particularly in developing countries. NCC has worldwide distribution and is endemic in Latin America, Indian subcontinent, China, and most of the African and Asian countries. It is absent in Israel and certain Asian countries where pig rearing is unacceptable for religious reasons. In the United States and European countries, NCC is becoming more common as a result of infected immigrants. Seroprevalence in villages of Mexico, Guatemala, Bolivia, Peru, and Ecuador is between 4.9% and 24%. In India it is between 2% and 3% in the general population. The high incidence of epilepsy in Latin America is attributed to rampant NCC. According to the Commission of Tropical Diseases of International League Against Epilepsy, age-adjusted prevalence of epilepsy in tropical countries is 10–15 per 1000 population and is largely caused by NCC. Seizures in people older than 25 years in endemic areas are caused by NCC in 50–70% of cases. Globally, it causes about 50,000 deaths annually. In India, 40% of focal seizures are caused by NCC, calcified NCC, and granuloma or single enhancing CT lesion consistent with cysticercal granuloma.

The disease is most common where there is close contact with pigs and where poor sanitation and personal hygiene exist. Humans, the definitive host, harbor the adult tapeworm in the intestines. Gravid proglottids containing highly infective fertile eggs are shed in the feces. NCC is acquired through the fecal-oral route by consuming contaminated food (raw vegetables or water) or even through infected fingers of self or food handlers. On the other hand, tapeworms are acquired by eating raw or undercooked infected pork. After ingestion, the eggs hatch into invasive larvae that penetrate the gut wall and lodge in various tissues including brain, muscles, subcutaneous tissue, liver, eyes, and spinal cord, through hematogenous spread. In tissues they mature into the fluid-filled larval form, the cysticercus, with an invaginated scolex.

Pathogenesis and Pathology   By necessity the survival of cysticerci in pigs depends on absence of significant inflammatory response on the part of the host. Cysticerci appear as thin-walled oval cysts, about 1 cm in diameter, with an invaginated scolex, which appears as a white nodule attached to one side of the cyst. The cyst wall consists of an outer smooth white eosinophilic layer, an inner cellular layer, and an innermost layer of loose connective tissue. The parasite escapes the host's immune surveillance mechanisms by secreting a serine protease inhibitor called *teniastatin*, which inhibits complement activation, lymphocytic migration, and cytokine formation. The presence of cysts is not always associated with symptoms. Approximately 3–8% of individuals dying of other causes show viable cysticerci in their brains on autopsy in endemic areas. It is only when the cysticerci undergo degeneration that the inflammatory response starts and symptoms such as seizures occur. This is especially true for the patient with single enhancing CT lesions. On the other hand, when the infection load is high, patients present with features of raised ICP and deteriorating mental status.

Different stages of natural evolution of cysticerci are described. Viable cysts have a minimal associated inflammatory response (vesicular stage). Inflammation, especially by the mononuclear cells around the cyst, results in the colloidal stage, which is followed by gradual replacement by fibrotic tissue and collapse of cyst wall (granular nodular stage). Finally replacement by fibrotic tissue and mineralization of the parasite results in the calcific stage. Whereas parenchymal cysts are small (about 1 cm diameter) in the cortical-subcortical area, larger extraparenchymal cysts may be present in the ventricles or the subarachnoid space. Parenchymal cysts are generally associated with seizures, raised ICP, and deteriorating mental status. When parasite load is high, inflammation around the cysts gives rise to a fulminant meningoencephalitis picture. Subarachnoid cysts generally attain large size with lobulations (grapelike appearance, the racemose variety), lose the scolices, and are usually seen at the base of the brain or the Sylvian fissure. Intraventricular NCC results in persistent or intermittent raised ICP caused by blockage of aqueduct of Sylvius or foramina of Luschka and Magendie. Inflammation of these cysts results in ependymitis and arachnoiditis with resultant meningitis, communicating hydrocephalus, or vasculitis with stroke.

Clinical Features The clinical symptoms occur 1–35 years after exposure and several years after CNS infestation by cysticerci. NCC has protean clinical manifestations depending on number, site, stage, duration of the cysts, and whether an inflammatory response is present. Seizures, both generalized and partial, are the most common symptom, occurring in about 92% of patients with parenchymal NCC in the active (colloidal and nodular-granular) and inactive (calcific) stages. The acute encephalitic form is common in children and is associated with rapid deterioration in neuropsychological status, recurrent seizures, intracranial hypertension, and coma. This form of presentation is usually seen in patients with high infection load with an inflammatory response. Focal neurological signs, such as hemiplegia and cerebellar ataxia, usually occur following the inflammatory reaction (meningoencephalitis), vasculitis, and stroke caused by NCC in the subarachnoid space. NCC is a common cause of stroke in young patients in Latin American countries. The infarcts may be small (lacunar) or large involving the middle cerebral artery. The clinical picture of raised ICP with headache, vomiting, cognitive dysfunction, neuropsychiatric decline, and papilledema occurs with multiple parenchymal NCC, with or without acute meningoencephalitis, with intraventricular cysts causing obstructive hydrocephalus, or with subarachnoid cysts causing severe meningitis and CSF outflow obstruction. Patients harboring cysts in the brainstem present with a corresponding focal neurological deficit. Involvement of the spinal cord is associated with compressive myelopathy. Downward migration of a subarachnoid cyst from the posterior fossa may cause extramedullary compression, whereas intramedullary cysticercosis occurs from hematogenous spread. Root pain occurs in about 1–5% of patients. Ocular cysts occur in about 1% of patients with retro-orbital pain similar to migraine, proptosis, ptosis, and diplopia. Retinal, vitreous, or subconjunctival cysts present with visual loss, scotoma, floaters, orbital abscess, and panophthalmitis, occurring spontaneously or after initiating specific cysticidal therapy. Patients with cysticerci in muscles can present with painful muscular hypertrophy and weakness, especially of the proximal group of muscles. Subcutaneous nodules may provide a clue to the etiology of epilepsy.

Diagnosis In endemic areas, diagnosis of NCC should be considered in almost all patients with neurological or psychiatric complaints. Presence of nodules in subcutaneous or subconjunctival tissue helps in the diagnosis. Definite diagnosis depends on demonstration of larval forms of *T. solium*. Recently, diagnostic criteria of NCC have been proposed based on clinical, neuroimaging, serological, histopathological, and epidemiological criteria. Absolute criteria include histopathological demonstration of parasite in brain or spinal cord lesion, neuroimaging consistent with NCC (cystic lesion showing scolex), or direct visualization of subretinal parasite by funduscopy. Major criteria include neuroimaging highly suggestive of NCC (cystic lesion without scolex, enhancing lesion, or typical parenchymal brain calcification), resolution of intracranial cystic lesions after cysticidal therapy, or spontaneous resolution of a small single enhancing lesion. Minor criteria include lesions compatible with NCC on neuroimaging (hydrocephalus, abnormal leptomeningeal enhancement, myelogram showing multiple filling defect in the column of contrast medium), clinical manifestations suggestive of NCC, positive CSF ELISA for detection of anti-cysticercal antibodies or cysticercal antigens, and cysticercosis outside CNS (histological diagnosis of subcutaneous or muscle nodule, x-ray films showing "cigar-shaped" soft tissue calcification, and direct visualization of cysticerci in the anterior chamber of eye). Epidemiological criteria include evidence of household contact with *T. solium* infection, individuals living in or coming from endemic area, and history of frequent travel to disease-endemic area. The presence of one absolute criterion or two major, one minor, and one epidemiological criterion is required for definitive diagnosis. On the other hand, one major plus two minor, one major plus one minor plus one epidemiological, or three minor plus one epidemiological criteria constitute probable.

Among the serological tests, more widely used ELISA shows 50% sensitivity and 65% specificity in CSF. More recently, enzyme-linked immunoelectrotransfer blot (EITB) assay has been shown to be 98% sensitive and 100% specific. This test is, however, positive in only 28% of patients with single enhancing lesion. Patients with calcified lesions and single enhancing CT lesions are often serologically negative. A monoclonal antibody based antigen-detection assay is highly specific for viable and degenerating cysticerci.

Plain radiography of soft tissue may show classic cigar-shaped calcifications. Neuroimaging with CT scan is more sensitive in detecting calcified lesions. When there are numerous calcified lesions, it gives the appearance of "starry night." Vesicular cysts appear as hypointense lesions with an eccentric intramural nodule representing the scolex in MRI. In the colloidal stage, the cysts show ring enhancement with edema, whereas in the granular-nodular stage they show disc-enhancing lesion with perilesional edema. The racemose form of the neurocysticerci appears as a bunch of grapes on an MRI scan.

CSF examination is usually nonspecific and shows mononuclear, lymphocytic, or eosinophilic pleocytosis and positive cysticercal antibody titers. Differential diagnosis includes TB, echinococcosis, paragonimiasis, sparganosis, cryptococcosis, and cystic astrocytoma for parenchymal NCC and echinococcosis, coenurosis, CNS tumors, epidermoids, and arachnoid and colloid cysts for extra-axial cysts.

Treatment NCC is treated with antiparasitic drugs along with symptomatic therapy. Patients with inactive parenchymal NCC with evidence of calcified lesions or degenerating parasites on neuroimaging do not require antiparasitic treatment. Because seizures are common symptoms in these patients, chronic anticonvulsant therapy is required. Patients with inactive disease and hydrocephalus from prior subarachnoid or ventricular infection also do not require antiparasitic treatment, but ventriculoperitoneal shunt may be required. Shunt failure is uncommon in this group.

Patients with active parenchymal disease are treated with albendazole, a benzimidazole anthelminthic agent, or praziquantel. Albendazole is preferred because it is less expensive, has better penetration into subarachnoid cysts, and is unlikely to have pharmacological interference with corticosteroids and other anticonvulsant agents. The dose of albendazole is 15 mg/kg per day divided in two oral doses for 8–28 days along with dexamethasone. Recent reports of treatment with praziquantel in three oral doses of 25 mg/kg separated by 2 hours, followed 5 hours later by dexamethasone at 10 mg intramuscularly, then 10 mg intramuscularly on the next 2 days has also shown good results. Administration of dexamethasone a few hours after praziquantel allows uptake of the drug by the cyst. Earlier, praziquantel was given orally in doses of 50 mg/kg per day in three divided doses for 14 days. Adverse effects of antiparasitic drugs are worsening of neurological status (e.g., headache, vomiting, dizziness, seizures, coma, and increased ICP) and are believed to be caused by a host inflammatory response to dying parasite. Many cysts resolve spontaneously over time. There is no consensus regarding treatment of active extraparenchymal NCC. Until recently, surgical removal of intraventricular NCC was done with or without ventriculoperitoneal shunt. Ventriculoperitoneal shunt in this group is complicated with frequent shunt failures. Neuroendoscopic removal of intraventricular NCC as an alternative method is less invasive. In patients with single ring-enhancing CT lesions presenting with epilepsy, treatment with anticonvulsant drugs alone is advocated because most of these resolve spontaneously. Treating them with anthelminthic agents does not improve the resolution of these lesions.

Prevention Improving sanitation, eliminating intestinal tapeworms, improving sewage disposal system, surveillance of pork farming, preventing pigs from entering human dwellings, and eating properly cooked clean vegetables and pork are some of the methods to prevent the occurrence of NCC.

ECHINOCOCCOSIS   Hydatid disease is caused by the cestode of the genus *Echinococcus*, found in the intestines of canines. The disease is common in people who live in close contact with dogs and cats. The highest incidence of echinococcal disease is seen in Greece, Lebanon, and Turkey. It is also reported from Australia, South Africa, east Africa, Canada, North America, Asia, and parts of Russia. The larval cysts of the parasite, the metacestodes, cause the hydatid disease in the intermediate hosts. Common sites are liver (50–70%), lungs (20–30%), bones, heart, and the spleen. CNS involvement is seen in fewer than 2% of patients and involves brain parenchyma and intraventricular and subarachnoid spaces.

Human hydatidosis can be caused by four species, causing different types of cysts. *Echinococcus granulosus* infection is the most common and it causes simple hydatid cyst. Dogs, cats, and other canines are the definitive hosts. The eggs, containing the *Echinococcus* larvae, are excreted in the feces of the host, which are accidentally ingested by the intermediate hosts (humans). The larvae penetrate the intestinal wall and are spread hematogenously to liver, brain, and other sites where they develop into the hydatid cysts.

Clinical Features   The latent period is 2–20 years. Involvement of liver and lungs causes abdominal pain, hepatosplenomegaly, or cough. Rupture of cyst causes an acute abdomen syndrome, dyspnea, hemoptysis, or a hypersensitivity reaction (60–70%). In the brain, cysts grow at a rate of about 1 cm per year. Patients with CNS cysts generally present with focal neurological deficits, seizures, or signs of raised ICP. The rupture of the cysts can cause an acute allergic response. Rarely, involvement of basal ganglia, cerebellum, cavernous sinus, and intrasellar and intraorbital spaces can be seen. Other sites of involvement are intraventricular, subdural, or spinal canal. Cord compression also occurs because of vertebral collapse caused by hydatid bone disease (hydatid Pott's disease).

Diagnosis The first clue to the diagnosis comes from plain x-ray films of the abdomen showing a calcified lesion or peripheral or CSF eosinophilia. X-ray film of the skull shows no abnormalities, or it shows evidence of bone erosion because of a large cyst. Neuroimaging with CT and MRI reveals a large spherical, smooth cystic lesion filled with fluid of CSF intensity with ventricular distortion and midline shift. The cyst wall is isodense or hyperdense to the brain tissue and does not show contrast enhancement unless ruptured or infected. On MRI, the cyst appears hypointense on T1-weighted images with a slightly hyperintense rim. On T2-weighted images the cyst wall appears hypointense and the fluid hyperintense. Daughter cysts usually accompany the main cyst. *E. granulosus* gives rise to single solitary cyst, whereas *E. multilocularis* is associated with multichambered complex cysts. The Casoni's test is now obsolete, but the serological tests such as hemagglutination test and ELISA using arc −5 antigen of the parasite are more sensitive.

Treatment The treatment of choice is surgical resection of the cyst. During the resection, care must be taken not to spill the contents of the cyst, because this causes anaphylaxis and the formation of innumerable daughter cysts in the surrounding tissues. Intracystic instillation of 20% saline, formalin, cetrimide, or silver nitrate and topical applications of 20% saline or silver nitrate to the surrounding tissues avoid this complication. The size of the cyst can be shrunk by pretreatment with albendazole (15 mg/kg per day for 40 days) or mebendazole (50 mg/kg) for 3 months. In patients in whom only partial resection of the cyst is possible, lifelong treatment is required.

Nematodes

ANGIOSTRONGYLIASIS *Angiostrongylus* or the rat lung worm can cause eosinophilic meningitis or meningoencephalitis in humans. The parasite is widespread in distribution and has been reported from practically every part of the world including Asia, Pacific region, Africa, and the Caribbean.

Transmission and Pathogenesis Rats are the definitive hosts for the parasite *A. cantonensis*, and the parasite is present in their pulmonary circulation. The intermediate hosts are freshwater snails, including grand African snails (*Achatina julica*), prawns, and crabs. Humans become infected if they consume mollusks containing the third-stage larvae. Once the larvae gain entry into the human brain, spinal cord, meninges, eyes, and other tissues, the parasites die and result in eosinophilic meningitis. The leptomeninges are more intensely affected with dense eosinophilic infiltrates along with mononuclear cells and neutrophils.

Clinical Features The latent period is 1–36 days. Severe headache, neck rigidity, varying degrees of altered mentation with vomiting, papilledema, optic neuritis, cranial nerve deficits, brisk reflexes, and seizures are common clinical features. Paresthesia, impaired vision, and generalized weakness are other common symptoms.

Diagnosis The CSF is helpful in diagnosis and reveals raised ICP, pleocytosis between 150 and 2000/µl with predominantly eosinophilic leucocytosis, and raised protein and near-normal sugar levels. Rarely, larvae can be seen on CSF examination. Neuroimaging findings on MRI scans include prominence of Virchow-Robin spaces, subcortical enhancing lesions, and abnormal high T2-signal lesions in the periventricular regions.

Treatment Treatment is generally supportive and analgesic and anti-inflammatory drugs are used. Corticosteroids have no significant role. Larvicidal drugs are generally avoided because they exaggerate CNS symptoms.

GNATHOSTOMIASIS Gnathostomiasis (Yangtze river edema, Shanghai's rheumatism, nodular eosinophilic panniculitis, consular disease, woodbury bug) is caused by *G. spinigerum*, a nematode found in the gut of dogs and cats. It usually causes cutaneous larva migrans and orbital masses, but rarely CNS involvement in the form of eosinophilic meningitis and radiculomyelopathy can occur. *Larva migrans* refers to a condition of protracted migration of larvae in tissues. The disease is common in Southeast Asia, Japan, Thailand, and Israel.

Dogs and cats are the primary hosts, and freshwater fish and cyclops are the intermediate hosts. The eggs passed in the feces contaminate freshwater where cyclops and other aquatic animals ingest them. Consuming undercooked intermediate hosts infects humans. The larvae migrate actively through various tissues producing symptoms.

Clinical Features Patients present with firm, red, itchy subcutaneous nodules, or urticarial rash, fever, and eosinophilia about 3 weeks after exposure. At times the parasite pierces the skin and appears externally on the skin surface where it can be removed for diagnosis and treatment. CNS involvement is the most serious complication and presents with meningoencephalitis, headache, cranial nerve palsy, depressed consciousness, subarachnoid and intracerebral hemorrhage, focal neurological deficits, and spinal cord involvement. Painful myeloradiculopathy with segmental pain and paraparesis is one of the most characteristic presentations. The CNS involvement may occur in isolation without concomitant skin involvement. Eosinophilic meningitis occurring in gnathostomiasis has a more serious course than that caused by *Angiostrongylus*. Orbital involvement results in uveitis, retinal hemorrhage, and detachment.

Diagnosis The diagnosis is based on the typical clinical picture, CSF findings, and history of exposure. CSF is hemorrhagic or xanthochromic with eosinophilic pleocytosis. CT and MRI scans reveal ring- or disc-enhancing lesions and evidence of intracerebral or subarachnoid hemorrhage. Serological tests are unreliable. Hemorrhagic CSF, painful radiculomyelopathy, and diffuse neurological involvement help differentiation from angiostrongyliasis.

Treatment The treatment is symptomatic with analgesics forming the mainstay of treatment. Albendazole in doses of 400–800 mg per day for 21 days has been tried with variable results. Ivermectin has been used in a single dose as an effective alternative. Systemic corticosteroids can be given in severe cases. The prognosis is not good and mortality is between 8% and 25%. About one third of patients are left with permanent neurological deficits. Surgical removal of the worm is possible if it migrates to accessible locations.

TRICHINOSIS Trichinosis or trichinellosis is caused by the nematode *Trichinella spiralis*. Other species known to cause the disease are *Trichinella nativa* (of Arctic bears) and *Trichinella nelson* (of scavengers of Africa). Trichinosis is seen all over the world except Australia. *Trichinella* cysts have been found in Egyptian mummies from 1200 BC.

The adult worm is an intestinal inhabitant, but the larvae localize in the skeletal muscles eliciting an eosinophilic inflammatory response and they transform there into cysts. Eating undercooked pork (*T. spiralis*), bears, or walrus in Arctic regions and "bush meat" in the tropics causes trichinosis. CNS involvement results in an intense inflammatory reaction by the parasite. The meninges in the fatal cases are intensely hyperemic with dense eosinophilic infiltrate in the perivascular regions. The CSF remains free of a significant inflammatory response. Inflammation of the vessels causes endarteritis and infarctions or hemorrhages in the involved regions of brain.

Clinical Features   Gastrointestinal symptoms with fever are the first symptoms occurring 1–2 days after ingestion of infected pork. Dissemination of the larvae by the hematogenous route causes fever, muscle pain, conjunctival chemosis, periorbital edema, subconjunctival hemorrhage, and eosinophilia about 5 days after infection. Localization of larvae in muscles leads to pain, swelling, and weakness of extraocular, neck, diaphragmatic, intercostal, limb, and paraspinal muscles. The larvae can invade heart, lungs, brain, and meninges. Involvement of brain occurs in about 10% of patients with eosinophilic meningitis, meningoencephalitis, seizures, delirium, coma, brain infarction, hemorrhage, and venous thrombosis. Peripheral neuropathy and necrotizing arteritis with mononeuritis multiplex are reported in less severe cases. Death is rare and occurs as a result of respiratory failure or massive involvement of myocardium with cardiac failure.

Diagnosis   In the appropriate clinical setting, eosinophilia, raised muscle enzymes, and raised serum IgG levels clinch the diagnosis. Muscle biopsy is diagnostic and a fresh muscle sample can reveal the larvae. Serological tests are available. The differential diagnosis includes inflammatory myopathies, eosinophilic myalgia syndrome, and systemic vasculitis.

Treatment   Oral mebendazole at 20 mg/kg is given every 6 hours for treatment of the intestinal nematode, which also prevents the larval stage. The efficacy of this drug against the tissue-invasive form is not established. The allergic symptoms secondary to tissue invasion can be managed by corticosteroids, analgesics, and antipyretics.

STRONGYLOIDIASIS   *S. stercoralis* is a free-living nematode found in warm and moist climates all over the world. Adult worms are passed in human feces and are found in soil where they lay eggs, which hatch to liberate rhabditiform larvae. In the indirect cycle, the rhabdiform larvae, under favorable conditions, transform into infective filiform larvae, pierce the skin of the host, and gain access to the lungs by the hematogenous route. Adult worms develop in the lungs and travel to the trachea where they make their way into the gastrointestinal tract. Occasionally rhabdiform larvae transform into infective filiform larvae and gain entry into the systemic circulation. The parasite lodges in the lungs, lymph nodes, spleen, muscle, heart, and brain.

High-risk individuals include: (1) residents and immigrants from countries where strongyloidiasis is common, (2) residents of Appalachian region of the United States, and (3) institutionalized individuals. The parasite can multiply in the host, especially by an autoinfection cycle. This is called *hyperinfection*.

Clinical Features Gastrointestinal symptoms include epigastric pain, tenderness, anorexia, nausea, vomiting, diarrhea, and malabsorption. Lungs are affected in the migratory phase and result in bronchospasm, cough, and hemoptysis. An inflammatory reaction at the site of skin penetration causes cutaneous larva migrans. Gram-negative septicemia and disseminated strongyloidiasis are serious manifestations. CNS involvement is in the form of polybacterial pyogenic meningitis and meningoencephalitis caused by gram-negative enteric bacteria, which ensheathe the surface of the parasite during its transit from the gastrointestinal tract. The most common organisms involved in these cases are *Klebsiella*, *E. coli*, and *Serratia*. Other manifestations are eosinophilic meningitis, encephalitis, vasculitis, and infarcts. The worms are identified in the CSF only rarely.

Diagnosis The disease is difficult to diagnose antemortem but should be suspected in immunocompromised individuals with features of sudden febrile encephalopathy or frank polymicrobial meningitis. Rarely, patients have eosinophilic meningitis. The CSF shows polymorphonuclear or eosinophilic pleocytosis with hypoglycorrhachia and raised protein level. Diagnosis is based on finding adult worm, larvae, or eggs in stool.

Treatment If diagnosed in time, treatment for the immunocompetent host is with albendazole at 400 mg once or twice daily for 3 days, ivermectin in a single dose of 200 mg/kg, or thiabendazole at 25 mg/kg twice a day for 3 days. Bacterial meningitis and septicemia associated with the disease should be managed with appropriate antibiotics. In the immunocompromised host, treatment with thiabendazole at 50 mg/kg twice a day for 2–4 weeks is recommended.

TOXOCARIASIS Toxocariasis is caused by larvae of *T. canis* (dogs), *T. catis* (cats), and *Baylisascaris procyonis* (raccoons). Larva migrans occurs in skin, viscera, and neural tissue.

Ingestion of food contaminated by eggs from the feces of cats and dogs results in human infection. It is common in children with a history of pica and geophagia. It is also contacted on beaches where cats and dogs deposit their feces. The larvae hatch from the eggs in the small intestine, penetrate the intestinal wall, and migrate to various tissues.

Clinical Features Cutaneous larvae migrans show serpiginous creeping tracts, which are itchy and get secondarily infected. Visceral larva migrans is characterized by pronounced eosinophilia (100%), hepatomegaly (85%), pulmonary symptoms (50%), and fever. Involvement of the nervous system causes encephalitis, meningoencephalitis, and spinal cord compression resulting in headache, disturbance of consciousness, seizures, childhood dementing syndromes, infarcts from vasculitis, eosinophilic granuloma, and paraplegia or quadriplegia. Ocular larva migrans results in retinal inflammatory mass.

Diagnosis Diagnosis of neural larva migrans is suspected by a history of exposure to dogs or cats and peripheral eosinophilia in a child with an encephalitic or a dementing illness. CSF shows eosinophilic pleocytosis and normal sugar and protein levels. ELISA and Western blot technique to detect IgG against larval secretory and excretory antigen can confirm the diagnosis. The differential diagnosis of neural larva migrans includes loiasis, gnathostomiasis, and strongyloidiasis. Ocular larvae migrans must be differentiated from retinoblastoma, toxoplasmosis, histoplasmosis, optic neuritis, and Coat's disease.

Treatment Anthelminthic agents, including thiabendazole (25 mg/kg twice daily for 5 days), mebendazole (100 mg three times a day for 7 days), or albendazole (15 mg/kg per day for 5 days), are useful. Diethylcarbamazine also shows good results. Laser photocoagulation to kill the larvae can be used if they are away from the macula or disc in the retina.

Trematodes

SCHISTOSOMIASIS Schistosomiasis, caused by the trematode *Schistosoma mansoni*, is seen in Africa, Brazil, and the West Indies. The adult worm infects humans. Ova of different schistosomes are passed in urine (*Schistosoma hematobium* and *S. mansoni*) or feces (*Schistosoma japonicum* and *S. mansoni*) of the infected mammals. They gain access to freshwater, hatch, and penetrate freshwater snails and cyclops. The larvae pierce the infected host and are liberated into the water. Humans get infected by bathing in or wading through the infected water. After entering the human body, larvae reach the circulation where they develop into adult worms that produce eggs. Oviposition takes place in the urinary venous plexus in *S. hematobium* and in the mesenteric and hepatic venous system in *S. japonicum* and *S. mansoni*.

Clinical Features A pruritic papular rash, or swimmer's itch, develops after exposure, and signs of acute toxemic schistosomiasis in the form of fever, myalgia, headache, urticaria, and lymphadenopathy (Katayama's fever) develop 11–50 days later. At this stage a mild transient meningoencephalitis or generalized vasculitis may occur in infection with *S. mansoni*.

The chronic stage of disease occurs when the worms complete intravascular migration and settle in the venules of mesentery, portal system, and bladder depending on the species. At this stage, symptoms are related to portal hypertension, hepatic cirrhosis, hepatosplenomegaly, variceal bleeding, intestinal polyps, diarrhea, cystitis, and hematuria.

Involvement of spinal cord, cauda equina, and conus medullaris, resulting in cord infarction, transverse myelitis, and granulomatous cauda equina compression, is associated with *S. mansoni* and *S. haematobium* infection. These are thought to be caused by ectopic eggs or worms in the spinal canal or cord parenchyma via arterial egg embolization or through the valveless intravertebral venous plexus, causing cord infarction or inflammatory granuloma. Cerebral involvement commonly occurs with *S. japonicum* infection (60%) and it may be in the form of cerebral inflammatory masses or vasculitis resulting in seizures, confusion, coma, focal neurological signs (e.g., hemianopic field defects, hemiplegia, and ataxia), and papilledema.

Diagnosis In endemic areas or in individuals with a history of travel to endemic areas, schistosomiasis should be considered in the differential diagnosis of painful cauda equina or spinal cord syndromes. Examination of stool and urine for ova and peripheral eosinophilia are not helpful. Liver or rectal biopsy may show granuloma with a centrally located ovum. CSF examination may show eosinophilic pleocytosis with CNS involvement. CT and MRI scans may demonstrate granuloma with edema in the brain and enlargement of the spinal cord with granulomatous cord disease. Multiple serological tests are described to detect antibodies to eggs, larvae, or adult worm, but they lack sensitivity and specificity. ELISA using keyhole limpet hemocyanin is helpful to distinguish acute from chronic antibody responses.

Treatment Praziquantel is effective against all species of schistosomes. A single oral dose of 40 mg/kg is sufficient for *S. japonicum*, *S. mansoni*, and *S. hematobium*. *S. mekongi* requires three doses of 20 mg/kg separated by 4 hours. Corticosteroids are needed during the treatment with antiparasitic therapy to reduce reaction and edema. Metrifonate and oxamniquine are effective against *S. hematobium* and *S. mansoni*, respectively. Neurological involvement during the acute phase is self-limiting and does not require treatment. Masses in the brain and spinal cord require surgical decompression.

PARAGONIMIASIS The causative agent is the oriental lung fluke of the *Paragonimus* species. The adult worms inhabit lungs, but the larvae rarely gain entry into ectopic sites, of which the brain is the most common leading to meningoencephalitis, seizures, and focal neuralgia syndromes.

The parasite is found in Southeast Asian countries (Japan, Taiwan, Philippines, India, and China), the United States, and west Africa. The most common etiological agents are *Paragonimus westermani, Paragonimus mexicanus,* and *Paragonimus miyazakii.* The intermediate hosts are freshwater fish, snails, and crabs. Humans get infected by consuming infected and partially cooked crabs and fish, contaminated water, or water plants. Adult worms migrate from the gastrointestinal tract to the lungs. The brain is affected when the parasite passes through the sheaths around the jugular veins, internal carotid arteries, or the nerve trunks.

Clinical Features Acute infection is characterized by cough, fever, pleural effusion, and hepatosplenomegaly. The chronic stage is associated with a cough productive of brown sputum, chest discomfort, recurrent hemoptysis, and night sweats. Migrating larvae and worms localize in the brain or spinal cord and present as a space-occupying lesion, raised ICP, epilepsy, meningitis, subacute encephalitis, infarction, headache, cranial nerve paresis, focal neurological deficits, papilledema, optic atrophy, mental retardation, and depressed consciousness.

Diagnosis Diagnosis is made by examination for eggs in the sputum, ELISA, intradermal test, chest x-rays, and peripheral eosinophilia. CSF findings are nonspecific. CT or MRI scans reveal characteristic conglomerate, multiple ring-shaped contrast-enhancing lesions, 1–3 cm in diameter located most commonly in temporal or occipital lobes. In chronic stages the CT and the plain radiographs of the skull may show evidence of characteristic soap bubble appearance and dilatated ventricles.

Treatment The most widely used drug for the treatment of paragonimiasis is praziquantel in doses of 25 mg/kg thrice daily for 2 days. Longer treatment may be required in resistant cases. Niclofalan in a single dose of 2 mg/kg is an alternative. Cerebral and spinal masses require surgical decompression. Corticosteroids or ventriculoperitoneal shunt may be indicated in some cases.

DISEASES CAUSED BY ECTOPARASITES Tick paralysis is an ascending flaccid paralysis caused by a large number of species. These are *Dermacentor andersoni* (North American wood tick),

Dermacentor variabilis (dog tick), *Amblyomma maculatum* in North America, *Ornithodoros lahorensis* in the Russian Republic, *Otobius megnini*, *Ixodes rubicundus*, *Rhipicephalus simus* in South Africa, *Ixodes tancitarus* in Mexico, *Amblyomma cyprium aeratipes* in the Philippines, and *Ixodes holocyclus* in eastern Australia. The tick is removed by pulling it out from the point of attachment with the help of forceps; it is induced to release its hold by paralyzing it with chloroform or lighter fluid. Tick paralysis may be severe and fatal. The agent injected by the tick that produces paralysis has yet to be fully characterized. Paralysis resolves within a few hours of removing the tick.

For a more detailed discussion, see Chapters 59A, 59B, 59C, 59D, 59E, 59F, and 59G in Neurology in Clinical Practice, 4th edition.

Multiple Sclerosis and Other Inflammatory Demyelinating Diseases of the Central Nervous System

29

MULTIPLE SCLEROSIS

Multiple sclerosis (MS) is the most common inflammatory demyelinating process in the central nervous system (CNS) and the leading cause of disability in young adults. Multifocal areas of demyelination with relative preservation of axons, loss of oligodendrocytes, and astroglial scarring characterize the disease.

Etiology

Autoimmunity
Low levels of autoreactive T cells and B cells are present in normal individuals. Autoimmunity develops when these cells lose tolerance, and a complex process of immune reactivity in target tissues begins. Myelin basic protein (MBP) is the primary candidate for the target tissue attacked.

Infection
The epidemiology of MS suggests an exogenous or environmental factor of some type. Human herpesvirus type 6 (HHV-6), Epstein-Barr virus (EBV), and *Chlamydia pneumoniae* have been recently investigated as potential triggers for MS. A definite relationship is not established.

Epidemiology

The median age at onset is 23.5 years. The peak age at onset is approximately 5 years earlier for women than for men. Auto-immune diseases in general and MS in particular affect women than men. The female-to-male ratio is 1.77:1.00. High-frequency areas of the world, with a current prevalence of 60 per 100,000 or more, include all of Europe including Russia, southern Canada, the northern United States, New Zealand, and the southeastern portion of Australia.

Clinical Features

The varied clinical features reflect the multifocal areas of CNS myelin destruction (MS plaques).

Cognitive Impairment

Frank dementia occurs in fewer than 5% of patients and only in severely affected individuals. However, patients frequently complain of a poor memory, a decreased capacity for sustained mental effort, and distractibility. Total lesion load based on magnetic resonance imaging (MRI) scans correlates with impairment on neuropsychological testing. Depression is the most common affective disorder and is in part secondary to the burden of having to cope with a chronic incurable disease. Aphasia, neglect syndrome, cortical blindness, or marked behavioral problems are rare.

Cranial Nerve Dysfunction

Optic neuritis (ON) is the most common type of involvement of the visual pathways. Bilateral ON occurs but is usually sequential rather than simultaneous. Acquired pendular nystagmus and internuclear ophthalmoplegia (INO) are more common features than individual ocular motor nerve palsies. Bilateral INO and vertical nystagmus on upward gaze often occur together. Ocular pursuit movements are typically saccadic rather than smooth. One form of nystagmus particularly characteristic of MS is acquired pendular nystagmus, in which rapid small-amplitude pendular oscillations of the eyes occur in primary position. Impairment of facial sensation is a relatively common finding, and trigeminal neuralgia in a young adult suggests the diagnosis of MS. Almost half of patients report vertigo.

Impairment of the Sensory Pathways

Sensory abnormalities are a common initial feature and occur in almost every patient at some time. The common symptoms are numbness, tingling, pins and needles, tightness, coldness, or swelling of limbs or trunk. Radicular pains, unilateral or bilateral, can be present, particularly in the low thoracic and abdominal regions. An intensely itching sensation, especially in the cervical dermatomes, usually unilateral, suggests MS.

Impairment of Motor Pathways

Corticospinal tract dysfunction is a common feature. A common pattern of disease evolution in the spinal form of MS is an ascending weakness that first involves the legs and then spreads to involve first one arm and then the other, beginning in the intrinsic hand muscles.

Impairment of Cerebellar Pathways

Cerebellar pathway impairment results in gait imbalance, difficulty in performing coordinated actions with the arms, and slurred speech. Examination reveals dysmetria, decomposition of complex movements, and hypotonia, affecting the arms more often than the legs. An intention tremor affects the limbs and head. Truncal ataxia impairs walking. Ocular findings include nystagmus, ocular dysmetria, and usually refixation saccades. Speech can be scanning or explosive in character.

Impairment of Bladder, Bowel, and Sexual Functions

The extent of sphincter and sexual dysfunction often parallels the degree of paraparesis. The most common complaint related to urinary bladder dysfunction is urgency, usually the result of uninhibited detrusor contraction. Constipation is more common than fecal incontinence and reflects upper and lower motor neuron impairment in addition to decreased general mobility. Approximately 50% of patients become completely sexually inactive secondary to their disease, and an additional 20% become less active.

Clinical Features Distinctive of Multiple Sclerosis

Some clinical phenomena are characteristic of but not unique to MS (Table 29.1). *Lhermitte's sign* is a transitory sensory symptom described as an electric shock radiating down the spine or into the limbs on flexion of the neck. *Uhthoff's phenomenon* is worsening of vision or other clinical feature by small increases in the body temperature. Fatigue is a characteristic finding in MS, usually described as physical exhaustion that is unrelated to the amount of activity performed.

Diagnostic Criteria

The neurological history and physical examination remain the cornerstone of diagnosis. New diagnostic criteria have been proposed, which include stringent guidelines for MRI and timing

Table 29.1: Common clinical features of multiple sclerosis

Clinical Features Suggestive of Multiple Sclerosis	Clinical Features Not Suggestive of Multiple Sclerosis
Onset between ages 15 and 50	Onset before age 10 or after 60
Relapses and remissions	Steady progression
Optic neuritis	Early dementia
Lhermitte's sign	Rigidity, sustained dystonia
Internuclear ophthalmoplegia	Cortical deficits such as aphasia, apraxia, alexia, neglect
Fatigue	Deficit developing within minutes
Worsening with elevated body temperature	

intervals to determine possible or definite MS (Table 29.2). The outcome of a diagnostic evaluation is MS, possible MS, or not MS.

Differential Diagnosis

The differential diagnosis of MS is quite limited in the setting of a young adult with two or more clinically distinct episodes of CNS dysfunction with at least partial resolution. Problems arise with atypical presentations, monophasic episodes, or progressive illness. Features that alert the clinician to the possibility of other diseases include: (1) family history of neurological disease, (2) a well-demarcated spinal level in the absence of disease above the foramen magnum, (3) prominent back pain that persists, (4) symptoms and signs that can be attributed to one anatomical site, (5) patients who are older than 60 years or younger than 15 years at onset, and (6) progressive disease.

Course

The most characteristic clinical course of MS is the occurrence of relapses, defined as the acute or subacute onset of clinical dysfunction that reaches its peak from days to several weeks, followed by a remission during which symptoms and signs resolve to a variable extent. The minimum duration for a relapse is 24 hours. Approximately 15% of patients never experience a second relapse.

Four categories of disease define the pattern and course of illness:

Relapsing remitting MS. Clearly defined relapses with full recovery or with sequelae and residual deficit on recovery. Lack of disease progression characterizes the periods between disease relapses.

Table 29.2: McDonald et al. (2001) diagnostic criteria for multiple sclerosis

Clinical Presentation	Additional Data Needed for MS Diagnosis
Two or more attacks; objective clinical evidence of 2 or more lesions	None
Two or more attacks; objective clinical evidence of 1 lesion	Dissemination in space, demonstrated by MRI **plus** two or more MRI-detected lesions consistent with MS Plus positive CSF **or** await further clinical attack implicating a different site
One attack; objective clinical evidence of 2 or more lesions	Dissemination in time, demonstrated by MRI **or** second clinical attack
One attack; objective clinical evidence of 1 lesion (monosymptomatic presentation; clinically isolated syndrome)	Dissemination in space, demonstrated by MRI **or** second clinical attack **or** two or more MRI-detected lesions consistent with MS Plus positive CSF **and** dissemination in time, demonstrated by MRI
Insidious neurological progression suggestive of MS	Positive CSF **and** dissemination in space, demonstrated by (1) nine or more T2 lesions in brain or (2) 2 or more lesions in spinal cord or (3) 4–8 brain lesions plus one spinal cord lesion **or** abnormal VEP associated with 4–8 brain lesions, or with fewer than 4 brain lesions plus 1 spinal cord lesion demonstrated by MRI **and** dissemination in time, demonstrated by MRI **or** continued progression for 1 year

Positive CSF–oligoclonal bands (detected preferably by isoelectric focusing) or raised IgG index. MRI parameters as listed in Table 60.4.1 and Table 60.4.2.

Primary progressive MS. Disease progression from onset with occasional plateaus and temporary minor improvements.

Secondary progressive MS. Initial relapsing-remitting disease course, followed by progression with or without occasional relapses, minor remissions, and plateaus.

Progressive relapsing MS. Progressive disease occurs from onset. Clear acute relapses occur, with or without full recovery. Continuing progression characterizes the periods between relapses.

Two severity outcomes are also described, as follows: (1) Benign MS is disease in which the patient remains fully functional in all neurological systems 15 years after the disease onset, and (2) malignant MS is disease with a rapid progressive course, leading to significant disability in multiple neurological systems or death in a relatively short time after disease onset.

Prognosis

Several factors are identified as possible prognostic indicators. MS follows a more benign course in women than in men. Onset at an early age is a favorable factor, whereas onset at a later age carries a less favorable prognosis. The relapsing form has a better prognosis than progressive disease. Impairment of sensory pathways and cranial nerve dysfunction, particularly ON, are favorable prognostic features, whereas pyramidal and particularly brainstem and cerebellar symptoms have a poor prognosis.

Diagnostic Studies

Although the diagnosis of MS remains clinical, several ancillary laboratory tests can aid in its diagnosis. The tests used most often are neuroimaging, particularly MRI, analysis of cerebrospinal fluid (CSF), and to a lesser extent, evoked potential studies. MRI has significantly changed the approach to MS and is now the modality of choice as an aid to the diagnosis. MS plaques occur in the periventricular region, corpus callosum, centrum semiovale, and to a lesser extent, deep white matter structures and basal ganglia. Features typical of MS plaques have an ovoid appearance and are arranged at right angles to the corpus callosum as if radiating from it. Patients with clinically definite MS have white matter lesions typical of MS in more than 90% of cases. The extent of cranial MRI abnormalities (and even pathology) does not necessarily correlate with the degree of clinical disability.

CSF findings alone cannot make or exclude the diagnosis of MS, but they can be useful adjuncts to clinical criteria. The CSF is grossly normal in MS, being clear, colorless, and under normal pressure. Total leukocyte count is normal in two thirds of patients, exceeding 15 cells/µl in fewer than 5% of patients and only rarely exceeding 50 cells/µl (a finding that should raise suspicion of another cause). The predominant cell type is the lymphocyte, the vast majority of which are T cells. CSF protein (or albumin) level is normal in most patients with MS. Albumin determinations are preferable because albumin is not synthesized in the CNS and thus gives a better indication of blood-brain barrier disruption than total protein, some of which may be synthesized within the CNS (i.e., immunoglobulin). Albumin levels are elevated in 20–30% of patients, although fewer than 1% of patients have a level twice the normal level. A common finding in MS is an elevation of CSF immunoglobulin level relative to other protein components, implying intrathecal synthesis. The immunoglobulin increase is predominantly IgG, but IgM and IgA are also increased.

Variants of Multiple Sclerosis

Several inflammatory demyelinating disorders bear an unknown relationship to MS. They are listed here as variants of MS, rather than as separate illnesses, because after long follow-up it is often found that the disease has reverted to a more standard variety of MS.

Recurrent Optic Neuropathy

Sequential affection of one nerve and then the other or simultaneous bilateral vision loss is uncommon in MS. Children and preadolescent patients are more likely than adults to have recurrent or simultaneous optic neuropathies.

Devic Disease (Neuromyelitis Optica)

Devic is the combination of bilateral optic neuropathy and myelopathy. The myelopathy tends to be more severe, with less likelihood of recovery. In some, the optic neuropathy and the myelopathy occur simultaneously, whereas in others one or the other component is delayed. The longer the interval, the more the pathology will be like typical MS.

Slowly Progressive Myelopathy

Slowly progressive myelopathy is a diagnosis of exclusion and refers to a small group of patients with only progressive myelopathy and no other diagnosis established. Progressive myelopathy caused by MS is part of the primary progressive MS group and carries the poor prognosis typical of that group. The choice of therapy is difficult. Some patients do better for a time with monthly intravenous corticosteroid therapy.

Acute Tumor-like Multiple Sclerosis (Marburg Variant)
The presenting feature of some patients with demyelinating disease is an acute large lesion of one hemisphere or the spinal cord. The prognosis is good, and most patients recover well clinically and their lesion volume rapidly clears.

Treatment and Management

Treatment of MS is directed toward relief or modification of symptoms, shortening the duration or limiting the residual effects of an acute relapse, preventing progression or slowing its pace, and supporting family and patient. Table 29.3 summarizes treatment strategies.

Spasticity
Spasticity slows voluntary movement, impairs balance and gait, and may cause painful flexor or extensor spasms. Partial control is often possible, although recovery of motor power is rare. Baclofen (20–80 mg every day) is a γ-aminobutyric acid agonist that relieves spasms. Intrathecal baclofen is delivered by use of an implanted pump. Tizanidine (2 mg qhs), a centrally active α_2-noradrenergic agonist, may be used alone or in combination with baclofen because the mechanism of action is different. Benzodiazepines and botulinum toxin type A are useful in selected patients.

Tremor
Tremors are usually seen in action or intention and may limit activities of daily living. Weighted wrist bracelets and specially adapted utensils are nonpharmaceutical options. Isoniazid, 800–1200 mg per day, with pyridoxine, 100 mg per day, may have marginal success. Useful anticonvulsants for tremor are primidone, carbamazepine, and gabapentin. Other drugs are clonazepam, propranolol, and ondansetron. Surgical thalamotomy or deep brain stimulation may be used in patients with refractory disease.

Fatigue
Fatigue must be separated from depression, medication side effects, or physical exhaustion from gait alterations. Amantadine has relatively few side effects and is well tolerated by most patients. Modafinil (Provigil) is a wakefulness-promoting agent recently approved for use in narcolepsy. Oral doses start at 200 mg in the morning and can be increased to 400 mg.

Table 29.3: Multiple sclerosis treatment strategies

Disease Course/Stage	Treatment Options	Evidence
Monosymptomatic (e.g., optic neuritis)— Acute attack	IV methylprednisolone, 1000 mg for 5 days, without oral taper	Class I evidence
Relapsing-remitting, no disease activity for several years, and/or no activity on MRI	IV corticosteroids if acute attack occurs	Class I evidence
Relapsing-remitting, current disease activity and/or activity on MRI	IV corticosteroids for acute attacks, plus for prevention (1) interferon β-1b (Avonex), 30 µg IM weekly; or (2) interferon β-1b (Betaseron), 1 mL SC qod; or (3) interferon β-1a (Rebif), 22 or 44 µg SC 3×/wk or (4) glatiramer acetate (Copaxone), 20 µg SC daily	Class I evidence for Avonex, Betaseron Rebif and Copaxone, All four are FDA approved
Relapsing-remitting, disease activity while on interferon or glatiramer acetate	Add monthly bolus of IV methyl-prednisolone OR oral immuno-suppressants	Class I and II evidence
Relapsing-remitting, accumulating disability (interferon/glatiramer acetate/ corticosteroid nonresponders)	IV monthly cyclophosphamide and pulse therapy OR IV mitoxantrone (Novantrone)	Class I evidence for Novantrone, which is FDA approved
Rapidly progressing disability	IV cyclophosphamide and cortico-steroid 8-day induction, followed by pulse maintenance	Class III evidence

Continued

Table 29.3: (continued)

Disease Course/Stage	Treatment Options	Evidence
Very rapidly progressing disability	Plasma exchange	Empiric
Secondary progressive	IV corticosteroid monthly pulses	Empiric
	IV cyclophosphamide/corticosteroid monthly pulses	Class III evidence
	Methotrexate, oral or SC, 7.5–20 mg/wk, with or without monthly corticosteroid pulses	Class I evidence
Primary progressive	IV corticosteroid monthly pulses	Empiric
	Methotrexate, oral or SC, 7.520 mg/wk, with or without monthly corticosteroid pulses	Empiric
	Cladribine, IV or SC	Empiric
	Consider mitoxantrone	Empiric

Bladder and Sexual Dysfunction
Bladder and sexual dysfunction are discussed in Chapter 21.

Depression
Selective serotonin reuptake inhibitors are the medication of choice for depression.

ACUTE DISSEMINATED ENCEPHALOMYELITIS

Acute disseminated encephalomyelitis (ADEM) is a uniphasic disorder, occurring in association with an immunization (postvaccination encephalomyelitis) or systemic viral infection (parainfectious encephalomyelitis) (Table 29.4). The pathological characteristics include perivascular inflammation, edema, and demyelination within the CNS. The clinical syndrome consists of rapid development of focal or multifocal neurological dysfunction followed by partial or near complete recovery. The diagnosis is uncertain in cases not preceded by either immunization or infection.

Table 29.4: Acute disseminated encephalomyelitis and related disorders

---

Acute disseminated encephalomyelitis
Uniphasic parainfectious or postvaccination inflammatory
   demyelinating disorder of the central nervous system
Acute hemorrhagic leukoencephalitis
Hyperacute form of acute disseminated encephalomyelitis,
   usually occurring after upper respiratory infections, with
   more tissue-destructive pathology
Site-restricted forms of monophasic acute inflammatory
   demyelinating disorders that may occur after viral illness
   or vaccination
Transverse myelitis
Optic neuritis
Cerebellitis
Brainstem encephalitis
Chronic or recurrent forms of parainfectious or postvaccination
   encephalomyelitis
Relationship with multiple sclerosis?
Combined peripheral and central nervous system inflammatory
   demyelinating disorders
Postvaccination: rabies, influenza?
Postinfectious: measles

Postvaccination Acute Disseminated Encephalomyelitis

The occurrence of neuroparalytic syndromes as a consequence of the original Pasteur rabies vaccine, prepared in the spinal cords of mature rabbits inoculated with fixed rabies virus, is well established. The Semple rabies vaccine, also grown in the nervous system of mature animals, had similar consequences. The present rabies vaccine, grown in human diploid cells, is not associated with ADEM. No vaccine used in the United States is known to cause demyelinating disorders of the CNS.

Measles-induced Acute Disseminated Encephalomyelitis

The overall experience suggests that acute monophasic neurological sequelae complicate 1 in 400–1000 cases of measles infection. The introduction of measles vaccination has greatly reduced the incidence of measles and its neurological complications, but the disease continues to occur in large epidemics in specific geographical areas.

Idiopathic Acute Disseminated Encephalomyelitis

Cases of acute encephalomyelitis occurring in the setting of nonspecific viral illness are difficult to diagnose with certainty and to distinguish from episodes of MS. Cases occurring in children, at an age too young to overlap with MS, are perhaps the most readily delineated. Tentative associations with ADEM have been made with several viral and bacterial infections: rubella, mumps, herpes zoster, herpes simplex, influenza, Epstein-Barr virus, coxsackievirus, *Borrelia burgdorferi*, *Mycoplasma*, and *Leptospira*.

The hallmark clinical feature of the disorder is the development of a focal or multifocal neurological disorder following exposure to virus. A prodromal syndrome of fever, malaise, and myalgias usually occurs. The onset of the CNS disorder is usually rapid, with peak dysfunction within several days. Recovery can begin within days, with complete resolution noted on occasion within a few days, but more often over the course of weeks or months. Corticosteroids are the current favored therapy.

For a more detailed discussion, see Chapter 60 in Neurology in Clinical Practice, 4th edition.

Hypoxic/Anoxic and Ischemic Encephalopathies

30

Hypoxic and ischemic states result from several conditions that range from cardiac arrest to carbon monoxide intoxication or septic shock. Immediate corrective action is required to ensure survival and minimize residual central nervous system damage. The four causes of hypoxic states are (1) insufficient cerebral blood flow, (2) reduced oxygen availability, (3) reduced oxygen carriage by the blood, and (4) metabolic interference with the use of available oxygen. These mechanisms often coexist, causing hypoxic-ischemic encephalopathy (HIE) (Table 30.1).

SYNCOPE AND CONFUSIONAL STATES

Syncopal attacks (see Chapter 1) are brief episodes of global cerebral ischemic anoxia. An almost immediate return of full awareness follows the brief loss of consciousness when assuming the recumbent position. More prolonged but still brief episodes of global hypoxia may be followed by minutes to hours of confusion and potentially the appearance of a fixed amnestic syndrome that resembles Korsakoff's psychosis. The predominantly anterograde amnesia may persist for weeks and occasionally is permanent. The presence of persistent anterograde amnesia presumably reflects the selective vulnerability of hippocampal neurons to anoxic insult.

Certain agents, such as carbon monoxide and cyanide, injure cells by damaging their mechanisms for carrying and using oxygen. The resulting nervous system damage is virtually identical to that resulting from ischemic or anoxic hypoxia. Prolonged states of marginal perfusion or reduced oxygen availability, as from respiratory failure, high-altitude exposure, or profound hypotension, initially result in mild cognitive deficits

Table 30.1: Clinical syndromes of central nervous system hypoxia and ischemia

"Mild" sustained hypoxia
 Cognitive impairment
  Confusional states
  Delirium
Brief anoxic-ischemic events
  Syncope
  Abortive or actual generalized seizure activity
Sustained severe hypoxia
  Coma with residual neurological deficits
   Dementia
   Vegetative state
   Brain death
  Seizure activity
  "Watershed" infarction of cerebrum, cerebellum, spinal cord
  Infarction distal to a pre-existing arterial stenosis or
   occlusion
  Postanoxic demyelination

Source: Adapted from Caronna, J. J. & Finklestein, S. 1978, "Neurological syndrome after cardiac arrest," *Stroke*, vol. 9, pp. 517-520.

that may progress to confusion. If the state is more severe and prolonged, a typical delirium with fluctuating levels of alertness, hallucinations, and delusions occurs.

FOCAL CEREBRAL ISCHEMIA

Prolonged hypotensive episodes associated with delirium or impaired levels of consciousness may cause cerebral infarction. Focal neurological deficits may then coexist with the diffuse dysfunction caused by generalized neuronal injury. Several mechanisms of infarction (hemodynamic, embolic, and thrombotic) are involved. Failure of perfusion pressure can result in areas of infarction in the arterial watershed zones, the end-arteriolar territories lying at the boundary of brain areas supplied by a single major intracranial artery, such as the middle cerebral artery. Watershed infarctions are associated with certain characteristic clinical states, including transcortical aphasias, cortical blindness (with varying degrees of fluent aphasia and anosognosia), bi-brachial paresis with gait dysfunction (*person in the barrel syndrome*), cerebellar dysmetria, and midthoracic anterolateral spinal cord infarction.

POSTANOXIC COMA

The specific duration of anoxia necessary to produce prolonged loss of consciousness and profound cerebral damage is unknown. Individual variation is significant and may depend on variables such as blood glucose levels, trickle reperfusion, preischemic medications, and body temperature.

After resuscitation, the severely anoxic patient is in deep coma, often transiently, without even the pupillary light reflex present. Survivors regain brainstem functions during the initial 1–3 hours but generally require ventilation support. Initially flaccid, the patient subsequently shows decerebrate or decorticate posturing. Seizure activity occurs in almost one third of patients within the first few days. The diagnosis of nonconvulsive status epilepticus is a consideration in patients who plateau in a stuporous state or experience a secondary decline in level of alertness.

Recovery rates vary. With time, initial flaccidity is replaced by reflex motor posturing, followed by avoidance movements, reflex grasping, eye opening, and finally arousal. Patients arousing within 24 hours are typically agitated and confused for a period of hours to days but ultimately recover most cognitive functions. Recent memory function is particularly sensitive to hypoxia. Patients whose coma persists beyond 4 or 5 days slowly become responsive to the environment, if only in a limited fashion. Structured environments, neuroleptic medication, bladder and bowel programs, and rehabilitative therapy help optimize functioning.

Persistent Vegetative State

A vegetative state develops in some patients with postanoxic coma. They open their eyes within a few days but make no apparent contact with the environment. The only motor responses are abnormal posturing. Brainstem reflexes recover quickly and sleep-wake cycles appear. With eye opening, other behaviors emerge, such as yawning, bruxism, smiling, crying, sneezing, and blinking when the examiner's hand is thrust toward the eyes. Consistent nonreflexive responses to stimulation are not established. Consistent following of moving people or objects does not occur. Persistence of this condition for a month after resuscitation is a *persistent vegetative state*. Pathological examination shows a necrotic forebrain and a preserved brainstem. Electroencephalographic findings are severely abnormal. The distinction of such patients from those with ventral pontine infarctions is imperative. The latter are *locked in*, lacking efferent responses but have normal cognition and preserved awareness.

Delayed Postanoxic Deterioration

Occasionally, patients seem to arouse early and begin to recover well from anoxic coma, only to relapse. They appear apathetic and confused. Examination reveals gait disturbance, spasticity, incontinence, movement disorders, and dysarthria. With supportive care, incomplete recovery occurs. Individuals older than 30 years are at greater risk for delayed deterioration. Carbon monoxide poisoning is often the initial cause of coma.

Other Sequelae

Recovery of cognitive functions generally proceeds rapidly during the first several weeks after anoxic injury and plateaus by 3 months. Moderate to severe biparietal dysfunction (acalculia, apraxia) occurs in one of three survivors. Almost half have moderate to severe memory impairment. Problems with planning and organizational skills, as well as depression, are common. Movement disorders frequently emerge during recovery from severe hypoxic events. Epilepsy is uncommon in surviving postanoxic patients.

Prognosis of Anoxic Coma after Cardiopulmonary Arrest

Cardiopulmonary arrest (CPA) is associated with a high rate of morbidity and mortality and is the most common cause of severe anoxic injury (Table 30.2). Hospital mortality among those who survive until hospital admission ranges from 50% to 90%. Of those surviving to hospital discharge, 20% die in 1 year and 40% within 3 years; of the remaining patients, 75% have severe neurological impairment, often with severe memory deficits (Table 30.3).

BRAIN DEATH

See Chapter 2 for a discussion on brain death.

Management of Coma due to Hypoxic-Ischemic Encephalopathy

HIE after CPA is a coma with a static or improving course, frequently complicated by seizure activity. New factors, such as sepsis and drug effects, may come into play during the patient's

Table 30.2: Cranial nerve reflex abnormalities and survival after cardiopulmonary arrest

Time After Cardiopulmonary Arrest	Number of Cranial Nerve Reflex Abnormalities*	Survivors (%)
<3 hrs	0	80
	1	46
	2	29
	3	0
<6 hrs	0	80
	1	37
	2	27
	3	0
<24 hrs	0	81
	1	38
	2	21
	3	0
24–48 hrs	0	76
	1	21
	2	0
	3	0

*Absent pupillary light reflex, absent corneal responses, absent spontaneous conjugate roving gaze; each count as one abnormal finding.
Source: Adapted from Snyder, B. D., Gumnit, R. J., Leppik, I. E., et al. 1981, "Neurologic prognosis after cardiopulmonary arrest: IV. Brainstem reflexes," *Neurology*, vol. 31, pp. 1092–1097.

prolonged illness. Primary intracranial disease can resemble anoxic states and may coexist with them. Patients who present with cardiac arrhythmias may have sustained a primary intracranial insult, such as a subarachnoid or intracerebral hemorrhage. Inspection of the optic fundi for papilledema or hemorrhages is essential. Any focal neurological finding should lead to a search for other intracranial pathology.

Patients may benefit from the induction of mild hypothermia for 12–24 hours postarrest. Parenteral histamine H_2-receptor blockers, such as ranitidine, are the most useful agents to prevent stress ulceration of the stomach. Other aspects of routine coma care involve preventing decubitus ulcers, ensuring suitable bladder drainage, and maintaining nutrition. No specific treatment reverses HIE. Rapidly reestablishing circulation and maintaining a normal or somewhat increased systemic arterial pressure are essential. Hyperthermia and seizure activity increase central nervous system metabolic activity and should be controlled.

Table 30.3: Guidelines that identify patients with poor or good prognosis after cardiopulmonary arrest

Time After Cardiac Arrest Clinical Sign	Patients with Virtually No Chance of Regaining Independence	Patients with Best Chance of Regaining Independence
Initial examination	No pupillary light reflex[*]	Pupillary light reflexes present; motor response decorticate posturing or decerebrate posturing; spontaneous eye movements conjugately roving or orienting
1 day	1-day motor response no better than decorticate posturing; spontaneous eye movements neither orienting nor conjugate; roving	1-day motor response withdrawal or better; 1-day eye opening to noise or spontaneously
3 days	3-day motor response no better than decorticate posturing	Motor response withdrawal or better; spontaneous eye movements normal
1 wk	Not obeying commands; spontaneous eye movements neither orienting nor conjugate	Obeying commands

[*]In the absence of some other cause.

Source: Adapted with permission from Levy, D. E., Caronna, J. J., Singer, B. H., et al. (1985), "Predicting outcome from hypoxic-ischemic coma," *JAMA,* 253, pp. 1420–1426.

The indication for anticonvulsant therapy is seizure activity that does not respond to correction of metabolic factors. Intravenous phenytoin loading is the mainstay for treating generalized tonic-clonic or partial complex status epilepticus. Phenobarbital loading may be safer for patients with certain types of cardiac arrhythmias or persistent hypotension but further depresses consciousness. Axial myoclonus can be very difficult to control. Benzodiazepines or valproic acid may be effective, but neuro-muscular blockade or deep sedation with morphine is more likely to prevent disruption of ventilation and interfere with nursing care. Glucocorticoids and calcium-channel blockers are of no value in treating HIE.

For a more detailed discussion, see Chapter 61 in Neurology in Clinical Practice, 4th edition.

Toxic and Metabolic Encephalopathies

31

Toxic and metabolic encephalopathies are characterized by altered mental status caused by the failure of organs other than the nervous system or by the presence of an endogenous or exogenous toxin or drug. Although the brain is isolated from the rest of the body by the blood–brain barrier, the nervous system often is affected severely by organ failure that leads to the buildup of toxic substances normally removed by other organs, especially the liver and kidney. Damage to homeostatic mechanisms that alter the internal milieu of the brain, such as the abnormalities of electrolyte and water metabolism associated with renal failure or the syndrome of inappropriate secretion of antidiuretic hormone (SIADH), is one mechanism of metabolic encephalopathy. In some cases, deficiency of a critical substrate after the failure of an organ, such as hypoglycemia due to fulminating hepatic failure, is the precipitating factor. In patients with coma of unknown etiology, nearly two thirds ultimately are found to have a metabolic cause. The history and physical examination usually define the affected organ system, but in many cases the cause is established only by laboratory investigations.

CLINICAL MANIFESTATIONS

Encephalopathies that develop insidiously may be difficult to detect because of the slowness with which abnormalities evolve. Abnormalities of mental status are always present and may range from delirium to coma (see Chapters 2 and 3). Initial impairments are often in the spheres of selective attention and the ability to process information. The neuro-ophthalmological examination is helpful when examining patients with metabolic disorders. Reflex constriction of the pupils to light and the oculovestibular responses are usually slowed but preserved, even in comatose patients. The eyes may be aligned normally in patients with mild encephalopathy; however, with more severe encephalopathy, dysconjugate roving movements are common.

Motor system abnormalities are common, particularly slight increases in tone. Other signs and symptoms of metabolic disorders may include spasticity with extensor-plantar signs (in liver disease), multifocal myoclonus (in uremia and hypoxia), cramps (in electrolyte disorders), Trousseau's sign (in hypocalcemia), tremors, and weakness. Generalized seizures occur in patients with water intoxication, hypoxia, uremia, and hypoglycemia but only rarely with liver failure. Focal seizures, including epilepsia partialis continua, are seen in patients with hyperglycemia.

TOXIC ENCEPHALOPATHIES

Hepatic Encephalopathy

Liver disease causes encephalopathy by two mechanisms: hepatocellular failure and the diversion of toxins from the hepatic portal vein into the systemic circulation. Usually, one mechanism predominates, although both coexist to some degree. This is particularly true in patients with cirrhosis in whom shunts are common and encephalopathy waxes and wanes. The term *portal systemic encephalopathy* is applied to patients with cirrhosis with shunts. Patients with *fulminant hepatic failure*, a disorder occurring in patients with previously normal livers who exhibit neurological signs within 8 weeks of developing liver disease, have pure hepatocellular dysfunction; few patients with congenital abnormalities or surgical portacaval shunts have symptoms due only to the shunt.

Clinical Features

The features that differentiate patients with fulminant hepatic failure from those with the much more common portal systemic encephalopathy are shown in Table 31.1. The diagnosis of hepatic encephalopathy is based on the signs and symptoms of cerebral dysfunction in a setting of hepatic failure. Sixty percent or more of all patients with cirrhosis with no overt evidence of encephalopathy show significant abnormalities when tested. Tests of attention, concentration, and visuospatial perception are the most likely to be abnormal. Hepatic encephalopathy may be precipitated by the use of sedatives, gastrointestinal hemorrhage, excessive dietary protein, hypokalemia, constipation, and infection.

Table 31.1: Features distinguishing fulminating hepatic failure from chronic hepatic encephalopathy or portal systemic encephalopathy

Feature	Fulminating Hepatic Failure	Portal Systemic Encephalopathy
History		
Onset	Usually acute	Varies; may be insidious or subacute
Mental state	Mania may evolve to deep coma	Blunted consciousness progresses to coma
Precipitating factor	Viral infection or hepatotoxin	Gastrointestinal hemorrhage, exogenous protein, drugs, uremia
History of liver disease	No	Usually yes
Symptoms		
Nausea, vomiting	Common	Unusual
Abdominal pain	Common	Unusual
Signs		
Liver	Small, soft, tender	Usually large, firm, no pain
Nutritional state	Normal	Cachectic
Collateral circulation	Absent	Present
Ascites	Absent	May be present
Laboratory tests		
Transaminases	Very high	Normal or slightly high
Coagulopathy	Present	Often present

Laboratory Features
Usually, standard laboratory test results, including those of serum bilirubin and hepatic enzymes, are abnormal. Products of normal hepatic function, including serum albumin and clotting factors, often are low, leading to prolongation of the prothrombin time. Measuring the arterial ammonia level may help in diagnosing hepatic encephalopathy. Electroencephalography (EEG) is useful in determining the severity of encephalopathy. The three stages in the EEG evolution are (1) a theta stage with diffuse 4- to 7-Hz waves, (2) a triphasic phase with surface-positive maximum deflections, and (3) a delta stage, characterized by random arrhythmic slowing with little bilateral synchrony.

Magnetic resonance imaging studies show high-signal abnormalities in the pallidum of patients with hepatic encephalopathy when T1 and inversion-recovery pulse sequences are used. In addition to these abnormalities, the T1 signal abnormality is widespread and found in the limbic and extrapyramidal systems and generally throughout the white matter. They regress or disappear after successful treatment or a liver transplant.

Treatment
Practice guidelines published by the American College of Gastroenterology identify four goals: (1) provide supportive care, (2) identify and treat precipitating factors, (3) reduce the nitrogenous load from the gut, and (4) assess the need for long-term therapy. Initial diagnostic and therapeutic efforts should be directed at the identification and mitigation of precipitating factors and reducing the nitrogenous load arising from the gastrointestinal tract. This is accomplished by a brief withdrawal of protein from the diet and the administration of cleansing enemas, followed by the use of lactulose. Antibiotics may be used as an alternative to lactulose. After the acute phase of hepatic encephalopathy, patients should receive the maximum amount of protein that is tolerated. Prolonged periods of protein restriction should be avoided.

Complications and Prognosis
Although hepatic encephalopathy is potentially completely reversible, prolonged or repeated episodes risk transforming this reversible condition into non-wilsonian hepatocerebral degeneration, a severe disease with fixed or progressive neurological deficits, including dementia, dysarthria, gait ataxia with intention tremor, and choreoathetosis. Some patients may develop evidence of spinal cord damage, usually manifested by a spastic paraplegia. Severe hepatic coma carries a substantial risk of death.

Uremic Encephalopathy

Many of the disorders that lead to the development of renal failure, such as hypertension, systemic lupus erythematosus, and diabetes mellitus, also cause disorders of the nervous system. It may be difficult to determine whether new neurological problems are caused by primary disorders of the nervous system or are secondary to uremia. Another difficulty is distinguishing neurological problems caused by the progression of renal disease from those caused by its treatment.

Clinical Features
The most notable difference between patients with renal encephalopathy and those with other forms of metabolic encephalopathy is the common coexistence of signs of obtundation (suggesting nervous system depression) and of twitching, myoclonus, agitation, and occasionally seizures (suggesting neural excitation).

Treatment
Dialysis is the primary treatment for uremic encephalopathy. Usually, hemodialysis is chosen, although occasionally peritoneal dialysis is used alternatively. After stabilization on dialysis, renal transplantation may be required.

METABOLIC DISTURBANCES

Disorders of Glucose Metabolism

Glucose is normally the exclusive fuel for the brain. The brain, unlike other organs, stores only trivial quantities of glucose (as glycogen), making it highly vulnerable to interruptions in the supply of glucose; the cerebral metabolic rate for glucose is high, but brain glucose concentrations are only 25% of the plasma concentration. The brain tolerates hyperglycemia better than hypoglycemia, but hyperglycemia also produces neurological impairment, largely because of osmotic effects.

Clinical Aspects of Hypoglycemia
The diagnosis of hypoglycemia, based only on clinical features, is difficult. Although most symptoms of hypoglycemia are attributable to nervous system dysfunction, they are nonspecific and variable even when blood glucose levels are very low. The term *neuroglycopenia* is sometimes used to refer to symptomatic hypoglycemia. Three syndromes are recognized, as follows:

1. The *acute syndrome* is usually caused by the action of short-acting insulin preparations or sulfonylureas. The initial

features are vague symptoms of malaise, feeling detached from the environment, restlessness associated with hunger, and nervousness that may lead to panic, sweating, and ataxia. The patient may recognize these symptoms and respond with oral glucose. Attacks may terminate spontaneously or proceed rapidly to generalized seizures and coma, with the attendant risk of permanent brain injury. Such patients are likely to arrive in the emergency department in coma with no history available.

2. The *subacute syndrome* is the most common form, with spontaneous hypoglycemia occurring in the fasting state. Instead of the symptoms of the acute syndrome, a slowing of thought processes and a gradual blunting of consciousness with retention of awareness develop. Amnesia for the episode is common. The diagnosis is difficult. Hypothermia is common, and unexplained low body temperatures should always indicate a blood glucose measurement.

3. *Chronic hypoglycemia* is rare and if confirmed suggests a probable insulin-secreting tumor or obsessive control of a diabetic. The characteristic features are insidious changes in personality, memory, and behavior that may be misconstrued as dementia. Unlike with the acute and subacute forms of hypoglycemia, glucose does not promptly relieve the symptoms, suggesting the presence of neuronal injury.

The detection of hypoglycemia in neonates and children is complicated by the nonspecificity of the symptoms (e.g., pallor, irritability, and feeding difficulties) and by the variable sensitivities of individual children to a given plasma glucose concentration.

Hypoglycemia is a medical emergency, and all patients suspected of being hypoglycemic, including those with coma of unknown cause, should be treated with parenteral glucose after adequate blood samples are obtained for laboratory testing. It is prudent to draw extra blood so that insulin and C-peptide levels can be measured if indicated by the patient's subsequent course.

Clinical Aspects of Hyperglycemia

The most important causes of hyperglycemia are diabetic ketoacidosis (DKA), nonketotic hyperosmolar coma (NKHC), and iatrogenic factors, such as parenteral hyperalimentation. DKA, a relatively common disorder in type I diabetics, is often precipitated by infection in a patient who was otherwise stable. It develops over several days and is heralded by polyuria and polydipsia due to the osmotic diuresis produced by glucosuria. These symptoms are followed by anorexia, nausea, disorientation, and coma. Sustained hyperventilation is common, especially in patients with severe acidosis. The diagnosis is frequently suspected on the basis of clinical findings; however, laboratory data, including measuring the plasma glucose levels, arterial blood gas levels, and electrolyte levels, and testing for ketone bodies are essential for confirmation and management. DKA is an insulin-deficient state, and administering insulin is the cornerstone of therapy. Replacing fluid and electrolytes and treating precipitating factors are required.

In contrast, NKHC is a feature of type II diabetes and mainly occurs in older patients, commonly as the first manifestation of the disease. This syndrome evolves more slowly than DKA, and the period of polyuria is more prolonged, leading to severe dehydration. The clinical features are those of hyperosmolality, hypovolemia, and cerebral dysfunction, with epileptic seizures, often focal, occurring in some individuals. Precipitating factors include infection, gastroenteritis, pancreatitis, and occasionally treatment with glucocorticoids or phenytoin.

Neurologists may become involved in the diagnosis and management of patients with NKHC when patients with no history of diabetes are brought to the emergency department with unexplained coma or seizures. Because hyperosmolality and the associated hypovolemia are usually much more severe in this condition than in DKA, maintaining an adequate blood pressure and cardiac output is the first priority. One or 2 liters of normal saline is given rapidly to restore blood volume and to reduce plasma osmolality. Additional fluid and insulin therapy are given as indicated by laboratory and clinical data.

Complications of Treatment
Patients with DKA experience rapid neurological and then cardiovascular deterioration. The mortality from DKA is still appreciable. Death is from cardiovascular collapse or complications of the infection that precipitated DKA.

DISORDERS OF WATER AND ELECTROLYTE METABOLISM

Patients with abnormalities of water and electrolyte metabolism often exhibit altered states of consciousness or epileptic seizures as an initial feature. The vulnerability of the central nervous system to abnormalities of water and electrolyte balance is mainly attributed to brain swelling. The role played by electrolytes is also important in maintaining transmembrane potentials, neurotransmission, and a variety of metabolic reactions, such as those involving the role of calcium and calmodulin.

Disordered Osmolality

Osmotic Homeostasis
The serum and hence whole-body osmolality are regulated by complex neuroendocrine and renal interactions that control thirst and water and electrolyte balance. When serum osmolality increases, the brain loses volume; when osmolality falls, the brain swells.

Hypoosmolality
Hypoosmolality is almost always associated with hyponatremia, and laboratory testing establishes the diagnosis. In patients with hyponatremia, serum osmolality must be measured to differentiate true from pseudo-hypoosmolality. Pseudo-hypoosmolality is encountered with lipemic serum or in neurological patients treated with mannitol.

Several neurological conditions are associated with hyponatremia because of its association with SIADH. In SIADH, hyponatremia occurs despite normal or increased blood volume, normal renal function, and the absence of factors that normally operate to produce antidiuretic hormone release. The syndrome may be relatively asymptomatic. In such cases, water restriction is the treatment of choice. The rapid correction of hyponatremia may cause *central pontine myelinolysis*.

Hyperosmolality
Hyperosmolality may be associated with intracranial bleeding caused by the tearing of veins that bridge the space between the brain and dural sinuses. Usually, hyperosmolality is diagnosed by laboratory findings of an elevated serum sodium concentration or hyperglycemia in diabetics. It is often caused by dehydration, especially in hot climates, by uncontrolled diabetes with or without ketosis, and less frequently by central lesions that reset the osmotically sensitive regions of the brain.

Disorders of Calcium

Hypercalcemia
Hypercalcemia is associated with hyperparathyroidism, granulomatous diseases, especially sarcoidosis, treatment with drugs including thiazide diuretics, Vitamin D, calcium itself, tumors that have metastasized to bone, and thyroid disease. Many cases are idiopathic. Severe hypercalcemia affects the brain directly,

causing coma in extreme cases. Less severe hypercalcemia may cause altered consciousness with a pseudodementia syndrome and weakness. Gastrointestinal, renal, and cardiovascular abnormalities also may be present. Severe hypercalcemia is life threatening. Initial treatment consists of a forced diuresis using saline and diuretics. Once the initial phase of treatment is accomplished, further management is determined by the cause of the hypercalcemia.

Hypocalcemia

Hypocalcemia usually is associated with hypoparathyroidism. The neurological symptoms are caused by the enhanced excitability of the nervous system. Symptoms include paresthesias around the mouth and fingers, cramps caused by tetanic muscle contraction, and epileptic seizures. In more chronic hypocalcemia, headache caused by increased intracranial pressure may occur, as may extrapyramidal signs and symptoms such as chorea or parkinsonism. Computed tomographic scans may show calcification of the basal ganglia. The physical examination should include attempts to elicit the Chvostek and Trousseau signs. Cataracts and papilledema may be seen. Severe hypocalcemia should be treated with infusions of calcium to treat or prevent epileptic seizures or laryngeal spasms, both of which are life threatening but unusual complications. Chronic therapy usually involves the administration of calcium and Vitamin D.

Disorders of Magnesium

Hypermagnesemia is unusual. Normal kidneys act to preserve magnesium homeostasis. Infusions of magnesium to treat eclampsia are the most common cause of hypermagnesemia. Hypocalcemia potentiates the effects of excess magnesium. Severe hypermagnesemia is life threatening, and concentrations in excess of 10 mEq/L must be treated. Magnesium deficiency usually occurs in patients with deficiencies of other electrolytes. Magnesium deficiency is usually part of a complex electrolyte imbalance, and accurate diagnosis and management of all aspects of the state are necessary to ensure recovery.

Disorders of Manganese

Manganese poisoning occurs primarily in manganese ore miners and causes parkinsonism.

DRUG INTOXICATION

The tentative diagnosis of intentional or accidental drug overdose must be considered during the course of the evaluation of

Table 31.2: Characteristics of drug overdose

1. Toxicity predicted by drug level—specific therapy determined by toxicology
   Acetaminophen, digoxin, ethylene glycol (not detected by most systems), lithium, salicylates, theophylline
2. Toxicity parallels drug level—supportive care required
   Barbiturates, ethanol, phenytoin
3. Toxicology confirms only clinical impression—clinical decisions determined by direct patient evaluation
   Cyanide, narcotics, organophosphates, tricyclic antidepressants
4. Toxicity correlates poorly with drug level—clinical decisions determined by direct patient evaluation
   Amphetamines, benzodiazepines, cocaine, hallucinogens, neuroleptics, phencyclidine, phenylpropanolamine

Source: Based on Mahoney, J. D., Gross, P. L., Stern, T. A., et al. 1990, "Quantitative serum toxic screening in the management of suspected drug overdose," *Am J Emer Med*, vol. 8, pp. 16-22.

almost all emergency department patients with altered behavior. Most overdoses are attributable to the following drugs in order of decreasing frequency: ethanol, benzodiazepines, salicylates, acetaminophen, barbiturates, and tricyclic antidepressants. Table 31.2 classifies drugs into four groups based on the usefulness of toxicological information and the relationships between drug levels and symptomatology.

For a more detailed discussion, see Chapter 62 in Neurology in Clinical Practice, 4th edition.

Deficiency Diseases of the Nervous System

32

Undernutrition causes several neurological disorders, ranging from isolated optic neuropathy to diffuse involvement of the peripheral nervous system and central nervous system. Deficiency of the B vitamins (thiamine, pyridoxine, nicotinic acid, and Vitamin B12) and of Vitamin E is most likely to produce neurological disease. The usual cause of dietary insufficiency in developed countries is chronic alcoholism or malabsorption states. Most dietary or malabsorptive causes of nutritional deficiency do not selectively deplete any single vitamin. One exception is pernicious anemia, in which malabsorption is restricted to Vitamin B12. Table 32.1 summarizes the common neurological manifestations of deficiency diseases.

VITAMIN DEFICIENCY

Vitamin B12 Deficiency

Vitamin B12 deficiency is one of a few nutritional diseases regularly seen in the United States. Dietary Vitamin B12 binds to intrinsic factor and absorbed into the circulation. Once absorbed, Vitamin B12 binds to transcobalamins for transport to tissues. As much as 90% of total body Vitamin B12 (1–10 mg) is stored in the liver. Even when vitamin absorption is severely impaired, depletion of the body store takes years. A clinical relapse in pernicious anemia after interrupting Vitamin B12 therapy takes an average of 5 years. Nitrous oxide anesthesia can precipitate acute illness in patients with subclinical deficiency.

Clinical Features
Paresthesias in the hands and feet are the usual initial features of Vitamin B12 deficiency. Weakness and unsteadiness of gait follow. Other features include mental slowing, depression, confusion, delusions, hallucinations, dyspepsia, and altered

Table 32.1: Neurological manifestations in deficiency diseases

Neurological Manifestations	Associated Nutritional Deficiencies
Peripheral neuropathy	Thiamine, Vitamin B12, Vitamin E, pyridoxine, folate
Dementia, encephalopathy	Vitamin B12, nicotinic acid, thiamine, folate
Seizures	Pyridoxine
Myelopathy	Vitamin B12, vitamin E, folate
Myopathy	Vitamin D, vitamin E
Optic neuropathy	Vitamin B12, thiamine, folate, and probably others
Spinocerebellar degeneration	Vitamin E

bowel habits. Examination shows signs of polyneuropathy, myelopathy, or both. Loss of vibration or position sense in the legs is the most consistent abnormality. Decreased tendon reflexes are absent in the legs and motor impairment ranges from clumsiness of gait to spastic paraplegia. Bilateral visual loss, optic atrophy, and centrocecal scotomas often antedate other clinical features.

Laboratory Studies
Imaging studies exclude structural causes. Magnetic resonance imaging (MRI) shows treatment-reversible T2 enhancement and spinal cord swelling in the lateral or posterior columns. Clinical features may precede MRI changes by at least 2 weeks and are most prominent at 3–5 months. MRI improvement occurs within a few months of starting treatment, although clinical normalization occurs over a few years. Macrocytic anemia is an inconstant feature and may be absent at the time of neurological presentation. Radioassay or a chemiluminescence assay measure serum cobalamin. The latter yields a higher normal reference range (250–1100 pg/ml as compared with 170–900 pg/ml for radioassay). Abnormally low serum Vitamin B12 or elevated metabolite levels confirm deficiency in the presence of an appropriate neurological picture. A normal serum cobalamin level does not exclude a deficiency state. A Schilling test further documents the underlying cause of malabsorption.

Management
In cases of uncertain diagnosis, institute a therapeutic trial of parenteral cobalamin while monitoring serum levels of homocysteine and methylmalonic acid before and after treatment. In cobalamin-deficient patients, homocysteine and methylmalonic

acid levels typically normalize within 7–10 days after treatment. Treat all patients with clinically overt Vitamin B12 deficiency with intramuscular injections of 100 μg daily or 1000 μg twice weekly for 2 weeks and then with weekly injections of 1000 μg for another 2–3 months. Lifelong maintenance therapy with monthly 1000-μg injections of Vitamin B12 treats vitamin malabsorption.

Folate Deficiency and Homocysteine

Clinical Features
Overt neurological features are rare. Folate deficiency may result in mild cognitive impairment or increased stroke risk in adults and increased frequency of neural tube defects in babies born to folate-deficient mothers. In 1998, the U.S. Food and Drug Administration mandated fortification of grain products with folate. The level of supplement on average increases the dietary folate intake of adults by 100 μg per day. The impact of this policy is unknown.

Diagnosis
Direct measurements of plasma and erythrocyte folate concentrations are available. Erythrocyte level is generally more reliable than plasma level.

Treatment and Management
Prospective studies on the use of folate in the prevention of vascular disease are in progress. Prophylaxis against neural tube defects in women with epilepsy requires daily folate supplements of 0.4 mg or more. In documented folate deficiency, the initial dose is 1 mg of folate three times per day, followed by a maintenance dose of 1 mg per day. The parenteral dose for acutely ill patients is 1–5 mg. Oral doses as high as 15 mg per day are not toxic. Large doses of folate can correct the megaloblastic anemia of Vitamin B12 deficiency without altering the neurological abnormalities.

Vitamin E Deficiency

Clinical Features
Vitamin E deficiency states usually occur in patients with significant fat malabsorption. A rare familial form of fat malabsorption is abetalipoproteinemia (Bassen-Kornzweig syndrome). The initial features of Vitamin E deficiency are usually weakness or gait unsteadiness. Examination shows a syndrome of spinocerebellar degeneration, often accompanied by a peripheral neuropathy. The most consistent abnormalities are

limb ataxia, areflexia, and severe loss of vibration and position sense. Cutaneous sensation is less affected. Many patients have nystagmus, ptosis, or partial external ophthalmoplegia. Mild to moderate proximal weakness is common but may be distal or diffuse.

Laboratory Studies

Low serum Vitamin E concentration establishes the diagnosis. Nerve conduction studies usually show a mild axonal neuropathy, with diminished or absent sural nerve action potentials and normal or slightly slow motor nerve conduction.

Treatment and Management

The recommended daily requirement of Vitamin E in healthy adults is 10 mg (equivalent to 10 IU) of D,L-α-tocopherol acetate, a commonly available form of the vitamin. The initial treatment is with an oral preparation of water-miscible tocopherol at a dose of 200–600 mg per day. Use higher oral dosages or parenteral administration if improvement does not occur.

Pellagra (Nicotinic Acid Deficiency)

Dietary deficiency of nicotinic acid (niacin) has largely disappeared in countries that mandate niacin enrichment of grains.

Clinical Features

Pellagra affects the gastrointestinal tract, skin, and nervous system (diarrhea, dermatitis, and dementia). Early symptoms of irritability, apathy, depressed mood, inattentiveness, and memory loss may progress to stupor or coma. In addition to the confusional state, examination shows spasticity, extensor-plantar responses, gegenhalten, and startle myoclonus.

Treatment

Oral nicotinic acid in doses of 50 mg three times a day is usually sufficient to treat symptomatic patients. The parenteral dose is 25 mg two to three times a day. Nicotinamide has similar therapeutic efficacy in pellagra, but it does not have niacin's vasodilatory and cholesterol-lowering activities.

Vitamin B6 (Pyridoxine) Deficiency

Although the terms *pyridoxine* and *Vitamin B6* are used synonymously, two other naturally occurring compounds, pyridoxal and pyridoxamine, possess biological activities similar to pyridoxine. All three compounds convert to pyridoxal phosphate, the coenzyme important for the metabolism of many amino acids.

Clinical Features

Sporadic cases of infantile seizures from dietary Vitamin B6 deficiency still result from breast-feeding by malnourished mothers. Birth is normal and the child healthy until the development of hyperirritability and an exaggerated auditory startle. Recurrent convulsions occur until correcting the dietary insufficiency. Another form of pyridoxine-responsive seizure occurs in infants with a congenital dependency on pyridoxine. They develop symptoms despite a normal dietary supply of pyridoxine. Most have seizures within days of birth and require 5–100 mg of pyridoxine to control their convulsions. Long-term administration of 10 mg per day is required. Seizures often reappear within days of pyridoxine withdrawal.

Vitamin B6 deficiency is unusual in adults and may be asymptomatic. Isoniazid, hydralazine, and penicillamine are probably responsible for most adult cases of Vitamin B6 deficiency. It is especially a problem in slow inactivators of isoniazid. Fifty percent may develop peripheral neuropathy on treatment. The initial features are numbness, tingling, and occasionally burning pain in the feet. If the drug is continued, symptoms spread proximally. Burning pain is disabling in some instances. Examination shows distal weakness, depressed tendon reflexes, and impaired distal sensation.

Prolonged use of moderate to high doses of pyridoxine (500 mg per day or more) may cause neuropathy. The patients have a predominantly sensory syndrome, with impaired cutaneous and deep sensation, areflexia, Romberg's sign, and sensory ataxia.

Management

The neurotoxicity of isoniazid and hydralazine is dose dependent. Even with high doses of isoniazid, pyridoxine supplements of 50 mg per day can prevent the development of neuropathy in nearly all patients.

Beriberi (Thiamine Deficiency Polyneuropathy)

Beriberi affects the heart and peripheral nerves, producing congestive cardiomyopathy, sensorimotor polyneuropathy, or both. The *wet* and *dry* forms refer to the presence or absence of edema. Beriberi is rare in developed countries.

Clinical Features

The neuropathy progresses over several weeks. Affected patients complain of paresthesias and weakness of the legs. Walking becomes difficult, and muscle tenderness and cramps, especially of the calves, are prominent. Most patients have tachycardia, palpitation, dyspnea, and fatigue, and half develop edema at the ankle or in the face.

The striking neurological finding is a stocking-glove distribution of cutaneous sensory loss. Weakness, when present, occurs first in the distal extensor muscles, giving rise to the characteristic symmetrical footdrop and wristdrop. Tendon reflexes are lost in the legs. Laryngeal nerve paralysis, producing hoarseness and weakness of voice, is a rare complication.

Laboratory Studies
Serum and urine thiamine concentrations may be decreased but do not reliably reflect tissue concentrations. Erythrocyte transketolase activity depends on thiamine and provides an assay of functional status. Elevated serum pyruvate concentrations provide additional confirmation. Electrodiagnostic studies show an axonal neuropathic pattern with normal or mildly reduced conduction velocity and neurogenic changes on the electromyogram. Cerebrospinal fluid examination is usually normal.

Treatment
A balanced diet supplemented with thiamine hydrochloride, 50–100 mg per day, treats the deficiency. Parenteral administration is required when gastrointestinal absorption is questionable. Gradual return of sensory and motor function occurs after a few weeks of treatment. Improvement in severely affected patients takes several months and may be incomplete.

Infantile Beriberi

An acute syndrome of thiamine deficiency in infants occurs in the rice-eating populations of Asia, most frequently in breast-fed infants younger than 1 year. Thiamine is often deficient in breast milk from mothers who eat primarily polished rice. Although called *infantile beriberi*, it bears little resemblance to the adult form. Acute cardiac symptoms are common, often preceded by a prodrome of anorexia, vomiting, deficient weight gain, and restlessness. Dyspnea, cyanosis, and signs of heart failure follow and can lead rapidly to death. Arytenoid edema and recurrent laryngeal neuropathy give rise to hoarseness, dysphonia, and eventually aphonia. Early warning signs of coughing and choking may be mistaken for respiratory tract infections. Central nervous system manifestations include drowsiness, ophthalmoplegia, and convulsions. These symptoms begin abruptly and have a grave prognosis. Parenteral administration of 5–20 mg of thiamine can be lifesaving.

Wernicke Syndrome

Although chronic alcoholism is the most common cause, cases occur in other conditions with a poor nutritional state (Table 32.2). Intravenous glucose administration or carbohydrate loading may precipitate Wernicke's encephalopathy in at-risk patients.

Clinical Features

The main features of Wernicke's encephalopathy are confusion, ophthalmoplegia, and ataxia. The confusional state develops over days or weeks, with inattention, apathy, disorientation, and memory loss. Stupor or coma is rare. Most patients have horizontal nystagmus on lateral gaze, and many have vertical nystagmus on upgaze. Ophthalmoplegia, when present, involves both lateral recti, either in isolation or with other extraocular muscle palsies. Sluggish reaction to light, light-near dissociation, or other pupillary abnormalities occur. Truncal ataxia is common, but limb ataxia is not. Other findings are hypothermia and postural hypotension, reflecting involvement of hypothalamic and brainstem autonomic pathways. Signs of nutritional deficiency and complications of alcoholism, such as peripheral neuropathy, tongue redness, skin changes, and liver abnormalities, are associated. Many patients also show signs of acute alcohol withdrawal, with tremor, delirium, and tachycardia.

Untreated Wernicke's encephalopathy is progressive. The mortality is 10–20%, even with thiamine treatment. With treatment, the ocular signs resolve within hours, although a fine nystagmus often persists. Apathy and lethargy improve over

Table 32.2: Associated conditions in nonalcoholic patients with Wernicke's encephalopathy

Hyperemesis of pregnancy
Systemic malignancy
Gastrointestinal surgery
Hemodialysis or peritoneal dialysis
Prolonged intravenous feeding
Refeeding after prolonged fasting or starvation
Anorexia nervosa
Dieting and gastric plication
Acquired immunodeficiency syndrome

weeks. Gait improves slowly and may be abnormal even months after treatment. As the global confusional state recedes, some patients show a Korsakoff syndrome.

Laboratory Studies

Wernicke's encephalopathy is a clinical diagnosis. MRI may show signal abnormalities on T2-weighted, fluid-attenuated inversion recovery and diffusion-weighted images in the periaqueductal regions, medial thalami, and bilateral mamillary bodies. The lesions sometimes show contrast enhancement. The signal abnormalities typically resolve completely with prompt treatment, but shrunken mamillary bodies are a late residual finding. The cerebrospinal fluid is either normal or shows a mild elevation in protein. Serum thiamine level and erythrocyte transketolase activity may be depressed, and serum pyruvate may be elevated.

Treatment

Patients suspected of Wernicke's encephalopathy should receive thiamine before administration of glucose to avoid precipitation of acute symptom worsening. Thiamine is the only effective treatment. Parenteral thiamine, 50–100 mg, is used in the acute stage because intestinal absorption is unreliable in debilitated and alcoholic patients

Korsakoff Syndrome

Korsakoff syndrome and Wernicke's encephalopathy are different stages of one disease process (Wernicke-Korsakoff syndrome). Korsakoff syndrome typically follows Wernicke's encephalopathy, emerging as ocular symptoms and encephalopathy subside.

Clinical Features

Both anterograde and retrograde amnesia are characteristic features of the memory impairment. Severe difficulty establishing a new memory couples with a limited ability to recall events that antedate the onset of illness by several years. Disorientation as to place and time are typical. Alertness, attention, social behavior, and most other aspects of cognitive functions are relatively preserved. Confabulation can be a prominent feature, especially in the early stages. Memory function is slow and usually incomplete despite treatment with thiamine.

Treatment

Except for the initial thiamine administration, treatment usually is limited to social support. Many patients require at least some form of supervision, either at home or in a chronic care facility.

Table 32.3: Neurological complications associated with alcohol abuse

Nutritional deficiency
   Wernicke's encephalopathy
   Korsakoff syndrome
   Pellagra
Direct effects of alcohol
   Acute intoxication
   Fetal alcohol syndrome
Abnormalities of serum electrolytes and osmolality
   Central pontine myelinolysis
Alcohol withdrawal
   Delirium tremens
Diseases of uncertain pathogenesis
   Alcoholic polyneuropathy
   Alcoholic myopathy
   Amblyopia
   Cerebellar degeneration
   Marchiafava-Bignami disease

Other Nutritional Diseases Associated with Alcoholism

Table 32.3 lists the neurological consequences of alcohol abuse. Neuropathy is the most common neurological complication. Most affected patients are between 40 and 60 years of age, and essentially all have a history of chronic and heavy alcohol intake.

For a more detailed discussion, see Chapter 63 in Neurology in Clinical Practice, 4th edition.

Effects of Toxins and Physical Agents on the Nervous System

33

OCCUPATIONAL AND ENVIRONMENTAL AGENTS

Recognition of Neurotoxic Disorders

A close temporal relationship between the clinical onset and prior exposure to a chemical agent helps the recognition of neurotoxic disorders. Single case reports that an agent is neurotoxic are unreliable, especially when similar neurological symptoms are common in the general population. Laboratory test results often are not helpful in confirming that a specific agent causes a neurological syndrome, either because the putative neurotoxin is not measurable in body tissues or because the interval since exposure makes the measurements meaningless.

Exposure to neurotoxins may lead to dysfunction of any part of the central, peripheral, or autonomic nervous systems and the neuromuscular apparatus. The neurological disorder is typically monophasic. Although progression may occur for several weeks after discontinuation of exposure, it eventually arrests and improvement may follow, depending on the severity of the original disorder. Prolonged or progressive deterioration long after cessation of exposure, or the development of neurological symptoms months to years after exposure, suggests that a neurotoxic disorder is not responsible.

Organic Chemicals

Acrylamide
Most cases of acrylamide toxicity occur by inhalation or cutaneous absorption. Acute high-dose exposure results in confusion, hallucinations, reduced attention span, drowsiness, and other features of encephalopathy. Peripheral neuropathy and cerebellar ataxia are consequences of either acute high-dose or

prolonged low-level exposure. The neuropathy is a length-dependent sensorimotor axonopathy. When exposure ends, the neuropathy arrests and slowly reverses. Measurement of hemoglobin-acrylamide may be useful in predicting the development of peripheral neuropathy.

Allyl Chloride
The industrial use of allyl chloride is the manufacturing epoxy resins, certain insecticides, and polyacrylonitride. Exposure leads to a mixed sensorimotor distal axonopathy. Recovery follows cessation of exposure.

Carbon Disulfide
Acute inhalation of high concentrations leads to an encephalopathy with symptoms that vary from mild behavioral disturbances to drowsiness and ultimately to respiratory failure. Long-term exposure to carbon disulfide may lead to extrapyramidal or pyramidal deficits, absent pupillary and corneal reflexes, optic neuropathy, peripheral neuropathy, and a characteristic retinopathy. Specific treatment is not available.

Carbon Monoxide
Occupational or environmental exposure to carbon monoxide occurs mainly in miners, gas workers, and garage employees. The neurotoxic effects of carbon monoxide relate to intracellular hypoxia. Carbon monoxide binds to hemoglobin with high affinity to form carboxyhemoglobin; it also limits the dissociation of oxyhemoglobin and binds to various enzymes. Acute toxicity leads to headache, disturbances of consciousness, and behavioral changes. Pyramidal and extrapyramidal disorders and seizures may occur. Treatment involves administration of pure or hyperbaric oxygen. Recurrence of motor and behavioral abnormalities may occur several weeks after partial or apparently full recovery from the acute effects. The degree of recovery from this delayed deterioration is limited, and some lapse into a persistent vegetative state.

Ethylene Oxide
Acute exposure to high levels produces headache, nausea, and a severe reversible encephalopathy. Long-term exposure to ethylene oxide or ethylene chlorohydrin may lead to a peripheral sensorimotor axonopathy and mild cognitive changes. Recovery generally follows cessation of exposure.

Hexacarbon Solvents
The hexacarbon solvents *n*-hexane and methyl-*n*-butyl ketone are both metabolized to 2,5-hexanedione, which is responsible for neurotoxicity. Exposure to either of these chemicals by

inhalation or skin contact leads to a progressive, distal, sensorimotor axonal polyneuropathy. Optic neuropathy or maculopathy and facial numbness have followed *n*-hexane exposure.

Acute inhalation exposure may produce feelings of euphoria, associated with hallucinations, headache, unsteadiness, and mild narcosis. Inhalation of glues for recreational purposes causes euphoria in the short term but may lead to a progressive motor neuropathy and symptoms of dysautonomia after high-dose exposure. An insidious sensorimotor polyneuropathy follows chronic usage.

Methyl Bromide

Several hours or more may elapse before the onset of symptoms follows acute high-level exposure to methyl bromide. Acute methyl bromide intoxication leads to an encephalopathy with convulsions, delirium, hyperpyrexia, coma, pulmonary edema, and death. Long-term low-level exposure causes polyneuropathy, visual disturbances, optic atrophy, and upper motor neuron deficits. Gradual improvement occurs with cessation of exposure. Treatment is symptomatic. Hemodialysis may help remove bromide from the blood.

ORGANOPHOSPHATES

Organophosphates are used mainly as pesticides and herbicides, but also as petroleum additives, lubricants, antioxidants, flame retardants, and plastic modifiers. Organophosphates inhibit acetylcholinesterase production by phosphorylation, resulting in acute cholinergic toxicity. Toxicity affects both the central and the peripheral nervous system. Treatment involves intravenous administration of pralidoxime (1 g) together with atropine (1 mg) subcutaneously every 30 minutes until sweating and salivation are controlled. Pralidoxime accelerates reactivation of the inhibited acetylcholinesterase, and atropine is effective in counteracting muscarinic effects, although it has no effect on the nicotinic effects such as weakness or respiratory depression. Ventilatory support is started before atropine is given.

The organochlorine pesticides include aldrin, dieldrin, lindane, and dichlorodiphenyltrichlorethylene (*DDT*). Tremor and convulsions may follow acute high-level exposure, but the effects of chronic low-level exposure are uncertain. Chlordecone may produce a neurological disorder characterized by "nervousness," tremor, clumsiness of the hands, gait ataxia, and opsoclonus.

Minor cognitive changes and benign intracranial hypertension may occur. Carbamate insecticides also inhibit cholinesterases but have a shorter duration of action than organophosphate compounds. The symptoms of toxicity are similar but milder. Treatment with atropine is usually sufficient.

SOLVENT MIXTURES

Styrene

Acute exposure to high concentrations of styrene leads to cognitive, behavioral, and attentional disturbances. The consequences of exposure to chronic low levels of styrene are not established. Described effects are abnormal psychomotor performance and visual abnormalities (impaired color vision and reduced contrast sensitivity).

Toluene

Chronic high exposure may lead to cognitive disturbances, upper motor neuron, cerebellar, brainstem, and cranial neuropathies, and tremor. An optic neuropathy may occur, as may ocular dysmetria and opsoclonus. MRI shows cerebral atrophy and cerebral white matter abnormalities.

Trichloroethylene

Recreational abuse of trichloroethylene occurs because it induces feelings of euphoria. Acute low-level exposure may lead to headache and nausea. Higher levels of exposure lead to trigeminal dysfunction characterized by progressive sensory impairment starting in the nose and spreading outward. Increasing exposure causes facial and buccal numbness followed by weakness of the muscles of mastication and facial expression. Ptosis, extraocular palsies, vocal cord paralysis, dysphagia, and encephalopathy may occur. The clinical deficits generally resolve with discontinuation of exposure.

Vacor

Ingestion of vacor, a rodenticide, leads to severe autonomic dysfunction and a milder sensorimotor axonopathy. Acute diabetes mellitus results from necrosis of the beta-islet cells of the pancreas.

METALS

Arsenic

Acute or subacute exposure to arsenic leads to nausea, vomiting, abdominal pain, diarrhea, hypotension, tachycardia, and vasomotor collapse. Obtundation is common and an acute confusional state may develop. A distal axonopathy develops within 2–3 weeks of acute or subacute exposure. Symptoms may worsen over weeks despite lack of further exposure. Detection of arsenic in urine is diagnostically useful within 6 weeks of a single large dose exposure or during ongoing low-level exposure. Chelation therapy with either water-soluble derivatives of dimercaprol (DMSA or DMPS) or penicillamine controls the systemic effects of acute arsenic poisoning and may prevent the development of neuropathy.

Lead

The toxic effects of inorganic lead salts on the nervous system differ with age. In children with lead poisoning, an acute gastrointestinal illness is followed by behavioral changes, confusion, drowsiness, reduced alertness, focal or generalized seizures, and coma with increased intracranial hypertension. In adults, lead produces a predominantly motor neuropathy, sometimes accompanied by gastrointestinal disturbances and a microcytic hypochromic anemia. Blood levels exceeding 70 µg/100 ml confirm lead intoxication. Lead encephalopathy is managed supportively, but corticosteroids are given to treat cerebral edema, and chelating agents (dimercaprol or 2,3-dimercaptopropane sulfonate) are useful.

Manganese

Manganese miners develop neurotoxicity following prolonged inhalation (months or years) of dust containing manganese. Headache, behavioral changes, and cognitive disturbances ("manganese madness") are followed by development of an extrapyramidal syndrome, with bradykinesia, rigidity, tremor, and dystonic posturing. The response to L-dopa is poor and the extrapyramidal syndrome may progress over several years. Myoclonic jerking may occur, sometimes without extrapyramidal dysfunction.

Mercury

The toxic effects of elemental mercury (mercury vapor), inorganic salts, and short-chain alkyl-mercury compounds predominantly involve the central nervous system and dorsal root ganglion sensory neurons. Clinical consequences of exposure include cutaneous erythema, hyperhidrosis, anemia, proteinuria, personality changes, intention tremor ("hatter's shakes"), and muscle weakness. The characteristic features of chronic methyl-mercury poisoning are sensory disturbances, constriction of visual fields, progressive ataxia, tremor, and cognitive impairment. The diagnosis of elemental or inorganic mercury intoxication usually can be confirmed by assaying mercury in urine.

Tellurium

The uses of tellurium include the manufacture of alloys; the coloring of glass, ceramics, and metalware; the production of rubber; and the manufacture of thermoelectric devices. Inhalation of volatile tellurium compounds leads to headache, drowsiness, a metallic taste, hypohidrosis, skin rash, and a curious odor resembling garlic in the breath. Recovery generally occurs spontaneously.

Thallium

Thallium salts cause severe neuropathy and central nervous system degeneration, causing discontinuation of their use as rodenticides and depilatories. Vomiting, diarrhea, or both occur within hours of consumption. Limb pain and severe distal paresthesias are followed by progressive limb weakness within 7 days. Cranial nerves are involved. In severe cases, ataxia, chorea, confusion, and coma, as well as ventilatory and cardiac failure, ensue. Alopecia, which appears 2–4 weeks after exposure, provides only retrospective evidence of acute intoxication. A chronic progressive, mainly sensory neuropathy develops in patients with chronic low-level exposure. Oral potassium ferric ferrocyanide (Prussian blue), which blocks intestinal absorption, together with intravenous potassium chloride, forced diuresis, and hemodialysis are successful in treating acute thallium intoxication.

EFFECTS OF DRUG ABUSE ON THE NERVOUS SYSTEM

Drug dependence refers to either a psychological or a physical dependence. In the former, drug-craving or drug-seeking behavior emerges when the drug is not available. Physical dependence implies the appearance of physiological symptoms and signs during drug withdrawal. *Drug tolerance* is defined as a diminished response to the same dosage of a drug and may reflect either increased metabolism of the drug or reduced physiological response to the drug at its normal cellular target.

Acute intoxication often leads to delirium, stupor, or coma, sometimes accompanied by myoclonus, seizures, and cardiorespiratory depression. *Chronic use* leads to drug tolerance or dependence. Abrupt abstinence of a habitually used drug causes an acute withdrawal syndrome. The *indirect nervous system* affects are from the infectious and embolic consequences of intravenous drug use and by hypersensitivity or immunological mechanisms. Urine screening of drugs of abuse is widely used in the diagnostic evaluation of patients.

Cocaine is the most commonly abused drug that results in emergency room visits. Next in frequency are heroin, marijuana, and methamphetamine. The so-called *club drugs*, frequently used in dance clubs, include γ-hydroxybutyrate), ketamine, MDMA (3,4-methylenedioxymethamphetamine, or *ecstasy*), lysergic acid diethylamide (LSD), and methamphetamine. Aside from the biological effects, forensic data link these drugs to causing many vehicular accidents, blunt trauma, gunshot and other penetrating injuries, and deaths. All substances of abuse have acute and chronic effects on the nervous system. The neurological consequences result from three mechanisms: (1) Acute intoxication or overdose leads to delirium, stupor, or coma, sometimes accompanied by myoclonus, seizures, or serious systemic consequences such as respiratory depression and cardiovascular collapse. (2) Chronic use often leads to drug tolerance or dependence. Abrupt abstinence of a habitually used drug produces an acute withdrawal syndrome. (3) Drug abuse may affect the nervous system indirectly, via infectious and embolic consequences of intravenous drug use, hypersensitivity or immunological mechanisms, or some other manner that is not yet understood. Urine screening of drugs of abuse is widely used in the diagnostic evaluation of patients.

Opioid Analgesics

Development of drug tolerance and dependence is an unavoidable physiological consequence of repeated use of opioids. Both morphine and heroin produce a sense of *rush*, accompanied by either euphoria or dysphoria. Hallucinations may occur. Other effects include pruritus, dry mouth, nausea and vomiting, constipation, and urinary retention. Overdose of heroin causes coma, respiratory suppression, and pinpoint pupils.

Hypotension and hypothermia may also occur, but seizures are rare. Naloxone is a safe and effective opioid antagonist and is used for treatment and diagnosis because it induces immediate reversal of both coma and respiratory depression in patients with opioid overdose. Two milligrams of parenteral naloxone may be repeated as needed up to 10–20 mg. The half-life of naloxone (1–4 hours) is shorter than most opioid agonists and repeated boluses are needed.

With development of drug dependence, symptoms and signs of withdrawal appear hours after the last opioid use. Drug craving appears first, followed by restlessness and irritability. Autonomic symptoms such as sweating, lacrimation, and rhinorrhea emerge. Still later, piloerection, aching, nausea, abdominal cramps, diarrhea, and coughing develop. With methadone, symptoms appear in approximately 12–24 hours, peak at 6 days, and last approximately 3 weeks. Opioid withdrawal in adults, though unpleasant, is not in itself life threatening. In contrast, opioid withdrawal in neonates is sometimes accompanied by myoclonus, seizures, or even status epilepticus.

Oral methadone, a long-acting opiate, is used to relieve opioid withdrawal symptoms. A dose of 20 mg once or twice a day is sufficient in opioid-dependent patients. The dose is then gradually reduced, with the hope of eventually achieving detoxification.

Sedatives and Hypnotics

Sedatives and hypnotics have calming effects and induce sleep when taken in sufficient doses. The group includes the benzodiazepines, barbiturates, and other less commonly used agents. The benzodiazepines account for more than one half of overdoses in the United States and are among the most frequently prescribed medications in Western countries. Heroin addicts often use benzodiazepines and barbiturates in conjunction with heroin. Alcoholics also use them to alleviate symptoms of alcohol withdrawal.

Benzodiazepines
Benzodiazepines are prescription drugs used to promote sleep or as tranquilizers. The acute effects are lassitude, drowsiness, confusion, amnesia, euphoria, and impairment of other psychomotor functions. Sufficiently severe overdose leads to coma, but not respiratory or cardiovascular depression. Overdose is rarely fatal, unless other drugs are used concurrently. Flumazenil is a specific antagonist for benzodiazepines. A dose of 0.2–5.0 mg given intravenously over 2–10 minutes is sufficient to reverse

benzodiazepine overdose. A lack of response is strong evidence that another drug is involved.

Chronic use of benzodiazepines may lead to tolerance and physical dependence. Withdrawal symptoms typically occur within 24 hours of cessation of use of a short-acting benzodiazepine and approximately 3–7 days after stopping a long-acting agent. Withdrawal symptoms include irritability, increased sensitivity to light and sound, sweating, tremor, tachycardia, headache, and sleep disturbances. In more severe withdrawal states, delirium, hallucinations, and seizures may occur.

Barbiturates

The acute symptoms of barbiturate use, like alcohol, include euphoria, sedation, slurred speech, and gait ataxia. Severe intoxication leads to coma, hypotension, and hypothermia. Breathing may be slow or rapid and shallow. Cheyne-Stokes breathing, respiratory depression, and eventually apnea occur with sufficient intoxication. Treatment is supportive. As a general rule, ingestion of more than 10 times the hypnotic dose is dangerous. Early gastric lavage may be useful, because barbiturates reduce gastric motility. Hemodialysis or hemoperfusion is rarely necessary. Withdrawal symptoms of barbiturates and alcohol are similar and include insomnia, irritability, tremor, tachycardia, nausea, and vomiting. Short-acting barbiturates withdrawal causes symptoms within 36 hours and long-acting barbiturates withdrawal occurs after several days. Treatment of withdrawal is reinstitution of the barbiturates, followed by gradual tapering.

Other Sedatives and Hypnotics

Other sedatives and hypnotics are less often abused than barbiturates and benzodiazepines. Methaqualone overdose is characterized by delirium, myoclonus, and seizures, sometimes followed by coma and acute congestive heart failure. Glutethimide overdose leads to coma, hypotension, and less frequently respiratory depression. Abuse recognition is by the anticholinergic effects and dilated unreactive pupils. Treatment includes diuresis, peritoneal or hemodialysis, or hemoperfusion with activated charcoal or resin.

Psychomotor Stimulants

Psychomotor stimulants have sympathomimetic effects on the central nervous system. Cocaine is most commonly abused. It may be administered intranasally or parenterally or it may be smoked ("crack"). Amphetamine, dextroamphetamine, methamphetamine, and methylphenidate also have significant abuse potential. MDMA, or *ecstasy*, is a hallucinogen in addition to its stimulant properties. In moderate doses, stimulants produce mood elevation, increased alertness, reduced fatigue, decreased appetite, and enhanced performance in various tasks. Some patients develop paranoia, delusions, hallucinations, agitation, and violence while others may be depressed or lethargic. Systemic symptoms include palpitation, pupillary dilation, tachycardia, and hypertension. More severe complications of cocaine are hyperthermia, dehydration, rhabdomyolysis, and myocardial infarction. Of the abused stimulants, cocaine is the most likely to cause seizures. This occurs more often when cocaine is smoked (crack cocaine) or given intravenously. Both acute ischemic and hemorrhagic strokes have been reported in association with stimulant use, especially cocaine and amphetamine.

Treatment of overdose includes supportive measures such as oxygen, cardiac monitoring, cooling for hyperthermia, antihypertensives, and blood pressure and ventilatory support as necessary. Sedatives may be used to treat agitation, and benzodiazepines and phenytoin to treat seizures.

OTHER SUBSTANCES OF ABUSE

Marijuana

Tetrahydrocannabinol is the primary active ingredient of marijuana and has effects on mood, memory, judgment, and sense of time. A sense of relaxation, subjective slowing of time, euphoria, or depersonalization occurs. Variable degrees of anxiety, paranoia, sedation, or sleepiness may occur. High doses of tetrahydrocannabinol produce hallucinations, paranoia, or a panic reaction. Treatment generally requires only calm reassurance. Tolerance develops with chronic usage. Irritability, restlessness, and insomnia are typical after abrupt discontinuation.

Phencyclidine and Ketamine

Phencyclidine and ketamine were developed as anesthetics. Analgesia, anesthesia, stupor, and coma develop at progressively increasing dosages. Euphoria, dysphoria, relaxation, paranoia, and hallucinations occur at moderate doses. Psychosis, agitation, bizarre behavior, and catatonia are common. Physical signs of fever, hypertension, sweating, miosis, and nystagmus may accompany the behavioral disturbances. Treatment is largely supportive. Rhabdomyolysis is common with overdose, and myoglobinuria should be looked for and treated.

Anticholinergics

Abuse of prescription drugs and plants containing the belladonna alkaloids, atropine, and scopolamine cause delirium and hallucinations. The psychoactive effects are accompanied by mydriasis, dry and flushed skin, tachycardia, urinary retention, and fever. Severe overdose may lead to myoclonus, seizures, coma, and death. Acute treatment employs intramuscular or intravenous injection of 1 mg of physostigmine.

Inhalants

Many hydrocarbons, nitrites, and nitrous oxide are present in common household and industrial products. At low to moderate doses, they induce a sense of euphoria, relaxation, incoordination, and slurred speech that resemble alcohol intoxication. Higher doses produce psychosis, hallucinations, and seizures. The duration of action is typically only 15–30 minutes, but the effects may be sustained by continual use.

Hallucinogens

The hallucinogens cause alteration of mood, perception, and thought processes, without significantly changing alertness, memory, and orientation. The synthetic ergot LSD is the best example and remains popular. In addition, a wide range of plants and mushrooms are known to be hallucinogenic. Acute ingestion rapidly leads to dizziness, blurred vision, nausea, and weakness. Visual hallucinations follow, associated with depersonalization and time distortion. Some experiences are terrifying (*bad trips*), resulting in injuries to self or others. Physical signs include fever, tachycardia, hypertension, mydriasis, seizures, and coma.

INDIRECT NEUROLOGICAL COMPLICATIONS

Stroke

The sources of embolism include valvular disease secondary to infective or marantic endocarditis, mural thrombi of cardiomyopathy, right-to-left shunt, aortic or other arterial dissection, and foreign materials injected during intravenous drug abuse. Vasospasm and vasculitis are mainly associated with the psychostimulants such as cocaine, amphetamines, methylphenidate, and phenylpropanolamine. Among stroke patients ages 15 to 44 years, drug abusers accounts for 12–31% of cases, and drug abuse is the most important risk factor for stroke in those younger than 35 years. The evaluation of patients with drug-related strokes should include a search for endocarditis or other source of embolization, a full cardiac evaluation, erythrocyte sedimentation rate, and antiphospholipid antibody assay. Cerebral angiography may be necessary, especially when vasculitis, aneurysms, or vascular malformations are suspected.

Cocaine is the most important cause of drug-related stroke and accounts for 50% of all cases. Neurological symptoms typically develop within hours of cocaine use. Seizures sometimes accompany the strokes.

Myelopathy

An acute myelopathy may develop after heroin and cocaine abuse. The syndrome resembles an anterior spinal artery syndrome, sudden onset of paraparesis, urinary retention, and a segmental sensory level with sparing of posterior column function.

Rhabdomyolysis and Myopathy

Muscle abnormalities range from asymptomatic elevation of serum creatine kinase to myoglobinuria and renal failure. This is usually associated with the abuse of heroin, cocaine, amphetamine, MDMA (ecstasy), and phencyclidine. Possible mechanisms include trauma, crush injury, hypotension, hypertension, fever, seizures, and excessive muscular activities. Repeated intramuscular injections of meperidine, pentazocine, or heroin sometimes lead to focal fibrosis and weakness of the injected muscles.

Neuropathy and Plexopathy

Compressive or stretch injuries to peripheral nerves and plexuses may result from drug abuse of any kind. Focal neuropathies develop secondary to compartment syndrome and secondary nerve ischemia. Many drug abusers have a distal sensory or sensorimotor polyneuropathy, but it is difficult to distinguish a direct drug effect from coexistent alcohol abuse and systemic diseases.

NEUROTOXINS OF ANIMALS AND PLANTS

Neurotoxins of Animals

Injuries and deaths resulting from snake and spider bites and scorpion stings occur in most parts of the world. In the United States, approximately 45,000 snake bites occur each year. Venomous snakes inflict 8000, but deaths are rare.

Snake Bite

A snake bite's overall effect depends on the type and size of snake involved, the length of time since the snake last ate, the type of bite, and the snake's ability to inject venom. Elapids and colubrids, like hydrophids, generally possess potent neurotoxins in their venom that can kill a human within minutes. The clinical syndrome is a rapid neuromuscular paralysis, respiratory distress, and in severe cases death. All snake-bite cases are medical emergencies until significant envenomation is ruled out. First-aid measures are to retard the absorption of venom and to remove it from the tissues. Early administration of antivenin, preferably intravenously, is critical. The choice and amount of antivenin to be given depend on the species of snake involved, the degree of envenomation, the patient's size, and the initial clinical response.

Spider Bite

In the United States, only the female black widow spider (*Lactrodectus mactans*) causes serious envenomation and neurological dysfunction. The toxic fraction in the spider venom causes enhanced release of acetylcholine-containing vesicles from the motor nerve endings, leading to neurotransmitter exhaustion and paralysis. Treatment consists of supportive measures and antivenin therapy in serious envenomation.

Scorpions

Bites by poisonous scorpions are generally more dangerous than spider bites. Scorpion envenomation is a public health problem in warm climates. In Mexico, there are 100,000–200,000 scorpion bites annually, resulting in 400–1000 fatalities. Small children in particular are prone to developing neurological sequelae. In the United States, more than 14,500 scorpion bites were reported in 2001, with no mortality. Toxic effects are exerted through alteration of voltage-gated ion channels, particularly sodium ionophores. Paresthesias are common and are usually associated with autonomic symptoms of sympathetic overdrive (tachycardia, hypertension, and hyperthermia). With severe envenomation, encephalopathy may result from direct central nervous system toxicity or secondary to uncontrolled hypertension. Treatment is symptomatic.

Neurotoxins of Plants and Mushrooms

Pharmacologically active agents are present in thousands of plants and mushrooms species. Although fatal poisoning is relatively rare, some species induce serious neurological symptoms. Approximately 75% of cases occur in children younger than 6 years. The best treatment is usually empirical, including gastric lavage or catharsis, supportive measures, and control of symptoms. With the exception of anticholinergic poisoning, there are few specific antidotes.

MARINE TOXINS

Toxic syndromes occur from the consumption of contaminated fish and shellfish, some of which have neurological consequences. See Table 33.1.

EFFECT OF PHYSICAL AGENTS ON THE NERVOUS SYSTEM

Ionizing Radiation

Radiation therapy affects the nervous system by causing damage to exposed regions or to blood vessels supplying neural structures. It may also produce brain tumors. Neurological injury is proportional to both the total dose and the daily fraction of radiation that were received.

Encephalopathy
Acute radiation encephalopathy, caused by cerebral edema, occurs within a few days of exposure and is characterized by headache, nausea, and a change in mental status. Treatment with high-dose corticosteroids usually provides relief. *Early delayed radiation encephalopathy* is probably caused by demyelination and occurs between 2 weeks and 3 or 4 months after irradiation. Headache and drowsiness are features, as is an enhancement of previous focal deficits. Symptoms resolve after several weeks without specific treatment. A brainstem encephalopathy may develop, which also recovers over a few weeks. *Delayed radiation encephalopathy* occurs several months or longer after cranial irradiation. It is characterized by diffuse cerebral injury (atrophy) or focal neurological deficits with signs of increased

Table 33.1: Fish and shellfish poisoning

Syndrome	Principal Toxins	Toxin Source	Transvector	Pathophysiology
Ciguatera fish poisoning	Ciguatoxins; maitotoxin; others	Dinoflagellates (*Gambierdiscus toxicus* and others)	Fish (multiple species of reef fish)	Na^+ and Ca^{++} channel activation
Pufferfish poisoning	Tetrodotoxins	Presumed bacteria (*?Vibrios* spp., *?Pseudomonas* spp.)	Various (pufferfish, salamanders, newt, and others)	Na^+ channel blockade
Scombroid fish poisoning	Histamine	Presumed bacterial (*?Vibrios* spp.)	Scombroid fish (tuna, mackerel, skipjack, etc.) and non-scombroid fish (mahi-mahi, sardines, etc.)	Histaminergic effects
Paralytic shellfish poisoning (PSP)	Saxitoxin and derivatives	Dinoflagellates (*Alexandrium* spp., *Gymnodium catenatum*, *Pyrodinium bahamense*)	Shellfish	Na^+ channel blockade
Neurotoxic shellfish poisoning (NSP)	Brevetoxins	Dinoflagellates (*Gymnodinium breve*)	Shellfish	Transforms fast Na^+ channels into slower ones
Amnestic shellfish poisoning (ASP)	Domoic acid and its congeners	Diatoms (*Pseudo-nitzschia* spp., *Nitzschia actydrophila*, *Amphora coffeiformis*)	Shellfish; fish (?)	Glutamate receptor activation
Diarrhetic shellfish poisoning (DSP)	Okadaic acid and derivatives; dinophysistoxins	Dinoflagellates (*Dinophysis* sp., *Prorocentrum* spp., *Proceratium reticulatum*, *Coolia* sp.)	Shellfish	Serine/threonine protein phosphatase inhibition

intracranial pressure. The disorder may result from focal cerebral necrosis caused by direct radiation damage or by vascular changes.

Myelopathy

A *transitory radiation myelopathy* occurs within the first year after incidental cord irradiation in patients with lymphoma and other neoplasms. It is self-limited and probably relates to demyelination of the posterior columns. A *delayed severe radiation myelopathy* may occur 1 year after completion of radiotherapy. The cause is necrosis and atrophy of the cord, with an associated vasculopathy. A focal neurological deficit progresses over weeks or months to paraplegia or quadriplegia. Corticosteroids may lead to temporary improvement, but no specific treatment exists. Recovery does not occur. Occasionally patients develop sudden back pain and leg weakness several years after irradiation, and MRI reveals hematomyelia; symptoms usually improve with time.

Plexopathy

A radiation-induced plexopathy may occur soon after treatment and must be distinguished from direct neoplastic involvement of the plexuses. A plexopathy also may develop 1–3 years after irradiation of the brachial or lumbosacral plexuses. Lack of pain, lymphedema, induration of the supraclavicular fossa, and the presence of myokymic discharges on electromyography all favor a radiation-induced plexopathy. The plexopathy is associated with small-vessel damage (endarteritis obliterans) and fibrosis around the nerve trunks.

Nonionizing Radiation

Nonionizing radiation is transformed to heat when striking matter. The heat may lead to tissue damage. The sun, incandescent and fluorescent light sources, welding torches, electrical arc furnaces, and ultraviolet radiation lamps produce ionizing radiation. Short-term exposure to ultraviolet light damages the retina and optic nerve fibers. Exposure to laser radiation can induce ocular damage.

High-intensity noise may lead to pain in the ear, tinnitus, vertigo, and hearing impairment. Chronic exposure to high-intensity noise of any frequency leads to focal cochlear damage and impaired hearing.

Concern has been raised that occupational or environmental exposure to high-voltage electrical power lines may lead to neurological damage from exposure to high-intensity electromagnetic fields. However, the effects of such exposure are uncertain and require further study. Nonionizing radiation at the radio frequency used by cellular telephones has caused concern with regard to sleep disturbances, headache, and brain tumors. A case–control study failed to identify any major increased risk associated with short-term use of cellular telephones.

Electrical Current and Lightning

The severity of electrical injury depends on the strength and duration of the current and the path in which it flows. Electricity travels along the shortest path to ground. Its passage through humans can be determined by identifying entry and exit burn wounds. When its path involves the nervous system, direct neurological damage is likely among survivors. In addition, neurological damage may result from circulatory arrest and trauma related to falling or a shock pressure wave.

A large current passing through the head leads to immediate unconsciousness, sometimes associated with ventricular fibrillation and respiratory arrest. Confusion, disorientation, seizures, and transitory focal deficits are common in survivors. Recovery generally occurs within a few days. Some survivors develop a cerebral infarct attributed to thrombotic occlusion of cerebral blood vessels. Residual memory and other cognitive disturbances are also common. Weaker current leads only to headache or other mild symptoms for a brief period.

Currents that involve the spinal cord cause a transverse myelopathy immediately or during the first week and may progress for several days. Peripheral or cranial nerve injury in the region of an electrical burn is often reversible, except when high-tension current is responsible, in which case thermal coagulation necrosis is likely.

Vibration

Exposure to vibrating tools such as pneumatic drills is associated with both focal peripheral nerve injuries and vascular abnormalities. The mechanism of production is uncertain but presumably reflects focal damage to nerve fibers.

Hyperthermia

Exposure to high external temperatures may lead to heat stroke. Disturbances of thermoregulatory sweating may be contributory. Hyperthermia leads to thirst, fatigue, nausea, weakness, muscle cramps, and eventually to confusion, delirium, obtundation, or coma. Coma can develop without any prodrome. Seizures are common, focal neurological deficits are sometimes present, and papilledema may occur. The prognosis depends on the severity of hyperthermia and its duration before initiation of treatment. Treatment involves control of the body temperature by cooling, rehydration of the patient, correction of the underlying cause of the hyperthermia, and prevention of complications.

Hypothermia

A core temperature less than 35°C may occur in very young or elderly persons and with environmental exposure, coma, hypothyroidism, malnutrition, severe dermatological disorders, and alcoholism. Alcohol promotes heat loss by vasodilation and may lead to coma directly or from environmental exposure to cold after trauma. Hypothermia also occurs in persons exposed to low temperatures in the working environment, such as divers, skiers, and cold-room workers. The usual compensatory mechanism for cooling is shivering, but this fails at body temperatures less than approximately 30°C. As the temperature declines, respiratory requirements diminish, cardiac output falls, and significant hypotension and cardiac arrhythmias ultimately develop. Neurologically, there is increasing confusion, psychomotor retardation, and obtundation until consciousness is eventually lost. At core temperatures less than 32°C, the appearance of brain death may be simulated clinically and electroencephalographically, but complete recovery may follow appropriate treatment. Management involves slow rewarming of patients and the prevention of complications such as aspiration pneumonia and metabolic acidosis.

Burns

The term *thermal burn* refers to a burn caused by direct contact with heat or flames. Patients with severe burns may have associated disorders such as anoxic encephalopathy from carbon monoxide poisoning, head injury, or respiratory dysfunction from smoke inhalation. Central neurological disorders may occur later during hospitalization and are secondary to systemic complications. Nerves may be damaged directly by heat, leading to coagulation necrosis from which recovery is unlikely.

For a more detailed discussion, see Chapters 64A, 64B, 64C, 64D, and 64E in Neurology in Clinical Practice, 4th edition.

Brain Edema and Disorders of Cerebrospinal Fluid Circulation

34

The brain and spinal cord lie within the rigid bony compartments of the skull and spinal canal. The total volume of fluid and tissue contained in the rigid skull is constant. Changes in volume of blood, cerebrospinal fluid (CSF), or brain compartments produce compensatory changes in the others.

CEREBROSPINAL FLUID

Choroid Plexuses and Production of Cerebrospinal Fluid

Choroid plexuses are secretory structures in the cerebral ventricles that interface between CSF and blood. The choroid plexus is the main producer of CSF. The rate of CSF production is 0.35 mL per minute. Acetazolamide inhibits carbonic anhydrase and reduces CSF production. Osmotic agents, such as mannitol and glycerol, lower CSF production by about 50%. However, none of these measures is effective in the long-term reduction of CSF production.

Arachnoid Granulations and Absorption of Cerebrospinal Fluid

Arachnoid granulations (pacchionian granulations) are the main sites for the drainage of CSF into the blood. They protrude through the dura into the superior sagittal sinus and act as one-way valves. As CSF pressure increases, more fluid is absorbed. When CSF pressure falls below a threshold value, the absorption of CSF ceases.

Cerebrospinal Fluid Pressure

Lumbar puncture is the traditional method to measure CSF pressure. Small fluctuations from the cardiac pulse and larger fluctuations from respirations take place in the fluid in the manometer. As intracranial pressure rises, tissue compliance falls and reserve capacity of the intracranial contents is lost. At that point, small changes in fluid volume may lead to large increases in intracranial pressure.

BRAIN EDEMA

Excess fluid can accumulate in the intracellular or extracellular spaces. *Cytotoxic edema* is cellular swelling, *vasogenic edema* is blood vessel leakage, and *interstitial edema* is transependymal flow in hydrocephalus. An overlap between the various types of edema usually occurs. Vasogenic edema expands the extracellular space in the white matter. Cytotoxic edema constricts the extracellular spaces.

Cytotoxic Brain Edema

Stroke, trauma, and toxins induce cytotoxic edema. After a stroke, brain water increases rapidly because of energy failure and loss of adenosine triphosphate. Cytotoxic edema worsens for 24–48 hours, during which there is a danger of brain herniation. Intracerebral hemorrhage causes brain edema, both around the hemorrhagic mass and in distant regions. Besides the cytotoxic edema at the site of injury, vasogenic edema can spread to other regions when the mass lesion is large.

A posterior edema syndrome involving occipital white matter is associated with hypertensive encephalopathy. The changes are transitory unless hemorrhage or infarction occurs. Rapid reduction in blood pressure is necessary. The reason for the predilection for the posterior circulation in this syndrome is uncertain. Edema may occur secondary to changes in osmolality. Patients treated for diabetic ketoacidosis, with rapid reduction of plasma glucose and sodium, are at risk for edema secondary to water shifts into the brain.

Treatment of Brain Edema

Blood volume can be reduced with hyperventilation, which lowers carbon dioxide. However, it is also detrimental because it constricts blood vessels, causing a worsening of the ischemia. Intraventricular drainage lowers the CSF volume. Agents that reduce the production of CSF, such as acetazolamide or diuretics, may be useful. Osmotic treatment with mannitol reduces brain volume and CSF production and improves blood flow. Corticosteroids lower intracranial pressure primarily in vasogenic edema but are less effective in cytotoxic edema and are not recommended in the treatment of edema secondary to stroke or hemorrhage.

IDIOPATHIC INTRACRANIAL HYPERTENSION

Idiopathic intracranial hypertension (IIH) was previously called *pseudotumor cerebri.*

Clinical Features

IIH occurs more frequently in women than in men. Obesity and menstrual irregularities are often present. Headache, often worse in the morning, is the main complaint. Sudden movements aggravate the headache. Some patients complain of dizziness. Transitory loss of vision can occur with change of position. Visual fields show an enlarged blind spot. Prolonged papilledema may lead to sector scotomas and rarely vision loss. Sixth cranial nerve palsies occur. Drugs associated with IIH are summarized in Table 34.1.

Diagnosis

Diagnosis requires ruling out other causes of increased intracranial pressure. All patients require a computed tomographic (CT) or magnetic resonance imaging (MRI) scan to exclude hydrocephalus and mass lesions. Lumbar puncture is needed, but only after imaging studies have ruled out a space-occupying lesion as

Table 34.1: Drugs frequently associated with idiopathic intracranial hypertension

Minocycline
Isotretinoin
Nalidixic acid
Tetracycline
Trimethoprim-sulfamethoxazole
Cimetidine
Prednisolone
Methylprednisolone
Tamoxifen
Beclomethasone

Source: Schutta, H. S. & Corbett, J. J. 1997, "Intracranial hypertension syndromes," in *Clinical Neurology,* 12th ed, eds R. J. Joynt & R. C. Griggs, Lippincott, Philadelphia.

the cause of the papilledema. Characteristic findings in the CSF include normal or low protein, normal glucose, no cells, and elevated CSF pressure.

Treatment

The initial spinal tap is therapeutic, lowering the raised intracranial pressure and reducing headache, as well as diagnostic. Acetazolamide is given in a starting dose of 250 mg twice daily, increasing to 1 g per day. Electrolytes must be monitored to avoid metabolic acidosis. Visual fields should be measured and the size of the blind spot plotted. Lumboperitoneal shunting has a reportedly high success rate. Fenestration of the optic nerve sheath to drain CSF into the orbital region reduces the papilledema without usually decreasing the intracranial pressure.

HYDROCEPHALUS

Hydrocephalus is defined as enlargement of the ventricles of the brain with an abnormal increase in the CSF volume relative to brain tissue. *Noncommunicating (obstructive) hydrocephalus* is caused by obstruction of the CSF outflow tracts so that the ventricles do not communicate with the subarachnoid space. *Communicating hydrocephalus* is usually caused by failure of spinal fluid reabsorption in the subarachnoid space. Cerebral atrophy resulting in compensatory ventricular enlargement is called *hydrocephalus ex vacuo* to distinguish it from excess fluid caused by obstruction of CSF outflow.

Acute hydrocephalus develops rapidly, reaching 80% of maximal ventricular enlargement within 6 hours. A slower phase of enlargement follows the initial rapid expansion, and ventricular enlargement plus continual production of CSF causes interstitial cerebral edema in the periventricular white matter. When the hydrocephalus stabilizes and enters a chronic phase, the CSF pressure may decrease, resulting in a normal pressure recording on random measurements.

Hydrocephalus in Children

Before the age of 2 years, when the cranial sutures are open, the diagnosis of hydrocephalus is suspected when serial measurements of head circumference fall above the normal developmental curves. Bulging of the anterior fontanelle may be seen, along with thinning of the skull and separation of the sutures. If the diagnosis is delayed, abnormal eye movements and optic atrophy may develop. Spasticity of the lower limbs may be observed at any stage. Acute enlargement of the ventricles is associated with nausea and vomiting.

Premature infants weighing less than 1500 g at birth have a high risk of intraventricular hemorrhage, and approximately 25% of these infants develop progressive ventricular enlargement, as shown by CT or ultrasound scans (see Chapter 55).

Adult-Onset Hydrocephalus

In adults, the features of hydrocephalus are headaches, papilledema, diplopia, and mental status changes. Sudden death may occur with severe increases in pressure. Rarely, hydrocephalus causes akinetic mutism as a result of pressure on the structures around the third ventricle. Other symptoms include temporal lobe seizures, CSF rhinorrhea, endocrine dysfunction (e.g., amenorrhea, polydipsia, and polyuria), and obesity, suggesting third-ventricle dysfunction. Gait disturbances are reported in patients with aqueductal stenosis, but hyperreflexia with an extensor-plantar response is uncommon.

Normal-Pressure Hydrocephalus

Normal-pressure hydrocephalus (NPH) is a term used to describe chronic, communicating adult-onset hydrocephalus. The triad of mental impairment, gait disturbance, and urinary incontinence is diagnostic. Ventricular enlargement is seen on CT or MRI scan. By definition, lumbar puncture reveals a normal CSF pressure. *Normal pressure* is an unfortunate term because patients who have undergone long-term monitoring with this syndrome have intermittently elevated pressures, often during the night.

Clinical Features

NPH can develop secondary to trauma, infection, or subarachnoid hemorrhage, but in about one third of cases, no cause is found. The presenting symptoms may be related to gait or mental function. When gait is the presenting factor, the prognosis for treatment is better. NPH causes an apraxic gait, which is an inability to lift the legs as if they were stuck to the floor. NPH leads to a reduction in intellect, which may be subtle. The dementia involves slowing of verbal and motor responses with preservation of cortical functions, such as language and spatial resolution.

Diagnosis
Diagnosis of NPH and selection of patients for placement of a ventriculoperitoneal shunt is difficult. CT and MRI scans have aided in separating Parkinson's disease, lacunar state, and NPH, although NPH may occasionally coexist with these diseases. Improvement in gait occurs after removal of CSF. Cisternography is a useful procedure that involves the injection of a radiolabeled tracer into the CSF with monitoring of its absorption for 3 days. Normally, the labeled material fails to enter the ventricles, moving over the convexity of the brain and leaving the CSF space within 12–24 hours. In patients with NPH, there is reflux of the tracer into the cerebral ventricles by 24 hours and retention in the ventricles for 48–72 hours.

Treatment
None of the available tests by themselves identify patients who will benefit from shunting. Most helpful is a combination of clinical signs and judiciously chosen laboratory tests. Success rates vary. Some describe improvement in 80% of treated patients. Others report that 36% had a poor response and 28% had major complications, including a high rate of infection and subdural hematomas after shunt placement.

For a more detailed discussion, see Chapter 65 in Neurology in Clinical Practice, 4th edition.

Developmental Disorders of the Nervous System

35

The events of neural maturation after initial induction and formation of the neural tube are each predictive of specific types of malformation of the brain and of later abnormal neurological function. Table 35.1 summarizes the features of major malformations of the brain.

MITOTIC PROLIFERATION OF NEUROBLASTS (NEURONAGENESIS)

After formation of the neural tube, the proliferation of neuroepithelial cells in the ventricular surface generates neurons and glial cells. The rate of division is greatest during the early first trimester in the spinal cord and brainstem and during the late first and early second trimester in the forebrain. Active mitoses cease well before birth, except for the periventricular region of the cerebral hemispheres and the external granular layer of the cerebellar cortex.

Disorders of Neuronagenesis

Inadequate mitotic proliferation of neuroblasts results in hypoplasia of the brain. The entire brain may be affected, or portions may be selectively involved. Every part of the nervous system normally produces excess neurons that a programmed process of cell death (*apoptosis*) reduces. Spinal muscular atrophy and pontocerebellar hypoplasia are examples of human diseases caused by programmed cell death not stopping at the proper time.

NEUROBLAST MIGRATION

All mature human brain cells migrate from their site of generation to their mature site. Migration of neuroblasts begins at

Table 35.1: Summary of clinical features of major malformations of the brain

	Micro-cephaly	Enceph-alocele	Dysmorphic Facies	Hydro-cephalus	Seizures	Vision Impair-ment	Mental Retar-dation	Hypotonia	Spasticity	Ataxia	Myopathy	Endo-crinopathy
Holoprosencephaly, alobar, semilobar*	+++	++	+++	+	++	+	++++	+++	+	++	0	++
Holoprosencephaly, lobar, middle interhemispheric variant*	+	0	+	++	++	0	+++	++	+	+	0	+
Septo-optic-pit. dysplasia	+	0	+	+	++	+++	+++	+	+	+	0	+++
Callosal agenesis, complete or partial	0	0	++	+	+++	+	+++	+	+	0	0	+
Callosal agenesis, Aicardi's syndrome	++	0	++	0	++++	+	++++	+	+	+	0	0
Callosal agenesis lipoma	0	0	+	+	++++	0	+	0	0	0	0	0
Colpocephaly, primary	++	0	++	+	++	+	+++	+	+	0	0	0
Lissencephaly or pachygyria (Miller-Dieker)	+	0	++++	0	+++	+	++++	+++	+	++	0	+

Lissencephaly or pachygyria (Walker-Warburg)	+++	++	++++	++	+++	+++	++++	++	+++	++++	++	++++	++
Pachygyria (Fukuyama)	+++	0	++	0	+++	+++	++++	0	+++	+++	++	+++	++
	++	0	+++	+	++	++	++++	0	+++	+++	0	+++	+
Cerebrohepatorenal disease (Zellweger)	0	0	++++	++	++++	++++	++	++	++++	0	+	+++	0
Tuberous sclerosis (Bourneville's disease)	+												
Hemimegalencephaly	+	0	++	+++	+++	+++	0	0	+++	0	0	0	+
Chiari malformations	+	+	+++	+++	+	+++	+++	+++	+++	+	+++	+++	+
Dandy-Walker malformation	0	+	+++	+	0	+++	++	++	0	0	0	0	0
Aqueductal stenosis/atresia	0	0	+	0	0	++	0	++	+	++	0	0	0
Cerebellar hypoplasias	0	0	+	0	+	++++	0	++++	++++	++++	0	0	0

Note: 0 = <5% of patients; + = 5–25%; ++ = 26–50%; +++ = 51–75%; ++++ = >75% of patients involved.

*In holoprosencephaly, anatomical varieties do not correspond to genetic defect and correlate poorly with midfacial hypoplasia.

about 6 weeks of gestation in the human cerebrum and is completed at 34 weeks or later. Glioblasts migrate until early in the postnatal period. Cerebellar external granule cells continue migrating throughout the first postnatal year.

Disorders of Neuroblast Migration

Nearly all malformations of the brain either are a direct result of faulty neuroblast migration or involve a secondary impairment of migration. Imperfect cortical lamination, abnormal gyral development, subcortical heterotopia, and other focal dysplasias result from factors that interfere with neuronal migration. The most severe migrational defects occur in early gestation, causing disturbances in the gross formation of the neural tube and cerebral vesicles. Heterotopia of brainstem nuclei also occurs. Later defects of migration cause disorders of cortical lamination or gyration, such as lissencephaly, pachygyria, and cerebellar dysplasias. Disordered neuroblast migration may be caused either by defective genetic programming or by acquired lesions that destroy or interrupt radial glial fibers.

Lissencephaly
Lissencephaly is a condition of a smooth cerebral cortex without convolutions. Gyri and sulci develop between 20 and 36 weeks of gestation, and the mature pattern of gyration is evident at term. In lissencephaly type 1 (*Miller-Dieker syndrome*), the cerebral cortex remains smooth. The histopathological pattern is that of a four-layer cortex. In lissencephaly type 2 (Walker-Warburg syndrome), the brain is smooth with a few poorly formed sulci containing disorganized and disoriented neurons.

Other Gyral Disturbances
Pachygyria signifies abnormally large, poorly formed gyri. *Polymicrogyria* refers to excessively numerous and abnormally small gyri. Schizencephaly is a unilateral or bilateral deep cleft usually in the general position of the sylvian fissure. In closed-lip schizencephaly, the cerebral cortical walls on either side of the deep cleft are in contact; *open lip* indicates a wide subarachnoid space between the two walls.

DISORDERS OF NEURULATION (1–4 WEEKS OF GESTATION)

Incomplete or defective formation of the neural tube from the neural placode is the most common type of malformation of the human central nervous system.

Anencephaly (Aprosencephaly with Open Cranium)

Anencephaly is a failure of the anterior neuropore to close or to remain closed at 24 days of gestation. Most forebrain structures, including the basal ganglia, do not develop. The cranium, meninges, and scalp do not close in the sagittal midline, and the remaining brain tissue is exposed to the surrounding amniotic fluid. Death occurs shortly after birth. An elevated concentration of α-fetoprotein in the amniotic fluid suggests the prenatal diagnosis, which sonography confirms at 12 weeks of gestation.

Cephalocele (Encephalocele; Exencephaly)

Most encephaloceles are midline parietal or occipital cranial defects that contain supratentorial tissue, cerebellar tissue, or both. Frontal encephaloceles are less common in North America and Europe but are common in Southeast Asia. They usually include olfactory tissue. The *Meckel-Gruber syndrome* is a large occipital encephalocele and lissencephaly. The encephalocele contains disorganized neural tissue, angiomatous malformations, focal hemorrhages, and zones of infarction.

The cerebral tissue in an encephalocele sac is usually extremely hamartomatous and may include heterotopia from an unexpected site, such as cerebellar tissue in a frontal encephalocele. The remaining intracranial brain is often dysplastic as well. Clinical neurological handicaps may be severe because even if the herniated tissue within the encephalocele is small and easily excised, concomitant intracranial malformations of the brain often result in epilepsy, mental retardation, motor impairment, and cortical blindness.

Meningomyelocele (Spinal Dysraphism, Rachischisis, Spina Bifida Cystica)

Failure of the posterior neuropore to close at 26 days causes a range of spinal defects that include failure of vertebral closure without herniation of neural elements (*spina bifida occulta*), herniation of meninges alone (*spina bifida cystica*), herniation of cord elements and nerve roots (*meningomyelocele*), and extensive dysplasia of the parenchyma of the spinal cord (*myelodysplasia*). Most defects are lumbosacral in location but may occur in the thoracic or cervical regions, usually as a rostral extension of lumbosacral lesions. The type II Chiari malformation (see the discussion on disorders of cerebellar development later in this chapter) is always associated with meningomyelocele; coexisting aqueductal stenosis with hydrocephalus is common. The level of the lesion and the extent of neural involvement determine the clinical features. Paraplegia is the rule and those with hydrocephalus usually have intellectual impairment.

The cause of these defects is not established, but dietary supplementation with folic acid (400 µg per day) before and during pregnancy is clearly prophylactic. An elevated concentration of α-fetoprotein in the amniotic fluid suggests the prenatal diagnosis, which fetal ultrasound establishes. Intrauterine surgery to close the defect is available at several centers. Preventing exposure of the cord to amniotic fluid may reduce much of the damage and preserve function.

The most important immediate complications of large meningomyeloceles in newborns are hydrocephalus and infection from leaking cerebrospinal fluid. Long-term complications include chronic urinary tract infections, decubiti, hydrocephalus, paraplegia, and other neurological deficits. Mental retardation is common but may be mild. Early closure of the open defect is desirable. Hydrocephalus requires ventriculoperitoneal shunt.

Diastematomyelia

Diastematomyelia is a spinal cord split into two halves along the sagittal plane, with each half having at least one dorsal and one ventral horn. A strand of fibrous tissue running from the dorsal to the ventral dura and occasionally a central bony spur between the two spinal cords may be present but is not the cause. The clinical features are those of a slowly evolving spinal cord syndrome with prominent sphincter disturbances. The leg involvement may be asymmetrical.

MIDLINE MALFORMATIONS OF THE FOREBRAIN (4–8 WEEKS OF GESTATION)

Developmental malformations of the prosencephalon relate to failure of the lamina terminalis differentiating into telencephalic structures. The lamina terminalis is the rostral membrane of the primitive neural tube that forms with closure of the anterior neuropore.

Holoprosencephaly

This malformation dates to 33 days of gestation, when the cerebral vesicle cleaves into two symmetrical hemispheres.

Magnetic resonance imaging (MRI) identifies three variants of holoprosencephaly.

1. *Alobar* holoprosencephaly is a single midline telencephalic ventricle with continuity of the cerebral cortex across the midline frontally. The corpus striatum and thalamus of the two sides are fused, and the third ventricle may be absent.
2. *Semilobar* holoprosencephaly has an incomplete interhemispheric fissure at least posteriorly. The occipital lobes and occipital horns of the ventricular system may approach a normal configuration, but fusion of the frontal lobes occurs across the midline.
3. *Lobar* holoprosencephaly is the least severe form. The hemispheres, although formed, remain in continuity through a band of cortex at the frontal pole or the orbital surface. The corpus callosum does not form completely.

Holoprosencephaly is part of the trisomy 13 phenotype. It also occurs as a genetic disorder transmitted by autosomal dominant or recessive inheritance in infants of diabetic mothers. Most commonly, it is a sporadic anomaly of unknown cause.

Midline facial defects, ranging from hypotelorism to midline facial aplasia with fusion of the eyes, occur in at least 90% of newborns with holoprosencephaly. Malformations of the viscera and musculoskeletal system occur in one third. The characteristic clinical course is severe developmental delay, mental retardation, and intractable seizures.

Arrhinencephaly

Absence of olfactory bulbs, tracts, and tubercles is often associated with holoprosencephaly and septo-optic dysplasia but also occurs with callosal agenesis or as an isolated cerebral anomaly. *Kallmann's syndrome* is an X-linked or autosomal dominant condition limited to males in which anosmia secondary to arrhinencephaly without other forebrain malformations is associated with lack of gonadotropic hormone secretion.

Septo-Optic Dysplasia

Septo-optic dysplasia is a common malformation consisting of a rudimentary or absent septum pellucidum with hypoplasia of the optic nerves and chiasm. Underdevelopment of the corpus callosum and anterior commissure and disturbances of the hypothalamic-pituitary axis are associated. The clinical features are impaired pituitary function, impaired vision, and mental retardation.

Agenesis of the Corpus Callosum

Agenesis of the corpus callosum is usually an isolated finding but is often associated with other midline malformations of the forebrain and aplasia of the cerebellar vermis. Isolated agenesis may involve the entire commissure or just affect the rostral fibers. Hypoplasia or partial agenesis is much more common than total agenesis. The clinical features of isolated agenesis may be minimal and shown only by tests of interhemispheric transfer.

Absence of the corpus callosum displaces the lateral ventricles laterally, and the third ventricle rises between them. Imaging studies easily reveal this configuration. Callosal agenesis is a component of trisomies 8, 11, and 13. *Andermann's syndrome* is autosomal recessive transmission of callosal agenesis, mental deficiency, and peripheral neuropathy. *Aicardi's syndrome* is X-linked transmission of callosal agenesis, chorioretinal lacunae, vertebral anomalies, mental retardation, and myoclonic epilepsy. A rare genetic form of callosal agenesis is associated with defective neural crest migration causing aganglionic megacolon (Hirschsprung's disease)

Colpocephaly

Colpocephaly is the opposite of semilobar holoprosencephaly. Symmetrical dilatation of the occipital horns of the lateral ventricles is associated with normal frontal horns. The optic nerves may be hypoplastic, and the corpus callosum is usually absent. Deficiency of callosal fibers from the deep white matter of the occipital lobes may explain the expanded occipital horns. Possible causes include infarction and cystic degeneration of the deep white matter of the posterior third of the cerebral hemispheres during the last trimester or a developmental disorder of neuronal migration. The clinical features of colpocephaly are mental retardation, spastic diplegia, epilepsy, and visual loss. Imaging studies are diagnostic.

DISORDERS OF EARLY NEUROBLAST MIGRATION (8–20 WEEKS OF GESTATION)

Lissencephaly (Agyria)

Lissencephaly is a failure of development of convolutions in the cerebral cortex because of defective neuronal migration.

The migrations of the cerebellum and the brainstem are usually involved, but the thalamus and basal ganglia are normal. Type 1 lissencephaly (*Miller-Dieker syndrome*) has characteristic features that include microcephaly, micrognathia, high forehead, thin upper lip, short nose with anteverted nares, and low-set ears. Affected children are mentally retarded, lack normal responsiveness to stimuli, initially exhibit muscular hypotonia that later evolves into spasticity and opisthotonos, and develop intractable seizures. Death before 1 year of age is common. A microdeletion at the 17p13.3 locus is usual. Type 2 lissencephaly is associated with several closely related genetic syndromes: Walker-Warburg syndrome, Fukuyama type muscular dystrophy, muscle-eye-brain syndrome of Santavuori, and Meckel-Gruber syndrome.

Subcortical Laminar Heterotopia (Band Heterotopia, Double Cortex) and Bilateral Periventricular Nodular Heterotopia

Subcortical laminar heterotopia and bilateral periventricular nodular heterotopia both result from X-linked recessive traits that occur almost exclusively in females. The initial features are severe seizure disorders, often associated with mental retardation. In subcortical laminar heterotopia, a heterotopic band of gray matter within the subcortical white matter lies parallel to the overlying cerebral cortex. The transcription product of the defective gene is called *double cortin*. In *bilateral periventricular nodular heterotopia*, islands of neurons and glial cells occur in the subependymal regions around the lateral ventricles. These neuroepithelial cells have matured in their site of origin without migrating.

Schizencephaly

The presence of a cleft in the region of the sylvian fissure, with open or closed lips, is termed *schizencephaly*. Schizencephaly is associated with defective expression of the gene *EMX2*. It may be associated with lissencephaly/pachygyria and may be unilateral or bilateral.

Hemimegalencephaly

Hemimegalencephaly, a severe dysgenesis, is either limited to one cerebral hemisphere or includes the ipsilateral cerebellar hemisphere and brainstem. Some are isolated malformations, and others are syndromic and associated with *epidermal nevus syndrome*, *Proteus' syndrome*, and *Klippel-Trenaunay-Weber syndrome*.

DISTURBANCES OF LATE NEUROBLAST MIGRATION (AFTER 20 WEEKS OF GESTATION)

A few neuronal precursors continue to migrate to the cerebral cortex after 20 weeks of gestation. Perinatal disorders, especially in premature infants, may interfere with late neuronal migrations. The clinical features are seizures and intellectual impairment.

DISORDERS OF CEREBELLAR DEVELOPMENT (32 DAYS OF GESTATION TO 1 YEAR POSTNATALLY

The cerebellum has the longest period of embryological development of any major structure of the brain. Therefore it is especially susceptible to the toxic effects of drugs, chemicals, viral infections, and ischemic-hypoxic insults. Malformations of the cerebellum may be confined to the cerebellum or be associated with brainstem or cerebral dysplasias. Selective hypoplasia or aplasia of the vermis, with intact lateral hemispheres, occurs in several genetic disorders. The clinical features are developmental delay, hypotonia, truncal titubation, and ataxia.

Dandy-Walker Malformation

The Dandy-Walker malformation is a ballooning of the posterior half of the fourth ventricle. It is often associated with failure of the foramen of Magendie to open. Associated malformations are aplasia of the posterior cerebellar vermis, heterotopia of the inferior olivary nuclei, and pachygyria of the cerebral cortex. Hydrocephalus almost always develops, but the prognosis is good if promptly treated.

Chiari Malformations

The Chiari malformation is a displacement of the tonsils and posterior vermis of the cerebellum through the foramen magnum, compressing the spinomedullary junction (*Chiari type I*). *Chiari type II* is a constant feature of lumbosacral meningocele. It involves the additional downward displacement of a distorted lower medulla. *Chiari type III* is actually a cervical spina bifida with cerebellar encephalocele. Hydrocephalus is commonly associated with all Chiari malformations. The pathogenesis is best explained by a molecular genetic hypothesis. Ectopic expression of a segmentation gene in the rhombomeres explains not only the Chiari malformation, but also the brainstem anomalies, the myelodysplasia, and the defective basioccipital and supraoccipital bone formation that results in a too small posterior fossa.

Cerebellar Hypoplasia

Chromosomal and genetically determined diseases are the main causes of global cerebellar hypoplasia. The most constant clinical features are developmental delay and generalized muscular hypotonia. Focal dysplasias and hamartomas of the cerebellar cortex are often asymptomatic.

Craniosynostosis

More than 100 syndromes include a component of craniosynostosis. Several have a genetic basis. Some are related to fibroblast growth factor receptor defects. The genetic bases of isolated craniostenoses of the coronal and sagittal sutures are not established.

For a more detailed discussion, see Chapter 66 in Neurology in Clinical Practice, 4th edition.

Developmental Disabilities | **36**

Five percent to ten percent of children have developmental disabilities. The definition of developmental disabilities is a disturbance in the acquisition of cognitive, motor, language, or social skills with a significant and continuing impact on developmental progress.

CEREBRAL PALSY

Clinical Features

Cerebral palsy (CP) is a static encephalopathy of prenatal or perinatal origin that affects motor tone and function, resulting in spasticity, hypotonia, ataxia, and dyskinesias. More than half of cases occur in preterm infants. The diagnosis requires a history of delayed motor milestones and a static motor disturbance. The likelihood of associated intellectual impairment and seizures is directly proportional to the severity of motor impairment.

Etiology and Evaluation

Brain imaging is extremely useful in determining the cause and the prognosis of CP. In full-term babies, the causative factor is prenatal in half and perinatal in half. Brain malformations are relatively common. CP in preterm newborns has a strong correlation with intraventricular hemorrhage and periventricular leukomalacia (see Chapter 55). Most genetic disorders with a phenotype suggesting CP ultimately cause progressive disability. Atypical features of CP and a history of other affected family members should suggest a genetic disorder.

Prevention and Management

Prevention of CP has focused on prevention of prematurity, optimal treatment during the perinatal period, and the development of neuroprotective agents (see Chapter 55). The main goals of treatment are to improve the child's motor function and to modify the environment to improve mobility. Orthopedic surgery is sometimes required. Dorsal rhizotomy is used to decrease spasticity and improve gait or make children who are wheelchair confined more comfortable. Botulinum toxin also has a role in the treatment of spasticity. The factors that decrease life expectancy in CP are immobility, profound retardation, and the need for special feeding. Otherwise, children with CP may live well into adult life.

MENTAL RETARDATION

Diagnosis

The American Association of Mental Retardation (AAMR) defines mental retardation (MR) not as an absolute condition but a construct that assists in educational planning and determines activities of daily living needs. The diagnosis therefore requires both a low intelligence quotient (IQ) (<70) and difficulties in at least two areas of adaptive functioning: communication, self-care, home living, social skills, community use, self-direction, health and safety, functional academics, leisure, and work. The definition therefore links the severity of MR to the degree of community support required to achieve optimal independence. Mild MR (IQ of 55–70) indicates intermittent support, moderate MR (IQ 45–55) limited support, severe MR (IQ 24–40) extensive support, and profound MR (IQ <25) pervasive support.

Evaluation and Etiology

In general, severe retardation is more likely to have a definable biological cause, whereas persons with mild MR tend to come from socially disadvantaged backgrounds and often have a family history of borderline IQ or mild retardation. The ratio of boys to girls with MR, especially with mild MR, is 1.4:1. Male excess is present in autism, undiagnosed nonsyndromic mental retardation, and X-linked monogenic disorders. The inheritances of more than 150 mental retardation syndromes are in an X-linked fashion with a frequency of 25 per 100,000.

Management

The management of children with MR focuses on finding the appropriate educational setting for children with mild MR, vocational training for those with moderate MR, and determining home or institutional placement for those with severe and profound MR.

AUTISTIC SPECTRUM DISORDERS

Diagnosis

The basis for diagnosis of autistic spectrum disorders (ASD) is on the early onset of a triad of deficits: impaired sociability, impaired verbal and nonverbal communication skills, and restricted activities and interests. Asperger disorder probably represents the high-functioning end of the ASD spectrum. The high concordance in monozygotic twins, the increased risk for recurrence in siblings, a broader autistic phenotype in families, and the association with several genetic disorders support a hereditary basis in many cases.

Clinical Features

Diagnosis is often delayed until late childhood, adolescence, or even adulthood because early language development is normal. Nonverbal learning disabilities or attention-deficit/hyperactivity disorder (ADHD) may be the presenting complaint. Although 40% show overall improvement during adolescence, as many as one third may deteriorate. Approximately two thirds of adults with autism show poor social adjustment, and one half require institutionalization.

Intelligence and Cognition
The presence of language and social deficits, but not IQ level, defines ASD. Although most children with ASD are mentally retarded, some have average or even superior intellectual ability. IQ is a key predictor of long-term outcome in autism.

Language
The severity of the language deficit generally parallels IQ. Long-term prognosis correlates with language skills at age 5 to 6 years.

Social Skills
Social dysfunction is a hallmark of ASD. The aloof child most resembles the popular notion of autism. Such children do not follow their parents around, run to greet them, or seek comfort. These children tend to be of low intelligence, have poor verbal and nonverbal communication skills, and exhibit little symbolic play.

Restricted Range of Behaviors, Interests, and Activities
A restricted range of behaviors, interests, and activities is the third cardinal feature of autism. In lower functioning children, these tend to consist of repetitive, stereotyped behaviors like twirling, rocking, flapping, licking, and opening and closing doors. Many such children have difficulty making transitions. Not only do they often not focus, but they also become over-focused. Some children, for example, with exceptional mathematical talents may meet the criteria for a diagnosis of an ASD or ADHD and grow up to be single-minded, peculiar, asocial chess or mathematics geniuses.

Evaluation
The standard neurological examination is generally normal. Tuberous sclerosis is probably the most common definable cause of autism. Tests for hearing impairment and subclinical seizures are indicated.

Management
Preschool children with ASD should receive special education in a therapeutic nursery or in a home-based behavioral modification program. The treatment of behavioral disturbances is medication.

LEARNING DISABILITIES

Learning disabilities (LDs) occur in approximately 10% of school-aged children and can affect one or more cognitive skills. LDs involve reading (dyslexia), motor functions (dysgraphia, dyspraxia), nonverbal skills (mathematics, written composition, visuospatial skills, socioemotional abilities), and attention (ADHD).

Dyslexia

Developmental dyslexia is an unexpected difficulty in learning to read. The definition is reading at a level that is two grades behind the actual or expected grade level, despite normal intelligence and a social and educational environment conducive to learning to read. Spelling difficulties may be a mild form of dyslexia that persists into adulthood.

The assessment of reading itself is the pivot point of an evaluation. The standard neurological examination is generally normal. Routine imaging is unnecessary. Several techniques for reading remediation are available. Generally, if one technique is unsuccessful, another is tried.

DEVELOPMENTAL DISORDERS OF MOTOR FUNCTION

Motor skill disorders consist of clumsiness, apraxia, dysgraphia, adventitious movements, and anomalous dominance or handedness. The definition of clumsiness is a slowness and inefficiency in performing elemental fine motor movements and sometimes in performing gross motor movements. Developmental dyspraxia is difficulty with motor learning and motor execution, with or without clumsiness. Dysgraphia is difficulty with writing. It can be a manifestation either of clumsiness or of dyspraxia. Adventitious movements, which occur normally on a developmental basis, include synkinesis, chorea, tremor, and tics. The establishment of handedness is never before age 1 year and always before age 5 years.

NONVERBAL LEARNING DISABILITIES

Children with nonverbal learning disabilities (NVLDs) generally have a significantly higher verbal as compared with performance IQ scores. Other difficulties include: (1) emotional and interpersonal difficulties (overlapping with ASD children), (2) paralinguistic communication problems, (3) impaired visuospatial and organizational skills, (4) impaired visuomotor skills, (5) academic difficulties in mathematics (dyscalculia), higher order reading comprehension (with normal decoding skills), and written composition, (6) attentional deficits and/or ADHD, (7) difficulty dealing with novelty or change, (8) difficulty grasping the whole picture, (9) marked slowness of performance, and (10) motor and tactile-perceptual neurological signs often with a left-sided bias. In the management of NVLDs, verbal skills are used to compensate for nonverbal deficits. The emphasis is on systematic learning because of the difficulty dealing with novel or complex situations.

Attention-Deficit/Hyperactivity Disorder

The estimated prevalence of ADHD in school-aged children is 20%. Although complete recovery from ADHD in childhood was expected, it now appears that ADHD persists in 70% of adults. Significant social-emotional difficulties in adulthood occur in 40–50%. Serious psychiatric or antisocial disabilities occur in 10%.

Table 36.1: Treatment of attention-deficit/hyperactivity disorder

Stimulants	Methylphenidate (Ritalin), dextroamphetamine (Dexedrine, Adderall), Pemoline (Cylert)
Alpha agonists	Clonidine (Catapres), guanfacine (Tenex)
Antidepressants	Selective serotonin reuptake inhibitors; tricyclic antidepressants; bupropion (Wellbutrin); trazodone, venlafaxine (Effexor); monoamine oxidase, selegiline (Deprenyl)
Antimanics	Lithium
Mood stabilizers	Carbamazepine (Tegretol), divalproex sodium (Depakote)
Beta blockers	Propranolol (Inderal), atenolol (Tenormin)
Antianxiolytics	Buspirone (BuSpar); clonazepam (Klonopin)
Neuroleptics	Haloperidol decanoate (Haldol); risperidone (Risperdal); phenothiazines

ADHD is an inappropriate inattention, impulsivity, distractibility, and hyperactivity for chronological and mental age. Table 36.1 delineates the treatment of attention-deficit/hyperactivity disorder. Approximately 25% of the first-degree relatives of a child proband with ADHD also have or have had ADHD. Stimulants drugs are the mainstay of treatment (Table 36.1).

For a more detailed discussion, see Chapters 7 and 67 in Neurology in Clinical Practice, 4th edition.

Inborn Errors of Metabolism of the Nervous System

37

The inborn errors of metabolism (IEMs) are a heterogeneous group of disorders resulting from abnormalities of the synthesis, transport, and turnover of dietary and cellular components. Approximately 1 per 1000 individuals is born with a metabolic disorder. IEMs are estimated to account for 20% of all deaths from genetic diseases; hereditary, neurological, or storage disorders account for 38%. Early diagnosis and intervention may influence the patient's quality of life and lead potentially to health care cost savings.

Defects of intermediary metabolic pathways cause disease either by the accumulation of a toxic metabolite or by the depletion of a metabolic by-product required to maintain proper cellular function. When an enzyme deficiency blocks normal catabolic routes, the diversion of metabolism to alternative pathways may disrupt cellular integrity. Deficient enzyme activity may arise from the following: (1) mutations in the primary gene sequence for the protein, (2) abnormal processing, that is, defects of post-translational modification, or (3) mistaken intracellular localization or improper folding of the enzyme. Metabolic defects may also result from defects of a structural or transport protein.

Most IEMs are multiorgan disorders that usually involve the nervous system. The clinical course can be acute, subacute, or chronic. Disorders characterized by intoxication or energy depletion usually present acutely as altered mental status. Seizures and hypotonia may be associated. Other clinical features associated with acute intoxication are vomiting, hepatic dysfunction, and renal dysfunction. Some IEMs follow an insidious course characterized by developmental delay or mental retardation, sensory-motor impairment, or dementia. Three diagnostic groups categorize IEMs: (1) disorders involving complex molecules (e.g., *lysosomal storage disorders*, *peroxisomal diseases*, *congenital defects of glycosylation*, and *defects of cholesterol synthesis*),

407

(2) disorders involving "small molecules" (e.g., *amino* and *organic acidurias, hyperammonemias,* and *lactic acidemias*), and (3) disorders associated with disruption of cellular energy metabolism (e.g., *mitochondrial respiratory-chain defects, disorders of carbohydrate metabolism,* and *disorders of fatty acid oxidation* [FAO]). Chapter 38 discusses mitochondrial disorders.

Metabolic defects involving complex molecules are usually progressive and unrelated to food intake, whereas those involving small molecules and cellular energy metabolism are more likely to become symptomatic in temporal relationship to food intake. The latter relationship accounts for the importance of dietary manipulation in the management of patients with certain IEMs.

GENERAL CONSIDERATIONS

Diagnostic Approach

In the setting of an acute illness, IEMs should be considered along with more common disorders, even when the family history is uninformative. The blood and urine of patients with acute neurological deterioration should be examined for signs of acidosis, ketosis, hypoglycemia, and hyperammonemia. Other considerations are screening tests for abnormalities of amino or organic acids (Table 37.1). Abnormal metabolites may not be present during stable periods or after the acute illness is over.

Cerebrospinal fluid (CSF) analysis is useful in specific cases. Determination of CSF levels of biogenic monoamines and γ-aminobutyric acid (GABA) may have diagnostic value in severe neonatal/infantile epileptic encephalopathy due to neurotransmitter defects. These are suspected in infants and children with (fluctuating) extrapyramidal disorders, particularly parkinsonism-dystonia, athetoid cerebral palsy, and vegetative disturbances. Table 37.2 lists the clinical characteristics of the IEMs.

Neurological deterioration is a characteristic feature of acute intoxication disorders, such as certain *aminoacidopathies* (maple syrup urine disease [MSUD]), *organic acidemias* (MMA, PA, IVA, MCD), and the *urea cycle defects* (UCDs). Abnormal urine odor is associated with the excretion of volatile metabolites (maple syrup in *MSUD*, sweaty feet in *IVA*, and *glutaric acidemia type II*). Isolated seizures are often the initial features of vitamin-responsive disorders (e.g., defects of pyridoxine and folinic acid metabolism, biotin-responsive multiple carboxylase deficiency) and are a prominent feature in nonketotic hyperglycinemia, sulfite oxidase deficiency, and congenital malabsorption

Table 37.1: Tests for the evaluation of a patient suspected of having an inborn error of metabolism

Tests	Clinical Utility
Ammonia	Urea cycle defects, organic acidemia
Carnitine, plasma or serum total and free (unesterified) and urine levels	Deficiency may develop in carnitine transport defects, disorders of fatty acid oxidation and branched chain amino acid metabolism, and valproic acid treatment
Acylcarnitine profile	Normal plasma acyl/free carnitine ratio: < 0.25
Ceruloplasmin	Decreased in Wilson's and Menkes' disease, aceruloplasminemia
Cholesterol	Low plasma levels in Smith-Lemli-Opitz syndrome, cerebrotendinous xanthomatosis; abnormal profile in the dyslipidemia
Free fatty acids (FFAs); ketone bodies (KBs): 3-OH-butyrate, acetoacetate	Disorders of fatty acid oxidation and ketolysis; supervised fasting and assessment of FFA:KB ratio and glucose and ketone levels distinction of hypoketotic and hyperketotic disorder
Lactate*	Defects of glycogen metabolism, gluconeogenesis and fatty acid oxidation (often seen with hypoglycemia); defects involving the electron transport chain, Krebs' cycle, and pyruvate dehydrogenase (absence of hypoglycemic episodes) Lactate:pyruvate ratio (Nl < 20:1) provides insight into oxidation-reduction status Normal blood lactate < 1.8 mmol/L Normal CSF lactate < 2.2 mmol/L
Very-long-chain fatty acid; phytanic acid	Disorders of peroxisomal metabolism
Uric acid	Elevated in Lesch-Nyhan syndrome[†] and other defects of purine metabolism and glycogen storage disorders; decreased in molybdenum cofactor deficiency and defects of purine metabolism
CSF:plasma ratio Glucose Glycine Serine	< 0.35 glucose transport defect > 0.6 nonketotic hyperglycinemia < 0.2 serine synthesis deficiency

*Presence or absence of hypoglycemia can be a useful aid to differential diagnosis of disorders that lead to lactic acidemia.
[†]Hyperuricemia may lead to nephrolithiasis, obstructive nephropathy, and gout.

Table 37.2: Clinical findings that are characteristic of an inborn error of metabolism

Disorder	Acute Metabolic Encephalop-athy	Metabolic Acidosis	Hyper-ammonemia	Hypo-glycemia
Aminoacidopathies	+/−			+/−
Organic acidemias*	+/−	+	+/−	
Urea cycle defects	+/−	−	+	
THAN§			+	
Fatty acid oxidation defects†			+/−	+
Defects of ketolysis		+		+/−
Defects of pyruvate metabolism and respiratory chain‡		+	+/−	
Glycogen storage disorders		+		+
Defects of gluconeogenesis		+		+

*Additional findings include increased anion gap and ketonuria.
†Usually associated with hypoketosis and may lead to secondary carnitine deficiency.
‡Normal lactate:pyruvate ratio (≤ 25) found with defects of pyruvate dehydrogenase or gluconeogenesis; elevated ratio suggests pyruvate carboxylase deficiency or mitochondrial disorder.
§Transient hyperammonenia of the newborn.

of magnesium. Congenital lactic acidosis and central hypotonia are features of pyruvate carboxylase deficiency, pyruvate dehydrogenase (PDH) deficiency, disorders of the Krebs cycle, and disorders in the mitochondrial respiratory chain. Recurrent hypoglycemia typically occurs in the glycogen storage disorders (GSDs) and in defects of FAO. Signs of cardiac involvement (cardiomyopathy, arrhythmias) are also associated.

Ophthalmological examination often provides a clue to the diagnosis of IEMs. Evidence of coloboma (congenital malformation of the optic nerve head or iris) may suggest an underlying brain abnormality. Vertical supranuclear ophthalmoplegia is a feature of Niemann-Pick disease type C and congenital disorders of glycosylation (CDG). Saccadic initiation failure and defective optokinetic nystagmus are features of *Gaucher's disease* (GD) *type 3*. Kayser-Fleischer rings (orange or greenish deposit around the limbus of the cornea caused by copper deposition within the

Descemet membrane) are characteristic of *Wilson's disease*. Table 37.3 lists additional characteristic eye findings of IEMs.

Hepatosplenomegaly and other signs of storage (e.g., coarse facies, nonimmune hydrops fetalis, and dysostosis multiplex) occur with the *lysosomal disorders*. Liver dysfunction and hepatomegaly usually occur in defects of carbohydrate metabolism (galactosemia and hereditary fructose intolerance) and bile acid synthesis, as well as in tyrosinemia and CDG. Unconjugated hyperbilirubinemia associated with liver dysfunction and/or hemolysis in infancy may lead to permanent brain damage due to kernicterus.

Cardiomyopathy may develop in IEMs associated with infiltrative (storage) disorders and defects of energy metabolism. The presence of hepatomegaly and other signs of systemic involvement (e.g., cataracts, coarse facies, and dysostosis multiplex) suggest storage disorders of glycogen or glycosaminoglycans. Defects of energy metabolism may be associated with acute or chronic encephalopathy, hepatic dysfunction, and several biochemical abnormalities (e.g., hypoglycemia, lactic acidosis ± ketosis, and elevated liver transaminase levels).

Delay of diagnosis until adolescence or adulthood occurs in acid maltase deficiency (muscle weakness and respiratory problems in the absence of cardiomyopathy), FAO defects (myoglobinuria and rhabdomyolysis after extreme exercise), X-linked adrenomyeloneuropathy (spastic paraparesis secondary to demyelination of the spinal cord and peripheral nerves), glycogen brancher enzyme deficiency (adult polyglucosan body disease with progressive upper and lower motor neuron disease, sensory loss, neurogenic bladder, and dementia), and acute intermittent porphyria (abdominal pain, psychosis).

Assessments of total and esterified carnitine levels and urinary carnitine excretion patterns are useful when a primary or secondary carnitine deficiency is suspected. Carnitine plays an essential role in the transfer of long-chain fatty acids across the inner mitochondrial membrane, in the detoxification of acyl moieties and in the maintenance of free coenzyme-A (CoA) levels. Dietary intake is the main source of carnitine. *Primary carnitine deficiency* due to defective transport leads to increased urinary loss and cardiac and skeletal muscle disease. *Secondary carnitine deficiency* occurs in several IEMs and may be partially responsive to oral carnitine supplementation. Table 37.4 provides a differential diagnosis of disorders involving carnitine metabolism.

Table 37.3: Ophthalmological findings associated with inborn errors of metabolism

Cataracts	Cherry red spot	Lens dislocation
Cerebrotendinous xanthomatosis	Galactosialidosis	Homocystinuria
Cholesterol synthesis defects	GM$_1$ gangliosidosis	Molybdenum cofactor deficiency
Galactokinase deficiency	Niemann-Pick disease A	Sulfite oxidase deficiency
Galactosemia	Sandhoff's disease	Retinopathy
Lowe's syndrome	Sialidosis type I	Carbohydrate-deficient glycoprotein syndrome
Menkes' syndrome	Tay-Sachs disease	Neuronal ceroid lipofuscinosis
Mucopolysaccharidoses	Optic atrophy	Mitochondrial defects
Peroxisomal disorders	Adrenoleukodystrophy	Peroxisomal disorders
Serine deficiency disorders	Canavan's disease	
Tyrosinemia type II	Hyperornithinemia with gyrate atrophy	
	Lafora's disease	

Table 37.4: Useful measures as an aid in the differential diagnosis of inborn errors of metabolism involving carnitine

Disorder	Plasma Total (μmol/l)	Carnitine Esterified (% of Total)	Urinary Carnitine
Control	40–60	< 30	Normal
Carnitine transporter deficiency	< 5	< 30	Paradoxically high free
Carnitine palmitoyl transferase-1 (CPT-1) deficiency	60–100	< 20	Normal or high
Carnitine translocase deficiency	5–30	80–100	High ester
Carnitine palmitoyl transferase-2 (CPT-2) deficiency	10–40	40–80	Normal or high ester
Defects in β-oxidation	10–30	30–60	High ester
3-OH-3-methylglutaryl-CoA-lyase deficiency	10–30	30–60	High ester

Source: From Nyhan, W. L. & Ozand, P. T. *Atlas of Metabolic Diseases*.

Brain magnetic resonance imaging (MRI) has significantly advanced the diagnosis and management of patients with IEMs. MRI also allows visualization of structural brain anomalies in children with mental retardation and seizures. For example, MRI images of patients with *adrenoleukodystrophy* typically show symmetrical areas of hypomyelination in the occipital lobes that extend to the splenium of the corpus callosum. Disease progression is associated with extension of white matter involvement from central to peripheral and from posterior to anterior, contiguously within the centrum semiovale and internal and external capsule. Abnormalities of both white and gray matter are observed when *mitochondrial disorders* that affect the central nervous system (CNS).

Proton magnetic resonance spectroscopy (MRS) is a useful adjunct to brain MRI and allows the determination of specific metabolites (e.g., elevated levels of N-acetoacetate in *Canavan's disease* and lactic acid in *mitochondrial disorders*, *defects* of *gluconeogenesis*, and *biotin-responsive multiple carboxylase deficiency*). MRS is also useful in monitoring response to treatment. Recently, MRS has enabled definition of the *creatine deficiency syndromes* (secondary to *guanidinoacetate methyltransferase deficiency*), a newly discovered group of disorders causing mental retardation and other neurological problems (e.g., extrapyramidal movement abnormalities and hypotonia).

Histological examination of appropriate tissue samples provides clues to the nature of the storage materials found in certain IEMs (e.g., *lysosomal disorders*). Microscopic examination of skin biopsy samples may be diagnostic. Portions are grown in tissue culture for subsequent biochemical or molecular (genetic) testing. Disorders of amino and organic acid metabolism, although not associated with deposition of storage material, are usable for confirmatory diagnosis by enzymatic assays. For some disorders, biochemical testing is not accurate for carrier detection because residual enzyme activity in a significant proportion of carriers overlaps with values obtained from the general population. In certain IEMs, molecular assays may be available for diagnostic purposes and carrier testing.

The GeneTests Web site (www.genetests.org) lists diagnostic laboratories that perform specialized genetic tests. In cases where the diagnosis is already established, several Web sites, including Mendelian Inheritance in Man (OMIM), GeneClinics, and the National Organization for Rare Disorders (NORD), provide detailed information. Support and patient advocacy groups also provide information about community resources and ongoing clinical trials.

Mutation Analysis in the Diagnosis of IEMs
Molecular genetic techniques offer an alternative means for the diagnostic confirmation of IEMs. This is particularly true for diseases associated with common mutations in which one or a few alleles account for a significant proportion of cases. In disorders with a known mutation, testing of other family members permits accurate carrier identification. Further, DNA analysis for prenatal diagnosis provides a rapid means of diagnosis because the use of chorionic villi or amniocytes does not require culture.

DNA testing has proven useful in the following disorders: medium-chain acyl-CoA dehydrogenase (MCAD) deficiency, myophosphorylase deficiency (McArdle disease), and GD. Among patients with MCAD of northwestern European descent, 80% are homozygous for a single missense mutation (A985G) and 17% carry this mutation in combination with another less common defect. This finding has improved the reliability of *MCAD* carrier identification and diagnosis, particularly of siblings who may be affected but asymptomatic at the time of family screening. In *hereditary fructose intolerance*, screening for the disease mutation in blood obviates the need for liver biopsy. However, in mitochondrial myopathies, muscle biopsy is required because blood and skins fibroblast may not be express the mutant gene.

IEMs Associated with Abnormal Brain Development and Encephaloclastic Lesions

Several metabolic disorders can cause a disruption of the normal sequence of brain development and lead to encephalocele, dysgenic corpus callosum, and neuronal migration defects (Tables 37.5 and 37.6). For instance, cystic necrosis of white matter ($\pm$ basal ganglia involvement) occurs in *deficiencies of PDH, pyruvate carboxylase* (PC), and *molybdenum cofactor*. The mechanisms proposed to explain abnormal brain development and encephaloclastic lesions in IEM include the production of a toxic or energy-deficient intrauterine milieu, modification of the content and function of membranes, and disturbance of the normal expression of intrauterine genes responsible for morphogenesis.

Imminent Death in a Child with a Suspected IEM

Obtain samples for diagnosis when a child develops acute fatal metabolic decompensation. A correct diagnosis may help families as they cope with their loss and enables appropriate counseling and prenatal diagnosis for subsequent pregnancies. Freeze plasma (separated from whole blood) and urine. A skin sample should be obtained using a sterile technique (using alcohol swabs and not iodine, which interferes with cell growth) and stored at room temperature in tissue culture medium. Place a small snip of skin in glutaraldehyde for subsequent electron microscopic studies whenever a storage disorder is suspected.

Management Considerations

The appropriate management of a patient with an IEM is determined by the particular metabolic derangement. Therapeutic strategies may include one or more of the following approaches: (1) substrate reduction by dietary manipulation or precursor synthesis inhibition, (2) removal (or enhanced clearance) of the toxic metabolites, (3) replenishment of depleted metabolites and/or cofactor supplementation, (4) enzyme (replacement) therapy, and (5) cellular replacement (e.g., bone marrow, liver, or kidney transplantation). Gene therapy had been actively explored, but trials have been suspended because the unexpected death occurred in a study subject with *ornithine transcarboxylase* (OTC) *deficiency*. Other approaches under

Table 37.5: Developmental brain malformations associated with an inborn error of metabolism

Disease	Neural Tube Defects	Holoprosencephaly	Cerebellar Malformations	Hypoplastic Temporal Lobes
Mitochondrial Disorders				
Respiratory chain enzyme deficiency			+	
Fatty acid oxidation				
Glutaric acidemia 2*			+	+
Folic acid metabolism				
Methylenetetrahydrofolate reductase deficiency	+			
Organic aciduria				
Glutaric aciduria 1†				+
Ethylmalonic aciduria	+			
Cholesterol metabolism				
Smith-Lemli-Opitz syndrome		+		
Glycoprotein metabolism				
Congenital disorder of glycosylation type 1			+	
Trace element metabolism				
Menkes' kinky hair			+	

*Resulting from a defect of the mitochondrial electron transport chain at coenzyme Q. Magnetic resonance imaging (MRI) T2-weighted scans also reveal increased signal intensity in the basal ganglia, and proton magnetic resonance spectroscopy scans show high choline:creatine ratio (indicative of dysmyelination) and elevated lactate.

†Resulting from deficient activity of the mitochondrial enzyme glutaryl-coenzyme A dehydrogenase. T2-weighted MRI images also reveal increased signal intensity in the basal ganglia and atrophy with progression.

Source: From Nissenkorn, A., et al. 2001, *Neurology,* vol. 56, p. 1265.

Table 37.6: Migration disorders and dysgenetic corpus callosum associated with IEM*

Disease	Pachygyria Lissencephaly	Polymicrogyria	Cortical Heterotopia	Cerebellar Dysplasia	Olivary Nuclei Dysplasia	Dysgenetic Corpus Callosum
Peroxisomal disorders†						
Zellweger syndrome‡	+	+	+	+++	++++	+++
Infantile Refsum						
Neonatal Pseudo-ALD						
Bifunctional enzyme deficiency	+	+	+	+++		
Chondrodysplasia punctata						
Mitochondrial disorders						
Pyruvate dehydrogenase deficiency	+		+	++	+	+
Fumarase deficiency		+	+	+		+
Fatty acid oxidation			+			
Carnitine palmitoyl transferase deficiency	+					
Glutaric acidemia 2	+		+			+

Continued

Table 37.6: (continued)

Disease	Pachygyria Lissencephaly	Polymicrogyria	Cortical Heterotopia	Cerebellar Dysplasia	Olivary Nuclei Dysplasia	Dysgenetic Corpus Callosum
Amino aciduria						
Maternal PKU	+					
Nonketotic hyperglycinemia		+				+
Organic aciduria						
3-OHisobutyric aciduria	+			++		++
3-OHbutyl-CoA deacylase deficiency				++		
Cholesterol metabolism						
Smith-Lemli-Opitz syndrome	+	+	+			+
Glycoprotein metabolism						
Congenital disorder of glycosylation type 1						
Trace element metabolism						
Menkes kinky hair disease			+	+		+

*Nissenkorn, A., et al. Inborn errors of metabolism, *Neurology* 2001, 56:1265–1272.

†Pseudo-Zellweger and pseudo-neonatal adrenoleukodystrophy have normal appearing cortexes.

‡The perirolandic distribution of pachygyria in Zellweger syndrome may help in the differential diagnosis of infants with hypotonia. Pattern is mainly occipital in congenital muscular dystrophy.

consideration are liver repopulation, chaperon-mediated therapy for diseases associated with residual enzyme activity, and the transplantation of stem cells with directed differentiation along specific lines.

Special Diets

When using special diets, attention must be given to caloric requirements and balanced nutrition that includes needed minerals and supplements. Diseases managed with dietary restriction include the aminoacidopathies phenylketonuria, *MSUD*, and *homocystinuria*. In *classic Refsum's disease*, reduction in dietary phytanate results in normalization of the biochemical and clinical phenotype.

Alternative dietary sources are necessary in some disorders. Medium-chain triglycerides are used as a lipid source in patients with very long-chain acyl co-a dehydrogenase deficiency (VLCAD) and long-chain hydroxy-acl-CoA dehydrogenase deficiency (LCHAD). The use of a high-cholesterol diet (± bile acids) in children with *Smith-Lemli-Opitz syndrome* (deficient 7-dihydrocholesterol-delta-reductase activity) improves growth and neurodevelopmental status, although clinical response is variable. In children with a *GSD*, carbohydrates are given to prevent hypoglycemia and suppress secondary metabolic derangements (e.g., hyperlipidemia and hyperuricemia). In the *urea cycle disorders*, arginine or citrulline is given to make up for compounds that are not synthesized secondary to the metabolic block.

Excretion or Detoxification of Toxic Metabolites

Methods to enhance excretion or detoxification of toxic metabolites are employed when their accumulation cannot be corrected by dietary manipulation. In patients with *hyperammonemia*, sodium benzoate and sodium phenylbutyrate, which conjugate with glycine and glutamine, are given to facilitate nitrogen excretion. In *isovaleric acidemia*, oral glycine conjugates with the highly toxic isovaleric acid to form a harmless by-product excreted in the urine. Administration of cystamine to patients with *cystinosis* promotes the formation of cysteine, which is subsequently excreted in the urine. Carnitine supplementation is given to patients with *organic acidemia* to prevent *secondary carnitine deficiency* secondary to the formation and renal excretion of acylcarnitine compounds. During acute metabolic decompensation, dialysis and hemofiltration may be used to facilitate rapid clearance of toxic metabolites. These techniques have been applied in the treatment of *MSUD* and *carbamylphosphate synthetase deficiency*.

Substrate Synthesis Inhibitors

The use of substrate synthesis inhibitors is a novel therapeutic strategy directed at blocking the production of toxic metabolites. In *tyrosinemia type 1 (fumarylacetoacetate hydrolase deficiency)*, NTBC (2-nitro-4-trifluoro-methylbenzoyl-1,3-cyclohexanedione) reduces the production of tyrosine degradation metabolites of by inhibiting the enzyme 4-OH-phenylpyruvate dioxygenase. Improved hepatic and renal function was noted among 95% of 300 patients with *tyrosinemia type 1*. In *GD type 1*, NB-DNJ (N-butyldeoxynojirimycin) administration decreases liver and spleen volumes and gradually improves hematological parameters with a decline in the levels of disease activity markers. NB-DNJ inhibits glucosyltransferase, the first enzymatic step in glycosphingolipid (GSL) biosynthesis. Metabolic homeostasis is achieved by limiting the accumulation of substrate to a level that can be sufficiently catabolized by a mutant but partially active enzyme. Given this mechanism of action, NB-DNJ may be potentially useful for other disorders of GSL metabolism (e.g., *late-onset Tay-Sachs* and *Sandhoff's disease*).

Replenishing Depleted Substrates

Replenishing depleted substrates partially corrects the underlying defect in some IEMs. In *carnitine-transport defect*, the use of carnitine results in the resolution of cardiomyopathy and prevention of further episodes of hypoketotic hypoglycemia. In other disorders, the production or binding affinity of a cofactor required for enzyme activity is impaired. These defects can be corrected by administration of pharmacological doses of the required supplement. Biotin given to children with *biotinidase* or *holocarboxylase deficiency* leads to good clinical outcomes except in the severe form. A sustained decrease of toxic metabolites and a favorable developmental prognosis results when Vitamin B12 is given for late-onset forms of *methylmalonic acidemia (MMA)*. Suppression of gut microbial propionate production and dietary protein restriction are complementary approaches for children with *MMA*.

Tetrahydrobiopterin (BH_4) is used to treat *disorders of biopterin synthesis*. Although BH_4 reduces elevated plasma phenylalanine levels by its action on liver phenylalanine hydroxylase, access to the CSF is minimal. Response has been observed in those with a "peripheral" type of defect. Tetrahydrofolate prevents demyelination in children with *folate deficiency* and *dihydropteridine reductase deficiency*. Responsiveness to cofactor administration can be assessed by controlled enzyme assays using the patient's cultured skin fibroblasts. A list of the cofactors used in various

Table 37.7: Cofactors used in the management of various inborn errors of metabolism

Cofactor	Dose (mg/day)	Disorder
Biotin	10–20	Propionic aciduria
		Multiple carboxylase deficiency
		Hyperlacticacidemia due to pyruvate carboxylase deficiency
Carnitine	50–100 orally; 400 intravenously	Branched-chain organic aciduria (methylmalonic acidemia, PA, IVA)
		Primary hyperammonemia
		Hyperlacticacidemia
		Fatty acid oxidation defects
Cobalamin (B12)	1–2	Methylmalonic aciduria
Folinic acid	10–40	Folinic-responsive seizures
Pyridoxine (B6)	50–100	Pyridoxine-responsive seizures, hyperoxaluria type 1, aromatic L-amino acid decarboxylase
Riboflavin (B2)	20–40	Glutaric aciduria
		Fatty acid oxidation defects
Thiamine (B1)	10–50	Maple syrup urine disease
		Hyperlacticacidemia due to pyruvate dehydrogenase deficiency

metabolic disorders and the recommended dose is shown in Table 37.7.

Enzyme Replacement Therapy
Enzyme replacement therapy (ERT) reverses the hematological and visceral manifestations of *GD*. This approach has been considered for the treatment of lysosomal storage disorders (LSDs) due to single enzyme deficiencies. The relevant enzymes are produced from genetically manipulated mammalian cells in culture and subsequently modified to expose the appropriate sugar residues to facilitate targeted cell uptake. Once purified, the recombinant enzyme is given intravenously on a regular basis. Beneficial effects have been noted in patients with *Fabry's disease*, *MPS type 1 (Hurler-Scheie syndrome)*, and *GSD II (Pompe's disease)*. Enzyme therapy is also being explored for other LSDs including *Niemann-Pick disease type B*, *MPS II (the*

mild variant of *Hunter's syndrome*) and *MPSVI (Maroteaux-Lamy syndrome).*

Organ Transplant

Metabolic correction through cellular replacement by bone marrow transplant (BMT) has been performed in patients with LSD (e.g., *MPS-I, GD type 3*). In *X-linked adrenoleukodystrophy*, BMT has resulted in prolonged remission with reversal of MRI abnormalities and stabilization or improvement of motor function. BMT is not appropriate for disorders characterized by rapid neurodegeneration, such as *MPS II (severe Hunter's syndrome)* and *MPS III (Sanfilippo's syndrome).*

Organ transplantation may be appropriate for disorders in which the metabolic defect is confined to the liver (e.g., *Crigler-Najjar syndrome, hyperoxaluria type I*) or leads to single organ failure (e.g., end-stage renal insufficiency in *Fabry's disease* and *hyperoxaluria type I*, and liver failure in *OTC deficiency, tyrosinemia,* and *GSD-IV*). Orthotopic liver transplantation is the treatment of choice for patients with *tyrosinemia* who do not respond to NTBC therapy or have evidence of hepatic malignancy. Microchimerism (the migration of donor-derived cells from the allograft) has been reported in a few patients following liver transplantation. However, this technique is probably not sufficient to correct the systemic metabolic defect.

Symptomatic Treatment

Symptomatic treatment remains a vital component of patient care. Several palliative measures improve quality of life and reduce the incidence and severity of disease-related complications. For instance, L-dopa improves motor function in patients with *tyrosine hydroxylase deficiency* and deamino-arginine-vasopressin (DDAVP) reduces the tendency for abnormal bleeding during surgery of patients with *GSD type 1A (von Gierke's disease)*. The administration of granulocyte colony-stimulating factor (G-CSF) to patients with GSD type 1B and neutropenia minimizes the risk of recurrent bacterial infection and gastrointestinal tract ulceration. Steroid and mineralocorticoid replacement is essential in patients with *adrenoleukodystrophy* and adrenal insufficiency.

Genetic Counseling

Genetic counseling is an important aspect of dealing with disease management. Approximately 90% of the IEMs are inherited as autosomal recessive traits. Of the remaining 10%, approximately two thirds are X-linked traits and one third are autosomal dominant traits. Prenatal diagnosis is available for most IEMs. Most parents are receptive to future prenatal diagnosis, and 41% would choose to take measures to prevent another affected pregnancy.

Disorders Involving Complex Molecules

The metabolism of complex molecules in lysosomes and peroxisomes involves different biochemical pathways than those responsible for the processing of dietary constituents. Dietary manipulation and vitamin or cofactor supplementation are therefore ineffective. An overview of the distinctive characteristics of these organelles and the associated general features are summarized in Tables 37.8 and 37.9. LSDs involve tissues and organs that develop normally but later malfunction. In contrast, early-onset peroxisomal disorders are often expressed as severe developmental malformations.

Lysosomal Storage Disorders

The lysosome is a membrane-bound intracytoplasmic vacuole that contains enzymes required for the degradation of complex lipids, proteins, and nucleotides. Its acidic milieu (pH ~ 5.4) is required for optimal activity of the contained hydrolytic enzymes and their cofactors\activators. More than 40 LSDs are described.

Progressive lysosomal storage of incompletely metabolized substrates occurs because of primary hydrolase deficiency, deficiency of a protective protein that aids in the lysosomal targeting and prevention of premature degradation of enzymes, or the absence of an "activator protein" necessary for enzyme–substrate interaction and degradation. Additional disease mechanisms include abnormal protein\enzyme processing, defects of posttranslational modification in the endoplasmic reticulum, failure to attach the appropriate targeting signals (e.g., mannose-6-phosphate) in the Golgi apparatus, and defective removal or transport of the substrate from lysosomes (e.g., *Niemann-Pick type C* and *sialic acid storage disease*). Abnormalities in endocytosis, vesicle fusion, and the processing of autophagic elements are identified in Danon's disease from defects of lysosomal-associated membrane protein-2 (LAMP-2). LAMP-2 is an integral membrane protein of endosomes and lysosomes. Other syndromes of intracellular vesicle formation damage that cause abnormal lysosomal formation and storage are *Hermansky-Pudlak syndrome* and *Chediak-Higashi syndrome*.

Clinically, the LSDs are a heterogeneous group of disorders involving multiple organ systems. The onset of the rapidly progressive forms is in the newborn or in early infancy. With later-onset forms, the initial features are delayed until adolescence or

Table 37.8: Characteristic biochemical features of the major cellular organelles

Lysosome	Peroxisome	Mitochondria
Acidic compartment, actively maintained (proton ATPase)	Metabolic functions: β-oxidation of fatty acids and derivatives, ether phospholipid synthesis	Site of coupling of oxidation and phosphorylation
Terminal compartment in endocytic pathway	Increased very-long-chain fatty acids	Generation of adenosine triphosphate
Rich in acid hydrolases (protease, glycosidase, sulphatase)	Disease often classified based on loss of single or multiple peroxisomal enzyme function	Symptoms reflect tissue specificity for aerobic metabolism: brain > skeletal, cardiac muscle > kidney > eye
Enzymes use mannose-6-phosphate targeting into pre-lysosome	Due to defects of biogenesis and targeting thru PTS1 and 2	Has unique DNA, which replicates independently of nuclear DNA
Autosomal recessive, except Fabry's disease, Hunter's syndrome (MPD-II), and Danon's disease, which are X-linked traits	Autosomal recessive, except for X-linked adrenoleukodystrophy	Occurrence may be sporadic, matrilineal, or autosomal (dominant or recessive) inheritance

Table 39.9: Clinical diagnostic clues that should lead to consideration of an underlying organelle pathology

Lysosomal	Peroxisomal	Mitochondrial
Oligosystemic (CNS, RES)	Multisystemic	Multisystemic
Chronic course	Hypotonia	Failure to thrive
Behavioral changes	Failure to thrive	Lethargy
Seizures (late)	Developmental delay	Cerebral dysgenesis
Leukodystrophy	Abnormal craniofacies	Sensorineural hearing loss
Cerebellar atrophy	Rhizomelic short stature	Ophthalmoplegia
Macular red spot	Cerebral dysgenesis	Retinitis pigmentosa
Hepatosplenomegaly	Sensorineural hearing loss	Cardiomyopathy
Skin lesions (angiokeratoma)	Hepatocellular dysfunction	Myopathy
Bone disease (dysostoses multiplex)	Adrenal dysfunction	Diabetes

CNS = central nervous system; RES = reticuloendothelial system.

adult life and the course may be acute, subacute, or chronic. Acute and subacute courses are usually associated with primary CNS involvement, developmental delay, and mental retardation.

Unlike the small molecule diseases, the clinical features of LSD are characterized by a subacute or chronic encephalopathy. Myoclonic seizures are seen in the following disorders: GM_2-gangliosidosis, sialidosis type 1, Schindler disease (α-galactosidase B deficiency), GD types 2 and 3, and fucosidosis. Some LSDs do not have primary CNS involvement (e.g., Fabry's disease, GD type 1, Niemann-Pick type B, MPS I-Scheie's syndrome, MPS IV-Morquio's syndrome, and mild MPS VI-Maroteaux-Lamy syndrome).

Rare variants of some sphingolipid storage disorders are caused by defects in the enzyme cofactor\activator required for complete substrate hydrolysis rather than a primary enzyme defect. Two categories of sphingolipid activators exist. One represents the GM_2 activator and the other a group of four molecules (saposin A, B, C, and D) derived by proteolytic cleavage of a common precursor, prosaposin. The gene localization for D-prosaposin is chromosome 10. Deficiency of the GM_2 activator results in the *AB variant of GM_2 gangliosidosis*. Saposin B activates arylsulphatase A. Deficiency of saposin B gives rise to a variant of *metachromatic leukodystrophy* (*MLD variant*). Saposin C activates glucocerebrosidase and α-galactocerebrosidase; its deficiency leads to a clinical picture often referred to as an *atypical form of GD* because of the clinical overlap between GD and the type 3 variant (subacute neuropathic GD). Disorders resulting from cofactor deficiencies are characterized by normal enzymatic activities *in vitro* when using the synthetic (artificial) substrate. Therefore the diagnosis can be missed by routine biochemical testing unless the assay is performed using the natural glycosphingolipid substrates. Molecular analysis may reveal the presence of mutations in the relevant encoding genes.

LSDs are usually transmitted as autosomal recessive traits, except for *Fabry's disease*, *Hunter's syndrome* (MPS-II), and *Danon's disease*. These are inherited as X-linked recessive traits. Biochemical assays are generally available for prenatal diagnosis. Diagnostic confirmation is also available by molecular (DNA) testing. In families where the causal mutation is known, molecular testing enables accurate assignment of carrier or affected status. Prenatal diagnosis is possible for almost all LSDs.

Peroxisomal Disorders
The peroxisome is an organelle involved in beta oxidation of very-long-chain fatty acids (VLCFAs), the synthesis of plasmalogen and bile acids, and oxidation of pipecolic, phytanic, and dicarboxylic acids. Peroxisomal disorders are generally classified according to the presence of single or multiple enzyme deficiencies. Most peroxisomal matrix proteins are targeted using one of two targeting sequences, in a unique system allowing the importation of oligomerized proteins through a specific shuttle involving a receptor and its cargo. Defects of these cellular mechanisms lead to disruption of peroxisomal metabolic functions. Table 37.10 summarizes the spectrum of clinical findings in peroxisomal disorders. Measurements of plasma VLCFA concentrations and impaired erythrocyte plasmalogen synthesis are the best screening techniques for peroxisomal disorders. Increased phytanic acid levels are found in *Refsum's disease* and *rhizomelic chondrodysplasia punctata*.

Disorders Involving Small Molecules

Disorders of intermediary metabolism often result in the accumulation of compounds that cause acute progressive neurological disorders. The phrase *disorders of small molecules* is used because the compounds that build up proximal to the metabolic block are often elevated in blood and CSF and may be

Table 37.10: Peroxisomal disorders

Defects of biogenesis I	
Spectrum: Zellweger syndrome—severe	Craniofacial dysmorphic features: large anterior fontanel, high forehead
	Psychomotor retardation
	Hypotonia
Neonatal adrenoleukodystrophy	Neonatal seizures
Infantile Refsum's disease—relatively milder	Cortical dysplasia, neuronal migration defects
	Hepatomegaly with liver dysfunction
	Chorioretinopathy
	Sensorineural hearing loss
	Calcific stippling of the epiphysis
	Renal cysts
Defects of biogenesis II	Shortened proximal limbs
Rhizomelic chondrodysplasia punctata	Facial dysmorphic features
	Cataracts
	Psychomotor retardation
	Calcific stippling of the epiphysis (may disappear after age 2 years) and extraskeletal tissues
	Ichthyosis
Single function deficiency	
Adrenoleukodystrophy	Intellectual regression, behavioral problems,
Adrenomyeloneuropathy	spastic paraparesis, sphincter problems, adrenal insufficiency
Refsum's disease	Retinitis pigmentosa, polyneuropathy, cerebellar ataxia
Pseudo-Zellweger	
Pseudo-neonatal	
Adrenoleukodystrophy	
Pseudo-infantile RD	
Bifunctional protein deficiency	
Hyperpipecolic acidemia	Enzyme defect not definitively established
	Encephalopathy, seizures
	Hypocholesterolemia
	Vitamin E deficiency

Table 37.11: Disorders of small molecule and energy metabolism

Disorder	Incidence
Aminoacidopathy	
Phenylketonuria	1:10,000
Maple syrup urine disease	1:180,000
Homocystinuria	1:300,000
Tyrosinemia	
Organic acidemia	
Branched-chain (methylmalonic,	Methylmalonic acidemia
propionic, isovaleric)	1:20,000
Urea cycle	
Ornithine transcarbamylase deficiency	1:70 to 100,000
Arginase	< 1:100,000
Carbohydrate (sugar) intolerance	
Galactosemia	1:40,000
Glycogen storage disease type IA	1:100,000
(von Gierke's disease)	
Fatty acid oxidation defects	
Medium-chain acyl-CoA	$\sim$ 1:20,000
dehydrogenase deficiency	

excreted in the urine or potentially cleared by dialysis. Diagnosis is enabled by detection of these compounds in blood, CSF, and urine. Serial measurements can monitor the effectiveness of therapy. Treatment often requires the elimination of the accumulating toxic compounds by dietary restriction and/or the provision of vitamins or cofactors. During episodes of acute decompensation, metabolic homeostasis may be rapidly achieved by exchange transfusion or by peritoneal dialysis or hemodialysis. Chronic control necessitates the use of compounds that bind with the toxic molecules and facilitate alternative pathways of clearance. Included in this group are the aminoacidopathies, organic acidemias, and the UCDs. Examples for each category and their estimated incidence are listed in Table 37.11.

Disorders of Amino and Organic Acid Metabolism

The main clinical feature of these conditions is a symptom-free interval followed by an acute "catastrophic" event (e.g., vomiting, lethargy, and coma). The acute episodes are characterized by metabolic acidosis, hypoglycemia, and/or hyperammonemia. These metabolic disorders cause progressive developmental regression and spasticity. A specific diagnosis relies on the pattern of abnormalities displayed on the amino and organic acid screening profile and by detection of the relevant acylcarnitine compounds in plasma and urine. These disorders are usually treated by dietary restriction, elimination of the toxic compounds, and adjunctive treatments using specific cofactor or vitamin supplements and carnitine as indicated.

Hyperammonemia

Blood ammonia is derived from protein catabolism and as a metabolic by-product of bacterial reactions in the gastrointestinal tract. Ammonia is neurotoxic and promotes excessive glutamine production in the cytosol of astrocytes by its action on glutamine synthetase. Ammonia can promote cellular swelling and brain edema by its osmotic effect. Blood ammonia concentrations may be elevated from a primary defect of the urea cycle (UCD) or secondarily in disorders of amino and organic acid metabolism. In the organic acidemias, intramitochondrial accumulation of acyl-CoA esters causes secondary inhibition of the urea cycle enzymes. Assessment of the plasma amino acid and ammonia levels and analysis of urine organic acids establishes the diagnosis. Measurement of urinary orotic acid concentrations is useful in the differential diagnosis (Table 37.12). Defects of the urea cycle are all inherited as autosomal recessive traits except for ornithine transcarbamylase deficiency, which is inherited as an X-linked trait.

The clinical features are variable; newborns may exhibit rapidly progressive neurological deterioration, with irritability or lethargy, seizures, coma, and respiratory arrest. Affected newborns are managed with exchange transfusion and peritoneal dialysis. Later-onset clinical UCD manifestations include developmental delay, behavioral problems, hepatomegaly, and gastrointestinal symptoms. Affected children and adults may show behavioral problems, confusion, irritability, and cyclic vomiting. Mental status deteriorates during metabolic stress.

Two disorders of amino acid metabolism, *lysinuric protein intolerance* (LSI) and *hyperammonemia-hyperornithinemia-homocitrullinemia* (HHH syndrome), are associated with hyperammonemic encephalopathy. *LSI* presents with growth retardation, hepatic and renal dysfunction, and hematological and pulmonary abnormalities. *HHH syndrome* is associated with an elevation of plasma ornithine and increased urinary excretion of homocitrulline (a derivative of lysine). The clinical features include intolerance to protein feeding, vomiting, seizures, and developmental delay. Ornithine administration improves urea cycle function in the *HHH syndrome* by providing the required precursor for uninterrupted completion of the sequential metabolic steps. Progressive spastic paraparesis is a late complication.

Table 37.12: Defects of the urea cycle

Enzyme Deficiency	Plasma Amino Acid Profile	Urine Orotic Acid
Carbamoylphosphate synthase	Absent citrulline, decreased arginine; increased glutamine, alanine	Normal or low
Ornithine transcarbamylase	Absent citrulline, decreased arginine; increased glutamine, alanine	Elevated
Argininosuccinic synthase (citrullinemia)	Markedly elevated citrulline; decreased arginine	Increased
Argininosuccinic lyase	Moderately elevated citrulline, argininosuccinic acid decreased arginine	Increased
Arginase	Increased glutamine, alanine	Increased

Disorders of Energy Metabolism

The energy requirements of cellular metabolism are derived from carbohydrates in the nourished state and from glycogen and fatty acids stores during fasting. Cellular energy is stored in the form of adenosine triphosphate (ATP) and generated in the cytoplasmic and mitochondrial compartments from glucose and FAO. The relevant metabolic pathways are largely hormonally mediated. Tissues with high aerobic metabolic rates, in the brain, skeletal muscle, and cardiac muscle, are most vulnerable to defects of energy metabolism.

Several clinical presentations suggest an underlying defect of energy metabolism. Acute or recurrent exercise intolerance and myoglobinuria, with or without cramps, are features of the glycogen and FAO disorders. Progressive neuromuscular weakness and hypotonia are features of the glycogenoses (*acid maltase, debrancher enzyme,* and *brancher enzyme deficiencies*), FAO defects, involving carnitine uptake and carnitine acylcarnitine translocase defects, and mitochondrial disorders (*cytochrome oxidase deficiency*). Acute or chronic weakness occurs in long-chain or very-long-chain acyl-CoA-dehydrogenase, short-chain L-3-hydroxy-acyl-CoA dehydrogenase, and trifunctional protein deficiencies. Avoidance of fasting is an important consideration in the management of patients with disorders of carbohydrate metabolism (glycogenolysis), FAO, and ketogenesis. In some cases, the calories for energy metabolism must be maintained by nasogastric or gastrostomy tube feedings.

Glycogen Storage Disorders

The GSDs are caused by enzyme defects of glycogen degradation. A number designates the historical sequence of their clinical characterization. Several subtypes are designated in recognition of the individual who called attention to the condition (i.e., *Pompe's disease*).

Disorders of Gluconeogenesis

Recurrent hypoglycemia and lactic acidosis, with or without ketosis, are the result of defects of gluconeogenesis. Neurodegenerative features are found in *deficiencies of PC* and *phosphoenolpyruvate carboxykinase* (PEPCK).

Fatty Acid Oxidation Defects

The oxidation of fatty acids involves four components: the carnitine cycle, mitochondrial oxidation, electron transfer, and the synthesis of ketone bodies. Some tissues use fatty acids and ketone bodies as an alternative energy source to spare glucose consumption. In contrast to muscle, the brain is unable to fully oxidize fatty acids but can use ketone bodies synthesized by the liver. In early onset disease, the course is characterized by episodes of hypoketotic, hypoglycemic coma, and metabolic decompensation during prolonged fasting or periods of illness and stress. Rhabdomyolysis, cardiomyopathy, and skeletal muscle weakness are features of chronic late-onset cases. *MCAD deficiency* is the most common *FAO defect*. The initial crisis is fatal in up to 25% of cases.

Disorders of Ketogenesis and Ketolysis

The liver converts excess acetyl-CoA, a by-product of FAO, to ketones. These are subsequently oxidized in the peripheral tissues. Ketone utilization by the brain spares other tissues, such as erythrocytes, which cannot meet their energy requirements from nonglucose substrates. Ketoacidosis is a prominent secondary feature of several defects of intermediary metabolism. Primary disorders of ketogenesis and ketolysis are rare.

Miscellaneous Metabolic Disorders

Dyslipidemias

Lipids are transported in plasma on lipoproteins wrapped in an amphiphilic coating of apolipoproteins, phospholipids, and unesterified cholesterol. Diseases associated with abnormal lipid absorption and metabolism result in low blood levels of the fat-soluble vitamins (A, D, E, and K). This is correctable by oral or parenteral supplementation.

Abetalipoproteinemia and *hypobetalipoproteinemia* are disorders of reduced low-density lipoprotein (LDL)-cholesterol metabolism. In *abetalipoproteinemia*, plasma apolipoprotein-B (ApoB) levels are undetectable and total cholesterol levels are usually less than 50 mg/dl. The defect is caused by absence of microsomal triglyceride transfer protein (MTP), and not by mutations in the *apoB* gene. Patients with *abetalipoproteinemia* have fat malabsorption and neurological disturbances that include dysmetria, cerebellar ataxia, and spastic gait. Ocular disturbances include retinitis pigmentosa, impaired night vision, nystagmus, and ophthalmoplegia. Failure to thrive and steatorrhea occurs in infancy, and the neurological complications appear during adolescence. Other features include anemia (acanthocytosis) and arrhythmia. Acanthocytosis is a consequence of reduced erythrocyte membrane fluidity. It is also seen in Vitamin E deficiency and neuroacanthocytosis. *Hypobetalipoproteinemia*, due to mutations in the *apoB* gene, causes a clinical syndrome similar to Friedreich's ataxia (ataxia and peripheral neuropathy). It is transmitted as an autosomal dominant trait. Most patients have low LDL-cholesterol concentrations (usually < 60 mg/dl). Rare patients homozygous for the defect have clinical features indistinguishable from those of abetalipoproteinemia. Vitamin supplements (A and E) have a beneficial influence on the neurological and ocular symptoms. Care should be taken to avoid Vitamin A toxicity by serial monitoring of vitamin levels.

Tangier disease is a rare autosomal recessive disorder caused by mutations in a cell-membrane protein called ABCA1, which normally mediates the secretion of excess cholesterol from cells into the high-density lipoprotein (HDL) metabolic pathway. It belongs to a family of ATP-binding cassette (ABC) transporters. These proteins are involved in the recognition of substrate and their transport across, into, and out of cell membranes. Cystic fibrosis, age-related macular degeneration, and *X-linked adrenoleukodystrophy* are other disorders associated with defects of genes that encode this class of proteins. *Tangier disease* is characterized by severe deficiency of HDLs and tissue storage of cholesterol esters. Clinical features include enlarged orange-yellow tonsils, splenomegaly, and a relapsing sensorimotor neuropathy. Patients may develop distal weakness, hyporeflexia, and decreased pain and temperature sensations with relative preservation of position and vibration sense.

Smith-Lemli-Opitz syndrome is characterized by multiple malformations, growth and psychomotor retardation, and behavioral disturbances. Cholesterol biosynthesis is abnormal. The serum concentration of cholesterol is low and serum levels of 7-DHC are elevated. Sterol abnormalities that result from deficiencies of cholesterol biosynthesis also explain other recently recognized disorders of morphogenesis. Sterol synthesis (SS) takes place partly in the peroxisomes. This explains why SS defects show some overlap in clinical features with the *peroxisomal biogenesis disorders*.

Cerebrotendinous xanthomatosis (cholestanolosis) is transmitted as an autosomal recessive trait. The condition is caused by mutations in the sterol 27-hydroxylase gene. The primary feature is the formation of xanthomatous lesions in the brain and tendons. Neurological impairments include mental retardation, progressive spasticity, pseudobulbar palsy, and cerebellar dysfunction. Brain MRI shows hyperintense signals that involve the corticospinal tracts in the brainstem, the white matter of both internal capsules, and the peritrigonal white matter. Bilateral cataracts and chronic diarrhea may precede the neurological deterioration. Biochemical findings include elevated plasma and bile cholestanol levels and increased urinary excretion of bile alcohol glucuronides associated with diminished biliary cheno-deoxycholic acid (CDCA). Therapy with CDCA reverses the neurological features

Lowe's oculocerebrorenal syndrome is transmitted as an X-linked trait and is characterized by bilateral congenital cataracts, mental retardation, and a renal ion-transport defect (Fanconi's syndrome). Disease results from mutations in the *OCRL* gene. This gene encodes a Golgi-associated protein (inositol polyphos-phate-5-phosphatase) that regulates the cellular levels of a metabolite (phosphatidylinositol 4,5-biphosphate) involved in vesicular transport. Female carriers can be identified by detection by slit-lamp examination of lens opacities. Symptomatic treat-ment with phosphate and Vitamin D prevents the development of severe rickets. Patients are at risk for glaucoma and should have serial monitoring of intraocular pressure.

Nonketotic hyperglycinemia (NKH), or glycine encephalopathy, is caused by a defect in the P-protein (glycine decarboxylase) gene, which encodes a component of the mitochondrial glycine cleavage system. *NKH* is clinically characterized by a neonatal encephalopathy. Infants develop lethargy, hypotonia, myoclonic seizures, and apnea. The electroencephalogram shows a burst-suppression pattern. CSF glycine is elevated and the ratio of CSF to plasma glycine concentration (normally < 0.4) is higher than 0.6. Brain MRI reveals a hypoplastic or absent corpus callosum and gyral malformations; cerebellar hypoplasia is an associated feature. Dextromethorphan and ketamine inhibit receptor excitation and are used for treatment. Prognosis is poor, and most affected children are mentally retarded.

Molybdenum cofactor is essential for xanthine oxidase, sulfite oxidase, and aldehyde oxidase activity, and thus deficiency of the cofactor causes refractory seizures, axial hypotonia, and limb rigidity. Urinary excretion of xanthine and sulfite is increased. Brain imaging shows multiple cystic cavities in the white matter.

Disorders of copper metabolism: Copper is an essential element for the activity of several enzymes. *Menkes' disease* and *Wilson's disease* result from mutations in highly homologous copper transporters. Menkes' syndrome is transmitted as an X-linked trait. The membrane copper transporter ATP7A is defective, causing a functional copper deficiency and low levels of serum copper and ceruloplasmin. Progressive neurodegeneration and marked connective tissue abnormalities are characteristic. The disease is usually lethal in infancy or childhood. Daily intra-venous copper histidine administration restores serum copper and ceruloplasmin levels and has favorable clinical results when started before neurodegeneration. *Wilson's disease* is an autosomal recessive disorder caused by mutations in the copper transporter (ATP7B) gene. Excessive copper accumulates in the liver and brain. Neurological features include tremors, loss of fine motor control and poor coordination, rigid dystonia, dysarthria, and swallowing difficulties. Diagnostic findings include the presence of Kayser-Fleischer rings and increased urine copper excretion, with low serum ceruloplasmin and increased liver tissue copper content. Basal ganglia degeneration is evident on MRI as increased T2 intensity in the caudate and putamen. The results of therapy by liver transplantation has been mixed.

Disorders of purine and pyrimidine metabolism: Purine and pyrimidine nucleotides are essential cellular components involved in energy transfer and the regulation and synthesis of DNA and RNA. Defects of purine and pyrimidine metabolism can result from disruption of biosynthetic, catabolic, or salvage pathways. *Lesch-Nyhan syndrome* is transmitted as an X-linked recessive trait. Hypoxanthine-guanine phosphoribosyltransferase (HGPRT), required in the purine salvage pathway, is deficient, causing hyperuricemia. Clinical features include chorea and athetosis, dysarthria, hyperreflexia, hypertonia, cognitive impairment, and behavioral disturbances that include impulsive and self-injuring activity. Dopamine concentrations in the basal ganglia and CSF are reduced and may account for some of the neurological features. Patients with partial HGPRT deficiency always have hyperuricemia and often have neurological abnormalities but do not show self-injuring behavior and usually have normal intelligence.

Porphyrias: Porphyrins play an important role in the formation of metalloporphyrin complexes, including hemoglobin, myoglobin, cytochromes, peroxidases, oxidases, and catalases. The *porphyrias* are caused by deficiencies of specific enzymes involved in the heme biosynthetic pathway. This pathway occurs in bone marrow elements (85%) or in the liver. The porphyries are characterized by the accumulation and excess excretion of by-products of intermediary heme metabolism and their oxidized products. Consider a diagnosis of *porphyria* in patients with unexplained neuropsychiatric signs, visceral (gastrointestinal and hepatic) symptoms, or cutaneous photosensitivity. Cutaneous manifestations are prominent in *hereditary coproporphyria* and *variegate porphyria*, but the neurovisceral disturbances may be indistinguishable from those of *acute intermittent porphyria* (AIP). *Porphyrias* with neurological features have either a constant or an intermittent excretion of aminolevulinic acid and porphobilinogen. The elimination of precipitating factors is an important method to reduce the frequency and intensity of acute exacerbations.

AIP is transmitted as an autosomal dominant trait. Mutations occur in the porphobilinogen deaminase (PBD) gene. Deficient activity of erythrocyte PBD activity is used to confirm the diagnosis. Bouts of abdominal pain, paresthesias, seizures, and peripheral neuropathy are prominent clinical features. Neurotic or psychotic behavior is also reported. Certain drugs can precipitate acute attacks and patients should be provided with a list of medications to avoid. Carbohydrate loading and administration of heme analogues are used to manage the acute crises.

Congenital disorders of glycosylation: The carbohydrate-deficient glycoprotein (CDG) syndromes are a heterogenous group of autosomal recessive disorders resulting from defects of the N-linked glycosylation pathway. Many proteins are rendered functional by glycosylation. The initial features of CDG syndromes may include ataxia, strabismus, unusual fat distribution, severe liver dysfunction, seizures, and strokelike episodes. Almost all CDGs show some degree of developmental and psychomotor retardation and many have gastrointestinal dysfunction. Testing for abnormal protein glycosylation is done by isoelectric focusing analysis of serum transferrin. Treatment is not available.

Canavan's disease (CD) is caused by deficiency of aspart acylase. Clinical features include hypotonia, delayed development, optic atrophy, and seizures. *CD* shares several features (e.g., progressive macrocephaly, demyelination) with *Alexander's disease*, a rare, progressive, leukoencephalopathy characterized by the widespread accumulation of Rosenthal's fibers. However, *Alexander's disease* has a later onset and slower course. Patients with Alexander's disease have missense mutations in the coding region of the glial fibrillary acidic protein gene.

For a more detailed discussion, see Chapter 68 in Neurology in Clinical Practice, 4th edition.

Mitochondrial Disorders

38

Mitochondria are the energy generators of animal cells. The diseases included under the term *mitochondrial disorders* are diverse and involve many parts of the nervous system and other organs. Discussions of the individual disorders are in several other chapters of this book.

GENETICS OF MITOCHONDRIAL DISORDERS

Table 38.1 summarizes a simplified clinical and genetic classification of mitochondrial diseases. With rare exceptions, individuals inherit mitochondrial DNA (mtDNA) solely from their mothers. Therefore the mode of transmission of mtDNA follows maternal line inheritance. With rare exceptions, a mother carrying a mtDNA point mutation will pass it to all her sons and daughters, but only her daughters will transmit it further to their progeny. Each cell contains hundreds of mitochondria and thousands of mtDNA copies. Normally, all mtDNA molecules are identical (homoplasmy). However, pathogenic mtDNA mutations and normal (wild type) mtDNA can exist together (heteroplasmy), and in this way the lethal effect of mutant mtDNA may be partially rescued. Consequently, cells, tissues, and the whole individual harbor two populations (pathogenic and wild type) of the mtDNA. The degree of heteroplasmy varies in individual cells, tissues, and organ systems; the somatic load of mutant mtDNA can reach the clinical threshold in some tissues but not in others. The mtDNA mutation load needed for clinical expression is typically in the range of 70–90%. Tissues with high oxidative metabolism, such as brain, eye, myocardium, and skeletal muscle, are especially vulnerable.

Table 38.1: Major gene mutations in mitochondrial disorders

Defects of Mitochondrial DNA

Disease/Syndrome	Main Mutation	Gene Location	Mode of Inheritance
PEO/multisystem PEO		Single large deletion	Sporadic
		Deletion-duplication	Sporadic
	nt-A3243G	tRNA$^{Leu(UUR)}$	Maternal
	nt-C3256T	tRNA$^{Leu(UUR)}$	Maternal
KSS		Single large deletion	Sporadic
		Large tandem duplication	Sporadic
Pearson syndrome/KSS		Single large deletion	Sporadic
MELAS	nt-A3243G	tRNA$^{Leu(UUR)}$	Maternal
	nt-T3271C	tRNA$^{Leu(UUR)}$	Maternal
MERRF	nt-A8344G	tRNA^{Lys}	Maternal
Myopathy		Single large deletion	Sporadic
	nt-A3243G	tRNA$^{Leu(UUR)}$	Maternal
	nt-G15762A	Cytochrome b	Sporadic
	nt-C3254G	tRNA$^{Leu(UUR)}$	Maternal
MiMyCa	nt-T8993G	ATPase 6	Maternal
NARP/MILS	nt-G3460A	ND1	Maternal
LHON	nt-G11778A	ND5	Maternal
	nt-T14484C	ND6	Maternal
Diabetes, optic atrophy, deafness		Single large deletion	Sporadic
Tubulopathy, diabetes, ataxia		Large tandem duplication	Maternal
Sideroblastic anemia	nt-T6721C	COX	Sporadic

Defects in Nuclear DNA Affecting Mitochondrial DNA or Enzyme Complexes

Disease/Syndrome	mtDNA/Complex Defect	Nuclear Gene/locus	Mode of Inheritance
PEO	Multiple mtDNA deletions	Twinkle, ANT1, POLG	Autosomal dominant
MINGIE	Multiple mtDNA deletions	Thymidine phosphorylase	Autosomal recessive
Leigh's syndrome	Complex IV	SURF1	Autosomal recessive
	Complex I	NDUFS7,8	Autosomal recessive
Leukodystrophy/myoclonus	Complex I	NDUFV1	Autosomal recessive
Encephalopathy, tubulopathy	Complex IV	COX10	Autosomal recessive
Encephalopathy, hepatopathy	Complex IV	SCO1	Autosomal recessive
Encephalopathy/myocardiopathy	Complex IV	SCO2	Autosomal recessive
Encephalopathy, hepatopathy, myopathy	MtDNA depletion	unknown	Autosomal recessive?

Note: ANT1 (adenine nucleotide translocater), COX10 (cytochrome c oxidase), NUDFS and NUDFV (complex I components), POLG (DNA polymerase gamma), SCO1 and SCO2 (mitochondrial copper proteins), SURF (cytochrome c oxidase assembly protein), and Twinkle (mtDNA helicase) are nuclear DNA-encoded proteins that are required for mitochondrial biogenesis.

KSS = Kearns-Sayre syndrome; LHON = Leber's hereditary optic neuropathy; MELAS = mitochondrial encephalomyopathy, lactic acidosis, and strokelike episodes; MERRF = myoclonic epilepsy with ragged red fibers; MILS = maternally inherited Leigh's syndrome; MiMyCa = mitochondrial myopathy and cardiomyopathy; MINGIE = myoneurogastrointestinal encephalopathy; NARP = neuropathy, ataxia, and retinitis pigmentosa; PEO = progressive external ophthalmoplegia.

Source: Adapted from Servidei, S. 2003, "Mitochondrial encephalomyopathies: gene mutation," *Neuromusc Disord*, vol. 13, p. 109.

APPROACH TO THE DIAGNOSIS OF MITOCHONDRIAL DISORDERS

Clinical Findings

Clinical clues suggesting mitochondrial disease are: (1) maternal inheritance, (2) any combination of brain, heart, muscle, eye, ear, liver, and kidney involvement, (3) strokes in children or young adults, (4) the combination of neuropathy and myopathy, (5) severe fatigue with intercurrent illnesses, and (6) long-term regression of skills and functioning.

Laboratory Findings

The mitochondrial metabolic test battery includes blood creatine kinase, lactate and pyruvate, plasma carnitine, blood and urine amino acids, urine organic acids, and cerebrospinal fluid (CSF) lactate and pyruvate (if the central nervous system is involved). Urine metabolic screen provides limited information and is not useful in either supporting the diagnosis of or detecting multisystem problems in mitochondrial diseases.

Neuro-ophthalmology

The four most common neuro-ophthalmological abnormalities seen in mitochondrial disorders are bilateral optic neuropathy (Leber's hereditary optic neuropathy), external ophthalmoplegia, pigmentary retinopathy, and retrochiasmal visual loss.

Neuroradiology

Brain atrophy is common in children with mitochondrial disease; developmental delay and basal ganglia calcification are common in Kearns-Sayre syndrome (KSS) and mitochondrial, encephalopathy, lactic acidosis, and strokelike episodes (MELAS) syndrome; and diffuse signal abnormalities of the white matter is characteristic of KSS. The diagnosis of MELAS syndrome relies on radiographic observation of strokelike episodes. They are "strokelike" because they do not conform to the anatomical territories of blood vessels; cortical gray matter is involved and the signal changes may be evanescent and fleeting in character. The initial or predominant lesions in MELAS syndrome are characteristically in the posterior cerebral hemisphere, and new lesions generally appear with acute illness and elevated CSF lactate levels. Leigh's syndrome shows bilateral hyperintense signals on T2-weighted and fluid-attenuated inversion recovery magnetic resonance imaging scans in the putamen, globus pallidus, and thalamus.

Muscle Biopsy

The "ragged red fibers" (RRF) are the hallmark feature in muscle histopathology. In frozen sections stained with Gomori trichrome, subsarcolemmal and intermyofibrillar accumulation of mitochondria appears as bright red masses against the background of the blue myofibrils. RRFs only occur in affected muscle. Therefore absence of RRF does not rule out mitochondrial disease.

DNA-based Diagnosis

Many mtDNA and nDNA mutations are known to cause mitochondrial disorders and testing for all is impossible. The most common mutation associated with a specific syndrome can be tested (see Table 38.1).

For a more detailed discussion, see Chapter 69 in Neurology in Clinical Practice, 4th edition.

Channelopathies: Episodic and Electrical Disorders of the Nervous System

39

Channelopathies are disorders caused by inherited mutations in ion channels. Most channelopathies affect either muscle or the nervous system. Despite phenotypic heterogeneity, a striking feature is their association with paroxysmal dysfunction.

ION CHANNELS

Ion channels are transmembrane glycoprotein pores that underlie cell excitability by regulating ion flow into and out of cells. The channels are often composed of distinct proteins called *channel subunits*. Different genes encode each subunit. Two mutations within the same gene can result in different physiological defects. The concept that different mutations in the same gene can cause different phenotypes is termed *phenotypic heterogeneity*. For example, mutations in the same muscle sodium channel gene can result in hyperkalemic periodic paralysis, hypokalemic periodic paralysis (hypo-KPP), potassium-aggravated myotonia (PAM), or paramyotonia congenita. Genetic heterogeneity is when different genetic mutations result in the same disease phenotype. For example, different mutations in the skeletal muscle sodium channel cause the hyperkalemic periodic paralysis phenotype.

PERIODIC PARALYSIS AND NONDYSTROPHIC MYOTONIAS

The periodic paralyses and nondystrophic myotonias encompass several skeletal muscle disorders inherited as autosomal dominant traits. The general features of these disorders are episodic weakness or stiffness with interictal return to an asymptomatic state and responsiveness to acetazolamide.

Hypokalemic Periodic Paralysis   Na channel.

Clinical Features
The prevalence of hypo-KPP is 1:100,000. Onset is usually during adolescence. Episodes are characterized by generalized limb weakness and reduced or absent tendon reflexes associated with hypokalemia. Attacks usually occur in the morning and are often triggered either by the ingestion of a carbohydrate load and high salt intake or by rest following strenuous exercise. A feeling of heaviness or aching in the legs or back heralds an attack. Despite complete paralysis, consciousness and sensation are preserved. The need for medical intervention is rare because respiratory paralysis is mild. The frequency, length, and severity of attacks are variable. They may occur several times per week or at intervals of weeks or months. Attack duration can be minutes to days, but more often lasts several hours. Afterwards, strength is usually normal, although mild weakness may persist for several days. A progressive permanent myopathy may develop later in life. Reducing the number of prior attacks reduces or prevents the myopathy.

Diagnosis
An accurate medical history is essential for the diagnosis. Observed attacks are rare and patients are normal in between. Characteristics of hypo-KPP that distinguish it from hyper-KPP are paralytic attacks that are less frequent, longer-lasting, precipitated by a carbohydrate load, and occur during sleep. Potassium concentrations are usually low during an attack, although concentrations less than 2 mM should suggest a secondary form of periodic paralysis. Electrocardiogram (ECG) changes that suggest an underlying hypokalemia are increased PR and QT intervals, T-wave flattening, and prominent U waves.

Excluding secondary forms of hypokalemic paralysis is essential when serum potassium concentrations remain low between attacks. Renal, adrenal, and gastrointestinal causes of persistent hypokalemia are common causes of hypo-KPP. Other considerations are thiazide diuretic use and thyrotoxic hypo-KPP.

Treatment
Lifestyle modification includes dietary modification to avoid high carbohydrate loads and refraining from excessive exertion. Oral potassium (5–10 g load) reverses paralysis during an acute attack. Prophylactic use of acetazolamide decreases the

frequency and severity of attacks. Dichlorphenamide, a stronger carbonic-anhydrase inhibitor than acetazolamide, prevents attacks at an average dose of 100 mg a day. Reducing the frequency of paralytic attacks may provide protection against the development of myopathy.

Hyperkalemic Periodic Paralysis

Clinical Features
Episodic weakness precipitated by hyperkalemia characterizes hyperkalemic periodic paralysis (hyper-KPP). The weakness is generally milder than in hypo-KPP, and it can be sufficiently severe to cause flaccid quadriparesis. During an attack, respiratory and ocular muscles are unaffected and consciousness is preserved. Frequency of attacks varies from several per day to several per year. Attacks are usually brief, lasting 15–60 minutes. Serum potassium concentrations are usually normal during an attack, but hyperkalemia provokes attacks. Unlike hypo-KPP, myotonia is present between attacks. Onset is usually in infancy or childhood, and characteristic attacks occur by adolescence. Rest after vigorous exercise, foods high in potassium, stress, and fatigue precipitate an attack. In most patients, onset is subacute, and before attacks some describe paresthesias or a sensation of muscle tension. Mild exercise may abort or lessen the severity of the attack. Mild weakness may persist after the attack, and the later development of a progressive myopathy is common.

Diagnosis
A thorough medical and family history and physical examination are the best diagnostic tools. Genetic testing is not generally available. Serum potassium level is normal between attacks and even during many attacks. In the absence of provocative testing by potassium administration, the clinical features are the basis for the diagnosis. Between attacks, either spontaneous or percussion myotonia is common. Failure to produce myotonia or weakness with cooling discriminates hyper-KPP from hypo-KPP. Peaked T waves on ECG suggest hyperkalemia.

Treatment
Acute attacks are often sufficiently brief and mild so that acute intervention is not required. A diet of low potassium and high carbohydrate decreases attack frequency. Some patients can abort attacks with mild exercise or by eating a high sugar load (juice or a candy bar). Acute treatment consists of lowering extracellular potassium levels with thiazide diuretics and inhaled β-adrenergic agonists. Intravenous calcium gluconate may be useful when weakness is very severe. Oral dichlorphenamide,

acetazolamide (125–1500 mg a day), and thiazide diuretics are used as prophylactic agents. Reducing attack frequency does not clearly prevent the later onset of myopathy.

Paramyotonia Congenita   Na chamel.

Clinical Features

Paradoxic myotonia, cold-induced myotonia, and weakness after prolonged cold exposure are the characteristic features of paramyotonia congenita. Unlike classic myotonia in which repeated muscle contractions reduce myotonia, in paramyotonia congenita repeated muscle contraction often exacerbates myotonia. Symptoms are present at birth and usually remain unchanged throughout life. The predominant muscles affected are those of the face, neck, and hand muscles, with particular susceptibility of the orbicularis oris. The onset of weakness is often during the day, lasting several hours, and exacerbated by cold, stress, and rest after exercise. Many patients are asymptomatic when warm. However, cold-induced stiffness and percussion myotonia in the thenar eminence and tongue may persist for hours after warming the body.

Diagnosis

A family history of exercise and cold-induced myotonia strongly supports the diagnosis. Serum potassium concentration may be high, low, or normal during attacks, and serum creatine kinase concentrations may be elevated 5–10 times the normal concentration. Repeated forceful eye closures cause progressive difficulty with relaxation and eventual inability to open the eyes. Electromyography (EMG) reveals fibrillation-like potentials and myotonic discharges accentuated by muscle percussion, needle movement, and muscle cooling.

Treatment

Symptoms are generally mild and infrequent. Treatment, when required, is directed at either myotonia, weakness, or both. Sodium channel blockers, such as mexiletine, are effective in some patients to reduce the frequency and severity of myotonia. Patients with weakness often respond to thiazides and acetazolamide. Cold avoidance reduces the frequency of attacks.

Myotonia Congenita   Cl⁻ channel.

Clinical Features

Myotonia congenita can be inherited as either an autosomal dominant trait (Thomsen's disease) or an autosomal recessive trait (Becker's myotonia). The main feature is myotonia—bouts of delayed muscle relaxation after contraction. Initiating abrupt, forceful movement after several minutes of rest causes the most pronounced myotonic stiffness. The myotonia displays a warm-up phenomenon, where the myotonia decreases or vanishes completely when the same movement is repeated several times. The clinical onset is often within the first decade. The myotonia is more prominent in the legs than all other muscles. Occasionally, myotonia is severe enough to impede a patient's ability to walk or run. In rare cases, sudden noise causes sufficient generalized stiffness to make the patient fall to the ground and remain rigid for several seconds. Some clinical features help distinguish the recessive and dominant forms. In general, patients with Becker's myotonia experience transitory bouts of weakness after periods of disuse, progressive myopathy and muscle hypertrophy may develop, and disease severity is greater. The recessive form is more common than the dominant form.

Diagnosis
Tapping the belly of a muscle with a percussion hammer can elicit myotonia that lasts for several seconds. Cardiac abnormalities, cataracts, skeletal deformities, and glucose intolerance are not components of myotonia congenita, and their presence should suggest one of the dystrophic myotonias. Muscle strength and tendon reflexes are normal, but patients commonly display muscle hypertrophy, often giving these patients an athletic appearance. Paramyotonia congenita is distinguished from myotonia congenita by the EMG finding of decremental compound muscle action potentials with muscle cooling. EMG with myotonia congenita typically reveals bursts of repetitive action potentials with amplitude (10 µV to 1 mV) and frequency (50–150 Hz) modulation, so-called *dive bombers* in the EMG loudspeaker.

Treatment
Sodium channel blocking agents (mexiletine) are the mainstay of treatment for those with severe myotonia. Other sodium channel blockers such as tocainide, phenytoin, procainamide, and quinine are also used.

Potassium-Aggravated Myotonia

Clinical Features
Potassium-aggravated myotonia is a rare autosomal dominant disorder. Clinical features are similar to those of myotonia congenita, except that myotonia fluctuates and is exacerbated with potassium administration. Episodic weakness and progressive myopathy do not occur. Symptom severity varies; some

experience only mild fluctuating stiffness and others a more protracted painful myotonia. PAM now encompasses the conditions previously known as *myotonia fluctuans, myotonia permanens*, and *acetazolamide-sensitive myotonia*. Exercise or rest after exercise, potassium loads, and depolarizing neuro-muscular blocking agents aggravate myotonia, whereas cold exposure has no effect. Prominent myotonia of the orbicularis oculi and painful myotonia suggest the diagnosis.

Diagnosis
The clinical features are the basis of diagnosis. Distinguishing PAM from other episodic nondystrophic myotonias can be difficult. Unlike patients with hyper-KPP and paramyotonia congenita, those with PAM do not experience weakness. The lack of muscle response to cooling further distinguishes PAM from paramyotonia congenita.

Treatment
Carbonic anhydrase inhibitors markedly reduce the severity and frequency of attacks of myotonia. Acetazolamide, starting at doses of 125 mg and titrating up to as much as 1.5 g per day (titrated to patient response), is most commonly used.

Andersen's/Tawil Syndrome

Clinical Features   K CNJ2 mutation
Andersen's/Tawil syndrome (ATS) is a rare autosomal dominant disorder characterized by periodic paralysis, cardiac arrhyth-mias, and dysmorphic features (hypertelorism, micrognathia, low-set ears, high-arched or cleft palate, short stature, and clinodactyly). The periodic paralysis can be hypokalemic, nor-mokalemic, or hyperkalemic. The cardiac phenotype usually includes prolonged QT intervals, but bidirectional ventricular tachycardia is also common. Phenotypic expressivity is extremely variable. Only one or two features of the syndrome may be present and the severity of any one feature is extremely variable. Rare individuals are asymptomatic disease-gene carriers.

Diagnosis
Meeting two of the following three criteria classifies an indi-vidual as affected: paroxysmal weakness, prolonged corrected QT interval with or without ventricular dysrhythmias, or characteristic dysmorphic features. ATS should be included in the differential diagnosis of any individual with documented long QT syndrome, even in the absence of periodic paralysis or dysmorphism. All patients with suspected periodic paralysis

require an ECG study for careful measurement of the corrected QT interval.

Serum creatine kinase concentrations are often normal during episodes of weakness. Potassium concentrations during an attack are inconsistent and usually abnormally low. Avoid hypokalemic challenges in patients with ATS because hypokalemia may exacerbate pre-existing QT prolongation and potentially cause life-threatening ventricular arrhythmias.

Treatment

The direction of treatment is to control underlying cardiac arrhythmias while decreasing the frequency, severity, and duration of attacks of weakness. This may be difficult, because some treatments for arrhythmias can produce weakness and treatments for weakness may exacerbate cardiac dysrhythmias. The treatment of acute attacks is with oral potassium. Prophylaxis with daily sustained-release potassium tablets may prevent attacks of weakness. Maintaining a high serum potassium level (> 4.5 mEq/liter) also has the additional advantage of narrowing the QT interval, thereby reducing the likelihood of developing ventricular arrhythmias.

Treating the arrhythmias of ATS may be difficult because of the lack of response to antiarrhythmic agents, some of which may exacerbate muscle weakness. Treating the underlying prolonged QT interval is the primary aim of therapy. Beta blockers are one of the mainstays of treatment in long QT syndrome, and patients with ATS tolerate them well. Patients with sustained ventricular tachycardia benefit from placement of an implantable defibrillator.

MALIGNANT HYPERTHERMIA

Malignant hyperthermia is a relatively uncommon syndrome characterized by a hypermetabolic reaction to volatile anesthetics and depolarizing neuromuscular blocking agents. Inheritance is usually autosomal dominant. Also observed is a multifactorial inheritance pattern. A further complication in defining inheritance and incidence is that many people with malignant hyperthermia do not develop symptoms on all exposures, and some are never exposed.

Clinical Features

Tachypnea, tachycardia, acidosis, rhabdomyolysis, and hyperthermia rapidly develop with exposure to several anesthetic agents. Unfortunately, establishing the diagnosis rarely occurs before the onset of symptoms.

Diagnosis

The caffeine-contracture test remains the best available test for diagnosis. This test involves exposing a thin strip of muscle to caffeine after electrical stimulation to achieve maximal contraction. Explanted muscle from patients with malignant hyperthermia has an increased contracture to caffeine exposure. The test is useful but not perfect; results are dependent on who is performing the test.

Treatment

Dantrolene sodium, an inhibitor of calcium release from the sarcoplasmic reticulum, is the mainstay of treatment. Its use has significantly reduced operative mortality.

CONGENITAL MYASTHENIC SYNDROMES

The congenital myasthenic syndromes are a rare, heterogeneous, nonimmune group of disorders of neuromuscular transmission. Details of these disorders are in Chapter 53.

FEM 3 Na+channel, FHM1 } (CaV2·1
EA2
SCA6

FAMILIAL HEMIPLEGIC MIGRAINE

Familial hemiplegic migraine (FHM) is a genetically heterogeneous condition linked to two loci, chromosome 1q and 19p. Genetic transmission is by autosomal dominant trait inheritance.

Clinical Features

Symptoms include both typical migraine and motor weakness of variable intensity associated with typical aura symptoms. Attacks generally follow a progression of symptoms: visual, followed by sensory, aphasic, motor, and brainstem dysfunction (dysarthria, vertigo, diplopia, decreased hearing, and tinnitus). Episodes can last several days to weeks. Fever, meningismus, and impairments of consciousness, ranging from confusion to coma, may be associated. Recovery between attacks is usually complete, but some patients display interictal nystagmus.

Diagnosis

Genetic testing for the underlying mutation is not widely available and the diagnosis relies on recognizing the clinical features. Clinical elements of FHM that help to distinguish it from migraine with aura are the longer duration of headache and the prominent association of neurological symptoms.

Treatment

Anecdotal evidence suggests that acetazolamide reduces the frequency of migraine attacks, but a multicenter double-blind randomized trial failed to prove efficacy.

FAMILIAL EPISODIC ATAXIAS

The familial episodic ataxias (EAs) are rare dominantly inherited diseases characterized by episodes of ataxia with onset in childhood, with complete resolution between attacks. Two distinct forms exist: EA type 1 (EA-1) and EA type 2 (EA-2).

Clinical Features

The characteristic features of EA-1 are attacks of cerebellar ataxia, jerking limb movements, and slurred speech that last for seconds to minutes. The episodes can occur spontaneously, but exertion, infection, stress, and startle are common triggers. Between attacks, patients may show myokymia (muscle rippling) resulting from motor nerve hyperexcitability, especially in the hands and around the eyes. Symptom onset is in infancy with spontaneous resolution in the second to third decade. Frequency, duration, and intensity of attacks vary greatly among affected patients.

Patients with EA-2 experience episodes of truncal ataxia that last for hours to days. Exertion and stress precipitate attacks. Age at onset varies between childhood and young adult life, but most present in the second decade. Vertigo, nausea, and vomiting are present in more than half of patients. Many exhibit spontaneous nystagmus during attacks but not afterwards. The patient is normal between episodes but frequently displays gaze-evoked rebound nystagmus. A coarse, spontaneous downbeat nystagmus develops late in the disease. Approximately half of patients with EA-2 report headaches that meet criteria for migraine. These patients have a mutation in the same gene implicated in familial hemiplegic migraine.

EA-3 is a similar disorder, described in two separate families. The presence of gaze-evoked nystagmus, a deficit in smooth pursuits, and lack of response to acetazolamide distinguish EA-3 from EA-1 and EA-2. Another distinct clinical entity, EA-4, is characterized by episodes of generalized ataxia, vertigo, imbalance, and tinnitus. Neither EA-3 nor EA-4 has an identified gene locus.

Diagnosis

Family history is the most useful factor in diagnosis. Careful examination for interictal signs, described previously, is also helpful.

Treatment

Acetazolamide reduces the severity of attacks. In general, patients with EA-2 show a greater response than patients with EA-1. An initial dose of 125 mg is later titrated to an average effective dose of 500–750 mg a day.

HEREDITARY HYPEREKPLEXIA *glycine*

Clinical Features

Human startle disease, or hereditary hyperekplexia, is a rare hereditary disease characterized by an exaggerated startle reflex. Although usually inherited in an autosomal dominant manner, several recessive mutations have been identified. The normal startle response is a primitive reflex (the Moro reflex) characterized by a stereotyped sequence of blinking, grimacing, neck flexion, and arm abduction and flexion. In patients with hyperekplexia, an overreaction occurs to unexpected sensory stimuli, with sudden generalized myoclonic jerks followed by stiffness. The stiffness often results in uncontrolled falling during standing and walking. Patients often develop a characteristic slow, wide-based cautious gait. Preservation of consciousness during attacks helps distinguish this from startle epilepsy. Attack frequency may increase during times of stress, fear, lack of sleep, or the expectation of being frightened. Onset of symptoms may be as early as the neonatal period, with rigidity or generalized hypertonia, nocturnal limb jerking, and an exaggerated startle response. Attacks vary in severity and frequency but may be so severe to cause apneic episodes and even death. A slight delay in motor development may occur in affected children. Physical examination usually reveals diffuse hyperreflexia. The diffuse hypertonicity of infancy resolves with time, and adults have normal tone between attacks.

Diagnosis

Tapping on the forehead may elicit an exaggerated head-retraction reflex. Tapping the root of the nose downward with a reflex hammer elicits a brisk involuntary backward jerk of the head. This reflex is generally absent in nonaffected individuals.

Treatment

Treatment with benzodiazepines helps reduce neonatal hypertonia and significantly reduces the severity and frequency of startle-induced attacks in some patients.

For a more detailed discussion, see Chapter 70 in Neurology in Clinical Practice, 4th edition.

Neurocutaneous Syndromes

40

Neurocutaneous syndromes are disorders with lesions in both the nervous system and the skin (*phakomatosis*). These disorders may be inherited or sporadic.

TUBEROUS SCLEROSIS

Tuberous sclerosis complex (TSC) is a disorder of cellular differentiation and proliferation that can affect the brain, skin, kidneys, heart, and other organs. Many of the clinical features of TSC result from hamartomas; true neoplasms also occur, particularly in the kidney and brain. Abnormal neuronal migration plays a major additional role in neurological dysfunction.

Genetics

Transmission of TSC is as an autosomal dominant trait with variable penetrance. The spontaneous mutation rate varies from 66% to 86%. Two genes are responsible for TSC. One gene (*TSC1*) is located at chromosome 9q34, and the other (*TSC2*) is adjacent to the gene for adult polycystic kidney disease at chromosome 16p13.3. No obvious phenotypic differences exist between *TSC1* and *TSC2*. The gene product of *TSC1* is tuberin. *TSC1* probably accounts for familial cases and is generally less severe.

Population-based studies suggest a prevalence of 1 per 6000–9000 individuals. However, because of the striking variability of clinical expression and severity, the diagnosis of TSC can be difficult in individuals with subtle findings, and the true prevalence may be considerably higher. Cutaneous findings are usually the first clue that a patient has TSC, but other features may lead to the diagnosis. Table 40.1 lists the current revised criteria for TSC.

Cutaneous Features
Hypomelanotic macules (*ash leaf spots*), found in up to 90% of patients, are present at birth but are difficult to see in newborns without an ultraviolet light. Other pigmentary abnormalities include confetti lesions (an area with stippled hypopigmentation, typically on the extremities) and poliosis (a white patch or forelock) of the scalp hair or eyelids. Facial angiofibromas (*adenoma sebaceum*), made up of vascular and connective tissue elements, become apparent before age 5 years as small red papules on the malar region. They gradually become larger and more numerous, sometimes extending down the nasolabial folds or onto the chin. The *shagreen patch* is most often found on the back or flank area; it is an irregularly shaped, slightly raised, or textured skin lesion. *Ungual fibromas*, nodular or fleshy lesions that arise adjacent to or underneath the nails, are specific for TSC.

Neurological Features
Mental retardation, seizures, and behavioral abnormalities are the main features. Seizures occur in almost 90% of patients. Most mentally retarded patients have epilepsy. Some with epilepsy are not retarded. Patients who have numerous lesions of the cerebral cortex shown by magnetic resonance imaging (MRI) tend to have more cognitive impairment and more difficulty with seizure control. Computed tomography (CT) best demonstrates the calcified subependymal nodules that characterize TSC. Children with infantile spasms have more cortical lesions and are more likely to exhibit long-term cognitive impairment. Subependymal giant cell astrocytomas (SEGAs) develop in 10% of patients. They enlarge and cause focal neurological deficits and increased intracranial pressure. Contrast enhancement on either CT or MRI helps distinguish a SEGA from the other cerebral lesions seen with TSC.

Retinal Features
Retinal hamartomas are difficult to identify without pupillary dilation and indirect ophthalmoscopy. Retinal lesions vary from the classic mulberry lesions adjacent to the optic disc to the plaquelike hamartoma or depigmented retinal lesions.

Systemic Features
Approximately two thirds of patients have a cardiac rhabdomyoma. Some children later develop cardiac arrhythmias or cerebral thromboembolism from the rhabdomyomas. Causes of

Table 40.1: Revised diagnostic criteria for tuberous sclerosis complex

Major features
1. Facial angiofibromas or forehead plaque
2. Nontraumatic ungual or periungual fibroma
3. Hypomelanotic macules (more than three)
4. Shagreen patch (connective tissue nevus)
5. Multiple retinal nodular hamartomas
6. Cortical tuber*
7. Subependymal nodule
8. Subependymal giant cell astrocytoma
9. Cardiac rhabdomyoma, single or multiple
10. Lymphangiomyomatosis[†]
11. Renal angiomyolipoma[†]

Minor features
1. Multiple randomly distributed pits in dental enamel
2. Hamartomatous rectal polyps[‡]
3. Bone cysts[§]
4. Cerebral white-matter radial migration lines*,[§,‖]
5. Gingival fibromas
6. Nonrenal hamartoma[‡]
7. Retinal achromic patch
8. Confetti skin lesions
9. Multiple renal cysts[‡]

Definite tuberous sclerosis complex: either two major features or one major feature plus two minor features

Probable tuberous sclerosis complex: one major plus one minor feature

Possible tuberous sclerosis complex: either one major feature or two or more minor features

---

*When cerebral cortical dysplasia and cerebral white-matter migration tracts occur together, they should be counted as one rather than two features of tuberous sclerosis.

[†]When both lymphangiomyomatosis and renal angiomyolipomas are present, other features of tuberous sclerosis should be present before a definite diagnosis is assigned.

[‡]Histological confirmation is suggested.

[§]Radiographical confirmation is sufficient.

[‖]One panel member felt strongly that three or more radial migration lines should constitute a major sign.

Source: Reprinted with permission from Roach, E. S., Gomez, M. R., & Northrup, H. 1998, "Tuberous sclerosis consensus conference: revised clinical diagnostic criteria," *J Child Neurol*, vol. 13, pp. 624-628.

congestive heart failure are obstruction of blood flow by intraluminal tumor or lack of sufficient normal myocardium to maintain perfusion. Renal angiomyolipomas occur in up to three fourths of patients. Single or multiple renal cysts are a common feature.

NEUROFIBROMATOSIS

Neurofibromatosis (NF) includes two separate diseases, each caused by a different gene: NF type 1 (NF1) or *von Recklinghausen's disease* is the most common neurocutaneous syndrome (1 in 3000 people). One half of NF1 cases result from a spontaneous mutation. NF type 2 (NF2) is characterized by bilateral vestibular schwannomas and is often associated with other brain or spinal cord tumors. NF2 occurs in only 1 in 50,000 people.

Molecular Biology

The cause of NF1 is a mutation of exon-60 of the *NF1* gene on chromosome 17q. The *NF1* gene product, *neurofibromin*, is partially homologous to guanosine triphosphatase (GTPase)–activating protein. Somatic NF1 mutations are associated with signs of NF in only a limited region of the body. Individuals with gonadal mosaicism have no outward features of NF1 but have multiple affected offspring.

The cause of NF2 is a mutation of the *NF2* gene on chromosome 22. The NF2 protein product is *schwannomin*. The *NF2* gene suppresses tumor function, and its dysfunction accounts for the common occurrence of central nervous system (CNS) neoplasms.

Cutaneous Features of Neurofibromatosis Type 1

Cutaneous lesions of NF1 include café au lait spots, subcutaneous neurofibromas, plexiform neurofibromas, and axillary freckling. Café au lait spots are flat, light to medium brown areas that vary in shape and size. They are typically present at birth but increase in size and number during the first few years. Neurofibromas are benign tumors arising from peripheral nerves. Neurofibromas can develop at any time; the size and number often increase after puberty.

Systemic Features of Neurofibromatosis Type 1

Lisch nodules are pigmented iris hamartomas that are pathognomonic for NF1. They are often not apparent during early childhood. Dysplasia of the renal or carotid arteries occurs in a small percentage of patients with NF1. Dysplasia of the renal or carotid arteries and pheochromocytoma occur in a small percentage of patients with NF1.

Neurological Features in Neurofibromatosis Type 1

The neurological features of NF1 vary even among affected members of the same family. Tumors occur in the brain, spinal cord, and peripheral nerves, although not as frequently as with NF2. Optic nerve glioma is the most common CNS tumor caused by NF1. Precocious puberty is a common presenting sign of optic nerve tumors. Approximately three fourths of patients with NF1 have increased signal lesions within the basal ganglia, thalamus, brainstem, and cerebellum on T2-weighted MRI. Their origin and significance are unclear. Full-scale intelligence quotient (IQ) scores are within the low normal range, but 40% have a learning disability or behavioral problem.

Clinical Features of Neurofibromatosis Type 2

In addition to bilateral vestibular schwannomas, patients with NF2 have multiple tumors of the CNS and few cutaneous lesions. Café au lait spots are uncommon.

Diagnostic Criteria for Neurofibromatosis

Table 40.2 lists the diagnostic criteria for NF. Screening for the *NF1* gene is technically difficult because the gene is large and several mutations exist. Commercially available studies have a 30% false-negative rate.

EHLERS-DANLOS SYNDROME

The clinical features, inheritance pattern, and specific molecular defects define several subtypes of Ehlers-Danlos syndrome. More than 80% of patients have type I, II, or III. Together these syndromes are characterized by fragile or hyperelastic skin, hyperextensible joints, vascular lesions, easy bruising, and excessive scarring after injuries. Aneurysm and arterial dissection are the most serious threats to the nervous system. Most aneurysms become symptomatic in early adult life. The most common intracranial vessel to develop an aneurysm is the internal carotid artery, typically in the cavernous sinus or just after it emerges from the sinus. Rupture of the aneurysm within the cavernous sinus often creates a carotid-cavernous fistula.

Table 40.2: Diagnostic criteria for neurofibromatosis

Neurofibromatosis type 1 (any two or more)
Six or more café au lait lesions more than 5 mm in diameter before
  puberty and more than 15 mm in diameter afterward
Freckling in the axillary or inguinal areas
Optic glioma
Two or more neurofibromas or one plexiform neurofibroma
A first-degree relative with neurofibromatosis type 1
Two or more Lisch nodules
A characteristic bony lesion (sphenoid dysplasia, thinning of the
  cortex of long bones, with or without pseudarthrosis)

Neurofibromatosis type 2
Bilateral VIII nerve tumor (shown by magnetic resonance imaging,
  computed tomography, or histological confirmation)
A first-degree relative with neurofibromatosis type 2 and a unilateral
  eighth nerve tumor
A first-degree relative with neurofibromatosis type 2 and any two of
  the following lesions: neurofibroma, meningioma, schwannoma,
  glioma, or juvenile posterior subcapsular lenticular opacity

Source: Data from Neurofibromatosis. Conference statement. 1988, National
Institutes of Health Consensus Development Conference. *Arch Neurol*,
vol. 45, pp. 575-578.

Arterial dissection can occur in intracranial or extracranial
arteries. The clinical presentation depends primarily on which
artery is affected. Surgery is difficult because the arteries are
friable and difficult to suture, and handling the tissue leads to
tears of the artery or separation of the arterial layers.

OSLER-WEBER-RENDU SYNDROME

Hereditary hemorrhagic telangiectasia (HHT), also known as
Osler-Weber-Rendu syndrome, is an autosomal dominant
disorder characterized by telangiectasias of the skin, mucous
membranes, and various internal organs. One gene is located at
chromosome 9q33-34 (*HHT1*), which encodes for endoglin, a
transforming growth factor-β (TGF-β) binding protein. The
other gene is located at chromosome 12q13 (*HHT2*), which
encodes for activin receptor–like kinase. Up to 30% of cases
arise from spontaneous mutations. Neurological features include
headache, dizziness, and seizures. Less common complications
are paradoxical embolism with stroke, intraparenchymal or
subarachnoid hemorrhage, and meningitis or cerebral abscess.

Many of the neurological complications arise because of a pulmonary arteriovenous fistula. Fistula resection or occlusion is the recommended treatment.

FABRY'S DISEASE

Deficiency of α-galactosidase-A causes Fabry's disease. Transmission is by X-linked inheritance. Enzyme analysis in cultured leukocytes or fibroblasts confirms the diagnosis. Patients will develop dark red or purple papules that tend to occur in clusters around the umbilicus or on the buttocks, scrotum, hips, or thighs. The size and number of the cutaneous lesions gradually increase with age, although the lesions themselves are asymptomatic.

The onset of temperature-sensitive painful dysesthesias of the distal limbs is in the first decade. Pain predates the appearance of the characteristic cutaneous lesions. Both cerebral thrombosis and hemorrhage occur, although thrombosis is more common. Brain hemorrhage can occur even without systemic hypertension from renal failure. Most patients with cerebrovascular complications are in their third or fourth decade. Cerebral hemispheric lesions are more common than brainstem lesions. The painful dysesthesias result from a sensory neuropathy. A completely effective treatment is not available. Carbamazepine or phenytoin may offer symptomatic relief from the painful paresthesias but do not reduce the vascular complications. Bone marrow transplantation is a potentially useful treatment.

STURGE-WEBER SYNDROME

Sturge-Weber syndrome (SWS) is characterized by a facial cutaneous angioma (port-wine nevus) associated with leptomeningeal and brain angioma, usually ipsilateral to the facial lesion. Other features include mental retardation, contralateral hemiparesis and hemiatrophy, and homonymous hemianopia. The syndrome occurs sporadically and in all races.

Cutaneous Features

The nevus usually involves the forehead and upper eyelid but may affect both sides of the face and extend onto the trunk and extremities. The facial angioma is usually obvious at birth. Occasional patients have the characteristic intracranial angioma and no skin lesion. Only 10–20% of children with a port-wine nevus of the forehead have a leptomeningeal angioma. Bilateral brain lesions occur in at least 15% of patients, including some with a unilateral cutaneous nevus.

Ocular Features

Glaucoma is the main ophthalmological problem. The risk of developing glaucoma is highest in the first decade. Untreated glaucoma causes progressive blindness.

Neurological Features

Epileptic seizures, mental retardation, and focal neurological deficits are the principal neurological abnormalities of SWS. Seizures usually start in conjunction with hemiparesis. Onset of seizures before 2 years of age increases the likelihood of future mental retardation and refractory epilepsy. Seizures eventually develop in 72–80% of patients with unilateral lesions and in 93% with bihemispheric involvement. The first few seizures are often focal even in those who later develop generalized tonic-clonic seizures or infantile spasms.

The neurological impairment caused by SWS depends in part on the site of the intracranial vascular lesion. Because the occipital region is frequently involved, visual field deficits are common. Hemiparesis often develops acutely, in conjunction with the initial flurry of seizures and may be permanent. Early developmental milestones are usually normal, but mild to profound mental deficiency eventually develops in approximately one half of patients. Only 8% of the patients with bilateral brain involvement are intellectually normal.

Diagnostic Studies

Neuroimaging studies distinguish children with SWS from those with isolated cutaneous lesions. MRI with gadolinium contrast demonstrates the abnormal intracranial vessels and is best to determine intracranial involvement.

Treatment

The more extensive the intracranial lesion, the more difficult it is to fully control seizures with medication. Hemispherectomy sometimes improves seizure control and promotes normal intellectual development and is the treatment of choice when intractable seizures begin in infancy. Otherwise, hemispherectomy is best for patients with clinically significant seizures who fail to respond to an adequate trial of anticonvulsants. Corpus callosotomy is used for patients with refractory tonic or atonic seizures.

PROGRESSIVE FACIAL HEMIATROPHY

Progressive facial hemiatrophy (*Parry-Romberg syndrome*) occurs sporadically. The relationship of this disorder to *en coup de sabre*, morphea, and linear scleroderma is uncertain. Progressive facial hemiatrophy involves mainly the upper face, whereas *en coup de sabre* tends to affect the lower face as well. Scleroderma and morphea affect other parts of the body. As a rule, only patients whose upper face and head are affected are likely to develop cerebral complications.

Clinical Features

Unilateral atrophy of the skin, subcutaneous tissue, and adjacent bone characterizes the disorder. The atrophic area is characteristically oblong or linear and sometimes begins as a raised erythematous lesion. The lesion may begin after trauma to the area. The atrophy eventually stabilizes, leaving the patient disfigured. Epilepsy is the most common neurological problem and many patients develop a mild hemiparesis.

ATAXIA-TELANGIECTASIA

Ataxia-telangiectasia (AT) is a neurodegenerative disorder transmitted as an autosomal recessive disorder affecting both genders. The gene associated with AT (*ATM*) is a large gene located at chromosome 11q22-23. More than 100 *ATM* mutations occurring in patients with AT have been discovered.

Cutaneous Features

Telangiectases typically develop between the ages of 3 and 6 years. The skin findings of AT are distinctive telangiectases most prominently involving the sclerae, earlobes, and bridge of the nose. Less common sites of telangiectases include the eyelids, neck, and antecubital and popliteal fossae. The occurrence of these telangiectases in a child with progressive ataxia is pathognomonic. Two other dermatological features of AT that may be overlooked are hypertrichosis and occasional gray hairs.

Neurological Features

Ataxia is usually the first manifestation of AT, appearing around 12 months. Truncal ataxia predominates, so sitting balance and gait are primarily affected. Muscle strength is normal and attainment of early motor milestones is normal. The ataxia is slowly progressive, and a wheelchair is required by age 12 years. Choreoathetosis, rather than ataxia, may dominate the clinical picture in older children. Abnormal eye movements are nearly universal in children with AT. Voluntary ocular motility is impaired; nystagmus, apraxia of voluntary gaze, and limitation of upgaze are the most common abnormalities.

The neurological features in adult patients include progressive distal muscular atrophy and fasciculations, with relative preservation of proximal strength. The gradual loss of vibration and position sense indicates involvement of the spinal cord dorsal columns and a peripheral polyneuropathy.

Immunological Features

The most striking non-neurological feature of AT is an increased frequency of sinopulmonary infections and a dramatically increased risk for malignancy of the lymphoreticular system, especially leukemia and lymphoma. Approximately 10–15% of patients with AT develop a lymphoid malignancy by early adulthood.

Laboratory Diagnosis

Nearly all patients with AT have an elevated α-fetoprotein level and approximately 80% have decreased serum immunoglobulin A (IgA), IgE, or IgG. Especially characteristic is a selective deficiency of the IgG2 subclass.

KINKY HAIR SYNDROME

Kinky hair syndrome, also known as *Menkes' disease* or *tricho-poliodystrophy*, is an X-linked disorder of connective tissue and neuronal metabolism caused by inborn disorders of copper metabolism.

Cutaneous Features

Connective tissue abnormalities are a major feature, leading to symptoms such as loose skin, hyperextensible joints, bladder diverticula, and skeletal anomalies. The hair is light colored and brittle on microscopic examination.

Neurological Features

In early onset cases, infants are normal at birth except for temperature instability. Within a few weeks or months, affected infants become hypotonic, and poor feeding may lead to failure to thrive. Infants are unusually susceptible to sepsis and often intolerant of heat. Chronic diarrhea is common. Hypotonia gradually develops into spastic quadriparesis with clenched fists, opisthotonus, and scissoring. Seizures are a prominent feature.

Neuroimaging

Cranial MRI and CT studies show diffuse cerebral atrophy with secondary subdural fluid collections, which may be large enough to cause mild compression of the ventricular system. In older children, MRI studies typically reveal diffuse white matter signal abnormalities suggestive of demyelination and gliosis, whereas in infants the white matter may be only focally affected.

Treatment

Restoring copper to normal levels in brain and other tissues is the focus of treatment. Aggressive copper replacement beginning in early infancy may be necessary to improve neurological outcome.

CEREBROTENDINOUS XANTHOMATOSIS

Cerebrotendinous xanthomatosis (CTX) is an autosomal recessive disorder characterized by tendon xanthomas, cataracts, and progressive neurological deterioration. Deposits of cholesterol and cholestanol are found in virtually every tissue, particularly the Achilles' tendons, brain, and lungs.

Neurological Features

Personality changes and decline in school performance may be the earliest neurological manifestations of this syndrome. Progressive loss of cognitive function typically begins in childhood. Ataxia with gait disturbance, dysmetria, nystagmus, and dysarthria is common. Psychosis with auditory hallucinations, paranoid ideation, and catatonia may occur. Cranial MRIs typically show cerebral and cerebellar atrophy and diffuse abnormal signal of the cerebral white matter, presumably reflecting sterol infiltration with demyelination. Focal lesions of the cerebral white matter and globus pallidus are sometimes demonstrable on MRI. Peripheral neuropathy is a prominent feature of CTX, as evidenced by pes cavus deformities, loss of deep tendon reflexes, and loss of vibration perception.

Xanthomas

Achilles' tendon is the most common site of tendon xanthomas, but quadriceps, triceps, and finger extensor tendons can be involved. Tendon xanthomas usually appear after the age of 10 years but occasionally occur in the first decade of life.

Treatment

Treatment of CTX focuses on lowering cholestanol levels, primarily with chenodeoxycholic acid and other lipid-lowering agents. Long-term treatment with chenodeoxycholic acid can lead to striking improvement in neurological function, resolution of peripheral and intracranial xanthomas, and improvement of electroencephalogram (EEG) and peripheral nerve conduction abnormalities and visual and somatosensory evoked potentials.

EPIDERMAL NEVUS SYNDROME

The term *epidermal nevus syndrome* (ENS) refers to various disorders that have in common an epidermal nevus and neurological manifestations such as seizures or hemimeganencephaly.

Cutaneous Features

Epidermal nevi are linear or patchy, slightly raised lesions that are present at birth or in early childhood. The most common location is on the head or neck.

Neurological Features

Cognitive deficits are common, and many patients are mentally retarded. Seizures occur in more than half of patients. Other neurological symptoms associated with ENS include cranial nerve palsies, hemiparesis (especially in patients with hemimeganencephaly), microcephaly, and behavior problems. Focal epileptiform discharges and focal slowing are the most common EEG abnormalities. The EEG abnormality is usually ipsilateral to the nevus. Cranial nerves VI, VII, and VIII are most likely affected. Cerebrovascular anomalies occur in approximately 10% of patients.

Other Features

Limb anomalies include clinodactyly, limb reduction defects, syndactyly, polydactyly, bifid thumbs, and talipes equinovarus. Colobomas are the most common eye anomaly.

Diagnosis

Megalencephaly ipsilateral to the epidermal nevus is the most common finding on neuroimaging. Focal pachygyria is the most common type of cortical dysplasia. The surface of the affected hemisphere may be smooth, the cortical mantle thickened, and the adjacent white matter abnormal.

HYPOMELANOSIS OF ITO

Hypomelanosis of Ito (HI) is a heterogeneous and complex neurocutaneous disorder affecting the skin, brain, eye, skeleton, and other organs. HI affects both genders equally and is usually a sporadic disorder with minimal recurrence risk.

Cutaneous Features

The skin findings are distinctive and are the only constant feature of HI; hypopigmented whorls, streaks, and patches are present at birth and tend to follow Blaschko lines. Blaschko lines form a V-shaped pattern over the back, an S-shaped pattern over the anterior trunk, and linear streaks over the extremities. The degree or distribution of skin depigmentation does not correlate with either the severity of neurological symptoms or the associated organ pathology.

Neurological Features

Seizures and mental retardation are the most common neurological abnormalities. Macrocephaly is more common than microcephaly. MRI studies show abnormalities of cerebral architecture that are stable over time.

VON HIPPEL–LINDAU SYNDROME

Von Hippel–Lindau syndrome (VHL) is an autosomal dominantly inherited disorder characterized by hemangioblastomas arising in the retina and CNS and visceral cysts and tumors. The VHL gene is a tumor suppressor gene located on chromosome 3.

Clinical Features

The most common pattern of VHL findings includes retinal and CNS hemangioblastomas and pancreatic cysts. Childhood onset of symptoms is unusual. Retinal hemangioblastomas may be asymptomatic, especially if they occur in the periphery of the retina. In the CNS, the most common site of hemangioblastomas is the cerebellum, followed by spinal and medullary sites. The frequency of cerebellar hemangioblastomas increases with age so 84% of patients with VHL have at least one such tumor by age 60 years. Pheochromocytomas occur in about 10% of patients with VHL and may be the only clinical feature, even in carefully screened individuals. Other neoplasms are renal cell carcinoma and endolymphatic sac tumors. Cerebellar hemangioblastomas are imaged with contrast-enhanced MRI.

Treatment

Careful screening is the most important aspect of management of patients with VHL. All first-degree relatives in a family with VHL or pheochromocytoma require evaluation.

WYBURN-MASON SYNDROME

Wyburn-Mason syndrome is a rare neurocutaneous syndrome characterized by retinal, facial, and intracranial arteriovenous malformations (AVMs). In contrast to VHL, in which intracranial vascular malformations are also prominent, Wyburn-Mason syndrome is not genetic.

Clinical Features

The vascular malformations of the retina and intracranial blood vessels may occur independently.

Approximately 25% of patients with retinal lesions also have intracranial vascular malformations. Retinal lesions range in magnitude from small asymptomatic lesions to massive vascular anomalies that involve most of the retina. Neurological and visual symptoms may begin at birth but usually develop in adulthood. Proptosis and catastrophic or slowly progressive visual loss are presenting symptoms of retinal AVMs. Retinal vascular malformations are demonstrated by fluorescein angiography. Vascular malformations of the face and brain can be demonstrated with conventional arteriography or with MR angiography.

Treatment

Treatment of the AVMs in Wyburn-Mason syndrome is the same as that for vascular malformations that occur sporadically. Photocoagulation of a retinal AVM is possible, but results are not encouraging. Treatment options for intracranial vessels include surgical resection, endovascular embolization, and radiosurgery.

XERODERMA PIGMENTOSUM

Xeroderma pigmentosum (XP) is a group of uncommon neurocutaneous disorders characterized by susceptibility to sun-induced skin disorders and variable but typically progressive neurological deterioration. XP is inherited in an autosomal recessive manner and occurs in from 1 in 30,000 to 1 in 250,000 population. Several gene mutations have been associated with XP and related syndromes such as Cockayne's syndrome, trichothiodystrophy, and De Sanctis–Cacchione syndrome. The principal neurological symptoms in XP-A are progressive dementia, sensorineural hearing loss, tremor, choreoathetosis, and ataxia. Progressive dementia begins in patients with XP-A during early childhood and IQ scores after 10 years are less than 50. Most patients older than 10 years have hearing impairments. Cerebellar signs develop at approximately the same time as the hearing loss. Microcephaly is present in approximately one half of patients. Cancer surveillance and avoidance of precipitating factors are the most important aspects of health screening of individuals with XP.

For a more detailed discussion, see Chapter 71 in Neurology in Clinical Practice, 4th edition.

The Dementias

41

The essential features of dementia are an acquired and persistent compromise in multiple cognitive domains that are severe enough to interfere with everyday functioning (Table 41.1). This definition stands in contrast to delirium or acute confusional states (ACSs), in which deficits or fluctuations in attentional processing are transient. Dementia syndromes *tend* to be chronic, progressive, and irreversible, whereas ACS *tends to* be acute to subacute, fluctuating, and reversible (Table 41.1). A symptomatic conceptualization of dementia is that of cortical versus subcortical dementia (Table 41.2).

ALZHEIMER'S DISEASE

Epidemiology

Alzheimer's disease (AD) prevalence increases exponentially between the ages of 65 and 85 years, doubling in every 5-year age-group. Most studies indicate prevalence by age 85 years in the range, or 30–40%. Demographic factors increasing risk include apoE4 allele, gender (women are perhaps more susceptible than men), lower education, family history of AD, coronary artery disease, and significant prior head trauma. Midlife hypertension and elevated homocysteine and fat levels in the diet are also reported risk factors. Nonsteroidal anti-inflammatory drugs, antioxidants, cholesterol-lowering agents, and hormonal replacement therapy in women may reduce the risk.

Clinical Features

AD is a progressive disorder of recent memory, language, visuospatial function, and executive function associated with a high frequency of neurobehavioral abnormalities at some point

Table 41.1: *DSM-IV* criteria for dementia

The development of multiple cognitive deficits include memory
impairment and at least one of the following:
  Aphasia
  Apraxia
  Agnosia
  Disturbance in executive functioning
The cognitive deficits must meet the following criteria:
  Be sufficiently severe to cause impairment in occupational or social
  functioning
  Represent a decline from a previous higher level of functioning
Diagnosis should not be made if the cognitive deficits occur
  exclusively during the course of a delirium. However, a dementia
  and a delirium both may be diagnosed if the dementia is present at
  times when the delirium is not present.
Dementia may be related etiologically to a general medical condition,
  to the persisting effects of substance abuse (including toxin
  exposure), or to a combination of these factors.

Source: Adapted with permission from *Diagnostic and Statistical Manual of
Mental Disorders (DSM-IV)*, 4th ed. 1994, American Psychiatric Association,
Washington, DC.

in the course. Characteristic behavioral and neuropsychiatric
symptoms develop during the midstages of the disease and
include psychosis (delusions and hallucinations), anxiety, sleep
disturbances, and depression. Onset at younger than 45 years
is usually associated with an autosomal dominant pedigree.
Typical cases have prominent early memory disturbance and subsequent language, visuospatial, and executive function impairment, but presentation and clinical course are variable.

Memory impairment is a *sine qua non* of AD. Patients with early
AD perform *immediate memory* (digit span) normally or have
only a mild deficit, compared with short-term memory. *Short-
term* or *recent memory*, assessed by remembering material over
intervals longer than 30 seconds, is more severely and earlier
affected. *Remote* or *long-term memory* (events in a person's past)
is better preserved in dementia.

Language disturbance, especially verbal fluency and word
finding, is an early feature of AD. Naming in semantic categories
(i.e., animals) is more impaired than words starting with a
particular letter. Difficulties with praxis usually occur later in the
course, after memory and language disturbances are evident.
Decline in visuospatial skills are a common symptom. Perceptual

Table 41.2: Characteristics of cortical and subcortical dementia

	Subcortical Dementia	Cortical Dementia
Severity	Mild to moderate	More severe earlier in course
Speed of cognition	Slow	Normal
Neuropsychological deficits	Frontal memory impairment (recall aided by cues)	Ophasia, apraxia, agnosia
Neuropsychiatric symptoms	Apathy, depression	Depression less common
Motor abnormalities	Dysarthria, extrapyramidal	Uncommon, gegenhalten
Pathology	Prominent changes in striatum and thalamus	Prominent changes in cortical association areas
Exemplary dementia	Progressive supranuclear palsy	Alzheimer's disease

deficits can be prominent early; some patients present with visual disorientation. Overt frontal lobe deficits such as intrusiveness or lack of self-care usually occur later.

Neuropsychiatric symptoms fall into four groups: affect or mood disturbances, psychoses (delusions and hallucinations), personality change, and disorders of behavior (agitation, wandering). Depression is common. Hallucinations and delusions are present in more than 30% of patients. Hallucinations are most commonly visual, occasionally auditory, and rarely olfactory. Subtle personality changes occur in 75% and include apathy, social disengagement, and disinhibition. Most behavioral disturbances occur in moderate to severe AD and may include verbal and physical aggression, wandering, agitation, inappropriate sexual behavior, uncooperativeness, urinary incontinence, binge eating, catastrophic reactions, and attempts at self-inflicted harm.

Although presentation most commonly involves deficits in memory, language, and visuospatial skills, judgment, insight, and motivation also decline. Final deterioration leads to a bedridden, mute, incontinent, and unresponsive state, which mimics the persistent vegetative state. Death is most commonly from infection or cardiac disease. Life expectancy of patients with AD is 8–12 years from onset, depending on the age when symptoms began. The neurological examination is normal outside of the mental status examination. At end stage, the patient is mute, incontinent, and bedridden, with flexion deformities of the limbs and impaired swallowing.

Laboratory Studies

Recommended laboratory studies include a complete blood cell count, electrolytes, glucose, blood urea nitrogen, creatinine, serum Vitamin B12 levels, thyroid function tests, and liver function tests. Electroencephalography (EEG) is not useful in the routine evaluation. Genetic testing for APP, for presenilin mutations, and genotyping for apolipoprotein E (apoE) are not routine. Cerebrospinal fluid (CSF) opening pressure, cell count, protein, and glucose concentrations are normal in AD. Lumbar puncture is performed only in the presence of metastatic cancer, suspicion of central nervous system (CNS) infection, reactive serum syphilis serology, hydrocephalus, age younger than 55 years, rapidly progressive or unusual dementia, immunosuppression, or suspicion of CNS vasculitis.

Genetics

A family history of AD is a major risk factor. Familial AD (FAD) has two forms: autosomal dominant, which has early onset (30s to 50s), and late onset FAD, which does not have an autosomal dominant pattern but has increased frequency in families. Mutations probably account for fewer than 1% of all FAD cases. Some late-onset FAD pedigrees are associated with inheritance of the E4 allele of apoE. Relative risk of AD is increased twofold to fourfold for a single E4 allele and sixfold to eightfold for homozygotes.

Neuroimaging

Perform an unenhanced magnetic resonance imaging (MRI) scan at least once during the symptomatic course. Generalized cerebral atrophy, greater than expected for age, is common with moderate or greater disease severity but in very early stages. Functional imaging studies such as single photon emission computed tomography (SPECT) and fluorine-18-fluorodeoxyglucose (FDG) positron emission tomography (PET) are not routinely used in diagnosis but may be useful in selected cases to differentiate among AD, vascular dementia (VaD), frontotemporal dementia (FTD), and corticobasal degeneration.

DOWN SYNDROME

More than 90% of patients with Down syndrome (DS) who die after the age of 30 years have the neuropathological and neurochemical features of AD.

Treatment and Management

Acetylcholinesterase Inhibitors

The primary pharmacological treatment of AD is with acetylcholinesterase inhibitors (AChEI). Three AChEIs are available—donepezil (Aricept), rivastigmine (Exelon), and galantamine (Reminyl). All three medications are effective as shown in double-blind placebo-controlled trials, by either stimulating or stabilizing performance. Provide progressively dosage increments until either a beneficial effect is noted or side effects interfere.

Medications for Behavioral and Neuropsychiatric Symptoms

Providing a quiet, familiar environment, with clear labels on doors and other objects throughout the house, reduces disorientation. Efficient lighting is important to reduce confusion at night. Intercurrent medical problems produce acute confusional states. Selective serotonin reuptake inhibitors treat depression and ease anxiety. Use short-acting benzodiazepines for sleep but not indefinitely.

FRONTOTEMPORAL DEMENTIAS

The FTDs are a group of neurodegenerative dementias affecting the frontal and/or temporal lobes relatively selectively, even into later stages of the disease. *Pick's disease* is one of the FTDs. Some are clinically distinct, but many develop more global dysfunction and become similar over time. To some extent, the clinical symptoms are referable to the anatomical distribution of pathology.

Clinical Features (Table 41.3)

FTD is primarily a neurobehavioral disorder that presents in middle or late life. The two general patterns of presentation and progression of FTD are progressive behavioral disturbance and progressive language disturbance. In the first, personality changes are prominent, executive function is impaired, and reasoning is altered. Patients pay less attention to their work or home responsibilities; behavior is purposeless and lacking in goals; planning, judgment, and mental flexibility are impaired; affect is shallow; and sympathy and empathy with others are lost. Some patients are disinhibited, overactive, and restless. Others are apathetic and lack motivation and initiative.

Males and females are equally affected. The mean duration of illness is approximately 8 years, although the range is from 2 to 15 years. Family history of a similar disorder in a first-degree relative occurs in approximately one half of cases, and some families will demonstrate autosomal dominant mode of inheritance.

Differential Diagnosis

Consideration of a diagnosis of FTD follows elimination of systemic causes. Other CNS cognitive/behavioral degenerative disorders are considered a cause by others because of the lack of social concerns by the patient.

Laboratory Studies

Blood and CSF studies are normal. The EEG may be normal until later stages, when anterior and frontal slowing emerges.

Table 41.3: Clinical criteria for frontotemporal dementia

Development of behavioral or cognitive deficits manifested by the following:

Early and progressive change in personality, characterized by difficulty modulating behavior, often resulting in inappropriate responses or activities, *or*

Early and progressive change in language, characterized by problems with expression of language or severe naming difficulty and problems with word meaning.

The deficits cause significant impairment in social or occupational functioning *and* represent a significant decline from a previous level of functioning.

The course is of gradual onset and continuing decline in function.

The deficits are not the result of other central nervous system, metabolic, or substance-induced conditions.

The deficits do not occur exclusively during the course of a delirium and are not better accounted for by a psychiatric diagnosis (e.g., depression, schizophrenia).

Source: Modified from McKhann, G. M., Albert, M. S., Grossman, M., Miller, B., et al. 2001, "Clinical and pathological diagnosis of frontotemporal dementia: report of the Work Group on Frontotemporal Dementia and Pick's Disease," *Arch Neurol,* vol. 58, pp. 1803-1809.

MRI may show frontal and temporal cortical atrophy, which may be asymmetrical and referable to prominent symptoms.

Management

Pharmacological control of disruptive symptoms or depression is the main treatment goal. Treatment with cholinesterase inhibitors has not been useful.

PROGRESSIVE APHASIAS

The progressive aphasias are a group of neurodegenerative syndromes with language dissolution as the primary presenting symptom. They are generally grouped with the FTDs and have been categorized as progressive focal cortical syndromes.

Primary Progressive Aphasia

The term *primary progressive aphasia* (PPA) originally referred to a syndrome of insidious onset and progressive nonfluent aphasia with anomia. Speech output requires manifest effort and is nonfluent and hesitant, with phonemic and semantic errors. Reading and writing are similarly affected. Word finding and repetition are impaired, and spelling is poor. Early on, preserved comprehension, insight, and nonlanguage cognitive skills including memory allow some patients to maintain employment and productivity for years after symptom onset. Initial neurological examination and EEG are normal. MRI shows left perisylvian atrophy.

Semantic Dementia

Semantic dementia is distinct from FTD and progressive aphasia but shares a common pathology. The prominent feature is profound loss of meaning, of both verbal and nonverbal information. Difficulties in naming and word comprehension are the initial symptoms, and then speech, although fluent, effortless, and grammatically correct, becomes increasingly empty and lacking in substantive words. Understanding gradually deteriorates, and conversation becomes constrained and stereotyped. Echolalia may ensue and progress to mutism. Early in the disorder, behavioral manifestations are variable. The primary finding is severe temporal lobe atrophy, particularly of the anterior aspects of the middle and inferior temporal gyri.

Motor Neuron Disease and Frontotemporal Degeneration

Frontotemporal degeneration associated with motor neuron disease (MND) presents as a frontal lobe syndrome or nonfluent aphasia. MND develops subsequently. This disease overlap of MND and FTD may result from differential spread of the degeneration from the frontal cortex to the motor cortex in FTD or in the other direction in cases of ALS that subsequently develop FTD symptoms.

Progressive Apraxia

Buccofacial apraxia is the initial feature in some patients with focal cerebral atrophy. It usually accompanies a fluent aphasia and left frontal lobe atrophy. Less often, a slowly progressive limb apraxia evolves. Object use is impaired, especially if both arms are needed for the tasks, such as using utensils to eat. The initial neurological examination is normal, but akinesia and rigidity emerge with time. EEG is normal, but PET or SPECT imaging shows loss of parietal function bilaterally.

PARKINSONIAN DEMENTIAS

Parkinsonian dementia syndromes are a heterogeneous combination of cognitive and motor features and encompass a broad range of causes (Table 41.4). The two main etiological categories are *primary degenerative*, representing disorders that are typically either sporadic or inherited, and *secondary parkinsonian syndromes* attributable to several different disorders, including drug-induced cognitive-motor syndromes. An intermediate (and less common) category of disorders that feature extrapyramidal dysfunction and associated cognitive alterations includes systemic metabolic derangements involving the excess accumulation of heavy metals or calcium in basal ganglia structures.

VASCULAR DEMENTIA

Vascular disease is the second most common cause of dementia after AD. Management focuses on prevention of subsequent vascular events (secondary prevention) and subsequent proper management of cerebrovascular risk factors (hypertension, diabetes mellitus, elevated serum lipids, heart disease).

White Matter Lesions (Leukoariosis) and Vascular Disease

CT or MRI (T2-weighted images) detects periventricular white matter lesions (WMLs). On CT, leukoariosis consists of ill-defined regions with low attenuation values around the frontal and occipital horns of the lateral ventricles, often extending into the frontal white matter and into the centrum semiovale. On T2-weighted MRI, the white matter changes have an increased signal. These nonspecific periventricular white matter abnormalities, termed *leukoariosis*, are a risk factor for dementia, although the relation between the two is not simple. Their presence in nondemented patients is of uncertain cognitive significance. WMLs are more common in pathological disorders that cause dementia, such as cerebral ischemic infarcts (VaD) and neurodegenerative disorders (e.g., progressive subcortical gliosis and FTD).

Cortical and Subcortical Vascular Dementia

Clinical manifestations of VaD may be either cortical or subcortical. Cortical manifestations include prominent neuropsychological and behavioral symptoms with or without sensory or motor deficits. Cortical VaD, also referred to as *multi-infarct*

Table 41.4: Classification and salient features of parkinsonian dementia syndromes

Etiology	Distinguishing Features
Degenerative (sporadic)	
Parkinson's disease with dementia	Motor signs initially, then onset of dementia
Dementia with Lewy bodies	Recurrent visual hallucinations; cognitive fluctuations
Progressive supranuclear palsy (PSP)	Early balance and bulbar deficits; down-gaze palsy
Corticobasal degeneration	Asymmetric limb signs (apraxia, myoclonus)
Multisystem atrophy	"Parkinson-plus" syndromes
Olivopontocerebellar atrophy	Brainstem/cerebellar atrophy; ocular dysmotility
Striatonigral degeneration	Pyramidal tract signs; laryngeal stridor
Shy-Drager syndrome	Marked orthostatic hypotension and dysautonomia
Degenerative (familial)	
Huntington's disease (HD)	Autosomal dominant; chorea, athetosis, personality changes
Neuroacanthocytosis	Autosomal dominant; HD-mimic; acanthocytic red blood cells
Machado-Joseph disease	Autosomal dominant; ataxia and dysarthria, cerebellar atrophy
Progressive subcortical gliosis	Autosomal dominant; white-matter gliosis, frontal atrophy
Familial frontotemporal dementia	Autosomal dominant; chromosome 17–linked, frontal atrophy

Secondary parkinsonian syndromes

Drug-induced encephalopathy/parkinsonism — Relevant drug exposure (neuroleptic, antiemetic)

Vascular parkinsonism — Multiple subcortical infarcts; may mimic PSP

Normal-pressure hydrocephalus — Prominent gait disturbance; urinary incontinence ± parkinsonism

Whipple's disease — May mimic PSP; mild cerebrospinal fluid pleocytosis; gastrointestinal symptoms prominent

Dementia pugilistica — Repetitive head trauma ± cavum septum pellucidum on MRI

Inherited metabolic disorders

Wilson's disease — Autosomal recessive; early-onset; impaired copper clearance;

Hallevorden-Spatz disease — early-onset; subcortical iron deposits

Idiopathic basal ganglia calcification — Autosomal dominant and recessive; subcortical calcium deposits *demantia* (MID), is usually caused by the accumulation of deficits through multiple bilateral supratentorial infarcts.

Unlike "cortical" VaD in which large cortical infarctions make up a predominant portion of the clinical presentation, *subcortical VaD* is usually associated with lacunar infarcts and WMLs. These patients have sensory and motor deficits, gait disorders (e.g., *marche à petits pas*; small hesitant steps), extrapyramidal signs, dysarthria, pseudobulbar palsy, urinary incontinence, depressed mood, apathy, and emotional lability. Patients have slowed mental processing and set-shifting task deficits. Subcortical arteriosclerotic encephalopathy (SAE), also known as *Binswanger's disease*, is a form of subcortical VaD. Gradual onset of cognitive difficulties is the initial feature in more than half of cases. Memory deficits, apathy, and slowed thinking are prominent. Motor abnormalities are found in later stages, with clumsiness, slowed actions, and gait disturbances.

Lesion Size and Strategically Localized Infarcts

It is clear that large ischemic lesions can cause VaD, especially those localized in frontal, temporal, or parietal regions. The size and number of lesions do not always explain the cognitive deficits. A threshold of tissue loss (e.g., 50–100 ml) may need to be exceeded. Thalamic and basal ganglia infarcts can produce significant motor and cognitive deficits severe enough to cause dementia.

Cerebral Amyloid Angiopathy

Deposits of β-amyloid can be seen in the cerebral blood vessels of all patients with AD. These deposits contribute to the development of leukoariosis in patients with AD. Familial cases of AD and cerebral amyloid angiopathy (CAA) are associated with multiple hemorrhages in the brain, spinal cord, and leptomeninges.

Cerebral Autosomal Dominant Arteriopathy with Subcortical Infarcts and Leukoencephalopathy

Cerebral autosomal dominant arteriopathy with subcortical infarcts and leukoencephalopathy is a hereditary disease associated with a mutation in the Notch3 gene on chromosome 19. The dominant clinical features are strokes and cognitive loss. It is diagnosed with skin biopsy and identification of the abnormality in the vascular basal membrane of blood vessels. It usually presents in the fifth decade with seizures, migraine type of headaches with aura, and clinical strokes. The dementia syndrome is a subcortical one, with memory and frontal lobe deficits. The course is progressive. MRI reveals significant ischemic lesions in the subcortical white and gray matter, especially in the internal capsule and basal ganglia, as well as lacunar infarctions.

Collagen Disorders And Vasculitis

Mild cognitive disorders are seen in up to 80% of patients with systemic lupus erythematosus. Memory and attentional deficits are more severe than language or visuoconstructional disorders. Psychiatric symptoms include major depression, anxiety, manic episodes, and psychosis.

Sjögren's syndrome (xerophthalmia and xerostomia) is associated with small-vessel arteritis, which can evolve to an acute meningoencephalitis. Patients with periarteritis nodosum can also develop a dementia syndrome following acute meningoencephalitis. The severity of the cognitive impairment may improve after treatment with steroids and cyclophosphamide. Dementia secondary to isolated cerebral vasculitis is rare.

OTHER CAUSES OF DEMENTIA

Several other chapters contain discussions of dementia. The dementia associated with cancer is discussed in Chapter 27, dementia associated with the human immunodeficiency virus and prion disorders in Chapter 28, dementia associated with deficiency diseases in Chapter 32, and dementia associated with toxins in Chapter 33.

Posttraumatic Dementia

Open or closed head trauma can cause neurological, psychiatric, and cognitive deficits. Five percent of patients with head trauma meet criteria for dementia. The clinical presentation is highly variable; some manifest clear signs of brain damage on neuroradiological examinations (e.g., hemorrhage or atrophy), and others have normal MRI or CT scans of the brain but have cognitive and affective disturbances. Posttraumatic dementia is often symptomatic as frontotemporal cognitive dysfunction, because of diffuse anterior subcortical axon shear that disrupts frontotemporal and cortical subcortical circuitry. Memory loss, deficits in mental processing speed, and difficulty with set-shifting functions are the most common cognitive symptoms.

Language can be preserved, although patients with extensive cortical damage can have language deficits.

NORMAL-PRESSURE HYDROCEPHALUS

The triad of gait apraxia, urinary incontinence, and progressive dementia characterizes normal-pressure hydrocephalus (NPH). Gait problems and urinary incontinence can precede the dementia syndrome in some cases. The gait problems resemble those observed in Parkinson's disease, although they improve after initiating gait. Cognitively, the predominant deficits are in speed of mental processing, abstract thinking, set-shifting tasks, and memory function; language test results can be normal in initial stages. CT and MRI showing ventricular enlargement (lateral, third, and fourth ventricles) associated with the clinical triad supports the diagnosis of NPH. The treatment of NPH is a ventricular peritoneal shunt.

For a more detailed discussion, see Chapter 72 in Neurology in Clinical Practice, 4th edition.

The Epilepsies

42

EPIDEMIOLOGY

Incidence and Prevalence

In most developed countries, incidence rates range from 40 to 70 per 100,000, but in developing countries the rates may be as high as 100 to 190 per 100,000. The prevalence of active epilepsy, defined as persons who take anticonvulsant drugs or who have had a seizure in the past 5 years, ranges from 4 to 10 per 10,000 in developed countries and up to 57 per 10,000 in developing countries. Approximately 1.5–5.0% of any population will have a seizure at some time. Traditionally, epilepsy has been more common in children than in adults. Recent studies suggest a shift to older age groups. The cause for epilepsy is identified in only one fourth to one third of cases.

Prognosis

The overall prognosis for remission is good but depends on the underlying cause. Among all people with epilepsy, 20–30% have benign genetic epilepsies that remit completely without treatment. Antiepileptic drugs easily control another 30–40%; remission is often permanent after discontinuing medications. Antiepileptic drugs are suppressive rather than curative in 10–20% of people with epilepsy, and in 20%, treatments, including surgery, reduce seizures only partially.

CLASSIFICATION OF SEIZURES AND EPILEPTIC SYNDROMES

The International League Against Epilepsy (ILAE) classification recognizes epilepsies and epileptic syndromes by incorporating

Table 42.1: The International League Against Epilepsy classification of epileptic seizures

I. Partial (focal, local) seizures
  A. Simple partial seizures (consciousness not impaired)
    1. With motor symptoms
    2. With somatosensory or special sensory symptoms
    3. With autonomic symptoms
    4. With psychic symptoms
  B. Complex partial seizures (with impairment of consciousness)
    1. Beginning as simple partial seizures and progressing to impairment of consciousness
    2. With no other features
    3. With features as in simple partial seizures
    4. With automatisms
  C. With impairment of consciousness at onset
    1. With no other features
    2. With features as in simple partial seizures
    3. With automatisms
  D. Partial seizures evolving to secondarily generalized seizures
    1. Simple partial seizures evolving to generalized seizures
    2. Complex partial seizures evolving to generalized seizures
    3. Simple partial seizures evolving to complex partial seizures to generalized seizures
II. Generalized seizures (convulsive or nonconvulsive)
  A. Absence seizures
    1. Absence seizures
    2. Atypical absence seizures
  B. Myoclonic seizures
  C. Clonic seizures
  D. Tonic seizures
  E. Tonic-clonic seizures
  F. Atonic seizures (astatic seizures)
III. Unclassified epileptic seizures (includes all seizures that cannot be classified because of inadequate or incomplete data and some that defy classification in hitherto described categories. This includes some neonatal seizures, such as rhythmic eye movements, chewing, and swimming movements.

the basic categories of partial and generalized seizures while taking into account seizure type, electroencephalographic (EEG) findings and prognostic, pathophysiological, and etiological information (Table 42.1 and Table 42.2). The most basic problem with present classifications is that they do not account for the underlying mechanisms of seizures.

Table 42.2: The International League Against Epilepsy classification of epilepsies and epileptic syndromes

I. Localization-related (focal, local, partial) epilepsies and syndromes
    A. Idiopathic (with age-related onset). At present, two syndromes are established:
        1. Benign childhood epilepsy with centrotemporal spike
        2. Childhood epilepsy with occipital paroxysms
    B. Symptomatic; this category comprises syndromes of great individual variability.
II. Generalized epilepsies and syndromes
    A. Idiopathic (with age-related onset, in order of age appearance)
        1. Benign neonatal familial convulsions
        2. Benign neonatal convulsions
        3. Benign myoclonic epilepsy in infancy
        4. Childhood absence epilepsy (pyknolepsy, petit mal)
        5. Juvenile absence epilepsy
        6. Juvenile myoclonic epilepsy (impulsive petit mal)
        7. Epilepsy with grand mal seizures on awakening
    B. Idiopathic, symptomatic, or both (in order of age of appearance)
        1. West's syndrome (infantile spasms)
        2. Lennox-Gastaut syndrome
        3. Epilepsy with myoclonic-astatic seizures
        4. Epilepsy with myoclonic absences
    C. Symptomatic
        1. Nonspecific cause: early myoclonic encephalopathy
        2. Specific syndromes: epileptic seizures may complicate many disease states
Under this heading are included those diseases in which seizures are a presenting or predominant feature.
III. Epilepsies and syndromes undetermined as to whether they are focal or generalized
    A. With both generalized and focal seizures
        1. Neonatal seizures
        2. Severe myoclonic epilepsy in infancy
        3. Epilepsy with continuous spikes and waves during slow-wave sleep
        4. Acquired epileptic aphasia (Landau-Kleffner syndrome)
    B. Without unequivocal generalized or focal features
IV. Special syndromes
    A. Situation-related seizures
        1. Febrile convulsions
        2. Seizures related to other identifiable situations, such as stress, hormones, drugs, alcohol, or sleep deprivation
    B. Isolated, apparently unprovoked epileptic events
    C. Epilepsies characterized by the specific modes of seizures precipitated
    D. Chronic progressive epilepsia partialis continua of childhood

Partial Seizures

The ILAE defines partial seizures as those in which the first clinical and EEG changes indicate activation of a system of neurons limited to one part of the cerebral hemisphere. A complex partial seizure is associated with impairment of consciousness and a simple partial seizure has no impairment of consciousness.

Simple Partial Seizures

Preservation of consciousness classifies a seizure disorder as simple partial. The clinical features depend on the brain region activated. The initial discharge is relatively localized, but the activity spreads to adjacent brain areas, causing progression of the clinical seizure pattern. The most common simple partial seizure patterns are those with either motor or sensory symptoms.

The ILAE classification divides simple partial seizures into four major categories: (1) those with motor signs, (2) those with somatosensory or special sensory symptoms, (3) those with autonomic symptoms or signs, and (4) those with psychic symptoms (see Table 42.1). The ictal onset may be clinically silent and all features of the seizure attributed to subsequent spread of ictal activity. Sensations that precede a seizure are termed *epileptic auras*. Auras are simple partial seizures that last seconds to minutes.

Complex Partial Seizures

Impaired consciousness without generalized tonic-clonic activity characterizes complex partial seizures. Individuals are usually either unaware that they had a seizure or unable to recall events that occurred during the seizure. Most complex partial seizures arise from the temporal lobe. As many as 30% of complex partial seizures arise from extratemporal locations, most commonly the frontal lobe but also the parietal and occipital lobes.

AUTOMATISMS Automatisms are more or less coordinated involuntary motor activity occurring during a state of impaired consciousness either in the course of or after an epileptic seizure and usually followed by amnesia. Several types are recognized. *De novo automatisms* are behaviors beginning spontaneously after the onset of the seizure and thought to be release phenomenon. *Reactive automatisms* also begin after the onset of the seizure but appear to be reactions to external stimuli. *Perseverative automatisms* are continuations of complex acts engaged in before the seizure started. Automatisms are often associated with temporal lobe seizures but also occur during complex partial seizures of extratemporal origin and with typical and atypical absence seizures.

TEMPORAL LOBE SEIZURES Complex partial seizures of temporal lobe origin may begin with impairment of consciousness or be preceded by a simple partial seizure or an aura. Auras vary in duration from seconds to several minutes before impairment of consciousness. Most complex partial seizures last longer than 30 seconds, usually 1–2 minutes; few last less than 10 seconds, which is a distinguishing characteristic from absence seizures. Postictal recovery is usually slow, with significant confusion that may last for several minutes or longer. A correlation of clinical features and site of seizure discharge is not universally accepted.

Distortions of memory include dreamy states, flashbacks, sensations of familiarity with unfamiliar events (*déjà vu*), or sensations of unfamiliarity with previously experienced events (*jamais vu*). Some patients experience a form of forced thinking, characterized by a rapid recollection of episodes from past life experiences (*panoramic vision*). Other possible seizure manifestations are alterations of cognitive state or affect. An initial behavioral arrest or brief motionless stare that precedes an epigastric sensation, emotional symptoms, and olfactory or gustatory hallucinations characterizes seizures of mesial temporal lobe onset. Auditory hallucinations or vertigo suggest neocortical onset.

FRONTAL LOBE SEIZURES Seizures of frontal lobe origin generally begin abruptly, are brief, show minimal postictal confusion, and often occur in clusters. Motor manifestations are prominent and the clinical features vary with the region of involved frontal lobe. The motor strip produces clonic activity of the contralateral arm or leg or the face. The spread of epileptic activity from one area of the motor cortex to contiguous regions produces progressive jerking of successive body parts (*jacksonian seizures*). The prerolandic area impairs speech and causes tonic-clonic movements of the contralateral face or repetitive swallowing. The supplementary motor cortex causes head turning with arm extension on the same side (fencer's posture). The dorsolateral prefrontal cortex causes forced turning of the eyes and head to the opposite side and speech arrest. The paracentral lobule causes tonic movement of the ipsilateral foot and often contralateral involvement of the legs. Cingulate seizures cause complex motor gestural automatisms with changes in mood and affect and autonomic signs. Anterior frontopolar seizures cause forced thinking, adversive movements of the head, and axial clonic jerks that may cause a fall. Orbitofrontal seizures cause motor and gestural automatisms and olfactory hallucinations and illusions.

PARIETAL LOBE SEIZURES Partial sensory seizures usually originate in the parietal lobe. Tingling or numbness, usually confined to one body region, can progress to adjacent parts. The likelihood that a specific body part is involved probably correlates with the size of its cortical representation. A desire to move a body part or a feeling that a part is moving characterizes other sensory seizures. Negative seizure phenomena are a sense that a body part is absent or that awareness is lost of a part or even a whole side of the body (asomatognosia). Seizures originating from other parts of the parietal lobe may cause a sensation of sinking, choking, or nausea; severe vertigo or disorientation in space; rudimentary vague sensations of pain or coldness; and receptive or conductive language disturbances.

OCCIPITAL LOBE SEIZURES Occipital lobe seizures are associated with visual symptoms. The epileptic images usually are elementary: flashes of light, scotomas, hemianopia, or amaurosis. Seizures from the occipital–temporal–parietal junction produce complex imagery including distortions of size (micropsia or macropsia), shape (metamorphopsia), or perceived distance from the individual. Visual hallucinations usually consist of previously experienced imagery. Occipital lobe seizures also may produce tonic or clonic contraversion of the eyes (oculoclonic or oculogyric deviation), clonic palpebral jerks, or forced closure of the eyelids.

VIOLENT BEHAVIOR Epileptic activity, particularly involving the temporal lobe, may cause emotional symptoms, such as fear, agitation, and, occasionally, undirected aggressive or violent behavior. Most violent behavior during a seizure is nonspecific and usually occurs in response to restraint. The following criteria should be met before concluding that a specific violent crime was the result of a seizure:

1. The diagnosis of epilepsy must be firmly established.
2. Epilepsy monitoring should verify the presence of aggression during epileptic automatisms.
3. The aggressive or violent act should be a difficult action with complex activity.
4. A clinical neurologist with special expertise in epilepsy should be involved in making the determination of whether the violence that occurred during the seizure could have contributed to the crime.

ELECTROENCEPHALOGRAPHIC CHARACTERISTICS OF PARTIAL SEIZURES The temporal lobe, usually the anterior temporal lobe, is the area of onset in approximately 80% of patients with partial seizures. During the interictal period, abnormalities of rhythm or transient epileptiform discharges suggest a seizure focus. Interictal epileptiform activity correlates fairly well with the site of ictal onset, but temporal sharp wave activity can be bilateral in one third of cases. Scalp EEG recordings during simple partial and even some complex partial seizures may be normal. The EEG patterns that occur during complex partial seizures of temporal lobe origin include (1) rhythmic 5–7 Hz activity without spike or sharp-wave activity, (2) rhythmic spike or sharp-wave activity, and (3) focal attenuation of normal activity. The localization of EEG activity is less defined during seizures from extratemporal foci, particularly those with frontal lobe onset.

Partial Epileptic Syndromes

The International Classification of the Epilepsies recognizes two "localization-related disorders": *benign childhood epilepsy with centrotemporal spikes* (benign rolandic epilepsy) and *childhood epilepsy with occipital paroxysms* (benign occipital epilepsy). The spectrum of benign childhood epilepsies is probably broader than just these two syndromes.

BENIGN CHILDHOOD EPILEPSY WITH CENTROTEMPORAL SPIKES

The characteristic seizure begins with sensory disturbance of the mouth, preservation of consciousness, excessive pooling of saliva, tonic or tonic-clonic activity of the face, and speech arrest when the dominant hemisphere is affected. The sensory or motor activity may spread to the arm. Secondary generalization may occur, especially when the seizures are nocturnal. Development, neurological examinations, and neuroradiological study results are normal. Seizures are typically nocturnal but can occur during the day. Headache and vomiting may be associated. Seizures usually stop in adolescence, and the outcome is favorable.

The EEG consists of a normal background with midtemporal and central, high-amplitude, often diphasic spikes and sharp waves with increased frequency during sleep. The spikes and sharp waves are usually unilateral. Because the overall prognosis for benign childhood epilepsy is good, treatment is not usually needed after the first or even the second seizure.

CHILDHOOD EPILEPSY WITH OCCIPITAL PAROXYSMS

Childhood epilepsy with occipital paroxysms is more heterogeneous than benign rolandic epilepsy. The seizures are partial motor or generalized tonic-clonic seizures that occur during sleep and visual seizures that occur during wakefulness. The visual symptoms are amaurosis, elementary or complex visual hallucinations, or illusions including micropsia, metamorphopsia, or palinopsia. The EEG shows high-voltage occipital spikes occurring in 1–3

Hz bursts or trains. The spikes disappear with eye opening and reappear 1–20 seconds after eye closure or darkness. The EEG shows high-voltage occipital spikes occurring in 1–3 Hz bursts or trains. The spikes disappear with eye opening and reappear 1–20 seconds after eye closure or darkness.

EPILEPSIA PARTIALIS CONTINUA *Epilepsia partialis continua* is a prolonged focal seizure. The typical features are repeated focal motor seizures occurring in clusters, which may secondarily generalize. Myoclonic activity may persist between attacks. The usual cause of epilepsia partialis continua is focal injury to the cortex from anoxia, inflammation, or a metabolic disturbance.

RASMUSSEN'S ENCEPHALITIS Rasmussen's encephalitis is a chronic progressive disorder of unknown etiology. Originally described in previously healthy children younger than 10 years, it also occurs in older children and adults. Partial motor seizures are limited to one hemisphere at onset but may become bilateral late in the course. The initial feature is frequent partial motor seizures of one limb. Episodes of secondary generalization are common. The seizures soon spread, and progressive hemiplegia is the rule. At first, the seizures respond to standard anticonvulsant therapy but then become refractory. Corticosteroids, intravenous immune globulin, and plasmapheresis are beneficial in some patients. Hemispherectomy is required for seizure control in most affected children.

Generalized Seizures

Generalized Tonic-Clonic Seizures
CLINICAL FEATURES Generalized tonic-clonic seizures have five phases, which do not occur each time:

1. *Premonition* is a vague sense that a seizure is imminent that may last for hours or days. Premonitions are not auras and do not have localizing value.
2. The immediate *pre–tonic-clonic phase* is characterized by a few myoclonic jerks, or brief clonic seizures, or deviation of the head and eyes.
3. The *tonic phase* usually begins with a sudden tonic contraction of the axial musculature and then the limbs, accompanied by upward eye deviation and pupillary dilation. Cyanosis develops as a result of restricted respiratory function.
4. The *clonic phase* evolves gradually from the tonic phase. Initially, the clonic activity is of low amplitude and

progressively increases. Incontinence of urine and occasionally stool may occur.

5. In the *postictal* phase, the individual is generally unresponsive, but respiration returns.

Some generalized seizures are only tonic or clonic. Clonic seizures carry no special significance compared with tonic-clonic seizures, but tonic seizures are more common with secondary generalized epilepsy than primary generalized epilepsy. Infants and children with tonic seizure often have other seizure types and mental retardation. Tonic seizures that develop in late childhood or in adults are usually a variant of generalized tonic-clonic seizures.

COMPLICATIONS OF SEIZURES   Generalized tonic-clonic seizures are associated with a higher rate of injury than other seizure types. Laceration of the tongue, cheeks, and lips is common, but additional injury occurs when observers attempt to place objects in the mouth. Unprotected falls cause head injuries and vertebral compression fractures occur in approximately 5–15% of people having seizures, usually older individuals. Aspiration pneumonia may occur. Mortality among patients with epilepsy is increased twofold to threefold compared to the general population. The term "sudden unexplained death in epilepsy" (SUDEP) is used when reasonable investigative measures cannot identify the cause of death in the absence of status epilepticus.

ELECTROENCEPHALOGRAPHIC CHARACTERISTICS OF GENERALIZED TONIC-CLONIC SEIZURES

Interictal. Approximately half of interictal EEGs in patients with generalized tonic-clonic seizures contain epileptiform activity. The epileptiform activity is usually one or more of four main patterns: (1) typical 3-Hz spike-and-wave complexes, (2) irregular spike-and-wave complexes, (3) 4–5 Hz spike-and-wave complexes, and (4) multifocal spike complexes.

Ictal. The EEG hallmark of idiopathic generalized tonic-clonic seizures is bihemispheric involvement at the onset. The tonic phase of a primary generalized tonic-clonic seizure usually begins with an abrupt decrease in the voltage lasting 1–3 seconds, accompanied by diffuse, low-voltage, 20–40 Hz activity (*desynchronization pattern*). After the desynchronization phase, as the tonic phase continues, the ictal sharp waves build in amplitude to rhythmic 8–10 Hz. High-amplitude repetitive polyspike-and-wave complexes gradually replace the desynchronization pattern. The clonic phase of the seizure develops when the polyspike-and-wave complexes slow to approximately 4 Hz. The ictal activity ends with diffuse suppression of EEG activity or low-voltage delta waves.

Absence Seizures

CLINICAL FEATURES   The simplest clinical feature of a typical absence seizure is the sudden onset of a blank stare, usually lasting 5–10 seconds. Ongoing activity may stop abruptly. The individual does not respond to external stimuli and is unaware of having had the seizure. Recovery is as sudden as the onset, and previous activity continues as though nothing had happened. Absence seizures accompanied by automatisms suggest a complex partial seizure.

ELECTROENCEPHALOGRAPHIC CHARACTERISTICS OF ABSENCE SEIZURES   The background rhythms are normal. The ictal pattern is a characteristic 3-Hz spike-and-wave pattern. Discharges lasting less than 3 seconds may not cause clinical seizures. The frequency of the spike-and-wave activity may be slightly faster than 3 Hz at seizure onset, slowing to 2.5–3.0 Hz as the seizure progresses. The EEG background is often abnormal in patients with atypical absence seizure because of diffuse slowing and focal or multifocal spike discharges. The ictal EEG consists of generalized slow spike-and-wave discharges in the range of 0.5–2.5 Hz.

Myoclonic Seizures

Myoclonus is a sudden, involuntary, shocklike muscle contraction arising from the central nervous system that causes a generalized jerk or a focal jerk. The jerks may be isolated or occur in clusters. Myoclonus can be epileptic or nonepileptic.

Tonic Seizures

Tonic seizures last an average of 10 seconds but can persist for up to 1 minute. The onset may be gradual or abrupt. A myoclonic jerk may occur at the beginning, followed by a generalized tonic contraction. Movement may be limited to the axial musculature (tonic axial seizure), extend to the proximal muscles of the arms and legs, or involve proximal and distal limb muscles in addition to axial muscles (global tonic seizure).

Atonic Seizures

Atonic seizures, commonly called *drop attacks*, occur abruptly and without warning and usually last 1–2 seconds. The main clinical feature is a sudden loss of tone, which may be limited to eye blinks or head drops but can involve the entire body. A severe atonic seizure poses a high risk of injury because of the suddenness and forcefulness of the fall. *Akinetic seizures* are similar to atonic seizures, except that tone is preserved; the patient is motionless but consciousness is impaired.

Generalized Epileptic Syndromes

The generalized epileptic syndromes are diverse in severity and etiology.

Benign Generalized Epileptic Syndromes

FEBRILE SEIZURES Febrile seizures occur in 2–5% of children. Many people with epilepsy have their first seizure during a fever, but *simple febrile seizures* are a distinct benign disorder that has a genetic basis. The mode of inheritance is not established. Most first febrile seizures occur between the ages of 6 months and 3 years (range, 1 month to 10 years) and may occur anytime during a febrile illness. They are usually single, generalized, and brief but may be complex (multiple, focal, and prolonged). Complex febrile seizures increase the risk of later nonfebrile seizures. Approximately one third of children with febrile seizures have at least one recurrence, but fewer than 10% have three or more.

The prognosis is excellent. Children who were neurologically normal before the seizures, even several febrile seizures, develop normally afterward. Febrile seizures do not require prophylactic anticonvulsant therapy.

BENIGN FAMILIAL NEONATAL CONVULSIONS Frequent brief seizures within the first few days of life are characteristic of benign familial neonatal convulsions, a rare dominantly inherited disorder. The seizures usually resolve by 6 months of age, but the risk of later epilepsy is about 15%.

BENIGN MYOCLONIC EPILEPSY OF INFANCY Benign myoclonic epilepsy of infancy develops in otherwise normal children before age 2 years. Brief generalized myoclonic seizures of variable intensity are the only seizure type. Head drops or eye blinks are the most characteristic seizure type. Attacks can last up to 10 seconds. Consciousness is not completely lost. The ictal EEG shows diffuse, irregular 3-Hz spike-wave or polyspike-wave discharges with the myoclonic jerks. The interictal EEG is usually normal. Generalized tonic-clonic seizures may develop later in life. Valproate controls the seizures, and the developmental outcome is good when treatment is started early.

JUVENILE MYOCLONIC EPILEPSY Juvenile myoclonic epilepsy (JME) is familial and presumed transmitted as an autosomal dominant trait. It accounts for 4–10% of all epilepsy. Age at onset is usually between 12 and 18 years. The characteristic feature is sudden mild to moderate myoclonic jerks of the shoulders and arms that usually occur after awakening. Generalized tonic-clonic seizures develop in 90% of cases, and approximately one third have absence seizures. The myoclonic seizures precede the generalized tonic-clonic seizures in approximately half of patients.

The interictal EEG in JME consists of bilateral symmetrical spike-and-wave and polyspike-and-wave discharges of 3–5 Hz, usually maximal in the frontocentral regions. The EEG correlate of the myoclonic jerks is a burst of high-voltage 10–16 Hz polyspikes followed by irregular 1–3 Hz slow waves and single spikes or polyspikes. Valproic acid usually controls seizures, but lifetime treatment is necessary. Lamotrigine or levetiracetam are used when valproic acid is not tolerated, with ethosuximide as the next option for uncontrolled absence seizures

EPILEPSY WITH GENERALIZED TONIC-CLONIC SEIZURES ON AWAKENING Epilepsy with generalized tonic-clonic seizures on awakening is probably distinct from JME. Onset is in the second decade, and 90% of seizures occur on awakening, regardless of the time of day. Seizures also occur with relaxation in the evening. Absence and myoclonic seizures may occur. The syndrome is genetic, but the mode of inheritance is unknown. The EEG shows a pattern of the idiopathic generalized epilepsies. Treatment is similar to that for JME.

ABSENCE SYNDROMES Several absence syndromes are recognized. The onset of *childhood absence epilepsy* is usually at 5–10 years of age but may be as early as 3 years of age. It is a hereditary disorder with a positive family history in 16–45% of cases. The exact mode of inheritance is likely to be multifactorial. The incidence in girls is greater than in boys. Up to 100 seizures may occur per day if untreated. EEG shows generalized 3-cps spike-and-wave complexes induced by hyperventilation. *Juvenile absence epilepsy*, with onset around puberty, may be a distinct but related syndrome. The absences are less frequent, but myoclonic and generalized tonic-clonic seizures are more frequent. Approximately half of the patients with absence epilepsy become seizure free 10 years after onset. Good prognostic factors include normal intelligence, normal neurological examination findings, male gender, and lack of hyperventilation-induced spike waves on the EEG.

Children who have stereotyped absences associated with bilateral rhythmic clonic jerking of the arms probably have a separate rare disorder, *epilepsy with myoclonic absences*. Age at onset is similar to that of childhood absence epilepsy, but the prognosis is worse; the seizures are often resistant to therapy and mental deterioration may occur.

Ethosuximide is the initial medication of choice to treat absence unless other seizure types also occur, in which case valproic acid is used. Some children require both drugs; others may benefit from the addition of clonazepam. Other treatments include lamotrigine, levetiracetam, topiramate, and zonisamide.

Severe Generalized Epileptic Syndromes

EARLY EPILEPTIC ENCEPHALOPATHIES WITH SUPPRESSION BURSTS. Two syndromes are identified in the category of early epileptic encephalopathies with suppression bursts; both with onset in the first 3 months of life: *early infantile epileptic encephalopathy* (EIEE) and *early myoclonic encephalopathy* (EME). These conditions are often difficult to distinguish. Tonic spasms, often in clusters, characterize EIEE, and myoclonic seizures are more typical of EME. Both disorders are associated with serious underlying metabolic or structural abnormalities. Some familial cases suggest an underlying genetic disorder. Psychomotor arrest and regression are constant features. Progression to infantile spasms and Lennox-Gastaut syndrome is common. EEG records a suppression pattern alternating with bursts of diffuse high-amplitude spike-wave complexes. Seizures are refractory to most anticonvulsant drugs. Vigabatrin may be beneficial for early infantile epileptic encephalopathy. Valproic acid and clonazepam are often used for myoclonic seizures, and carbamazepine is contraindicated.

WEST'S SYNDROME West's syndrome is the clinical triad of infantile spasms, arrest of psychomotor development, and hypsarrhythmia on EEG. The identified causes are divided into prenatal (cerebral dysgenesis, genetic disorders, intrauterine infection), perinatal (anoxic injury, head trauma, infection), or postnatal (metabolic disorders, trauma, infection). No cause (cryptogenic) is identifiable in up to 40% of cases.

The onset is usually before the age of 1 year, with peak onset between 3 and 7 months of age. The spasms occur in clusters and are characterized by sudden flexor or extensor movements of the trunk. Developmental arrest and regression begin with or before the spasms. On the waking record, hypsarrhythmia consists of disorganized high-voltage slow waves, spikes, and sharp waves that occur diffusely with a posterior predominance. The prognosis for children with infantile spasms is extremely poor, but the major determinant of outcome is the underlying cause of the spasms. Early treatment does not improve prognosis.

Vigabatrin, not yet available in the United States, has become the treatment of choice. Other effective drugs include valproic acid, clonazepam, and zonisamide. Corticosteroids (adrenocorticotropic hormone [ACTH], prednisone, or prednisolone) are useful when drug treatment fails. Some affected infants have focal brain abnormalities that may respond to surgical treatment.

LENNOX-GASTAUT SYNDROME The defining features of Lennox-Gastaut syndrome are (1) the presence of several seizure types, (2) a characteristic interictal EEG abnormality, and (3) diffuse cognitive dysfunction. The causes of Lennox-Gastaut syndrome are similar to those of West's syndrome and can be divided into the symptomatic and the cryptogenic. Abnormalities of the frontal lobe are more often associated with Lennox-Gastaut syndrome than any other region of the brain. The onset of seizures is between 1 and 7 years. Generalized seizures are the rule. Cognitive function is normal in 40% of children at the onset of the seizures but then deteriorates. The waking interictal EEG consists of an abnormally slow background with characteristic 1.5–2.5 Hz slow spike-and-wave interictal discharges, often with an anterior predominance. Bursts of rhythmic 10-Hz activity characteristically occur during sleep.

The seizures are often refractory to anticonvulsant drugs. Valproic acid and benzodiazepines are the mainstay of therapy. Lamotrigine and topiramate also may have a role. The addition of felbamate to existing therapy improves seizure control in approximately 30% of patients but risks aplastic anemia and hepatotoxicity. Corticosteroids and ACTH are beneficial in some cases, and the ketogenic diet may be useful.

EPILEPSY WITH MYOCLONIC-ASTATIC SEIZURES The age at onset of epilepsy with myoclonic-astatic seizures is usually between 1 and 6 years of age. Most individuals are neurologically normal at the onset of seizures. Absence and myoclonic-astatic seizures are the predominant seizure type. Generalized tonic-clonic seizures may occur, but tonic seizures are uncommon and usually occur only in sleep. One half of children exhibit cognitive deterioration, but overall the prognosis is better than that for Lennox-Gastaut syndrome. Early treatment with antiepileptic drugs effective against generalized seizures may be associated with a better prognosis.

LANDAU-KLEFFNER SYNDROME Age at onset of Landau-Kleffner syndrome is between 3 and 9 years. An acquired aphasia, usually associated with seizures, is the presenting feature. Several seizure types occur, including generalized tonic-clonic, partial, and myoclonic seizures. The severity of the seizure disorder does not correlate with the language loss. Characteristically, children exhibit word deafness in the face of otherwise normal hearing. The EEG may show spike activity over the temporocentral regions, often bilateral. Other EEG patterns occur, such as multifocal spike and slow waves. Standard antiepileptic drugs usually control the seizures, but recovery of language is variable. The efficacy of high-dose steroids is variable.

ELECTRICAL STATUS EPILEPTICUS DURING SLOW-WAVE SLEEP Neuropsychological regression, with or without seizures, is the presenting feature of children with electrical status epilepticus during slow-wave sleep. Age at onset is 1–12 years. This disorder is distinct from Landau-Kleffner syndrome. The EEG characteristically shows continuous spike and slow waves during non–rapid eye movement sleep. Several seizure types occur, which are commonly nocturnal. Seizures and EEG changes usually disappear in the second decade, but cognitive and language function often remain impaired.

PROGRESSIVE MYOCLONIC EPILEPSIES The progressive myoclonic epilepsies are a heterogeneous group of genetic disorders. Inborn errors of metabolism are usually the cause. The main features are myoclonus, epilepsy, cognitive impairment, and progressive neurological deterioration. The rate and degree of progression varies between disorders. As the underlying biochemical abnormalities are established, the disorders have been classified as inborn errors of metabolism rather than as progressive myoclonic encephalopathies.

Status Epilepticus
The definition of status epilepticus is a seizure continuing for longer than 30 minutes or seizures that recur over 30 minutes without the patient regaining consciousness between seizures. Status epilepticus is a medical emergency that requires prompt vigorous treatment.

CLINICAL FEATURES Any type of seizure can evolve into status epilepticus. The most commonly recognized form of status epilepticus is the generalized tonic-clonic, or convulsive, type. Most common are repeated tonic-clonic seizures lasting 2–3 minutes, without the individual regaining consciousness between seizures; however, continuous seizures also occur. Characteristic of generalized nonconvulsive (absence) status epilepticus is stupor, a confused state, or clouding of consciousness, and little or no motor activity.

EPIDEMIOLOGY The annual number of cases of status epilepticus in the United States is between 100,000 and 150,000.

Approximately one half occur in young children, but adults older than 60 years have a high risk. Status epilepticus occurs in three settings: (1) patients who sustain an acute process that affects the brain, such as metabolic disturbances, hypoxia, CNS infection, head trauma, or drug intoxication, (2) in epileptic patients having an exacerbation of seizures, often caused by abrupt reduction in antiepileptic medication, and (3) as a first unprovoked seizure, often heralding the onset of epilepsy.

MANAGEMENT The main goals of treatment are to maintain stable vital functions, prevent systemic complications, terminate seizure activity, and evaluate for and treat underlying causes of the prolonged seizures. Time is a critical factor in the treatment of status epilepticus. Evaluation and treatment should proceed quickly and in an organized manner. The initial steps are a rapid assessment and stabilization of cardiovascular and respiratory function. The intent of a brief history and physical examination is to identify an immediate and potentially treatable cause. Table 42.3 outlines the recommended method for managing status epilepticus. Table 42.4 lists the drugs available for treatment.

CAUSES OF SEIZURES

Almost all diseases and injuries of the brain can cause symptomatic epilepsy. This section is limited to conditions not fully discussed elsewhere.

Posttraumatic Epilepsy

Head trauma increases the susceptibility to subsequent seizures. The onset may be early (< 1 week) and late (> 1 week) after the injury. Risk factors for early seizures are the severity of the injury, frontoparietal location, depressed skull fracture, intracranial hematoma, and young age. Young children have the highest risk of early posttraumatic seizures, and the risk progressively decreases through adult life. Risk factors for late-onset posttraumatic epilepsy are the type and severity of injury, the occurrence of early posttraumatic seizures, and intracranial hematoma. A loading dose of phenytoin in the first 24 hours after injury, followed by maintenance therapy with phenytoin, decreases the rate of seizures within the first week but has no effect on the risk of later seizures.

Psychogenic Seizures

Psychogenic seizures are emotionally triggered, episodic non-epileptic events or spells that can be extremely difficult to

Table 42.3: A suggested timetable for the treatment of status epilepticus*

Time (min)	Action
0–5	Diagnose status epilepticus by observing continued seizure activity or one additional seizure.
	Give oxygen by nasal cannula or mask; position patient's head for optimal airway patency; consider any abnormalities as necessary; initiate ECG monitoring.
	Obtain and record vital signs at onset and periodically thereafter; control any abnormalities as necessary; initiate ECG monitoring.
	Establish IV access; draw venous blood samples for glucose level, serum chemistries, hematology studies, toxicology screens, and determinations of antiepileptic drug levels.
	Assess oxygenation with oximetry or periodic arterial blood gas determinations.
6–10	If hypoglycemia is established or a blood glucose determination is unavailable, administer glucose; in adults, give 100 mg of thiamine first, followed by 50 ml of 50% glucose by direct push into the IV line; in children, the dose of glucose is 2 ml/kg of 25% glucose.
5–20	Administer either lorazepam, 0.1 mg/kg IV at 2 mg/min, or diazepam, 0.2 mg/kg IV at 5 mg/min. If diazepam is given, it can be repeated if seizures do not stop after 5 minutes; if diazepam is used to stop the status, phenytoin should be administered next to prevent recurrent status.
10–30	If status persists, administer phenytoin, 15–20 mg/kg IV, no faster than 50 mg/min in adults and 1 mg/kg/min IV in children; monitor ECG and blood pressure during the infusion; phenytoin is incompatible with glucose-containing solutions; the IV line should be purged with normal saline before the phenytoin infusion. Alternatively, fosphenytoin, 20 mg/kg phenytoin equivalents at 150 mg/min in adults or 3 mg/kg/min in children, can be used.
20–40	If status does not stop after 20 mg/kg of phenytoin or fosphenytoin, give additional doses of 5–10 mg/kg of phenytoin or fosphenytoin to a maximum dose of 30 mg/kg.

Continued

Table 42.3: (continued)

Time (min)	Action
40–60	If status persists, give phenobarbital, 20 mg/kg IV at 50–100 mg/min; when phenobarbital is given after a benzodiazepine, the risk of apnea or hypopnea is great, and assisted ventilation is usually required. If seizures continue, give an additional 5–10 mg/kg of phenobarbital.
> 60–70	If status persists, give anesthetic doses of drugs such as midazolam (loading dose of 0.2 mg/kg by slow IV bolus, then 0.75–10.00 µg/kg/min), propofol (loading dose of 12 mg/kg IV, followed by 2–10 mg/kg/hr) or pentobarbital (5–15 mg/kg IV bolus over 1 hr, followed by 0.5–3.0 mg/kg/hr); ventilatory assistance and vasopressors are virtually always necessary. Continuous EEG monitoring is indicated throughout therapy, with the primary end point being suppression of EEG spikes or a burst-suppression pattern with short intervals between bursts.

*Time starts at seizure onset. Note that a neurological consultation is indicated if the patient does not wake up, convulsions continue after the administration of a benzodiazepine and phenytoin, or confusion exists at any time during evaluation and treatment.

ECG = electrocardiogram; EEG = electroencephalogram; IV = intravenous.
Source: Modified with permission from Dodson, W. E., Delorenzo, R. J., Pedley, T. A., et al. 1993, "Treatment of convulsive status epilepticus—recommendations of the Epilepsy Foundation of America's Working Group on Status Epilepticus," *JAMA*, vol. 270, pp. 854–859.

distinguish from epileptic seizures. They occur in people with and without epilepsy.

Diagnosis
Four patterns of behavior occur during psychogenic seizures: (1) sustained or repetitive muscular contractions that can be unilateral or bilateral, (2) muscle inactivity or loss of tone, (3) unresponsiveness without the presence of other observable behavioral phenomena, and (4) unresponsiveness in association with apparently purposeful or semipurposeful or apparently automatic or semiautomatic behaviors.

Although no rule works consistently, the following features are more likely to occur in psychogenic than in epileptic seizures: (1) gradual onset or progression from the initial symptoms to the complete episode, (2) symptoms such as palpitations,

Table 42.4: Major drugs used to treat status epilepticus: intravenous doses, pharmacokinetics, and major toxicity

	Diazepam	Lorazepam	Phenytoin	Phenobarbital
Adult IV dose in mg/kg (range [total dose])	0.15–0.25 (10 mg)	0.1 (48 mg)	15–20	20
Pediatric IV dose in mg/kg (range [total dose])	0.1–1.0 (10 mg)	0.05–0.50 (14 mg)	20	20
Pediatric per rectum dose in mg/kg	0.2–0.5 (20 mg maximum)			
Maximal administration rate in mg/min	5.0	2.0	50	100
Time to stop status in minutes	1–3	6–10	10–30	20–30
Effective duration of action in hours	0.25–0.50	> 12–24	24	> 48
Potential side effects				
Depression of consciousness	10–30 min	Several hours	None	Several days
Respiratory depression	Occasional	Occasional	Uncommon	Occasional
Hypertension	Uncommon	Uncommon	Occasional	Uncommon
Cardiac arrhythmia			In patients with heart disease	

Source: Modified with permission from Dodson, W. E., Delorenzo, R. J., Pedley, T. A., et al. 1993, "Treatment of convulsive status epilepticus—recommendations of the Epilepsy Foundation of America's Working Group on Status Epilepticus," *JAMA,* vol. 270, pp. 854–859.

malaise, choking, dizziness, or acral paresthesias, (3) quivering, side-to-side movements of the head, pelvic thrusting, and uncontrolled flailing, thrashing, or nonsynchronous rhythmic movements of the limbs, and (4) quasi-volitional speech or movements in response to observers during periods of apparent unresponsiveness. The presence of interictal epileptiform activity in the EEG does not rule out the diagnosis of psychogenic seizures because epileptic seizures and psychogenic seizures may coexist in the same patient. The ictal EEG, preferably with video monitoring, usually can distinguish psychogenic from epileptic seizures.

Treatment
Present the patient with an established diagnosis of pseudoseizures in an extended and supportive counseling session. During the session, explain the differential diagnosis, the psychogenic basis, and the treatment alternatives. Stop anticonvulsants if there is no evidence of epilepsy.

Catamenial Epilepsy

Catamenial epilepsy is the clustering of seizures in relation to the menstrual cycle. The physiological basis of catamenial epilepsy relates to the activating effects of estrogens on seizures and the suppressive effects of progesterone on epileptiform discharges. Seizure exacerbation occurs in three basic patterns: (1) during the perimenstrual phase, (2) during the periovulatory phase, and (3) during the entire second half of the menstrual period. Charting the frequency of seizures over the menstrual period helps to determine the pattern and to plan therapy. Progesterone is used for treatment, but other treatments can be considered.

EVALUATION OF SEIZURES

The goals of the evaluation of the individual who presents with paroxysmal episodes or events are to (1) determine whether the individual has epilepsy, (2) correctly characterize the type of seizures and, if possible, identify a specific syndrome, (3) identify potential causes of the seizures, (4) determine the course of treatment, if needed, and (5) provide the individual and interested parties a guide for the course of the disorder. The evaluation should proceed in a systematic fashion.

History and Physical Examination

Always obtain the history by direct contact with witnesses who saw the event. An inadequate or faulty description is the leading cause of misdiagnosis. A home video of the spell often provides the diagnosis. Thoroughly investigate a family history of seizures, often requiring contact with grandparents and children. Direct special attention toward examination of the skin for neurocutaneous disorders, dysmorphic features for chromosome disorders, and subtle impairments or asymmetries of fine motor skills and coordination.

Laboratory Studies

Electroencephalographic Monitoring

Routine EEG should be recorded during awake and sleep to maximize the chance of seeing epileptiform activity. When routine EEG findings are normal, recommend the use of ambulatory recordings. When the diagnosis remains in doubt, consider inpatient evaluation with continuous video/EEG monitoring.

Neuroimaging

Magnetic resonance imaging is the most important imaging technique in the evaluation of the patient with seizures, particularly the partial epilepsies. High-resolution structural scanning can assist in the detection of pathological abnormalities in up to 90% of patients with intractable epilepsy. It is particularly useful in the diagnosis of mesial temporal sclerosis and hippocampal atrophy ipsilateral to the epileptogenic region.

Functional Studies

Positron emission tomography and single-photon emission computed tomography permit physiological evaluation of patients with epilepsy. Hypometabolic areas in the interictal period correlate well with areas of seizure onset.

PRINCIPLES OF TREATMENT

Initiation of Therapy

Critical to the decision to treat is determining whether the individual has epilepsy. Some treatment failures result from the misdiagnosis of nonepileptic paroxysmal events. Once the diagnosis is established, correct identification of the seizure type and epileptic syndrome is critical to the choice of treatment. Other than the benign epilepsies of childhood, epilepsy usually is a chronic condition that does not remit spontaneously and requires treatment. On the other hand, depending on the clinical situation, lifelong treatment is not always necessary.

The following basic principals increase the likelihood of achieving seizure control without drug toxicity:

1. Use a single drug whenever possible.
2. Increase the dose of that drug to either seizure control or toxicity (decreasing the dose if toxicity occurs).
3. If a drug fails to control seizures without toxicity, switch to another appropriate drug used alone and again increase the dose until seizure control occurs or toxicity intervenes.
4. Remember that the "therapeutic drug range" is a guideline and not an absolute. Some patients achieve seizure control with blood concentrations below the range, and others tolerate concentrations above the range without toxicity.
5. Use two drugs only when monotherapy has failed. Some patients may have more seizures when taking two drugs, compared with one drug, because of drug interactions.
6. Be aware that the ability to metabolize anticonvulsant drugs is different in the young, the elderly, pregnant women, and people with certain chronic diseases, especially hepatic and renal disease, compared with healthy nonpregnant adults.
7. Routine schedules of laboratory monitoring are recommended for all antiepileptic medications in common use. Routine testing, however, does not detect or prevent severe reactions, most of which are idiosyncratic.

Choice of Medication

The primary basis for choosing an anticonvulsant drug is efficacy against a specific seizure type. Other considerations are expense, dosing schedule, and available preparations. Table 42.5 summarizes available drugs.

Surgery for Epilepsy

A subset of individuals with intractable seizures, estimated to be less than 5%, may be candidates for surgery. *Focal cortical resections*, usually involving the temporal lobe, are the most common surgical procedures for the treatment of epilepsy. The tissue removed is usually limited to only a portion of the temporal lobe, depending on the seizure focus and the underlying pathology. *Multiple subpial resections* are performed when a seizure focus is in or near a region of functional cerebral cortex. *Hemispherectomy* is useful when the seizure focus is not localized but is limited to one hemisphere. Examples are Sturge-Weber syndrome and Rasmussen's encephalitis. *Corpus callosotomy* is used to interrupt pathways of spread of seizure

Table 42.5: Antiepileptic drugs approved for use in North America, Europe, or Japan

Drug	F (%)	T_{max} (hr)	Protein Binding (%)	Route of Elimination	$T_{[1/2]}$ (hr)	T_{ss} (days)	Dose Range (mg/kg)	Target plasma drug concentration (range) mg/liter	µmol/liter
Carbamazepine	75–85	4–12	75	Hepatic	20–50 days† / 5–20 days†	20–30	10–30	3–12	12–50
Clobazam	>90	1–4	85	Hepatic	10–30		0.5–2.0	NA	NA
Norclobazam					36–46	10			
Clonazepam	>90	1–4	85	Hepatic	20–40	6	0.1–0.15	NA	NA
Ethosuximide	>90	1–4	<10	Hepatic	30–60	7	10–40	40–100	300–700
Felbamate	>90	2–6	25	Renal 90%	14–23	4	40–80	30–100	120–400
Gabapentin	35–60	2–3	0	Renal	5–9	1–2	30–40	4–16	20–100
Lamotrigine	>90	1–3	55	Hepatic	15–60	3–10	1–15	2–20	8–80
Levetiracetam	>90	0.6–1.3	<10	Renal	7	2	20–60	20–60	115–350
Lorazepam	>90	1.5–2.0	90	Hepatic	15	3	0.03	NA	NA
Oxcarbazepine	>95	1–2		Hepatic	2	2	15–30		
MHD*		3–5	40		10–15			5–50*	20–200*
Phenobarbital	>90	0.5–4.0	45	Hepatic	65–110	15–20	2–5	10–30	40–130
Phenytoin	>90	2–12	90	Hepatic	10–60§	15–20	5–10	3–20	12–80
Primidone	>90	2–4	<20	Hepatic	8–15	15–20	10–20		

Continued

Table 42.5: (continued)

Drug	F (%)	T_{max} (hr)	Protein Binding (%)	Route of Elimination	$T_{[1/2]}$ (hr)	T_{ss} (days)	Dose Range (mg/kg)	Target plasma drug concentration (range)	
								mg/liter	μmol/liter
Tiagabine	>90	1–2	96	Hepatic	2–9	1–2	0.1–1	5–70	12–170
Topiramate	>80	1–4	15	Renal 70%	12–30	3–5	5–9	2–25	6–75
Valproic acid	>90	1–8‡	70–93	Hepatic	5–15	2	15–30	50–100	350–700
Vigabatrin	80	0.5–2.0	0	Renal	5–7	2	40–100		
Zonisamide	>90	2–5	55	Hepatic	50–70	10–15	4–8	10–40	45–180

F = fraction absorbed, bioavailability; NA = not applicable; T_{max} = time interval between ingestion and maximal serum concentration;
$T_{[1/2]}$ = elimination half-life; T_{ss} = steady-state time.
*Monohydroxy derivative, 10-OH-carbamazepine.
†Concentration dependent.
‡Absorption of enteric coated tablet is delayed.
§Steady-state values for half-life and serum levels are reached only after complete autoinduction.

activity, rather than to eliminate the focus. Indications for callosotomy are not clearly defined.

Vagal Nerve Stimulation

Vagal nerve stimulation is an approved procedure for the adjunctive treatment of refractory partial onset seizures in adults and adolescents older than 12 years. The mechanism of action is unknown. Placement of the device is surgical and it is usually well tolerated. Adverse effects during stimulation include hoarseness or voice alteration, throat pain, coughing, dyspnea, paresthesia, and muscle pain.

For a more detailed discussion, see Chapter 73 in Neurology in Clinical Practice, 4th edition.

Sleep and Its Disorders

43

NORMAL SLEEP

The Normal Sleep-Wake Cycle

In adults, sleep is usually consolidated in one single episode during each day-night cycle. Night sleep consists of two main phases: non–rapid eye movement (NREM) and rapid eye movement (REM) sleep. The equivalent phases in infancy are quiet and active sleep. NREM sleep is divided into four stages characterized by a progressive increase in sleep depth and an increase in the strength of stimulus necessary to cause arousal: Stage 1 is drowsiness with loss of the posterior dominant rhythm; the occurrence of sleep spindles signals stage 2; stage 3 contains a greater abundance of slow waves; and stage 4 is characterized by more than 50% of delta activity.

NREM sleep stages occupy the first 60–90 minutes of sleep and are followed by the first REM sleep cycle of the night. During a complete nocturnal sleep cycle, approximately four to six NREM-REM cycles occur. Stages 3 and 4 of NREM sleep are most intense during early sleep cycles. REM stages last longer in the second half of the night. In REM sleep, electroencephalographic (EEG) findings look like those of wakefulness.

Evolution of Sleep Patterns with Age
Sleep requirements change dramatically from infancy to old age. Newborns have a polyphasic sleep pattern, with 16 hours of sleep a day. The sleep requirement decreases to approximately 10 hours a day by 3–5 years of age. In preschool children, sleep assumes a biphasic pattern. Adults exhibit a monophasic sleep pattern, with an average duration of 7.5–8.0 hours a night but changes back to a biphasic pattern in old age.

Sleep Habits
Two groups of individuals are recognized: evening types and morning types. Evening types (*owls*) have difficulty getting up

early and feel tired in the morning; however, they feel fresh and energetic toward the end of the day. These people perform best in the evening; they go to sleep late and wake up late. In contrast, morning types (*larks*) wake up early, rested and refreshed, and work efficiently in the morning. Owls and larks are determined by genetic factors.

Circadian Rhythm

The human body has an internal biological clock. Dysfunction of circadian rhythm results in several important human sleep disorders. The two types of sleepiness are physiological and subjective. Physiological sleepiness is the body's propensity to sleepiness. The two highly vulnerable periods of sleepiness are 2:00–6:00 AM and 2:00–6:00 PM. Physiological sleepiness depends on homeostatic factor and circadian phase. *Homeostatic factor* refers to a prior period of wakefulness and sleep debt. The circadian factor determines the body's propensity to maximal sleepiness, between 3:00 AM and 5:00 AM. The second period of maximal sleepiness (3:00–5:00 PM) is not as strong as the first.

CAUSES OF EXCESSIVE DAYTIME SLEEPINESS

Excessive sleepiness may result from both physiological and pathological causes. Sleep deprivation and sleepiness because of lifestyle and habits of going to sleep and waking up at irregular hours can be considered to result from disruption of the normal circadian and homeostatic physiology.

Neurological Causes of Excessive Sleepiness

Tumors and vascular lesions affecting the ascending reticular activating arousal system and its projections to the posterior hypothalamus and thalamus lead to daytime sleepiness. Lesions of this system often cause coma rather than just sleepiness. Symptomatic narcolepsy may result from craniopharyngioma and other tumors of the hypothalamic and pituitary regions. Cataplexy associated with sleepiness, sleep paralysis, and hypnagogic hallucinations occurs in patients with rostral brainstem gliomas with or without infiltration of the walls of the third ventricle. Other neurological causes of excessive daytime sleepiness (EDS) include bilateral paramedian thalamic infarcts, posttraumatic hypersomnolence, and multiple sclerosis.

CLASSIFICATION OF SLEEP DISORDERS

The International Classification of Sleep Disorders (ICSD) is used by sleep specialists. Sleep disorders are grouped into four broad categories: dyssomnias, parasomnias, sleep disorders associated with medical or psychiatric disorders, and proposed sleep disorders. *Dyssomnias* are subdivided into intrinsic, extrinsic, and circadian rhythm sleep disorders. Intrinsic disorders result from causes in the body, whereas extrinsic disorders are primarily caused by environmental factors. Circadian rhythm disorders result from disruption of sleep-wake schedule changes. Abnormal movements and behavior intruding into sleep without necessarily disturbing sleep architecture characterize *parasomnias*.

CLINICAL PHENOMENOLOGY

Insomnia

Insomnia is a symptom rather than a disease and is characterized by an inadequate amount of sleep or impaired quality of sleep. Insomnia is divided into transient (1 week), short term (1–3 weeks), and chronic (>3 weeks). The symptoms of insomnia often interfere with interpersonal relationships or job performance. Insomnia is a heterogeneous condition that results from various factors. Factors that result in transient or short-term insomnia are similar, but the disturbances that produce short-term insomnia are of greater magnitude. Causes of transient and short-term insomnia include a change of sleeping environment, jet lag, unpleasant room temperature, stressful life events, acute medical or surgical illnesses, stimulant medications, or withdrawal of central nervous system–depressant medications.

Chronic insomnia can be caused by the chronic use of drugs or alcohol; medical, neurological, or psychiatric disorders; or several primary sleep disorders. Insomnia commonly coexists with or precedes the development of several psychiatric illnesses. Some patients with chronic insomnia have either idiopathic or psychophysiological insomnia or insomnia as a symptom of another primary sleep disorder.

Idiopathic Insomnia
Idiopathic or primary insomnia, previously called *childhood-onset insomnia*, is defined as a lifelong difficulty in initiating and maintaining sleep, resulting in poor daytime functioning. The cause of this syndrome is unknown.

Psychophysiological Insomnia
Psychophysiological insomnia is defined as a chronic insomnia resulting from learned sleep-preventing associations and increased tension or agitation. Onset is in young adults and symptoms persist for decades.

Sleep-State Misperception
In sleep-state misperception, subjects complain of sleeplessness but without objective evidence. Despite complaints of no sleep or poor sleep over many years, studies document a normal sleep pattern.

Inadequate Sleep Hygiene
Good "sleep hygiene" includes avoidance of caffeinated beverages, alcohol, and tobacco in the evening, avoidance of intense mental activities and vigorous exercise close to bedtime, avoidance of daytime naps and excessive time spent in bed, and adherence to a regular sleep-wake schedule.

Insufficient Sleep Syndrome
Insufficient sleep is probably the most common cause of sleepiness in the general population. It results from various factors, such as lifestyle, competitive drive to perform that sacrifices sleep, and environmental light and sound. Chronic sleep deprivation may lead to daytime sleepiness, irritability, lack of concentration, decreased daytime performance, muscle aches and pains, or depression.

Altitude Insomnia
Altitude insomnia refers to sleeplessness that develops in some individuals on ascent to altitudes higher than 4000 m in conjunction with other features of acute mountain sickness, such as fatigue, headache, and loss of appetite.

Narcolepsy

Epidemiology, Genetics, and Family Studies in Narcolepsy
Both genetic and environmental factors contribute to the development of narcolepsy. The mode of inheritance is thought to be autosomal dominant in humans, recessive in Doberman pinschers (*canarc*-1) and Labrador retrievers, and multifactorial in poodles.

Clinical Features
The syndrome of narcolepsy is a lifelong neurological condition that generally begins in an adolescent or young adult with sleep attacks. Peak incidence occurs at ages 15–20 years. The typical sequence of symptom onset is (1) EDS and sleep attacks, (2)

cataplexy, and (3) sleep paralysis. *Sleep attacks* are an irresistible desire to fall asleep. The attacks may occur under inappropriate circumstances and in inappropriate places. They are generally brief, lasting for a few minutes to 15–30 minutes, and on awakening the patient usually feels fresh. *Cataplexy* is characterized by sudden loss of tone in the voluntary muscles, except for respiratory and ocular muscles. The cataplectic attacks are often triggered by emotional factors, such as laughter, rage, and anger. *Sleep paralysis* is a sudden unilateral or bilateral limb paralysis during sleep onset at night (*hypnagogic*) or while awakening (*hypnopompic*) in the morning. The patient is conscious but is unable to move or speak. *Hypnagogic hallucinations* occur either at the onset of sleep or while awakening early in the morning. The hallucinations are vivid, often fearful visual imagery. Disturbance of night sleep, together with the four major manifestations, may be termed the *narcoleptic pentad*. *Automatic behavior* is found in 20–40% of patients. During these episodes, the patient performs the same function repetitively, speaks or writes in a meaningless manner, drives on the wrong side of the road, or drives to a strange place and then forgets the episodes.

Diagnosis

Diagnosis depends primarily on clinical history. Sleep studies usually show REM activity occurring within 15 minutes of sleep onset, compared with 60–90 minutes in normal people. Human leukocyte antigen studies and decreased cerebrospinal fluid hypocretin-1 help to confirm the diagnosis.

Management

The administration of stimulants, such as modafinil, pemoline, methylphenidate, dextroamphetamine, or methamphetamine, is the treatment of choice for narcoleptic sleep attacks. Modafinil, a novel wake-promoting agent, is frequently used as the initial treatment. The treatment of cataplexy is with tricyclic antidepressants, such as protriptyline, imipramine, and clomipramine (10–200 mg per day). Sodium oxybate (γ-hydroxybutyrate) in 3–9 g nightly doses is effective for treating cataplexy and narcoleptic sleep attacks. Nonpharmacological treatment of narcolepsy includes general sleep hygiene measures, sodium, short daytime naps, and joining narcolepsy support groups.

Sleep Apnea Syndrome

Sleep apnea is cessation of breathing during sleep. Two main types of apnea are distinguished by respiratory measurements. *Obstructive apnea* (upper-airway apnea) is the more common variety. The diaphragm and chest wall move with changes in intrathoracic pressure, but obstruction prevents airflow at the nose or mouth. In *central apnea*, all respiratory movements are absent, and oronasal airflow is absent. Many apneic episodes have a central component followed by an obstructive component (*mixed apneas*).

Causes of Sleep Apnea

Mechanical obstruction to the upper airway is the most common cause of sleep apnea. Oropharyngeal narrowing may be caused by bone, joint, muscle, or soft tissue abnormality. *Failure of central respiratory motor neuron output* mechanisms with hypoventilation, sometimes accompanied by sleep apnea, occurs with brainstem lesions. Many neuromuscular disorders are accompanied by weakness or stiffness of respiratory muscles, as well as by obstruction of the upper airway. Severe sleep apnea, with both obstructive and central episodes, occurs in approximately one third of subjects with myotonic dystrophy. Failure of respiratory sensory mechanisms occurs with loss of chemoreceptor control systems. Subjects with the Shy-Drager syndrome, multisystem atrophy, and other dysautonomias and related degenerative brainstem disorders may develop sleep apnea.

Symptoms

The main features of obstructive sleep apnea are snoring, typically present for many years, and frequent arousals from sleep for which the subject is usually amnesic. A witness is necessary for diagnosis. The cardiovascular and cerebral consequences of obstructive sleep apnea range from hypoxia to sudden death. The main daytime symptom is EDS.

In central sleep apnea syndromes, snoring and restlessness are less marked or absent, although frequent apneas occur with or without arousal. The presenting complaint may be insomnia, not daytime sleepiness as in obstructive sleep apnea syndromes.

Signs

Physical examination should include assessment of respiratory, oropharyngeal, neurological, hematological, and cardiovascular functions. Examination of the oropharyngeal region may detect redundant oropharyngeal tissues, such as large edematous uvula, redundant mucosal folds of the pharyngeal walls, low-hanging long soft palate, or large tonsils and adenoids, especially in children. Other findings may include macroglossia, micrognathia, and retrognathia. Examination reveals obesity in about 70% of cases.

Management of Obstructive Sleep Apnea

The management of the obstructive sleep apnea syndrome involves the treatment of associated medical conditions, reduction of risk factors, and the use of mechanical appliances. The indications for treatment include disabling daytime sleepiness, sleep hypoxia with decreases in arterial oxygen saturation, the presence of pulmonary hypertension or cardiac arrhythmia, extremely heavy snoring with other symptoms, systemic hypertension, polycythemia, right ventricular failure, psychiatric problems, and impotence.

Nasal continuous positive airway pressure (CPAP) is an effective and common treatment, and many systems are available for long-term home use. Several airway patency devices are available that hold the jaw forward to prevent tongue prolapse or to increase nares diameter. The usefulness of these devices is limited. Surgical reconstruction of the palate and oropharynx can abolish snoring, but its benefits in sleep apnea are uncertain.

Restless Legs Syndrome

Restless legs syndrome (RLS) is idiopathic in most cases but may occur secondary to conditions such as iron deficiency, uremia, or polyneuropathy. The hallmark of idiopathic or primary RLS is intense, disagreeable creeping sensations (paresthesia or dysesthesia) in the legs that are relieved by moving. Symptoms are worse when lying down in the evening and occur most commonly at sleep onset. Affected patients generally have severe difficulty in initiating sleep because of paresthesias and restlessness of the legs. Severely affected individuals may also have paresthesias during the day when resting or sitting quietly. Neurological examination findings in the idiopathic form of RLS are generally normal. The condition may be exacerbated during pregnancy or by caffeine or iron deficiency. Family history is positive in 40–50% of the patients, which suggests a dominant mode of inheritance. The nonergot dopamine agonists, pramipexole and ropinirole, are safe and effective treatments for RLS.

Periodic Limb Movement of Sleep

Periodic limb movement of sleep (PLMS) is a polysomnographic finding and is characterized by periodically recurring limb movements during NREM sleep. Most patients dorsiflex the ankles and flex the knees and hips every 20–40 seconds. Most also experience RLS.

Circadian Rhythm Sleep Disorders

Circadian rhythm sleep disorders result from a mismatch between the body's internal clock and the geophysical environment either because of malfunction in the biological clock (primary circadian rhythm disorders) or because the clock is out of phase because of a shift in environment (secondary circadian dysrhythmias). Jet lag and shift work are two common sources of secondary circadian dysrhythmias resulting from exogenous factors.

Circadian rhythm sleep disorders may be treated by the use of chronotherapy, phototherapy, or both. *Chronotherapy* refers to the intentional delay of sleep onset by 2–3 hours on successive days until the desired bedtime has been achieved. After this, the patient strictly enforces the sleep-wake schedule.

Parasomnias

Parasomnias can be defined as abnormal movements or behavior intruding into sleep during the night intermittently or episodically without disturbing the sleep architecture. No special treatment is needed for most of the parasomnias. The subjects with partial arousal disorders (e.g., sleepwalking, sleep terrors, and confusional arousals) must be protected from injury to self or others by arranging furniture, using a padded mattress, and paying particular attention to doors and windows. If attacks of sleepwalking or sleep terrors occur frequently, treatment with an antidepressant (e.g., imipramine) or small doses of a benzodiazepine (e.g., clonazepam) may be tried for a short period.

Somnambulism (Sleepwalking)

Sleepwalking is common in children between 5 and 12 years of age. Sometimes it persists in adulthood or (rarely) begins in adults. Sleepwalking begins with abrupt motor activity arising out of slow-wave sleep during the first one third of sleep. Episodes generally last less than 10 minutes. Family history is often present. Injuries and violent actions have been reported during sleepwalking episodes, but generally individuals can negotiate their way around a room. Sleep deprivation, fatigue, concurrent illness, and sedatives may act as precipitating factors.

Sleep Terrors

Sleep terrors occur during slow-wave sleep. Peak onset is between 5 and 7 years of age. As with sleepwalking, familial cases are common. Episodes of sleep terrors are characterized by intense autonomic and motor symptoms, including a loud piercing scream. Patients appear highly confused and fearful.

Many also have a history of sleepwalking episodes. Precipitating factors are similar to those described for sleepwalking.

Hypnic Jerks

Hypnic jerks, or "sleep starts," occur at sleep onset in many normal individuals and are physiological phenomena without any pathological significance. The episodes are associated with sudden brief myoclonic jerks of the limbs or the whole body, lasting for a few seconds. Sometimes these are accompanied by sensory phenomena, such as a sensation of falling. These may be triggered by stress, fatigue, or sleep deprivation. "Sleep starts" may occur in up to 70% of the general population.

Rhythmic Movement Disorder

Rhythmic movement disorder is noted mostly before 18 months of age and is occasionally associated with mental retardation. It is a sleep-wake transition disorder with three characteristic movements: head banging, head rolling, and body rocking. Rhythmic movement disorder is a benign condition, and the patient outgrows the episodes.

Nocturnal Leg Cramps

Intensely painful sensations accompanied by muscle tightness occur during sleep. The spasms usually last for a few seconds but sometimes persist for several minutes. Cramps during sleep are generally associated with awakening. Many normal individuals have nocturnal leg cramps; the cause remains unknown. Local massage or movement of the limbs usually relieves the cramps.

Nightmares (Dream Anxiety Attacks)

Nightmares are fearful, vivid, and often frightening dreams, mostly visual but sometimes auditory, seen during REM sleep. Nightmares may accompany sleep talking and body movements. These most commonly occur during the middle to late part of sleep at night. Nightmares are mostly a normal phenomenon. Up to 50% of children, perhaps even more, have nightmares beginning at age 3–5 years. The frequency of nightmares continues to decrease as the child grows older, and the elderly have very few or no nightmares.

Rapid Eye Movement Sleep Behavior Disorder

REM sleep behavior disorder (RBD) is an important REM sleep parasomnia commonly seen in elderly persons. A characteristic feature of RBD is intermittent loss of REM-related muscle hypotonia or atonia and the appearance of various abnormal motor activities during sleep. Violent dream-enacting behavior occurs during REM sleep, often causing self-injury or injury to the bed partner. RBD may be idiopathic or secondary. Most cases are now thought to be secondary and associated with neurodegenerative diseases, especially parkinsonism.

Bruxism (Tooth Grinding)
Bruxism frequently presents between the ages of 10 and 20 years, but it may persist throughout life, often leading to secondary problems such as temporomandibular joint (TMJ) syndrome. Nocturnal bruxism is noted most prominently during NREM stages I and II and REM sleep. An episode is characterized by stereotypical tooth grinding and is often precipitated by anxiety, stress, and dental disease. Local injections into masseter muscles may be used to prevent dental and TMJ syndrome complications.

LABORATORY ASSESSMENT OF SLEEP DISORDERS

The two most important laboratory tests for diagnosis of sleep disturbance are polysomnographic (PSG) study and the multiple sleep latency test (MSLT). An overnight PSG study is the single most important laboratory test for the diagnosis and the treatment of patients with sleep disorders, particularly those associated with EDS. All-night PSG study is required rather than a single-day nap study. A daytime single-nap study generally misses REM sleep. A PSG study is routinely indicated for the diagnosis of sleep-related breathing disorders, for CPAP titration in patients with sleep-related breathing disorders, and for the evaluation of the presence of obstructive sleep apnea in patients before they undergo laser-assisted uvulopalatopharyngoplasty.

The MSLT is important for documenting excessive sleepiness objectively. The test has been standardized and is performed after an overnight PSG study. The test consists of four to five daytime recordings of EEG, electromyogram, and electro-oculogram at 2-hour intervals, each recording lasting up to 20 minutes. The test measures the average sleep-onset latency (timed to the first epoch of any sleep stage for the clinical purpose) and sleep-onset REMs.

For a more detailed discussion, see Chapter 74 in Neurology in Clinical Practice, 4th edition.

Headache and Other Craniofacial Pain

44

Population-based studies have estimated that the lifetime prevalence for any type of headache is in excess of 90% for men and 95% for women. A survey of a sample of 20,000 households in the United States revealed a prevalence rate of migraine of 18.2% in females and a 6.5% rate among males, resulting in an estimated 27.9 million migraine sufferers in the United States.

CLASSIFICATION

Table 44.1 lists the 14 main headache types. Until the actual pathogenesis of primary headache syndromes is determined, it will not be possible to develop a unitary classification of head pain.

HEADACHE ATTRIBUTED TO NONVASCULAR, NONINFECTIOUS INTRACRANIAL DISORDERS

Intracranial lesions that occupy space, often referred to as *mass lesions*, produce head pain by traction on, or compression of, pain-sensitive structures. The nature, location, and temporal profile of headache produced by an intracranial mass depend on many factors, including the location of the lesion, its rate of growth, its effect on the cerebrospinal fluid (CSF) pathways, and any associated cerebral edema. The intracranial mass lesion may be neoplastic, inflammatory, or cystic. Each type can result in either localized or generalized head pain. The type of headache is characteristic of raised intracranial pressure (ICP) but is not diagnostic of a particular underlying disease.

Table 44.1: Classification of headache

The Primary Headaches
    1. Migraine
    2. Tension-type headache
    3. Cluster headache and other trigeminal-autonomic cephalalgias
    4. Other primary headache disorders
The Secondary Headaches
    5. Headache attributed to head and/or neck trauma
    6. Headache attributed to cranial and/or cervical vascular disorder
    7. Headache attributed to nonvascular, noninfectious intracranial disorder
    8. Headache attributed to a substance or its withdrawal
    9. Headache attributed to infection
    10. Headache attributed to disturbance of homeostasis
    11. Headache or facial pain attributed to disorder of cranium, neck, eyes, ears, nose, sinuses, teeth, mouth, or other facial or cranial structures
    12. Headache attributed to psychiatric disorder
    13. Cranial neuralgias and central causes of facial pain
    14. Other headache, cranial neuralgia, central or primary facial pain

Source: Reprinted with permission from the International Headache Society Second Headache Classification Committee 2004. "The International Headache Classification, 2nd ed," *Cephalalgia*, vol. 24, suppl. 1, pp. 1-195.

The following features raise the possibility of an intracranial mass lesion:

1. Headache is subacute and progressive in nature.
2. Onset is at older than 40 years.
3. Change in headache pattern, such as increased intensity of pain, increased frequency of attacks, development of new features, or decreased response to treatment.
4. Association with any of the following: nausea or vomiting not explained by migraine or systemic illness; nocturnal occurrence or morning awakening; precipitation or worsening by changes in posture or Valsalva maneuver; confusion, seizures, or weakness.
5. Neurological examination findings are not normal.

Whether raised ICP, in the absence of a shift of intracranial structures, results in headache is uncertain. Factors that determine pain production are the rate of pressure elevation and its duration. Obstructive hydrocephalus results from lesions that prevent the free egress of CSF from the ventricular system. The pain is often worse on awakening, occipital in distribution, and associated with neck stiffness. Vomiting, blurred vision, and transitory obscuration of vision are caused by papilledema and failing vision by optic atrophy.

Low-Pressure Headache

The headache of lowered CSF pressure characteristically develops in the upright position and is rapidly relieved by recumbency. It most commonly occurs after lumbar puncture. An identical syndrome of headache caused by low CSF pressure can occur when fluid leaks through the cribriform plate, through the petrous bones, or through any basal skull defect.

Idiopathic Intracranial Hypertension

Headache, transitory visual obscuration, pulsatile tinnitus, and diplopia are the most common presenting symptoms of idiopathic intracranial hypertension (pseudotumor cerebri). The headache tends to be worse on awakening and aggravated by activity. The blurring and obscuring of vision result from raised ICP. Once magnetic resonance imaging (MRI) has excluded intracranial mass, lumbar puncture manometry confirms the high CSF pressure.

Transient Syndrome of Headache with Neurological Deficits and Cerebrospinal Fluid Lymphocytosis

A transitory syndrome characterized by recurrent episodes of headache accompanied by reversible neurological deficits and CSF pleocytosis was originally termed *migrainous syndrome with CSF pleocytosis*. One or more episodes of neurological deficits accompany moderate to severe headache and sometimes fever. Each episode lasts hours, with a total duration of the syndrome from 1 to 70 days. CSF abnormalities include a lymphocytic pleocytosis varying from 10–700 cells/mm^3, elevation of CSF protein concentration, and sometimes elevated opening pressure. MRI findings are normal, the etiology is unclear, and no treatment alters the self-limited course.

Headache Attributed to Infection

Inflammation of any pain-sensitive structures in the cranial cavity can produce headache. Meningitis and meningoencephalitis both have headache as a major symptom. The characteristics of the head pain depend on whether the infection is acute or chronic. Acute meningitis produces a severe headache with neck stiffness and other signs of meningismus, including photophobia and irritability. Pain is often retroorbital and worsened by moving the eyes. Chronic meningitis resulting from fungal or tuberculous infection can also lead to headache that may be severe and unrelenting. The headache of intracranial infection is nonspecific and is always a consideration, especially in those with a compromised immune state.

Sinusitis, mastoiditis, epidural or intraparenchymal abscess formation, and osteomyelitis of the skull can cause focal and generalized headache. The associated features suggest the diagnosis.

HEADACHE ATTRIBUTED TO CRANIAL AND/OR CERVICAL VASCULAR DISORDERS

Aneurysms, Arteriovenous Malformations, and Thunderclap Headache

Intracranial aneurysms and arteriovenous malformations (AVMs) are rarely responsible for headache unless they rupture. Rapid enlargement of an aneurysm may produce local pain by pressure on a cranial nerve or on other pain-sensitive structures. The term *thunderclap headache* describes a severe headache of instantaneous onset that may be a symptom of an expanded unruptured aneurysm or the sentinel bleed from an aneurysm or AVM. The cause is unknown in most patients. The headache reaches peak intensity by 30 seconds and lasts from hours to days. Headaches may recur over a 7-day period but do not recur regularly over subsequent weeks to months. Other conditions that present with thunderclap headache are cerebral venous sinus thrombosis, cervicocephalic arterial dissection, pituitary apoplexy, acute hypertensive crisis, and spontaneous intracranial hypotension.

Subarachnoid Hemorrhage

Rupture of an intracranial aneurysm or AVM results in a subarachnoid hemorrhage, with or without extension into the parenchyma of the brain. The headache of a subarachnoid hemorrhage is characteristically explosive and intense. Movement aggravates the headache; photophobia and phonophobia are associated. Relief of the intense headache generally requires parenteral analgesics.

Parenchymal Hemorrhage

A cerebral or cerebellar hemorrhage causes headache of rapid onset and increasing severity. The stretching and shifting of pain-sensitive fibers produce a traction headache. As the hematoma enlarges, it may obstruct the CSF circulation through the ventricular system and lead to increased ICP.

Cerebral Ischemia

Cerebral infarction, whether embolic or thrombotic, may cause head pain. Pain location does not predict the vascular territory involved. Cortical infarction is more likely associated with headache than deep cerebral hemisphere infarctions. It may be either steady or throbbing and is not as explosive or as severe as the headache of subarachnoid hemorrhage. Flashing lights, field defects, and other visual disturbances may represent symptoms of cerebrovascular disease and migraine. The migrainous aura tends to march across the visual field over the course of minutes and the headache follows a latent interval. The headache of cerebrovascular insufficiency or occlusion has a more variable relationship to the visual disturbances.

Carotid and Vertebral Artery Occlusion and Dissection

The combination of headache, ipsilateral Horner's syndrome, and contralateral hemiparesis is generally the result of carotid occlusion. The common clinical syndromes associated with carotid dissection include (1) hemicranial pain plus ipsilateral oculosympathetic palsy, (2) hemicranial pain and delayed focal cerebral ischemic symptoms, or (3) lower cranial nerve palsies, usually with ipsilateral headache or face pain. The most common symptom of vertebral dissection is headache and neck pain. The headache, with or without neck pain, is followed, after delay, by focal central nervous system ischemic symptoms.

Giant Cell Arteritis

Giant cell arteritis is a common and serious cause of headache in the elderly. It leads to permanent blindness if unrecognized and untreated. The clinical features of giant cell arteritis result from inflammation of medium and large arteries.

Clinical Features

Headache is the most common symptom, experienced by 72% of patients at some time, and is the initial symptom in 33%. It is sometimes associated with focal tenderness of the affected superficial temporal artery. More than one half of patients experience aching in proximal and axial joints, proximal myalgias, and often significant morning stiffness (*polymyalgia rheumatica*). This is the initial symptom in one fourth of patients. The onset of giant cell arteritis may be acute with sudden transitory or permanent visual loss.

Diagnosis

The best indicator of giant cell arteritis is elevation of the erythrocyte sedimentation rate (ESR), although it is occasionally normal. The diagnosis relies on confirmatory temporal artery biopsy results.

Treatment

Never withhold treatment pending the result of temporal artery biopsy. Initiate prednisone at 40–60 mg per day and continue for 1 month, then start a cautious taper of less than 10% of the daily dose per week. If ischemic complications are imminent or evolving, implement parenteral high-dose corticosteroids until these complications stabilize. Monitor disease activity by clinical assessment and determination of the ESR. Methotrexate, 10 mg per week, may be an effective adjunctive treatment that allows for more rapid tapering of the prednisone dose.

HEADACHE CAUSED BY DISEASE OF OTHER CRANIAL OR NECK STRUCTURES

Ocular Causes of Headache

In the absence of injection of the conjunctiva or other obvious signs of eye disease, headache and eye pain rarely have an ophthalmological cause. A white eye *is rarely* the cause of a monosymptomatic painful eye. Acute angle-closure glaucoma causes severe eye and frontal head pain and vomiting. The sclera is injected, the cornea steamy, the pupil fixed in midposition, and the globe stony hard. It is an ophthalmological emergency.

Cluster headaches, migraine, dissection of the carotid artery, and many other varieties of headache cause orbital and retroorbital pain. Of particular interest is SUNCT (short-lasting, *u*nilateral, *n*euralgiform, headache attacks with *c*onjunctival injection, *t*earing, rhinorrhea, and forehead sweating) syndrome because of its specific localization to the orbit and associated conjunctival injection and marked tearing. Sharp jabs of pain through the eye lasting 1 second or longer can occur as part of idiopathic stabbing headache that is indomethacin responsive. Most commonly seen in migraineurs, the sharp eye pain is occasionally felt in the ipsilateral occipital region simultaneously.

Nasal Causes of Headache and Facial Pain

Acute purulent sinusitis causes local and referred pain. The distribution of the pain depends on the sinuses involved. Maxillary sinusitis causes pain and tenderness over the cheek; frontal sinus disease causes frontal pain; sphenoid and ethmoidal sinusitis causes pain behind and between the eyes referred to the vertex. Acute rhinosinusitis is commonly associated with fever, purulent nasal discharge, and other constitutional symptoms. The pain is worse on bending forward and is often relieved as soon as the infected material drains from the sinus. Chronic rhinosinusitis is not a cause for headache or facial pain unless associated with a relapse into an acute phase. So-called "sinus headaches" without an underlying infection remain unsubstantiated. Malignant tumors of the sinuses and nasopharynx can produce deep-seated face and head pain before involving cranial nerves or otherwise becoming obvious.

Temporomandibular Joint Disorders

Mechanical disorders of the joint, alterations in the way the upper and lower teeth relate, and congenital and acquired deformities of the jaw and mandible can give rise to head and face pain and are occasionally responsible for the episodic and chronic pain syndromes seen by neurologists. Table 44.2 lists the criteria for identification and localization of temporomandibular joint (TMJ) disorders.

Headaches and the Cervical Spine

Degenerative joint disease and cervical disc herniation rarely give rise to headache in the absence of neck pain. Occipital headache and neck pain on awakening are common with arthritis of the cervical spine. With activity, the headache and associated stiffness of the neck subside. For patients with severe degenerative changes in the cervical facet joints, exercise, heat, and the use of simple analgesics can help both the neck and the head pain. Recommend surgical fusion or discectomy only if in the presence of bony instability or spinal cord or nerve root compression.

Other Headaches

Cough headache is a headache of sudden onset precipitated by a brief, unsustained Valsalva maneuver, such as coughing, laughing, sneezing, and bending. Transitory increased intrathoracic pressure triggers the headache. The pain is bursting or explosive,

Table 44.2: Criteria for identification and localization of temporomandibular joint disorders

Temporomandibular Pain	Temporomandibular Dysfunction
Pain should relate directly to jaw movements and mastication	Interference with mandibular movement (clicking, incoordination, and crepitus)
Tenderness in the masticatory muscles or over temporomandibular joint on palpation	Restriction of mandibular movement
Anesthetic blocking of tender structures should confirm presence and location of pain source	Sudden change in occlusal relationship of the teeth

lasting seconds to minutes. *Exertional headache* is a bilateral throbbing headache precipitated by sustained physical exercise, such as weightlifting, dancing, running, bowling, and football. The headache is not explosive in onset but builds in intensity and lasts between 5 minutes and 24 hours. Indomethacin, used shortly before exercise or on a regular basis, is usually effective. *Headache associated with sexual activity* is a severe occipito-nuchal headache during intercourse or at orgasm. Indomethacin or ergotamine tartrate taken several hours before intercourse may prevent headache.

MIGRAINE

Table 44.3 shows the current classification of migraine.

Clinical Aspects

The initial migraine attack usually occurs during the second decade of life; 90% of afflicted persons will have their first attack by age 40 years. After puberty, migraine is more common in females, whereas migraine affects both genders equally in pre-pubertal children. A family history of migraine is present in up to 90% of migraineurs. Although migraine classification distinguishes attacks with and without aura, many patients have attacks of both types. Migraine headache is never maximal at onset but builds to a peak over 30 minutes to several hours. The attack generally lasts several hours to a full day.

Table 44.3: Migraine

1.1. Migraine without aura
1.2. Probable migraine without aura
1.3. Migraine with aura
    1.3.1. Typical aura with migraine headache
    1.3.2. Typical aura with non-migraine headache
    1.3.3. Typical aura without headache
    1.3.4. Familial hemiplegic migraine
    1.3.5. Sporadic hemiplegic migraine
    1.3.6. Basilar type migraine
1.4. Probable migraine with aura
1.5. Childhood periodic syndromes that are commonly precursors of migraine
    1.5.1. Cyclical vomiting
    1.5.2. Abdominal migraine
    1.5.3. Benign paroxysmal vertigo of childhood
1.6. Retinal migraine
1.7. Complications of migraine
    1.7.1. Chronic migraine
    1.7.2. Status migrainosus
    1.7.3. Persistent aura without infarction
    1.7.4. Migrainous infarction
    1.7.5. Migraine-triggered seizures

Source: Reprinted with permission from the International Headache Society Second Headache Classification Subcommittee. "The International Headache Classification," 2nd ed, *Cephalalgia,* 2004.

Migraine without Aura
Focal cerebral or brainstem disturbances do not precede or accompany the headache. The attack may cause nocturnal awakening but more often begins after awakening at the normal time. At first, the pain may be unilateral and supraorbital or generalized. An initial unilateral headache may become generalized or switch to the contralateral side. A common pattern is for the headache to migrate posteriorly and become occipital and upper cervical pain. This process is probably the result of the development of sustained contraction of the scalp and upper cervical paraspinal muscles.

The quality of the pain is throbbing (pulsatile) but can be steady at rest and then become pulsatile with activity, after a Valsalva maneuver, or during the head-low position. The severity of pain varies during the attack and from episode to episode. Some are a mild inconvenience, and others are severe and incapacitating. Most migraineurs want to lie down during all but mild attacks. Associated symptoms are photophobia, phonophobia, and nausea.

Migraine with Aura
Migraine with aura is a recurrent periodic headache preceded or accompanied by an aura consisting of transitory visual, sensory, motor, or other focal cerebral or brainstem symptoms. The quality of headache is identical to that of migraine without aura but is more likely to be unilateral. The most common aura is the *scintillating scotoma*, a shimmering arc of white or colored lights in the homonymous part of one visual field.

Migraine Aura without Headache
A *migraine equivalent* is a characteristic aura not followed by a headache. The identity of migraine equivalents is easy when the attacks occur on a background of migraine with aura. In the absence of such a history, the disturbance may be difficult to distinguish from an episode of transient cerebral or brainstem ischemia. Acute episodes of confusion representing the aura can occur with migraine. *Acute confusional migraine* occurs most often in children or adolescents, but it can occur later in life.

Basilar Migraine
Basilar artery migraine usually occurs during adolescence. The headache is occipital and severe. The aura, which lasts 10–45 minutes, usually begins with typical migrainous disturbances of vision such as teichopsia, graying of vision, or actual temporary blindness. The visual symptoms are bilateral. Numbness and tingling of the lips, hands, and feet often occur bilaterally. Ataxia of gait and ataxic speech may lead to the suspicion of intoxication. Mild impairment of consciousness may occur as the other symptoms are subsiding. Arousal coincides with the onset of a severe throbbing occipital headache. The pain may generalize to the whole head and is often associated with prolonged vomiting. After sleep, the headache is usually gone.

Ophthalmoplegic Migraine
Ophthalmoplegic migraine is an uncommon condition with onset in childhood. Recurrent attacks are the usual pattern. Each episode begins with a unilateral orbital and retroorbital headache, often accompanied by vomiting, lasting 1–4 days. Either during the painful stage or occasionally as the headache subsides, ipsilateral ptosis occurs and within a few hours progresses to a complete paralysis of cranial nerve III. Cranial nerve IV or VI is rarely involved. MRI shows thickening and contrast enhancement of the nerve as it exits the midbrain. This disorder is probably best considered a cranial neuropathy. The prognosis is favorable for recovery unless attacks occur very frequently.

Complications of Migraine

Migraine associated with hemiparesis occurs sporadically or as a familial trait. In *familial hemiplegic migraine*, the weakness is more severe and prolonged. The diagnosis is suggested by a history of migraine with aura. Weakness may last for hours, days, or even weeks in rare cases. Recovery is usually complete, except in rare situations in which cerebral infarction is associated.

A facioplegic form of complicated migraine with recurrent episodes of upper and lower motor neuron facial palsy also occurs.

Migraine Genetics

Although prior familial migraine studies have shown no clear mendelian inheritance patterns, recent genetic studies support the hypothesis of a genetic contribution. Perhaps the most striking evidence of a genetic basis for migraine is familial hemiplegic migraine (FHM).

FHM is a rare autosomal dominant subtype of migraine with aura in which in the context of otherwise typical migraine attacks patients experience hemiplegia. The hemiparesis of FHM is in many cases prolonged beyond the customary time limit of 1 hour usually associated with migraine aura. FHM was mapped to chromosome 19p13 in linkage studies inspired by the association of migraine and cerebral autosomal dominant arteriopathy and with subcortical infarcts and leukoencephalopathy.

Management

Treatment can be directed at the acute attack or at the prevention of recurrences. Prophylactic therapy is rarely needed unless the frequency or duration of attacks seriously interferes with the patient's lifestyle. Avoidance of trigger factors is important in the management of migraine.

Symptomatic Treatment

Symptomatic treatment should be started as early in the development of an attack as possible. For many patients, a simple oral analgesic, such as aspirin, acetaminophen, naproxen, or ibuprofen, or an analgesic combination with caffeine may be effective.

Ergot

Dihydroergotamine (DHE) is administered by the parenteral and intranasal routes. This medication should be considered when nausea and vomiting limit the use of oral medications or when other medications are ineffective. Although the effect of DHE is slower than sumatriptan, it does have similar efficacy after

2 hours, and it is associated with a lower recurrence of headache in 24 hours. It is associated with increased nausea in some patients, and it may need to be combined with an antiemetic agent. When given intravenously in an acute medical care setting, the use of an antiemetic is mandatory.

Triptans
Triptans are highly selective at certain 5-hydroxytryptamine (5-HT) (serotonin) receptors and can be administered orally, intranasally, or subcutaneously (Table 44.4). All seven triptans that are available in the United States seem to have a beneficial effect on migraine-associated symptoms, including nausea, photophobia, and phonophobia, which also improves the patient's ability to return to normal functioning. The potential side effects of all the oral triptans are similar. They consist of tingling, flushing, and a feeling of fullness in the head, neck, or chest.

Prophylactic Treatment
When the attacks of migraine occur weekly or several times a month, or when they are less frequent but very prolonged and debilitating, a preventive program is appropriate. Attacks of migraine that occur in a predictable pattern can also respond to prophylactic medication.

β-Adrenergic blocking drugs are widely used for the prophylaxis of vascular headaches. Propranolol should be administered in doses of 80–240 mg per day and, if tolerated, should be given a 2–3 month trial. As with all β-adrenergic blocking agents, administration of propranolol should be discontinued slowly to avoid cardiac complications. It is contraindicated in those with an asthmatic history and should be used with caution in patients using insulin or oral hypoglycemic agents because it may prevent the adrenergic corrective responses to hypoglycemia. The main dose-related adverse effect is depression. Timolol, nadolol, atenolol, and metoprolol have approximately the same benefit in migraine as propranolol. When one of these agents is partially effective, the individual headaches that break through can be treated with analgesics, with or without ergotamine tartrate or sumatriptan, as described previously.

Amitriptyline and other antidepressants can be helpful in migraine prophylaxis, just as they are useful in the prevention of tension-type headaches. The benefit seems to be independent of their antidepressant action. Used in doses of 10–150 mg at night, amitriptyline, imipramine, or desipramine may provide some protection against frequent attacks of migraine and especially against the chronic daily headache that may have

Table 44.4: Serotonin (5-HT) agonists used in acute migraine treatment

Drug	Route(s)	Dose	May Repeat Doses if Headache Recurs	Maximum Dose per 24 hr
Dihydroergotamine (DHE-45)	IV	0.5, 1.0 mg	1 hr	3 mg
	IM	0.5, 1.0 mg	1 hr	3 mg
	SC	0.5, 1.0 mg	1 hr	3 mg
(Migranal)	Nasal spray	2 mg (0.5 mg/spray) one spray in each nostril, repeat in 15 min		3 mg
Almotriptan (Axert)	Oral	12.5 mg	2 hr	25 mg
Eletriptan (Relpax)	Oral	20, 40 mg	2 hr	80 mg
Frovatriptan (Frova)	Oral	2.5 mg	2 hr	7.5 mg
Naratriptan (Amerge)	Oral	1 mg, 2.5 mg*	4 hr	5 mg
Rizatriptan (Maxalt)	Oral	5 mg, 10 mg*	2 hr	30 mg
Sumatriptan (Imitrex)	Oral	25 mg, 50 mg, 100 mg	2 hr	300 mg
	SC	6 mg	2 hr	12 mg
	Intranasal	5 mg, 20 mg*		40 mg
Zolmitriptan (Zomig)	Oral	2.5 mg,* 5 mg	2 hr	10 mg
	Intranasal	5 mg	2 hr	10 mg

*These are the recommended starting dosages based on efficacy and tolerability.

evolved from more typical intermittent migraine. The optimal dose for migraine prophylaxis must be determined by titration of the dose.

The calcium-channel–blocking agents have limited benefit in migraine. Verapamil in doses of 80–120 mg three times a day reduces the frequency of migraine with aura, but it is not as useful in common migraine. Oral riboflavin, 400 mg per day, and oral magnesium, 600 mg of a chelated or slow-release preparation, have been shown in double-blinded, placebo-controlled, randomized studies to be effective in migraine prophylaxis. Methysergide, sodium valproate, and topiramate also have a beneficial effect in the prophylactic treatment of migraine.

CLUSTER HEADACHE

In *episodic cluster headache*, attacks of pain occur daily for days, weeks, or months before an attack-free period of remission occurs. This respite lasts from weeks to years before another cluster of attacks develops. In *chronic cluster headache*, attacks of pain occur for more than a year without a remission longer than 2 weeks. The chronic form may develop de novo or evolve from episodic cluster headache.

Clinical Features

Cluster headache occurs predominantly in males. Onset is usually in the third decade. The first cluster persists 4–8 weeks and is followed by a headache-free period of months to years. Eventually, the clusters become seasonal and then more frequent and longer lasting. During a cluster, one or more attacks occur per 24 hours, often at the same time of day. Onset during the night or 1–2 hours after going to sleep is common.

The attacks are similar in the episodic and the chronic phase. The pain is strictly unilateral and remains so from cluster to cluster, the location is in the retroorbital and temporal region but may be maximal in the cheek or jaw (*lower syndrome*). It is usually described as steady or boring and of terrible intensity (*suicide headache*).

Onset is usually abrupt or preceded by a brief sensation of pressure in the soon-to-be-painful area. The pain intensifies very rapidly, peaking in 5–10 minutes and then persisting for 45 minutes to 2 hours. After the attack, the patient is completely free from pain but exhausted; however, the respite may be transitory because another attack usually follows shortly. Unlike patients with migraine, people with cluster headaches do not lie down; they are restless and walk the floors. Other ipsilateral abnormalities during the attack are blockage of the nostril, overflow tears, conjunctival injection, and distention of the temporal artery.

Investigations

In most patients, the clinical features establish the diagnosis; special neurological investigations are unnecessary. However, an atypical episodic cluster headache warrants an imaging study. However, it may be advisable to obtain an imaging study to help reassure the patient that the attacks are not due to some major intracranial abnormality.

Treatment and Management

Care should be taken to reassure the patient that the syndrome, even though unbearably painful, is benign and not life threatening. Pain reduction but not cure should be promised. The frequency, severity, and brevity of individual attacks of cluster headache and their lack of response to many symptomatic measures necessitate the use of a prophylactic program for most patients. The treatment plan is determined by several factors, including whether the phase of the disorder is episodic or chronic and the presence or absence of other disease states, such as hypertension and coronary or peripheral vascular insufficiency.

Acute (Symptomatic) Pharmacological Therapy

Given the rapid onset and short time to peak intensity of the pain of cluster attacks, a fast-acting symptomatic treatment is imperative. Oxygen, subcutaneous sumatriptan, and subcutaneous or intramuscular DHE provide the most rapid, effective, and consistent relief for cluster headache attacks. Oxygen delivered at a flow rate of 8–10 liters per minute via a non-rebreathing face mask can dramatically abort an attack. Sumatriptan, 6 mg by subcutaneous injection, aborts an individual cluster attack. However, preemptive treatment before the anticipated onset of an attack does not prevent the attack. DHE-45 administered intravenously provides prompt and effective relief of a cluster attack.

Pharmacotherapy

Transitional prophylaxis involves the short-term use of corticosteroids, ergotamine, or DHE. This typically induces a rapid suppression of attacks while one of the maintenance agents can take effect.

Maintenance prophylaxis refers to the use of preventive medications throughout the anticipated duration of the cluster period. Start the preventive medication at cluster onset in conjunction with either corticosteroids or ergotamine derivatives and continue their use after the initial suppressive medications are discontinued. The calcium-channel blockers, methysergide maleate, and lithium are the agents of choice.

Surgical Treatment

Thirty to 50 years ago, injection of alcohol into the gasserian ganglion and trigeminal root section was used in the treatment of chronic migrainous neuralgia (cluster headache). These procedures did not gain widespread acceptance and were gradually abandoned because of the high incidence of complications, including neuroparalytic keratitis, postoperative herpes keratitis, and anesthesia dolorosa of the denervated area.

INDOMETHACIN-RESPONSIVE HEADACHE SYNDROMES

Indomethacin-responsive headache syndromes (IRHSs) represent a unique group of primary headache disorders characterized by a prompt, absolute, and often permanent response to indomethacin.

Paroxysmal Hemicranias

The paroxysmal hemicranias are primarily disorders of young adults. The female-to-male ratio is approximately 2:1. Chronic and episodic paroxysmal hemicrania differ predominantly in their temporal profile. *Chronic paroxysmal hemicrania* occurs daily, with multiple discrete attacks occurring throughout a 24-hour period. *Episodic paroxysmal hemicrania* is characterized by bouts of attacks separated by remission periods. The headache bouts can range from 2 weeks to 5 months, and remission periods can last 1–36 months. Both disorders are associated with daily attacks of severe, short-lived, unilateral pain, which is often maximally felt in the orbital-periorbital or temporal region. The characteristic attack frequency is five per day, each lasting 20 minutes. Each paroxysm is accompanied by at least one ipsilateral autonomic feature (lacrimation, ptosis, eyelid edema, conjunctival injection, nasal congestion, or rhinorrhea).

Hemicrania Continua

Hemicrania continua is characterized by a continuous unilateral headache of moderate intensity that may involve the entire hemicranium or simply be confined to a focal area. The female-to-male ratio is approximately 2:1, and the average age at onset is 28 years (range, 5–67 years). The continuous headache is often punctuated by painful unilateral exacerbations lasting 20 minutes to several days. Attacks may alternate sides, and unilateral attacks may rarely become bilateral. Stabbing head pains ("ice picks") are often a feature of this disorder, usually on the ipsilateral side and usually during a period of exacerbation. Indomethacin is effective in doses ranging from 25–300 mg daily. The usual starting dose is 25 mg three times daily with meals.

SUNCT

SUNCT is a moderately severe unilateral cephalalgia characterized by neuralgiform pain of very short duration (15–120 seconds). The paroxysms are usually felt in or around the eye and are sometimes triggered by cutaneous stimuli or neck movements. Attack frequency ranges from 1 or 2 per day, up to 30 per hour. Lamotrigine has been effective in several patients.

Primary Stabbing Headache

Persons describe brief, extremely sharp twinges of pain that occur without warning and that can be felt anywhere in the head, including the orbit. The pains are graphically described as being like a spike being driven into the skull, hence the term *ice-pick headache*. When stabs of pain occur frequently, the treatment of choice is indomethacin, administered in a regimen similar to that described for the paroxysmal hemicranias.

TENSION-TYPE OR MUSCLE CONTRACTION HEADACHE

Chronic headaches that are not associated with focal neurological symptoms and do not have the gastrointestinal features of migraine are often diagnosed as tension headaches and are ascribed to persistent contraction of the scalp, neck, and jaw muscles. Tension-type headaches, which can begin at any age, are generally bilateral (commonly occipitonuchal, bitemporal, or bifrontal). They are often described as being like a tight band around the head, a sense of pressure, or a bursting sensation. The pain may wax and wane throughout the course of a day or may be described as being present and steady for days, weeks, or even years at a time. Despite the complaint of a constant headache, sleep may be undisturbed. In general, tension-type headaches are not associated with nausea and vomiting and are much less commonly associated with light and sound sensitivity than migraine.

Chronic tension-type headache, especially when it becomes a daily event, can persist for years. It is difficult to manage and rarely responds completely to any therapeutic regimen. Spontaneous remissions may occur, and in some patients the condition subsides with age. Secondary depression, drug addiction, and chronic pain behavior are often the result of chronic headaches.

Techniques to promote relaxation of the scalp and neck muscles can be helpful; these methods include stretching exercises, the application of heat and massage to the neck, biofeedback conditioning, and relaxation training. For occasional mild tension-type headache, aspirin or acetaminophen may be sufficient treatment. The most effective prophylactic drug is amitriptyline.

CRANIAL AND FACIAL NEURALGIAS

Trigeminal Neuralgia

Clinical Features

Trigeminal neuralgia is a paroxysmal pain in the distribution of one or more divisions of the trigeminal nerve. It is triggered by an ipsilateral sensory stimulus to the skin, mucosa, or teeth. The pain is described as electric-like, shooting, or lancinating. Each attack lasts only seconds, but the pain may be repetitive at short intervals so one attack blurs into another. Most attacks are in the second and third divisions of the trigeminal nerve. Primary trigeminal neuralgia (*tic douloureux*) begins after age 40 years. It is not associated with sensory impairment and motor disturbances. Secondary trigeminal neuralgia caused by lesions involving the gasserian ganglion or its sensory root may be associated with sensory loss in the fifth cranial nerve distribution, weakness and atrophy of the muscles of mastication, and involvement of adjacent cranial nerves. Tic douloureux has no accompanying laboratory or radiographic abnormalities. Trigeminal neuralgia that has its onset in young women or is bilateral in distribution is often caused by multiple sclerosis.

Treatment and Management

Treatment of trigeminal neuralgia resulting from a focal lesion compressing the sensory root of the trigeminal nerve is surgical exploration and decompression of the nerve. Management of primary trigeminal neuralgia can be either medical or surgical. Carbamazepine is the most effective drug for the treatment of trigeminal neuralgia. Therapeutic doses generally range from 600 to 1200 mg per day. Second-line options for the management of trigeminal neuralgia include phenytoin, baclofen, and valproate. Other drugs that have been used include gabapentin, clonazepam, lamotrigine, oxcarbazepine, and topiramate.

For a young patient who does not respond to medical treatment, posterior fossa microvascular decompression should be considered. Stereotactic radiosurgery with the gamma knife is an effective therapy for trigeminal neuralgia and the least invasive surgical option.

Glossopharyngeal Neuralgia

Glossopharyngeal neuralgia is similar in quality and periodicity to trigeminal neuralgia. Unilateral pain is felt in the throat, the tonsillar region, the posterior third of the tongue, the larynx, the nasopharynx, and the pinna of the ear. Swallowing, chewing, speaking, laughing, or coughing usually triggers the pain.

Carbamazepine and phenytoin have been administered with mixed success in glossopharyngeal neuralgia. Intracranial section of the glossopharyngeal and upper rootlets of the vagus nerve is almost always successful in giving complete pain relief.

Occipital Neuralgia

A headache in the occipital region may be due to entrapment of the greater or lesser occipital nerves on one or both sides. The patient may have a history of trauma to the back of the head, but more commonly the condition develops spontaneously. Chronic contraction of the neck and posterior scalp muscles may be responsible for entrapment of the occipital nerves.

The pain is described as shooting from the nuchal region up to the vertex. In addition to the lancinating pains, dull occipital discomfort may be present. Percussion over the occipital nerves should reproduce the symptoms, and discrete tenderness should be evident in the area of the nerve low in the occipital region. Local anesthetic and corticosteroid can be infiltrated around the nerve as a diagnostic procedure. While the area remains anesthetized, the spontaneous pain should be relieved and pain should not be triggered by percussion over the nerve. In many instances, this treatment results in long-term relief. Avulsion or nerve section should be avoided because these procedures often do not give complete relief and may lead to formation of a neuroma.

For a more detailed discussion, see Chapter 75 in Neurology in Clinical Practice, 4th edition.

Cranial Neuropathies | *45*

Chapter 8 covers optic nerve disturbances, Chapter 10 covers auditory and vestibular nerve disturbances, and Chapter 11 covers olfactory nerve disturbances.

OCULOMOTOR NERVE

Brainstem Syndromes

Dysfunction of the third nerve can occur anywhere from its nuclear origins in the midbrain to its final terminations within the orbit. After the fascicles of the oculomotor nerve exit the brainstem, they fuse in the interpeduncular fossa. Any extra-axial mass in this area could involve one or both oculomotor nerves. Aneurysms of the posterior communicating artery and basilar bifurcation produce internal ophthalmoplegia. The initial feature is a dilated and relatively fixed pupil. Raised intracranial pressure produces transtentorial uncal herniation with extrinsic compression of the third cranial nerve (CN) on the margin of the tentorium. The peripheral location of the pupil-loconstrictor fibers makes them vulnerable to compression. Unilateral pupillary enlargement on the side of the lesion may be the earliest sign of increased intracranial pressure (Hutchinson's pupil).

Cavernous Sinus Syndromes

Disturbances inside the cavernous sinus cause dysfunction of the third, fourth, and sixth CNs. Most abnormalities in this location cause compressive injury. These include dissection or thrombosis of the carotid artery, thrombophlebitis, fungal infections, aneurysms, and primary and metastatic neoplasms. Infarction of the third CN in the cavernous sinus involves the central core of the nerve, sparing peripheral pupilloconstrictor fibers. A painful pupil-sparing palsy of CN III is characteristic.

Superior Orbital Fissure and Orbit

The clinical features of lesions of the third CN in the orbit or in the superior orbital fissure are difficult to distinguish. Coexisting optic nerve dysfunction suggests orbital involvement. Involvement of maxillary division facial sensation suggests that the lesion extends at least as far back as the midcavernous sinus. The *Tolosa-Hunt syndrome* usually appears in the fourth through sixth decades and manifests over several weeks as a steady, boring, unilateral orbital pain. Optic nerve involvement is unusual. Corticosteroid responsiveness is the rule.

Distal Branch Syndromes

The oculomotor nerve subdivides into superior and inferior branches as it enters the orbit. The superior branch supplies the superior rectus and levator palpebrae superioris muscle, and the inferior branch supplies the inferior and medial rectus and inferior oblique muscles. Orbital trauma selectively causes paralysis of these terminal branches. Isolated superior branch oculomotor palsy produces a characteristic picture of unilateral ptosis and weakness of the superior rectus, with preserved pupillary, medial, and inferior rectus muscle function. The cause is often idiopathic, but internal carotid artery aneurysms and myasthenia can produce similar findings.

TROCHLEAR NERVE

Diplopia, the main complaint in traumatic fourth nerve palsies, usually subsides in less than 1 year. Image tilting and vertical diplopia occur only in acquired cases of recent onset, not in congenital fourth CN paralysis. Trauma is the most common cause of trochlear nerve palsy in adults; 20% of traumatic cases are bilateral. Head impact at the time of trauma may disrupt the crossing fibers in the anterior medullary velum. Vascular ischemic disease from hypertension, diabetes, and atherosclerosis accounts for approximately one fifth of cases. Transitory ipsilateral trochlear nerve paresis may occur after anterior temporal lobectomy for intractable seizures. Fourth nerve palsies in children are either congenital or traumatic.

TRIGEMINAL NERVE

The trigeminal, or fifth, CN is a mixed motor and sensory nerve. Most of the lateral portion of the fifth nerve transmits sensation from sharply defined cutaneous fields on the face, oral cavity, and nasal passages. The smaller motor division travels with the third division of the sensory portion of the nerve and provides motor function to the muscles of mastication. Magnetic resonance imaging (MRI) shows atrophy and fatty replacement of muscle mass when the mandibular division has undergone motor denervation. Trigeminal sensory neuropathy presents with sensory disturbance in one or more divisions of the nerve. When associated with scleroderma and other connective tissue disease, the sensory neuropathy is bilateral and painful and the motor pathway spared.

Numb Chin and Cheek Syndromes

Numbness of the lower lip may be the initial feature of metastatic disease to the lower jaw, affecting primarily the inferior alveolar nerve. Numbness in the malar region suggests basal or squamous cell carcinomas of the face. Mandibular bone atrophy from aging causes paresthesias in the chin.

Trigeminal Neuralgia

See Chapter 20 for a discussion of trigeminal neuralgia.

Traumatic Neuropathies

Both cranial and facial trauma may affect the peripheral infraorbital and supraorbital branches of the trigeminal nerve. Trigeminal nerve branch injury rarely results from dental anesthetic injections. Lingual nerve injury follows surgery on the third molar and after laryngeal mask airway placement, causing paresthesias on the ipsilateral tongue surface.

Herpesvirus Infections

Herpes simplex and zoster viruses produce lifelong infections of the trigeminal ganglia. Activation of the latent viral infection causes recurring herpes simplex mucous membrane lesions (cold sores) and painful zoster infections.

ABDUCENS NERVE

Abducens nerve palsy is the most common of all oculomotor palsies. The cause is often indeterminate. Small-vessel ischemic infarction is the most likely cause in adults with a history of hypertension or diabetes. In children, tumors (13%) and trauma (40%) are the usual causes. The usual tumor is a brainstem glioma, and abducens nerve weakness may be the first sign of disease. Abducens nerve paresis in newborns is usually transitory.

Brainstem Syndromes

Lesions at different foci in the brainstem produce distinct syndromes. Infarctions in the territory of anterior inferior cerebellar artery cause the rare combinations of ipsilateral sixth CN palsy, gaze palsy, and peripheral seventh CN weakness (*Millard-Gubler syndrome*) and sixth CN palsy and contralateral hemiplegia (*Foville's syndrome*). A characteristic disorder, referred to as *one-and-a-half syndrome*, consists of preservation of abduction in only one eye, which also exhibits jerk nystagmus in the abducted position, while the other eye lies fixed in midline for all attempts at lateral movement.

Extra-Axial Posterior Fossa Syndromes

As the sixth nerve exits the pontomedullary junction, it travels along the base of the clivus before entering the cavernous sinus. Cerebellopontine angle tumors cause combinations of abducens, trigeminal, facial, and auditory nerve dysfunction. Basal tumors or infiltrating processes may compress the abducens nerve. The combination of ocular motor nerve palsies with trigeminal disturbances suggests cavernous sinus disease such as tumor or aneurysm. Both unilateral and bilateral abducens paresis occur in the syndrome of spontaneous intracranial hypotension.

FACIAL NERVE (VII)

The facial nerve is the longest and most complex of the CNs, consisting of six segments: intracranial, internal auditory canal, labyrinthine or petrous, tympanic, mastoid, and intraparotid. The labyrinthine, tympanic, and mastoid segments are in the fallopian canal. It supplies the muscles of facial expression, the salivary and lacrimal glands, and conveys taste sensation from the anterior two thirds of the tongue. Both congenital and acquired disease may damage the facial nerve from its brainstem nuclear origin to its peripheral terminations in the face.

Supranuclear lesions produce a different pattern of facial paralysis than infranuclear and nuclear lesions. The traditional explanation is that the lower face has primarily a contralateral innervation, whereas the upper face has both ipsilateral and contralateral innervation. However, a contributing factor is that the cortical representation of the upper face is in the anterior cingulate gyrus, and not the motor cortex. The explanation for the disparity between emotional facial mimetic expression and voluntary facial movement is that different pathways subserve these functions.

Clinical Evaluation

Factors that determine clinical features include lesion size, disorder severity, acuteness of onset, and unilateral versus bilateral. In determining the anatomical site of abnormality, one must first distinguish upper from lower motor neuron lesions (Table 45.1). With unilateral facial palsy, upper motor neuron disorders affect the voluntary movements of the lower face, with relative sparing of the orbicularis oculi, frontalis, and corrugator muscles because the upper face has bilateral corticobulbar innervation. Congenital hemiplegia always spares the entire face, suggesting that the lower face has bilateral corticobulbar innervation at birth.

A sudden severe unilateral infranuclear paralysis, as seen in Bell's palsy, produces (in addition to an obvious cosmetic embarrassment) significant dysarthria, pooling of saliva, drooling, and

Table 45.1: Clinical differential features of upper motor neuron versus lower motor neuron facial weakness

Upper Motor Neuron Lesions	Lower Motor Neuron Lesions
Unilateral paresis of voluntary movements of lower face with sparing of the frontalis muscle	Unilateral paresis of all mimetic muscles, including the frontalis muscle
Facial muscle weakness less apparent with emotional than with voluntary action	Degree of facial weakness similar with emotional and voluntary movements
Preservation or accentuation of facial reflexes	Suppression of facial reflexes
Preserved taste, anterior two thirds of tongue	Possible impairment of taste
Normal lacrimation	Possible abnormality of lacrimation

decreased tearing. Depending on the size of the lesion, taste perversion and hyperacusis may be associated. The moderate degree of weakness of the lower face seen with a unilateral corticobulbar lesion produces few complaints. Bilateral corticobulbar disease devastates speech and swallowing functions. Facial reflexes help establish or localize lesions of the facial nerve. Upper motor neuron disorders with unilateral facial paresis affect the voluntary movements of the lower face with relative sparing of the orbicularis oculi, frontalis, and corrugator supercilii muscles.

Congenital Disorders

The cause of congenital facial nerve palsies may be intrapartum nerve trauma or aplasia of the motor nucleus. The most common cause of facial asymmetry in newborns is unilateral absence of the depressor anguli oris muscle that depresses the corner of the mouth when the infant cries. The motor nucleus is aplastic. *Möbius' syndrome* occurs on a sporadic or familial basis. The main features are congenital paralysis of CNs VII and VIII with variable orofacial and limb malformation. Clues pointing to a congenital cause are other birth defects, especially microtia and external auditory canal atresia.

Traumatic Facial Palsy

A peripheral facial paralysis in the context of head trauma raises the possibility of basilar skull fracture. Transitory facial palsy occurs in up to 20% of patients undergoing sphenoidal electrode insertion for prolonged video-electroencephalographic monitoring.

Pregnancy

Facial palsy affects women of reproductive age three times more often than men of the same age, and pregnant women three times more often than nonpregnant women. Most cases occur in the third trimester or in the puerperium. Women developing facial palsy while pregnant are at increased risk of hypertensive disorders of pregnancy such as preeclampsia.

Bilateral Facial Palsy

Bilateral simultaneous peripheral facial weakness most often accompanies the Guillain-Barré syndrome. Bilateral facial weakness in the presence of aseptic meningitis suggests Lyme disease. *Bannwarth's syndrome* is the association of Lyme aseptic meningitis and facial weakness. Recurrent bilateral facial palsy suggests sarcoidosis and time of seroconversion in human immunodeficiency virus infection.

Bell's Palsy

Bell's palsy is the most common acquired disease of the facial nerve. The causes are mainly unknown but are probably of viral or immune-mediated origin. Both genders and all ages are equally affected. The initial feature is often pain in or behind the ipsilateral ear, suggesting an ear infection. Unilateral weakness follows within several days and achieves maximal paralysis within 3 days. Paresthesias on the involved side of the face sometimes occur early in the course. Impairment of taste and hyperacusis (from weakness of the stapedius muscle) are often present.

Eighty-five percent of patients recover completely within 3 months of onset. Incomplete paralysis at the onset is perhaps the most favorable prognostic sign. The prognosis is worse when facial nerve palsy is associated with geniculate herpes (*Ramsay Hunt syndrome*); pain and vesicles in the external auditory canal or soft palate establish the diagnosis. MRI shows contrast enhancement of the involved nerve.

Prednisone treats Bell's palsy in adults. However, its value is not established. Children always recover completely and do not require treatment. Acyclovir is the recommended therapy for all patients with geniculate herpes. It shortens the initial episode and reduces the chance of recurrence.

Aberrant regeneration may take several forms, the most prominent being involuntary tearing of the eye on the involved side when eating (*crocodile tears*) or synkinesis of the facial musculature when chewing. This often takes the form of *jaw winking* wherein lid closure on the involved side accompanies jaw opening. Bell's palsy in the elderly suggests the possibility of diabetes or hypertension. Recurrent Bell's palsy may be associated with a deeply furrowed tongue (lingua plicata) and recurrent facial edema (*Melkersson's syndrome*).

Hemifacial Spasm

Rapid irregular paroxysms of clonic twitching of one or more muscle groups innervated by the facial nerve characterize hemifacial spasm. Hypertension is a predisposing factor if the hemifacial spasm occurs on the left, but not the right, side of the face. The twitches usually begin unilaterally about the eye and then spread to the other facial muscles, especially the perioral muscles, but never beyond the domain of the facial nerve. The contractions persist for minutes and are often precipitated by stress, fatigue, or voluntary movements of the face and may persist in sleep.

Surgical decompression of an aberrant arterial loop compressing the facial nerve may be curative, but initial treatment is with carbamazepine, gabapentin, or botulinum injections.

GLOSSOPHARYNGEAL NERVE (IX)

Fibers of the glossopharyngeal nerve, or ninth CN, originate from several nuclear complexes (tractus solitarius [gustatory nucleus], nucleus ambiguus, and inferior salivatory nucleus) in the brainstem. They pass outward as several distinct subsets of fibers, to emerge from the medulla between the inferior olive and inferior cerebellar peduncle, caudal to the seventh CN and rostral to the tenth CN. CN IX exits the skull through the jugular foramen along with CNs X and XI and comes to lie between the internal jugular vein and the internal carotid artery.

Isolated lesions of the glossopharyngeal nerve are extremely uncommon. Almost invariably, involvement of this nerve occurs in conjunction with that of the vagus, accessory, and hypoglossal nerves. Isolated paralysis of the glossopharyngeal nerve produces slight and usually transitory dysphagia. Peripheral dysfunction of the nerve may be a result of blunt neck trauma, such as nonfatal suicidal hanging, diseases of the middle ear, and pharyngeal abscesses.

VAGUS NERVE (X)

The vagus is the longest of all the CNs. In many respects, its origins and functions are similar to those of the glossopharyngeal nerve. Vagal nerve dysfunction with vocal cord paresis may be the initial feature of multisystem atrophy. Primary thoracic disease may damage the recurrent laryngeal branches of the vagus nerve. Tumors of the mediastinum and lung are the most common causes of isolated vocal cord palsy.

The motor fibers of the vagus arise from the nucleus ambiguus and the dorsal motor nucleus of the vagus. The sensory portions have cell bodies of origin in the jugular and nodose ganglia. Exiting the skull through the jugular foramen, the vagus nerve travels within the carotid sheath between the internal jugular vein and the carotid artery, giving off pharyngeal branches and superior and inferior (recurrent) laryngeal nerves. Spontaneous dissection of the internal carotid artery may present with an isolated vagal neuropathy.

Brainstem Lesions

Supranuclear involvement of the vagus nerve is significant only when it is bilateral, producing a pseudobulbar type of syndrome with dysphagia and dysarthria. Nuclear involvement of the vagus nerve occurs as part of motor neuron disease in patients with progressive bulbar palsy. Vascular lesions within the medulla may involve the vagus nerve.

SPINAL ACCESSORY NERVE (XI)

The function of the spinal accessory (SA) nerve is motor. The cranial portion, with the vagus and glossopharyngeal nerves, supplies the musculature of the pharynx and larynx, whereas the spinal portion innervates the sternocleidomastoid and upper portions of the trapezius musculature.

The sternocleidomastoid draws the occiput toward the side of the contraction, rotating the face to the opposite side. Contracting together, the sternocleidomastoid muscles flex the cervical spine. Although the SA nerve is considered a purely motor nerve, the symptoms of its dysfunction are both motor and sensory, the latter being predominantly pain. In acute lesions, traumatic or inflammatory, the pain is steady, severe, and localized to the neck and top of the shoulder.

A unilateral lesion causes obvious drooping of the affected shoulder. Winging of the scapula is caused by paresis of the middle trapezius muscle, and loss of abduction is caused by weakness of the upper trapezius. Long thoracic nerve lesions increase winging.

The most common cause of eleventh CN palsies is secondary to nerve injury during surgery.

HYPOGLOSSAL NERVE (XII)

The hypoglossal nerve (CN XII) is purely motor, supplying innervation to the extrinsic and intrinsic muscles of the tongue. Arising from the hypoglossal nucleus beneath the floor of the fourth ventricle in the caudal medulla, it courses ventrally through the brainstem to exit between the pyramidal tract and the olivary eminence. A lesion of the hypoglossal nerve causes ipsilateral weakness and wasting of the tongue, which deviates to the weak side when protruded. Motor neuron disease and poliomyelitis may involve the hypoglossal nuclei, causing progressive tongue atrophy with fasciculations.

Jugular Foramen Syndrome

Clinical Features and Etiology

The most common causes of the jugular foramen and allied syndromes are primary and metastatic tumors, vascular lesions, trauma, inflammatory, and iatrogenic lesions. The most common primary tumors are schwannomas, glomus tumors, and meningiomas. Schwannomas constitute approximately 25% of all tumors in the head and neck, but schwannomas of nerves IX, X, and XI, in the absence of neurofibromatosis, constitute approximately 3% of all intracranial schwannomas.

Schwannomas of the jugular foramen present with hearing loss and dizziness indistinguishable from acoustic neuroma. Other presentations are the jugular foramen syndrome or a neck mass. The clinical signs indicate dysfunction of CNs IX, X, and XI in 80%, hearing loss in 70%, and facial palsy in 25%. Contemporary diagnosis of these tumors involves both computed tomography and MRI scanning.

Glomus jugulare tumor is a highly vascular tumor that may involve the glossopharyngeal nerve and the other nerves (vagus and accessory) traversing the jugular foramen and can enlarge sufficiently to damage the facial and hypoglossal nerves. The patient usually has pulsatile tinnitus followed by conductive hearing loss. The most common neoplastic causes of jugular foramen syndrome are primary nasopharyngeal tumors that spread locally to the cranial base or distant metastases from breast, lung, prostate, and lymph tissue.

For a more detailed discussion, see Chapter 76 in Neurology in Clinical Practice, 4th edition.

Movement Disorders | *46*

BASAL GANGLIA

No clear consensus exists on which structures are included in the basal ganglia. This chapter considers those structures in the striatopallidal circuits involved in modulation of the thalamo-cortical projection: the caudate nucleus, the putamen, the globus pallidus externa and interna, the two divisions (pars compacta and pars reticulata) of the substantia nigra (SN), and the subthalamic nuclei (STN). Disorders of the basal ganglia cause prominent motor dysfunction but not frank weakness.

PARKINSONIAN SYNDROMES

Parkinson's Disease (Idiopathic Parkinson's Disease, Paralysis Agitans)

The terms *Parkinson's disease* (PD) and *idiopathic PD* are reserved for the clinical syndrome of asymmetrical parkinson-ism, usually with rest tremor, in association with the specific pathological findings of loss of dopaminergic SN neurons with eosinophilic cytoplasmic inclusions (Lewy bodies). A genetic form of parkinsonism, clinically indistinguishable from PD, has been linked to missense mutations in the alpha-synuclein gene. PD is a syndrome with both genetic and environmental causes.

Epidemiology
PD accounts for more than 80% of all parkinsonism. The prev-alence is 360 per 100,000 and the incidence is 18 per 100,000 per year. The prevalence shows a gradual increase after the age of 50 years and a steeper increase after age 60 years. Disease onset before age 30 years suggests a hereditary form of parkinsonism.

Table 46.1: Hoehn and Yahr stage

Stage	
I	Unilateral involvement only, minimal or no functional impairment
II	Bilateral or midline involvement, without impairment of balance
III	First sign of impaired righting reflex, mild to moderate disability
IV	Fully developed, severely disabling disease; patient still able to walk and stand unassisted
V	Confinement to bed or wheelchair unless aided

Clinical Features

The onset and progression of PD are gradual. Resting tremor in one hand is the most common initial feature. The tremor is often associated with decreased arm swing and shoulder pain. Bradykinesia and rigidity are often detectable on the symptomatic side. Midline signs such as reduced facial expression or mild contralateral bradykinesia and rigidity may already be present. The disorder usually remains asymmetrical throughout much of its course. With progression, generalized bradykinesia causes difficulty with arising or turning in bed. The gait and balance are progressively affected and lead to falls. Sudden arrests in movement, called *freezing*, follow—first with gait initiation or turning and then during walking. Bulbar functions deteriorate, impairing communication and nutrition. The Hoehn and Yahr stage accurately outlines the natural course of disease (Table 46.1). Autonomic symptoms include reduced gastrointestinal transit time with postprandial bloating and constipation, urinary frequency and urgency, sometimes with urge incontinence, impotence, disordered sweating, and orthostatic hypotension. Cognitive changes include decreased attention and concentration, diminished working memory, planning, and organization, and sometimes global dementia. Anxiety and mood disorders are common. Sleep disturbance is nearly universal and includes restless legs syndrome, periodic leg movements of sleep, and rapid eye movement (REM) sleep behavior disorder (RBD).

Diagnosis

PD remains a clinical diagnosis. Routine laboratories are not helpful. The main value of neuroimaging is to exclude other similar conditions.

Treatment

Six types of medications are available for the symptomatic treatment of PD: anticholinergics, amantadine, L-dopa, monoamine

Table 46.2: Commonly used antiparkinsonian drugs

Drug	Usual Starting Dose	Usual Daily Dose
Anticholinergics		
Trihexyphenidyl	1 mg	2–12 mg
Benztropine	0.5 mg	0.5–6.0 mg
Biperidin	1 mg	2–16 mg
Amantadine	100 mg	100–300 mg
L-DOPA		
(with carbidopa)		
Immediate release	100 mg	150–800 mg
Controlled release	100 mg	200–1000 mg
Dopamine agonists		
Bromocriptine	1.25 mg	15–40 mg
Pergolide	0.05 mg	2–4 mg
Pramipexole	0.375 mg	1.5–4.5 mg
Ropinirole	0.75 mg	8–24 mg
Cabergoline	0.25 mg	0.25–4.0 mg
Catechol-O-methyl transferase inhibitors		
Entacapone	200 mg with each dose	200 mg with each dose
Tolcapone	300 mg	600 mg

oxidase inhibitors, catechol-O-methyltransferase inhibitors, and dopamine agonists (DAs) (Table 46.2). Symptomatic treatment begins when the patient notices functional, occupational, or social disability. About 70% of patients with PD require symptomatic therapy within 2 years of disease onset. Selegiline and amantadine are useful for initial therapy, but carbidupa/levadopa (CD/LD) or DAs are the choices when therapy that is more potent is required. CD/LD is the most potent and best-tolerated drug, but it promotes the development of motor fluctuations. Irrespective of initial treatment, all patients with PD experience an evolution of their response to L-dopa that includes wearing off and other motor fluctuations.

Wearing off is the predictable return of PD in advance of the next scheduled dose. *On off* is the unpredictable reappearance of PD when central levels of antiparkinsonian drugs are within the target therapeutic range. *Delayed on* is a prolongation of the time required for the central antiparkinsonian drug effect to appear. *Dose failure* is the complete failure to develop a favorable response to an incremental dopaminergic dose. *Protein-related offs* occur when the transport of L-dopa across the intestinal wall is impeded by competition for facilitated transport by large

Table 46.3: Management of drug-related motor fluctuations in Parkinson's disease

Wearing off
  Adjust L-dopa dose and interdose interval
    Shorter interval
    Smaller increment, especially if dyskinesia is a problem
    Liquid carbidopa/L-dopa
Add catechol-O-methyltransferase inhibitor
    Entacapone
    Tolcapone
Add dopamine agonist
  Add amantadine
  Add selegiline
Dyskinesia
  Adjust L-dopa dose and interdose interval
    Smaller increment
    Shorter interval, if needed
  Add dopamine agonist and reduce L-dopa dose
  Add amantadine
  Add atypical antipsychotic
Morning dystonia
  Chew or crush first dose, take with carbonated beverage
  Add dopamine agonist
  Add baclofen
  Add anticholinergic
On-off fluctuations
  Careful identification/management of predictable fluctuations
  Add dopamine agonist

amounts of neutral amino acids. *Peak-dose dyskinesias* are usually choreiform or stereotypical movements present at the peak of the therapeutic response; dystonic movements are seen less commonly. *Off-period dystonia* usually appears in the more severely affected foot in the morning before the first daily doses, sometimes reappearing during wearing off. *Diphasic dyskinesias* are usually large-amplitude dyskinetic movements of the lower body during the time of increasing and decreasing L-dopa levels. Armed with a few basic principles and a common sense approach, the clinician can usually smooth out fluctuations for most patients (Table 46.3).

Surgical Treatment
Palliative surgical approaches include stereotactic destruction of physiologically defined overactive brain nuclei (thalamotomy, pallidotomy), deep brain stimulation (DBS) using implanted

pulse generators, and the implantation of cellular sources of dopamine. Surgical approaches aimed more at the degenerative process itself include delivery of trophic factors using implanted pumps or by gene therapy, as well as cellular transplantation.

Dementia with Lewy Bodies

Fluctuating impairment of consciousness, disruption of attention and visuospatial abilities, visual hallucinations, and parkinsonism are the characteristic features of dementia with Lewy bodies (DLB). Patients are extremely sensitive to dopamine receptor antagonists and experience severe parkinsonism when treated with neuroleptics. Treatment is difficult. Use antiparkinsonian agents to treat parkinsonian signs and atypical antipsychotics for behavioral features.

Multiple System Atrophy

Multiple system atrophy (MSA) includes disorders with various combinations of pyramidal, extrapyramidal, cerebellar, and autonomic features. Within this category are subtypes named for their predominant clinical manifestations. The more purely parkinsonian MSA (*MSA-P*) replaces the term *striatonigral degeneration*. Cerebellar MSA (*MSA-C*) replaces the term *olivopontocerebellar atrophy*. Autonomic MSA (*MSA-A*) replaces the term *Shy-Drager syndrome*.

MSA is a rare disorder characterized by parkinsonism (87%), autonomic dysfunction (74%), cerebellar ataxia (54%), and pyramidal signs (49%). MSA-P usually presents with symmetrical parkinsonism, often without tremor. The response to L-dopa is generally short-lived. Many develop midline dystonia. Autonomic signs include orthostatic hypotension, incontinence, and impotence. MSA-C is parkinsonism with prominent cerebellar signs, especially wide-based ataxic gait. Autonomic signs are variable. MSA-A presents as autonomic failure. Early signs are incontinence in women and impotence in men. Orthostatic hypotension is the rule.

Clinical tests of autonomic dysfunction may be helpful in the diagnosis or treatment. Magnetic resonance imaging (MRI) brain scans differentiate MSA from PD but do not adequately distinguish among the subtypes of MSA. Treatment is difficult. Specific interventions are not available and symptomatic therapies provide only partial relief of disability. Orthostatic hypotension may improve with nonpharmacological measures such as liberal salt and water intake, compressive stockings, and sleeping with the head up, but most people require pharmacotherapy with fludrocortisone, midodrine, or other agents. Mean survival is 7–9 years.

Progressive Supranuclear Palsy

Progressive supranuclear palsy (PSP) is a progressive illness characterized by vertical supranuclear ophthalmoplegia, axial rigidity, pseudobulbar palsy, and mild dementia. Onset is in the sixth to seventh decade and more men than women are affected. Initial features are gait disorder and falling. An akinetic-rigid state with symmetrical signs and prominent axial rigidity follows. The trunk and neck are hyperextended. The characteristic facial appearance includes a wide-eyed stare, furrowing of the forehead, and deepening of other facial creases. Pseudobulbar palsy with dysarthria and dysphagia often leads to aspiration. Frontal lobe features and dementia are common. PSP is rapidly progressive, and by the fourth year half of patients need assistance walking and have dysarthria and visual symptoms. Clinical criteria establish the diagnosis. MRI signs of PSP include midbrain atrophy, increased signal in the midbrain, globus pallidus, and red nucleus, third ventricle dilatation, and atrophy of the frontal or temporal lobes. Response to treatment is variable; dopaminergic agents aid about 40% of patients. The prognosis of PSP is poor, with a median duration of survival of 10 years.

Corticobasal Degeneration

Corticobasal degeneration (CBD) is a rare disorder with onset after age 60 years. Characteristic features are akinetic rigidity, apraxia, dystonia, tremor, and aphasia. Its most recognizable form is predominantly a motor disease. Motor signs include parkinsonism with strikingly asymmetrical rigidity, asymmetrical dystonia, myoclonus, apraxia, alien limb, and cortical sensory loss. Cognitive signs range from subfluent aphasia in patients with predominantly right-sided motor signs to a generalized dementia. MRI shows cortical atrophy, with widening of the sylvian and interhemispheric fissures and dilatation of frontal, parietal, and temporal sulci. Treatment is not available.

Frontotemporal Degeneration with Parkinsonism Linked Chromosome 17

The frontotemporal dementias (FTDs) are a group of illnesses characterized by behavioral changes and neuropsychological evidence of frontal lobe dysfunction. They include Pick's disease, pallidopontonigral degeneration, disinhibition-dementia-parkinsonism-amyotrophy, familial multisystem tauopathy with presenile dementia, familial subcortical gliosis, FTD, FTD with ALS, FTD with inclusion body myopathy, and FTD with parkinsonism linked chromosome 17 (FTDP-17). Up to 60% of patients with FTD have affected family members.

Considerable phenotypic and genotypic heterogeneity exists in FTDP-17. The disorder most often begins in the fifties or sixties with personality and behavioral changes, including disinhibition and aggressiveness, as well as frontal executive dysfunction. Other common signs include social misconduct, stereotyped verbalizations, impaired recent memory, and parkinsonism. The prognosis is poor with death within 10 years.

Bilateral Striatopallidodentate Calcification (Fahr's disease)

Calcification of the basal ganglia has many causes. It is an incidental finding in up to 1% of all computed tomographic (CT) brain scans and occurs in infectious, metabolic, and genetic disorders. Familial and sporadic forms occur. Symptoms usually begin between ages 30 and 60 years. Common features include cognitive dysfunction, cerebellar signs, dysarthria, pyramidal signs, psychiatric illness, gait disorder, and sensory impairment. Half of patients have parkinsonism and/or chorea. Fewer than 10% of patients have tremor, dystonia, athetosis, or orofacial dyskinesia. The presence of symptoms correlates with the amount of calcification. Specific treatment is not available.

Parkinsonism-Dementia Complex of Guam

The Chamorros, an indigenous people of Guam, have a high incidence of an ALS-like illness. A smaller number have a syndrome of parkinsonism with dementia, the parkinsonism-dementia complex (PDC). Some people have both motor neuron disease and parkinsonism-dementia. Exposure to an environmental factor, the cycad nut, in adolescence or early adulthood is responsible. Ingestion of cycad nuts or bats that feed on the nuts is the source. Exposure to a dietary factor is also responsible for *Guadeloupean parkinsonism*.

Postencephalitic Parkinsonism

Between 1916 and 1927, there was a worldwide epidemic of encephalitis lethargica, which killed about 250,000 persons and left an additional 250,000 with chronic disability. The survivors of the acute illness developed parkinsonism, usually within 10 years of the infection. Postencephalitic parkinsonism (PEP) resembles PD, except behavioral and sleep abnormalities are more prominent, extraocular movements are often abnormal, and oculogyric crises are common. No records exist of subsequent epidemics of encephalitis lethargica. The symptoms of PEP tend to be L-dopa responsive, but behavioral complications limit therapy.

Drug-Induced Parkinsonism

Dopamine receptor–blocking drugs reproduce the major clinical features of PD. The signs are usually symmetrical, and the tremor is more often present during posture holding than at rest. The most common causes of drug-induced parkinsonism (DIP) are the typical neuroleptic antipsychotic drugs, antidopaminergic antiemetics, and drugs that deplete presynaptic nerve terminals of dopamine, such as reserpine and tetrabenazine. Among the newer or "atypical" antipsychotics, the relative propensity to cause DIP is as follows: risperidone $\geq$ ziprasidone > olanzapine > quetiapine > clozapine. This ranking reflects their respective affinity for the D_2 receptor. Although reversible, DIP resolves slowly over 6 months, and symptomatic treatment with anticholinergics may be required. Occasionally, parkinsonism does not resolve, suggesting the offending drug likely has unmasked an underlying parkinsonism.

Toxin-Induced Parkinsonism

Several drug addicts developed acute and severe parkinsonism following intravenous injection of a synthetic heroin contaminated by MPTP. Despite the 10-year interval from exposure to death, active neurodegeneration did not occur. MPTP-induced parkinsonism is L-dopa responsive but is complicated by the early development of motor fluctuations and dyskinesias and psychiatric complications. Cognitive function usually remains intact. Other toxins that induce parkinsonism are *acute carbon monoxide poisoning* and *manganese* toxicity.

TREMOR

Physiological Tremor

A fine tremor of the outstretched limbs is a universal finding. The frequency ranges from 7 to 12 Hz. The tremor is usually not noticeable, but fatigue, anxiety, fear, excitement, stimulant use, and hyperthyroidism accentuate its amplitude.

Essential Tremor

Clinical Features
Essential tremor (ET) is one of the most common movement disorders. The prevalence is higher in men than in women and in whites than in nonwhites. ET is a monosymptomatic illness characterized by a gradually increasing amplitude postural and kinetic tremor of the forearms and hands, in the absence of endogenous or exogenous triggers or other neurological signs. The median age at onset is 15 years. The patient becomes aware of a barely perceptible postural or action tremor of the distal arms and hands. The kinetic tremor is higher in amplitude and causes more disability than the postural tremor. Handwriting is particularly troublesome. The tremor worsens with time and causes disability. ET is a monosymptomatic illness and the remainder of the neurological examination findings are normal.

Genetics
Two thirds of patients give a positive family history of tremor, usually in a first-degree relative. Hereditary ET is genetically heterogeneous with loci on chromosomes 3 and 2 and a candidate locus on chromosome 4.

Treatment
Patients with mild ET whose main source of disability is tremor during meals often benefit from a premeal cocktail. β-Adrenergic blockers and primidone are the two most commonly used drugs. Primidone improves ET in about 50% of patients and is more effective for head tremor than other agents. Its effective dose range is 50–350 mg daily given as a single nighttime dose or in divided dose increments. Stereotactic thalamotomy suppresses contralateral tremor as much as 75% in up to 90% of cases.

Dystonic Tremor

Three types of tremor are associated with dystonia. Some family members of persons with hereditary dystonia have isolated tremor (*dystonia gene–associated tremor*). In others, a person with dystonia of one or more body parts may have pure tremor in other body parts (*tremor-associated with dystonia*). Lastly, tremor may be part of the dystonia, sharing body distribution and directional preponderance with the dystonic movement (*dystonic tremor*). The treatment of dystonia gene–associated tremor and tremor associated with dystonia are the same as ET, whereas treating dystonic tremor is as part of the underlying dystonia (see discussion later in this chapter).

Primary Writing Tremor

Primary writing tremor is a rare condition characterized by a 4–7 Hz tremor in the hand during the assumption of a writing posture or during the writing task itself. Most patients are men, and one third have a family history of writing tremor. A similar number improve after ethanol ingestion. The tremor may respond to β-adrenergic blockade, primidone, or anticholinergic medications. Botulinum toxin injections provide the most consistent relief. Thalamic DBS is effective in some cases.

Orthostatic Tremor

Orthostatic tremor is a high-frequency (14–18 Hz) isometric tremor that presents with tremor in the legs during quiet standing. Patients may be unaware of the tremor but complain of unsteadiness and sensory complaints in the legs. Unlike parkinsonian and ETs, orthostatic tremor shows significant side-to-side coherence, suggesting a central generator. Clonazepam is the most effective pharmacological treatment.

Palatal Tremor

Essential palatal tremor (PT) occurs in the absence of an underlying structural lesion. Symptomatic PT is secondary to an underlying structural lesion. Clinical features and neuroimaging distinguish essential from symptomatic PT. In essential PT, both genders are equally affected. Rhythmic movements of the tensor veli palatini muscle produce the tremor. Patients complain of audible ear clicks. The movements usually disappear during sleep. Symptomatic PT affects men more than women and is not associated with ear clicks. The levator veli palatini rather than the tensor veli palatini is involved. Simultaneous tremor of other regional structures with cranial nerve innervation may coexist (i.e., pendular nystagmus). Laryngeal involvement may interrupt speech or may cause rhythmic involuntary vocalizations. Brain MRI shows hypertrophy of the superior olive, associated with lesions in the brainstem and cerebellum. Phenytoin, carbamazepine, clonazepam, diazepam, trihexyphenidyl, and baclofen are first-line agents in the treatment of PT. Injections of botulinum toxin into the tensor veli palatini muscle are beneficial in essential PT.

CHOREA

Huntington's Disease

Huntington's disease (HD) is a highly penetrant autosomal dominant disease characterized by a progressive movement disorder associated with psychiatric and cognitive decline, culminating in a terminal state of dementia and immobility.

Clinical Features

The best prevalence figure for HD is 10 per 100,000. Age at onset is 30–55 years. About 5% of cases begin at younger than 21 years; the juvenile phenotype differs from the adult phenotype, and patients are frequently misdiagnosed. HD is a progressive degenerative disease that affects movement, behavior, and cognitive function. Table 46.4 outlines the common symptoms of the early, middle, and advanced stages of the illness. Intractable falls lead to wheelchair or bed confinement. Dysarthria and dysphagia progressively impair communication and nutrition. Most patients spend their last years in nursing homes. Mean survival is 17 years. Generally, patients with earlier onset have the largest number of CAG repeats and tend to progress more rapidly than older onset patients.

Diagnosis

The most cost-effective diagnostic procedure is genetic testing. HD is a dominantly inherited condition caused by an unstable expanded CAG trinucleotide repeat in exon-1 of the huntingtin gene on the tip of the short arm of chromosome 4. Normal alleles have fewer than 30 CAG repeats. Alleles with 30–35 repeats do

Table 46.4: Symptoms of Huntington's disease

Early	Middle	Late
Clumsiness	Unsteadiness	Weight loss
Chorea	Dropping things	Speech disorder
Irritability	Gait disorder	Swallowing disorder
Sadness	Sleep disorder	Bladder incontinence
Depression	Cognitive dysfunction	Bowel incontinence
Decreased motivation	Decreased memory	
Sexual dysfunction		

Source: Adapted with permission from Kirkwood, S.C., Su, J. L., Conneally, P., & Foroud, T. 2001, "Progression of symptoms in the early and middle stages of Huntington disease," *Arch Neurol* vol. 58, no. 2, pp. 273–278.

not cause clinical disease but may become unstable, particularly when transmitted by a man. Alleles with 36–39 repeats may cause disease, but with a reduced phenotype. Everyone with 40 or more CAG repeats in the huntingtin gene will develop the clinical illness.

Treatment
No treatment influences disease progression. Symptomatic treatment options include amantadine and tetrabenazine for chorea and atypical antipsychotics, such as olanzapine, for behavior control.

Dentatorubral-Pallidoluysian Atrophy (Haw River Syndrome)

Dentatorubral-pallidoluysian atrophy (DRPLA) is an inherited neurodegenerative disease that is rare outside Japan. Typical symptoms of DRPLA include chorea, ataxia, myoclonic epilepsy, dystonia, parkinsonism, psychosis, and dementia. Onset is usually in the patient's twenties, with death 20 years later. Anticipation occurs with paternal transmission of the gene. The nature and severity of symptoms guide the investigation and management.

Neuroacanthocytosis and the McLeod Syndrome

Acanthocytes are in peripheral blood smears of patients with three neurological syndromes: *abetalipoproteinemia*, *neuroacanthocytosis*, and the *McLeod syndrome*. Neuroacanthocytosis and the McLeod syndrome are associated with movement disorders.

Neuroacanthocytosis is an autosomal recessive disorder with onset at age 35 years. The predominant movements are chorea, dystonia, and tics; parkinsonism may occur in more advanced stages. Orofacial dystonia with dystonic tongue protrusion are prominent and interfere with eating. In addition, many patients exhibit lip and tongue biting and prominent dysarthria and dysphagia. Behavioral changes resemble those seen in HD. Subcortical dementia is a late feature. Other features include seizures, myopathy, and axonal neuropathy. In patients with neuroacanthocytosis, acanthocytes usually make up 5–20% of peripheral blood erythrocytes.

The McLeod syndrome is an X-linked recessive disorder. The syndrome begins around age 50 years and progresses slowly. The most common clinical feature is an axonal peripheral neuropathy. Some patients have myopathy, and all have elevations in serum creatine kinase. Limb chorea is a constant feature, facial tics are common, and some have dystonia and seizures. Subcortical dementia and behavioral changes occur later in the course in half of the cases. Cardiomyopathy and hemolytic anemia are common. Neuroimaging studies may show caudate atrophy with secondarily enlarged lateral ventricles. Treatment is symptomatic.

Rheumatic (Sydenham's) Chorea

Chorea appears months after the index infection. It is a disorder of childhood, affecting girls more often than boys. The chorea begins insidiously but progresses over weeks and generally resolves within 6 months. Chorea may start on one side of the body before generalizing. Restlessness, irritability, and emotional lability are common. The disorder usually lasts up to 6 months. About 20% of chorea cases recur. Enlargement of the basal ganglia may be seen on MRI brain scan. Valproic acid, pimozide, and carbamazepine are effective symptomatic treatments for the chorea. People with a history may have a recurrence in the presence of hormonal stress such as during pregnancy or estrogen treatment.

Ballismus

Ballismus is a proximal flinging movement. Ballism most commonly affects the limbs on one side of the body (hemiballismus) but may involve both legs (paraballismus). Ballism is a form of chorea. Both typically coexist, and with time chorea replaces ballistic movements. Hemiballismus is relatively rare. The mean age at onset is from 48 to 75 years and the underlying causes are often stroke or tumor. Dopamine antagonists and dopamine depleters effectively decrease choreiform movements. Beneficial results are reported using gabapentin and valproic acid.

Senile Chorea

Senile chorea is an idiopathic disorder characterized by the development in old age of continuous mouthing, chewing, or tongue movements. Treatment of patients with disabling movements is with antidopaminergic drugs, but their use requires close surveillance for the development of tardive dyskinesia (TD).

Tardive Dyskinesia

TD is a movement disorder that develops in the context of chronic dopamine receptor blockade. Typical patients are those chronically treated with neuroleptic drugs or antiemetics. TD usually requires a minimum of 6 weeks or more of dopamine receptor blockade, but onset can occur with the first dose. Reported risk factors include age, female gender, affective disorder, and edentulousness. The appearance of TD is repetitive stereotypical (e.g., chewing) movements of the mouth, tongue, and lower face (orobuccolingual dyskinesias). The most important intervention in TD is to prevent its occurrence. Discontinue neuroleptics and atypical antipsychotic substituted. Catecholamine-depleting drugs, particularly tetrabenazine, are often very useful in the treatment of severe TD.

DYSTONIA

Childhood Onset Generalized Primary Dystonia

Clinical Features
Most primary generalized dystonias begin in childhood. The most common childhood form is primary generalized dystonia (DYT1), an autosomal dominant disorder with relatively low penetrance. It is particularly common in persons of Ashkenazi Jewish descent. Onset is usually by age 9 years and onset after age of 40 years is rare. An action-induced leg dystonia is the earliest symptom. The condition generalizes over a period of 5 years. Patients with early onset or with leg dystonia are more likely to generalize than those with later onset or arm dystonia. Generalized dystonia produces severe disability and most patients become nonambulatory. Even in generalized disease, laryngeal and pharyngeal dystonia remains rare. Other childhood-onset generalized dystonias do not account for large numbers of cases. DNA testing is available for DYT1 dystonia, but the low penetrance of the disease limits the usefulness of this test for prenatal or presymptomatic diagnosis.

Treatment
A trial of dopaminergic therapy is reasonable in the absence of genetic confirmation of the DYT1 mutation. About 50% of patients younger than 20 years respond to high-dose anticholinergic therapy. Baclofen, clonazepam, benzodiazepines, and dopamine-depleting medications are useful in some patients. Chronic intrathecal baclofen helps some patients with dystonia, especially those with concomitant spasticity. Stereotactic thalamotomy benefits 66% of patients receiving the operation, but some worsen, and side effects are common. Thalamotomy may be most useful for patients with dystonia of the distal limb. Axial symptoms may improve after bilateral pallidotomy or pallidal DBS.

Adult Onset Primary Focal and Segmental Dystonia

Focal and segmental dystonias may have a genetic basis. About 25% of patients have a positive family history of dystonia.

Clinical Features
Cervical dystonia and blepharospasm are the most common adult-onset dystonias. The focal and segmental dystonias start in the hand, neck, or face. Cervical dystonia accounts for about half of focal dystonia cases. The initial complaint is neck pain, difficulty maintaining a normal head position, and sometimes tremor. Sensory tricks to break the dystonia include resting the head against a wall or high-backed chair or touching the chin or back of the head lightly with one hand. Spontaneous remissions occur in 20% of patients, although recurrence is very common. Focal dystonia of the eyelids, blepharospasm, is often preceded by an abnormal sensation in the eye. Increased blinking or eyelid spasm follows. Placing a finger alongside the eye induces improvement. Oromandibular dystonia (cranial dystonia) may accompany blepharospasm. Oromandibular dystonia typically consists of involuntary jaw opening or closing, tongue protrusion, dysarthria, and dysphagia. Eating and speaking activates the dystonia. Sensory tricks in oromandibular dystonia include touching the face or inserting something into the mouth.

The occupational or task-specific dystonias are those that arise in the context of repetitive or skilled use of a body part. The most common task-specific dystonia is writer's cramp, in which action dystonia of the arm and hand develops during writing. Players of wind instruments may develop dystonia of embouchure, with difficulty maintaining the proper mouth and lip posture. Isolated foot dystonia in an adult is rare and suggests an underlying structural lesion. Adult-onset primary focal or segmental dystonia is a clinical diagnosis.

Treatment
Medical treatment is difficult and employs those agents typically used in generalized dystonia. Botulinum toxin injections are very helpful in treatment. Overall, more than 75% of treated patients report moderate to marked improvement in dystonic pain or posture.

X-Linked Dystonia Parkinsonism (DYT3; Lubag's Syndrome)

X-linked dystonia parkinsonism (DYT3) is an X-linked condition of progressive dystonia and parkinsonism affecting Filipino males from the Panay island. Affected men may show dystonia, parkinsonism, tremor, chorea, or myoclonus. Lubag's syndrome affects men in the fourth or fifth decade.

Dopa-Responsive Dystonia (DYT5)

Dopa-responsive dystonia (DRD) is usually dominantly inherited with incomplete penetrance (DYT5). DYT5 results from mutations in the guanosine triphosphate cyclohydrolase-1 (*GTPCH-1*) gene on chromosome 14.

Clinical Features
Girls are preferentially affected. DRD is a childhood-onset generalized dystonia with a sustained complete response to low doses of L-dopa. The disorder begins in the first decade with an action dystonia in the foot. The fully formed illness ranges in severity from mild focal to disabling generalized dystonia. The most characteristic historical feature is prominent diurnal fluctuation. Affected patients may be almost normal in the morning and become progressively disabled over the course of the day. Peak disability is late in the evening. Parkinsonian symptoms become part of the clinical picture over time. DNA testing is not feasible.

Treatment
DRD responds to low doses of L-dopa (100–300 mg daily). Patients with DRD do not develop the motor fluctuations and dyskinesias associated with chronic L-dopa therapy in PD. Anticholinergic drugs may also be useful.

Myoclonus Dystonia (DYT11)

Clinical Features
Dystonia is the predominant symptom of myoclonus dystonia (MD), but tremor and myoclonus are present as well. Some patients have pure myoclonus. Symptoms begin in the first decade and predominantly affect the head, arms, and upper body. The involuntary movements may be exquisite sensitivity to ethanol. Psychiatric features include affective disorder, obsessive-compulsive disorder, substance abuse, anxiety, phobic or panic disorders, and psychosis. No other neurological deficits develop and the course is usually benign.

Treatment
MD responds poorly to medical therapy.

Rapid-Onset Dystonia Parkinsonism (DYT12)

Rapid-onset dystonia parkinsonism (RDP) is a rare disorder in which signs of parkinsonism and upper body dystonia develop subacutely. Onset ranges from childhood to adulthood. Dystonia preferentially affects bulbar muscles and progresses over days to weeks, and then remains stable. The majority of cases belong to a small number of families showing dominant inheritance with incomplete penetrance. A genetic locus is on chromosome 19. Symptoms do not improve with administration of levodopa.

Wilson's Disease (Hepatolenticular Degeneration)

Wilson's disease (WD) is an autosomal recessive disorder of copper metabolism related to mutations in the ATP7B gene on chromosome 13. Genetic testing is not available.

Clinical Features

WD is a rare heredodegenerative disorder in which abnormal copper deposition occurs in several organs. In childhood, copper accumulates in the liver causing cirrhosis and liver failure. Once cirrhosis has developed, extrahepatic copper deposits occur in the brain, eyes, and kidneys. Some patients present with hemolytic anemia, hypersplenism, or renal failure. Neurological signs usually present during adolescence or early adulthood. Neurological presentations include parkinsonism, postural and kinetic tremor, ataxia, titubation, chorea, seizures, dysarthria, and dystonia. A fixed stare with a smiling expression and drooling is typical. Dystonia is present at presentation in 37% of cases. Sensation is spared. Dementia is mild, but psychiatric features are common. In the presence of neurological signs, ophthalmological examination always demonstrates copper deposition in Descemet's membrane (*Kayser-Fleischer rings*).

Laboratory Studies

Liver function study results are abnormal, aminoaciduria is present, and serum uric acid is low. Bone is demineralized and brain MRI shows decreased signal intensity (hypodensity) in the striatum and superior colliculi and increased signal intensity in the midbrain tegmentum. Low serum ceruloplasmin, elevated 24-hour copper excretion, the presence of Kayser-Fleischer rings, and elevated hepatic copper confirm the diagnosis.

Treatment

The goal of treatment is to reduce the body burden of copper and to prevent its reaccumulation. Acute chelation began with D-penicillamine, but more recent treatment strategies stress the use of less toxic therapies such as trientine and zinc or tetrathiomolybdate. Measuring urine copper excretion and plasma copper levels monitors treatment. Trientine and zinc maintain chronic therapy.

Pantothenate Kinase–Associated Neurodegeneration, Hallervorden-Spatz Disease; Hypoprebetalipoproteinemia, Acanthocytosis, Retinitis Pigmentosa, and Pallidal Degeneration

Several disorders cause neurodegeneration with brain iron accumulation. Pantothenate kinase–associated neurodegeneration (PKAN), formerly Hallervorden-Spatz disease, is an autosomal recessive neurodegenerative disorder presenting in childhood with the insidious onset of dystonia and gait disorder. Virtually all families with typical PKAN have mutations in the pantothenate kinase gene (*PANK2*) on chromosome 20. Pantothenate kinase is an important regulatory enzyme in coenzyme A synthesis.

Clinical Features
Rigidity, dysarthria, spasticity, dementia, retinitis pigmentosa, and optic atrophy develop and progress relentlessly until death in early childhood. T2-weighted MRI brain scans show areas of reduced attenuation in the globus pallidus surrounding an area of hyperintensity, the *eye of the tiger* sign. Atypical forms of the illness begin later and are more slowly progressive. Patients frequently present with early speech disorder and often have personality changes suggestive of FTD. Although the MRI scan shows evidence of iron accumulation, the "eye of the tiger" sign is not seen and these patients do not have mutations in the *PANK2* gene. The *HARP* syndrome (*h*ypoprebetalipoproteinemia, *a*canthocytosis, *r*etinitis pigmentosa, and *p*allidal degeneration) is linked to mutations in the *PANK2* gene as well.

Posttraumatic Dystonia

Hemidystonia is the common presentation of traumatic dystonia, but cervical, segmental, axial, or spasmodic dysphonia also occurs. Most cases have occurred in children or adolescents who have survived severe head injury. Often, the dystonia emerges as a traumatic hemiparesis improves or resolves. There may be a latent period of 1 day to 6 years between the trauma and the development of dystonia. Neuroimaging shows focal lesions in the caudate, putamen, or thalamus contralateral to the dystonia. The prognosis is poor. Most cases are refractory to medical therapy. Botulinum toxin injections, DBS, or stereotactic thalamotomy may be helpful.

Tardive Dystonia

Clinical Features

Tardive dystonia (TDy) should be differentiated from transient acute dystonic reaction and from TDs. Men are more likely to develop TDy and at a younger age than women. All of the typical antipsychotics, as well as antiemetics with dopamine receptor–blocking properties, have been associated. Symptoms begin insidiously after days to decades of neuroleptic therapy. The median duration of exposure to neuroleptics at the time of onset is 5.1 years. TDy usually presents as focal or segmental dystonia, such as blepharospasm, or oromandibular or cervical dystonia, but the most typical presentation is a truncal dystonia associated with pronating movements of arms and extension of the elbows. Dystonic symptoms may improve over 5 years if the offending neuroleptic agent is withdrawn, although recovery is less common than in choreic patients with TD.

Treatment

The best management is prevention. Once TDy develops, atypical antipsychotics are substituted for the offending neuroleptic. Tetrabenazine, anticholinergics, benzodiazepines, and baclofen are reported to help TDy. Botulinum toxin injections can be particularly helpful.

Paroxysmal Kinesogenic Dyskinesia (DYT10)

Paroxysmal kinesogenic dyskinesia (PKD) is a childhood-onset disorder characterized by attacks of dystonia, chorea, or other hyperkinesias. Boys make up 80% of cases. Family history is common. Rapid movement, often in response to an unexpected stimulus, triggers the episode. The movements may be unilateral or bilateral. The spells last less than 1 minute and occur up to 100 times daily. Spells tend to decrease in adulthood. Diagnosis depends on history, the examination is normal, and diagnostic studies are normal. Two loci for PKD (DYT10) localize to chromosome 16. PKD usually responds to anticonvulsant medications.

Paroxysmal Nonkinesogenic Dyskinesia (DYT8)

Paroxysmal nonkinesogenic dyskinesia (PNKD) usually begins in infancy and affects boys more than girls. The spells of PNKD occur less frequently but are more prolonged than in PKD. Their frequency ranges from several episodes per month to several episodes per day and their duration is generally between 10 minutes and several hours. Action does not precipitate attacks, but ethanol, caffeine, fatigue, and stress serve as triggers. Genetic loci for PNKD (DYT8) are on chromosomes 1 and 2. Unlike PKD, PNKD does not respond to anticonvulsants. Some patients respond to clonazepam, other benzodiazepines, carbamazepine, gabapentin, anticholinergics, L-dopa, acetazolamide, and neuroleptics.

TICS

Tourette's Syndrome

Clinical evidence suggests that Tourette's syndrome (TS) is a hereditary disease. However, definite mendelian inheritance is not established and a genetic locus not identified.

Clinical Features
Prevalence estimates for TS vary from 10 to 700 per 100,000. Although the prevalence is greater among children in special schools, the vast majority of patients have normal intelligence. Boys more often than girls are affected. Onset is in childhood or early adolescence, most often between the ages of 2 and 10 years. Typical early signs of TS are cranial motor tics including eye blinks, stretching of the lower face, and shaking the head. Vocal tics include sniffing, throat clearing, grunting, whistling, chirping, and words, including profane words (coprolalia). The tics wax and wane, and new tics enter and leave the repertoire. Tics may be simple or complex and can resemble any voluntary or involuntary movement. Patients with TS have both motor and vocal tics. Symptoms increase throughout childhood, with peak expression in adolescence, and become somewhat less troublesome in adulthood. Attention-deficit/hyperactivity disorder (ADHD), conduct disorder, and obsessive-compulsive disorder are often associated. The diagnosis of TS rests entirely on the history and physical examination. The neurological examination findings are usually normal, as are neuroimaging and electrophysiological study results.

Treatment
The first step in treatment is to define the sources of disability. Children in whom tics are causing social or educational disability require treatment. Neuroleptic medications such as haloperidol and pimozide are first-line therapy. Fluphenazine and tetrabenazine are also effective with minimal side effects. Obsessive-compulsive disorder responds to selective serotonin reuptake inhibitors. Clonidine and methylphenidate are safe to use for comorbid ADHD.

Adult-Onset Tics

Adult-onset tics are much rarer than childhood-onset tics and usually represent recurrences of childhood onset tics. Many affected patients have childhood histories of obsessive-compulsive tendencies and family histories of tic disorders. Adult-onset tic disorders often develop after a triggering event and are more severe and socially disabling than the more typical young-onset disease. Tics in adults are relatively resistant to pharmacotherapy. Other causes of adult-onset tics include central nervous system stimulants, tardive tics, and neuro-acanthocytosis.

Postinfectious Autoimmune Neuropsychiatric Disorders Associated with Streptococcal Exposure

Postinfectious autoimmune neuropsychiatric disorders associated with streptococcal exposure (PANDAS) is a controversial entity linked to TS. Prepubertal children with PANDAS have an explosive onset of obsessive-compulsive disorder, tics, hyperactivity, and choreiform movements. An association exists with prior group A beta-hemolytic streptococcal infection, although the syndrome is distinct from rheumatic fever and Sydenham's chorea. Affected children have enlargement of the caudate, putamen, and globus pallidus by volumetric MRI. Intravenous immune globulin and plasmapheresis reduce obsessive-compulsive symptoms. Plasmapheresis improves tics.

MYOCLONUS

Essential Myoclonus

Myoclonus presents as an isolated neurological sign or is accompanied only by tremor or dystonia. Essential myoclonus (EM) can be sporadic or inherited. Dominantly inherited EM usually presents before age 20 years. Myoclonus is multifocal with upper body predominance. Alcohol may dramatically suppress the myoclonus. Myoclonus dystonia and EM are allelic disorders linked to the ε-sarcoglycan gene on chromosome 7.

Hereditary Geniospasm (Chin Tremor)

The characteristic feature of hereditary geniospasm is involuntary vertical movement of the tip of the chin and quivering and mouth movements. Geniospasm may be spontaneous or stress induced. Trembling becomes apparent in infancy or early life and last minutes. Attack frequency diminishes with age. The disorder is genetically heterogeneous, with linkage to chromosome 9q13-21 in some families. Geniospasm may be a form of hereditary EM.

Posthypoxic Myoclonus (Lance-Adams Syndrome)

Posthypoxic myoclonus (PHM) is a generalized myoclonus that occurs during recovery from acute severe brain hypoxia. The typical patient is in coma for several days to 2 weeks. Myoclonus and seizures may be present during the comatose phase. After the patient recovers from coma, myoclonic jerks become apparent, especially with voluntary movements, which trigger volleys of high-amplitude jerks and intermittent pauses in the activated body part. The myoclonic movements typically flow to body parts not directly involved in the voluntary movements. The amplitude of the myoclonus is directly proportional to the delicacy of the attempted task, producing extreme disability in the performance of activities of daily living. Gait is disturbed by positive myoclonic jerks, but also by negative myoclonus resulting in falls. Other neurological signs include seizures, dysarthria, dysmetria, ataxia, and cognitive impairment.

Some improvement occurs with time, but most patients have significant disability. Valproic acid and clonazepam provide improvement in about 50% of patients. Levetiracetam is also effective, but vigabatrin and gabapentin are not.

Startle and Hyperekplexia

Hyperekplexia (Hx) is a startle syndrome characterized by muscle jerks in response to unexpected stimuli. Both autosomal dominant and autosomal recessive inheritance exist. Two forms of startle exist. Characterizing the major form is continuous stiffness beginning in infancy, and exaggerated startle culminating in falls. Some patients have seizures and low intelligence. Only excessive startle and hypnic myoclonic jerks occur in the minor form. Startle in patients with Hx differs from normal startle because of the low threshold, the generalized response, and the failure to habituate with repeated stimuli. The origin of the pathological startle is in the lower brainstem, possibly the medial bulbopontine reticular formation. The disorder is genetically heterogeneous. Most defined mutations involve the α_1-subunit of the inhibitory glycine receptor. Symptomatic Hx results from infarction, hemorrhage, or encephalitis. Clonazepam is the treatment of choice.

Spinal Myoclonus and Propriospinal Myoclonus

Spinal myoclonus (SM) is a syndrome of involuntary rhythmic or semirhythmic myoclonic jerks in a muscle or group of muscles. The myoclonic jerks may be unilateral or bilateral. Some are stimulus sensitive. The jerks arise from spontaneous motor neuron discharge in a limited area, often a single segment of the spinal cord. Propriospinal myoclonus (PM) is a more widespread disorder in which myoclonic jerks are propagated up and down the spinal cord from a central generator. Most patients with PM have had minor spinal cord trauma with normal MRI findings. Other causes are severe spinal cord injury, multiple sclerosis, human immunodeficiency virus infection, Lyme infection, syringomyelia, spinal cord tumors, and spinal cord infarction. PM particularly occurs in the transition from wake to sleep.

Toxin- and Drug-Induced Myoclonus

Several drugs and environmental agents with central nervous system toxicity cause myoclonus. Criteria for drug- or toxin-induced myoclonus include verified exposure, temporal association, and exclusion of genetic or other causes. The myoclonus produced by drugs and toxins is often multifocal or generalized, stimulus and action sensitive, and accompanied by other nervous system signs. Treatment requires withdrawal of the causative drug and symptomatic treatment with clonazepam, valproic acid, or levetiracetam.

MISCELLANEOUS MOVEMENT DISORDERS

Hemifacial Spasm

The prevalence of hemifacial spasm is 14.5 per 100,000 in women and 7.4 per 100,000 in men.

Clinical Features

Twitching of the muscles supplied by the facial nerve characterizes the disorder. Onset is in adulthood, usually between 45 and 52 years. Women are affected more often than men. Most cases are sporadic. Twitching first affects the periorbital muscles but spreads to other ipsilateral facial muscles over a period of months to years. The spasms are synchronous in all affected muscles. In about 5% of cases, the opposite side of the face becomes affected, but when bilateral the spasms are never synchronous on the two sides. The spasms of hemifacial spasm may be clonic or tonic, and often a paroxysm of clonic movements culminates in a sustained tonic contraction. Although the spasms occur spontaneously, they may be precipitated or exacerbated by facial movements or by anxiety, stress, or fatigue. Affected muscles may be weaker than their contralateral counterparts. Detailed neuroradiological evaluation may demonstrate compressing vascular structures in most, if not all, patients with hemifacial spasm. Yet, serious underlying causes are rare, and many clinicians do not routinely image patients with typical hemifacial spasm unless surgery is a consideration.

Traditionally, the treatment of hemifacial spasm was with anticonvulsants, typically carbamazepine and more recently gabapentin. Botulinum toxin injected into the periorbital subcutaneous tissue is the treatment of choice. Clinically meaningful improvement occurs in almost all cases and side effects are mild and transient. Intracranial microvascular decompression of the nerve is successful in relieving spasms in up to 90% of patients, but complications such as facial nerve injury and hearing loss occur in up to 15% of patients.

Painful Legs–Moving Toes Syndrome

Painful legs–moving toes syndrome (PLMTS) is a rare condition characterized by pain in the legs and spontaneous movements of the foot and toes.

Clinical Features
The pain usually precedes the onset of involuntary movements and varies in constancy and intensity. The condition is sometimes painless. The toe and foot movements are complex and combine flexion, extension, abduction, and adduction in various sequences. Moving or repositioning the foot or toes precipitates or aborts the movements. Similar movements may occur in the arms, with or without accompanying pain. PLMTS has been associated with injuries to the spinal cord and cauda equina, spinal nerve roots, peripheral neuropathy, and soft tissue or bony limb trauma. EMG studies show that long bursts of normal motor unit firing with normal recruitment patterns produce the movement.

Treatment
Many medications, including baclofen, benzodiazepines, anticonvulsants, and antidepressants, have been tried, but none are effective. Lumbar sympathetic block or epidural stimulation may provide transient relief. Spontaneous resolution is unusual.

Stiff Person Syndrome

Stiff person syndrome (SPS) is a rare syndrome of progressive rigidity of axial and proximal appendicular muscles with muscle hypertrophy and extreme lumbar lordosis. Intense spasms superimpose on a background of continuous symptoms. Gait is slow and stiff legged. Some authors divide SPS into three syndromes: *stiff trunk syndrome, stiff limb syndrome*, and *rapidly progressive encephalomyelitis with rigidity*. EMG examination shows continuous firing of normal motor units.

SPS is associated with autoimmune disorders, such as type I diabetes, thyroiditis, myasthenia gravis, pernicious anemia, and vitiligo. High titers of antibodies to the 65-kd fraction of glutamic acid decarboxylase (GAD) are present. SPS may result from dysfunction of descending suprasegmental pathways, possibly secondary to immune-mediated inhibition of γ-aminobutyric acid synthesis. Paraneoplastic SPS occurs with breast and other cancers.

Untreated SPS progresses to extreme disability. Diazepam at doses between 20 and 400 mg per day is the most effective symptomatic treatment. Plasmapheresis and immunosuppression have variable effects on the condition. Intravenous immune globulin provides clinical improvement and decreases in anti-GAD antibody titers.

For a more detailed discussion, see Chapter 75 in Neurology in Clinical Practice, 4th edition.

Cerebellum and Spinocerebellar Disorders

47

ACQUIRED ATAXIAS

Ataxia with Gluten Sensitivity

Antigliadin antibodies bind to the Purkinje cells of the cerebellum. Individuals with gluten sensitivity may develop a slowly progressive ataxia associated with brisk tendon reflexes, peripheral neuropathy, and mild cognitive changes. Myoclonus and eye movement abnormalities are associated. The characteristic nervous system pathology includes Purkinje's cell loss, cerebellar infiltration by T lymphocytes, and posterior column degeneration. Some patients have typical celiac disease on duodenal biopsy, even when gastrointestinal symptoms are minor. Whether a gluten-free diet or immune therapy will improve ataxia associated with glutin sensitivity remains uncertain.

Ataxia and Glutamic Acid Decarboxylase Antibodies

Few patients with progressive ataxia have glutamic acid decarboxylase (GAD) antibodies. Most are middle-aged women. Ataxia is occasionally associated with peripheral neuropathy, slow saccades, and in some cases *stiff person syndrome*. Many have multiple organ-specific antibodies including those directed against thyroid cells, parietal cells, and pancreatic islet cells. Insulin-dependent diabetes is invariably associated. The antibody titers are higher than those found in patients with adult-onset diabetes and bind to presynaptic nerve terminals around cerebellar Purkinje's cells. GAD, the enzyme that synthesizes γ-aminobutyric acid (GABA) from glutamate, is potentially pathogenic because it binds to GABA terminals. Intravenous immune globulin (IVIG) may cause partial remission of symptoms.

Hypothyroidism

Few patients with hypothyroidism develop mild gait ataxia in conjunction with systemic symptoms. Thyroid hormone replacement can improve the neurological symptoms.

Infectious

Ataxia can be one of several neurological features of post-infectious encephalomyelitis. A restricted cerebellar syndrome occurs in children following some viral infections, especially varicella. In such cases, acute ataxia is the only feature of disease. A similar syndrome occurs in adolescence after having Epstein-Barr virus infection. Cerebrospinal fluid (CSF) analysis may show some elevation of protein concentration and a modest mononuclear pleocytosis. Magnetic resonance imaging (MRI) scans often reveal signal density changes in the cerebellum. Prognosis for recovery is excellent.

A combination of ataxia, ophthalmoplegia, and other lower cranial nerve palsies occurs with brainstem encephalitis (*Bickerstaff's encephalitis*). Human immunodeficiency virus (HIV) infection causes many neurological syndromes, including ataxia. Approximately 30% of patients with HIV-associated dementia have an ataxic syndrome at the onset of illness and before cognitive decline.

Creutzfeldt-Jakob disease (CJD) is part of the differential diagnosis of progressive ataxia. CJD is a rapidly progressive dementia secondary to the accumulation of mutant prion protein. Among patients with CJD, 17% have early ataxia and more than 60% have cerebellar pathology at death. The ataxic variant of CJD begins with minor behavioral symptoms followed by ataxia. Upper motor neuron signs are common, myoclonus occurs in 25%, and dementia is a late feature. These patients survive slightly longer than patients with typical CJD. The mean time to death is 16 months, with a range of 7 weeks to 8 years. Ataxia is the initial feature of both *Gerstmann-Sträussler-Scheinker* (GSS) syndrome, an autosomal dominant form of CJD, and growth hormone-related CJD. The new variant CJD may also present with cerebellar dysfunction.

Nutritional

Acquired Vitamin E deficiency, secondary to fat malabsorption, causes ataxia. Examples include cystic fibrosis and cholestatic liver disease.

Paraneoplastic Cerebellar Degeneration

Paraneoplastic cerebellar degeneration is a rapidly progressive pancerebellar syndrome that reaches its nadir within months of onset. The main features are ataxia, dysarthria, and oscillopsia. Other possible neurological features include dementia, extrapyramidal signs, hearing loss, and dysphagia. MRI scans show atrophy of the cerebellum. An autoimmune process triggered by cancer initiates the syndrome. The *anti-Yo antibody* is associated with ovarian cancer and causes a cerebellar syndrome. The *anti-Hu antibody*, associated with small cell lung cancer, typically causes a multifocal disorder. Sensory ganglionopathy is most common, but Purkinje's cell degeneration occurs in about 25% of patients. Detection of the *anti-Ri antibody* in patients with breast cancer predicts the development of truncal ataxia and opsoclonus. Patients with Lambert-Eaton syndrome secondary to small cell cancer of the lung develop ataxia but have no demonstrable antibodies.

Toxic

Alcohol
Alcohol is the main toxic agent causing ataxia. Many chronic alcoholics have midline cerebellar degeneration at autopsy. This condition is characterized by a progressive gait disturbance with little upper limb ataxia, speech difficulties, or eye movement abnormalities. This may reflect the relative sparing of the cerebellar hemispheres. Imaging studies reveal vermian atrophy.

Chemotherapy
Conventional doses of 5-fluorouracil (5-FU) used to treat breast and gastrointestinal tract cancer may cause cerebellar ataxia when pyrimidine metabolism is abnormal because of dihydropyrimidine dehydrogenase deficiency. Large doses of 5-FU cause a subacute pancerebellar syndrome. Excessive doses of cytosine arabinoside cause a cerebellar syndrome. Pathological examination reveals loss of Purkinje's cells, gliosis, loss of dentate neurons, and spongiform changes.

Metals
Contamination from mercury-containing fungicides has caused epidemics of organic mercury poisoning. Mercury is particularly toxic to cerebellar granule cells and the visual cortex. The toxic syndrome is characterized by paresthesias, ataxia, and restricted visual fields. Manganese poisoning causes ataxia and parkinsonism. Bismuth toxicity resulting from excessive intake of bismuth

subsalicylate (*Pepto-Bismol*) causes a syndrome of gait ataxia, confusion, and myoclonus.

Solvents

Chronic solvent abuse, especially toluene in spray paint and paint thinners, causes persistent neurological deficits that include ataxia, cognitive deficits, pyramidal tract dysfunction, and dysarthria.

Anticonvulsants

Transitory cerebellar signs are associated with high blood concentrations of several antiepileptic drugs. Persistent ataxia and Purkinje's cell loss occurred primarily in epileptics treated with toxic dosages of phenytoin for prolonged periods. The cerebellar atrophy that occurs secondary to phenytoin toxicity is not always associated with clinical ataxia.

INHERITED ATAXIAS

Autosomal Recessive Ataxias

Most autosomal recessive ataxias based on specific gene loci begin in childhood or early adulthood (Table 47.1). Single cases occur in many families. Typically, the heterozygous parent is normal. Identification of other affected family members is more likely if the sibship size is large or an extended pedigree is available. Both genders are affected. Parental consanguinity is more likely but not essential.

Friedreich's Ataxia

CLINICAL FEATURES The estimated prevalence of Friedreich's ataxia (FA) is 2 per 100,000. Age at onset is younger than 25 years, typically early in adolescence. Increasing gait difficulties bring the patient to medical attention. Neurological examination reveals gait ataxia and loss of proprioceptive sense in the legs. Tendon reflexes are absent, either in all limbs or only the legs. Most patients also exhibit signs of central nervous system (CNS) involvement, including dysarthria, extensor-plantar responses, and eye movement abnormalities. Few patients have cardiac disease or a spinal deformity and later develop neurological disease. Ambulation is lost 9–15 years after onset. At this stage, marked ataxia is present in all limbs, proprioceptive loss is profound, and all tendon reflexes are absent. Other features include paraparesis, dystonia, flexor spasms, and increasing dysarthria and dysphagia.

Table 47.1: Autosomal recessive ataxias with known gene loci

Disease	Gene Locus	Gene	Mutation
Friedreich's ataxia	9q13–21.1	X25	GAA expansion
Ataxia-telangiectasia *	11q22-23	ATM	Point mutations/deletions
Ataxia with oculomotor apraxia*	9p13	Aprataxin	Point mutations/deletions/insertions
ATLD*	11q21	MRE11	Point mutations
SCAN-1*	14q31	TDP1	Point mutations/deletions/insertions
AVED	8q	αTTP	Point mutations
ARSACS	13q11	SACS	Point mutations
Ataxia, neuropathy, high α-fetoprotein	9q33-34	Unknown	Unknown
IOSCA	10q24	Unknown	Unknown
Ataxia, deafness, optic atrophy	6p21-23	Unknown	Unknown
Unverricht-Lundborg disease	21q	Cystatin B	Repeat expansion

*These all involve mutations in DNA repair genes. Xeroderma pigmentosum and Cockayne's syndrome are other multiple system DNA repair defects in which one may see ataxia.

ARSACS = autosomal recessive spastic ataxia of Charlevoix-Saguenay; ATLD = ataxia-telangiectasia–like disorder; AVED = ataxia with isolated vitamin E deficiency; IOSCA = infantile onset spinocerebellar ataxia; SCAN-1 = spinocerebellar ataxia with axonal neuropathy 1; TDP = tyrosyl DNA phosphodiesterase; TTP = tocopherol transfer protein.

Systemic abnormalities include an abnormal electrocardiogram (ECG), hypertrophic cardiomyopathy, and diabetes. Spinal and foot deformities are common. The mean age at death is the fourth decade, usually of cardiac origin.

Nerve conduction studies show early absence or reduction of sensory nerve potentials. Brain MRI scans reveal no abnormalities in the cerebellum, but the upper cervical cord shows atrophy.

THE FA MUTATION   The FA mutation is an unstable expansion of a repeated trinucleotide (GAA) sequence within the first intron of the gene X 25 on chromosome 9q13-21.1. More than 80% of normal alleles have fewer than 10 GAA repeats. Long normal alleles with 12–40 repeats are believed to serve as a reservoir for expansion into mutations. Expanded alleles have 66 to more than 1000 repeats. Because disease inheritance is recessive, both gene copies must have mutations to produce disease. In nearly 95% of affected individuals, the GAA expansion occurs in both alleles (homozygous expansion), although the size of the expansion can be different. Patients with clinical findings compatible with FA but with only a heterozygous expansion of the GAA repeats have point mutations in the unexpanded allele. Commercially available FA mutation analysis cannot distinguish between such compound heterozygotes and unaffected carriers of the disease. No individual with FA has a homozygous point mutation.

Many individuals with a phenotype very atypical for FA carry the FA mutation but have variations in phenotype. These include age at onset later than 25 years (*late-onset FA* [LOFA]), retained or exaggerated tendon reflexes (*FA with retained reflexes* [FARR]), a later onset with retained reflexes, and a very late onset of mild gait ataxia, spastic paraparesis, and chorea. As with other trinucleotide repeat diseases, the GAA repeat size and the age at onset are inversely related. Cardiomyopathy and diabetes tend to occur with larger (>700) GAA repeats. Because the size of the GAA expansion exhibits somatic mosaicism, the severity of pathology in a particular tissue may depend to some extent on the repeat size in that tissue.

Approximately 5% of patients with FA have heterozygous GAA expansion in one copy of the gene and a point mutation in the second copy. Both missense and truncating mutations located in the carboxy-terminal half of the frataxin gene appear to be associated with a typical FA phenotype. Missense mutations in the amino-terminal half such as the G130V mutation appear to result in a milder phenotype with less ataxia, greater spasticity, and absence of dysarthria.

TREATMENT The supportive care of patients with FA includes adequate rehabilitation efforts aimed at better mobility by use of appropriate devices. Monitoring and caring for the systemic complications are also important. These include skeletal deformities, cardiomyopathy, and diabetes.

Ataxia-Telangiectasia
The discussion of ataxia-telangiectasia (AT) is in Chapter 40.

Ataxia with Isolated Vitamin E Deficiency
Mutations in the gene encoding the α-tocopherol transfer protein (α-TTP) on chromosome 8 are responsible for a childhood-onset recessive ataxia associated with isolated Vitamin E deficiency (AVED). The severity of the phenotype associated with these mutations depends on residual protein activity. The disease has some resemblance to FA, but age at onset is from 2 to 52 years, the incidence of cardiomyopathy is lower, and head titubation is more common. Patients with AVED typically have less than 1.8 mg/L of Vitamin E in serum. Treatment with large doses of Vitamin E will elevate the levels and perhaps slow progression of the disease.

Abetalipoproteinemia
Mutations in the microsomal triglyceride transfer protein are the cause of abetalipoproteinemia, a rare disease. The presence of retinopathy, malabsorption (including that of Vitamin E), low serum cholesterol levels, and acanthocytes establishes the diagnosis. Serum lipoprotein electrophoresis also establishes the diagnosis.

Autosomal Recessive Ataxia with Oculomotor Apraxia
Early onset of ataxia, autosomal recessive inheritance, and features resembling AT such as oculomotor apraxia, loss of deep tendon reflexes, and cerebellar atrophy characterize this disorder. Serum albumin is decreased and total cholesterol elevated. Unlike with AT, malignancies are not part of the phenotype. The gene mutation involves the *aprataxin* gene, which may be involved in DNA repair as well.

Other DNA Repair Defects Causing Ataxia
Mutations in MRE11 cause an AT-like disorder (ATLD) and mutations in the TDP1 gene cause spinocerebellar ataxia with axonal neuropathy (SCAN1). These patients do not have the systemic features that characterize AT and ATLD. *Cockayne's syndrome* and xeroderma pigmentosa are diseases caused by DNA repair defects in which systemic disease dominates the phenotype, but CNS features include ataxia. Mutations in genes

encoding components of the nucleotide excision repair pathway are responsible.

Other Genetically Defined Autosomal Recessive Ataxias

Other recessive ataxias have been genotyped in a limited number of families. These include an FA2 locus on chromosome 9p characterized by ataxia, neuropathy, and high α-fetoprotein (9q); ataxia, deafness, and optic atrophy (6p); and ataxia with increased saccadic speed (1p).

Ataxias with Defined Biochemical Errors

The cause of many childhood and young adult–onset ataxias are metabolic errors in which diagnosis requires specific laboratory tests rather than gene-based tests. Table 47.2 lists these diseases. Some are amenable to therapy.

Mitochondrial Diseases and Ataxia

Progressive ataxia is often an intrinsic feature of many mitochondrial cytopathies related to mutations in the mitochondrial DNA (mtDNA). The association of ataxia with myopathy, external ophthalmoplegia, or other features of mitochondriopathies suggests a mitochondrial disease (see Chapter 38).

Autosomal Dominant Ataxias

Autosomal dominant ataxias usually begin in adult life. The disease occurs in each generation of the pedigree. Genetic heterogeneity is common among the dominant ataxias (Tables 47.3 and 47.4). Progressive dominant ataxias are labeled spinocerebellar ataxia (SCA) followed by a number to denote the chromosomal locus.

Clinical Features

As a group, the progressive dominant ataxias have overlapping clinical features. Gradually progressive cerebellar ataxia is the core feature. Many are associated with clinical signs referable to pathology in other CNS structures. Oculomotor abnormalities unrelated to cerebellar dysfunction include gaze palsy, ptosis, blepharospasm, and an "ocular stare." Other patients have facial atrophy, facial fasciculations, tongue atrophy, and fasciculations. Brisk reflexes, with or without spasticity, and extensorplantar responses are common features. Extrapyramidal signs include akinetic-rigid syndromes, hypomimic facies, chorea, athetosis, and dystonia. Peripheral nerve disease occurs frequently and includes distal sensory loss and loss of deep tendon

Table 47.2: Ataxias in which specific biochemical abnormalities may confirm or point to the diagnosis (some also appear in Table 47.1)

Disorder	Laboratory Tests
AVED	Low vitamin E levels
Abetalipoproteinemia	Low vitamin E levels, high cholesterol, abnormal lipoprotein electrophoresis
AOA	Low albumin, high cholesterol
AT	High α-fetoprotein, low IgA
Cerebrotendinous xanthomatosis	High serum cholestanol
Adrenoleukodystrophy	Serum long chain fatty acids
Ataxia with CoQ deficiency	Low CoQ in muscle biopsy
Vanishing white matter disease	MRI, MRS
Late onset GM$_2$ gangliosidoses	Hexosaminidase in fibroblasts
CDG syndromes	Transferrin isoelectric focusing
Mitochondrial diseases	Lactic acid levels, RRF in muscle
Sialidosis	Neuraminidase
Maple syrup urine disease	Urine amino acids
Organic acidurias	Urine organic acids, ketone bodies
Urea cycle defects	Plasma ammonia
Pyruvate dehydrogenase deficiency	Lactate levels

AOA = ataxia with oculomotor apraxia; AT = ataxia-telangiectasia; AVED = ataxia with isolated vitamin E deficiency; CDG = carbohydrate-deficient glycoprotein; CoQ = coenzyme Q; MRI = magnetic resonance imaging; MRS = magnetic resonance spectroscopy; RRF = ragged red fibers.

reflexes and amyotrophy. The motor syndrome is inexorably progressive with loss of ambulation over 10–15 years. A faster rate of progression correlates with earlier onset of disease.

The episodic ataxia (EA) syndromes cause intermittent episodes of imbalance, dysarthria, vertigo, and abnormal eye movements that last from minutes to hours. At least two gene mutations give rise to EA. EA-1 is associated with brief episodes of ataxia and no interictal cerebellar abnormalities. In EA-2, the ataxic episodes are longer and may be associated with interictal abnormalities such as nystagmus. Some patients with EA-2 also develop progressive ataxia.

Diagnosis
Imaging and other laboratory studies are useful to exclude other disorders. DNA analysis provides definitive diagnosis.

Table 47.3: Autosomal dominant ataxias that have been genotypically defined

Disease	Locus	Gene	Mutation
SCA-1	6p22.3	Ataxin 1	CAG expansion
SCA-2	12q24.12	Ataxin 2	CAG expansion
MJD (SCA-3)	14q21	Ataxin 3	CAG expansion
SCA-4	16q22.1	Unknown	Unknown
SCA-5	11p11-q11	Unknown	Unknown
SCA-6	19p13.2	CACNA1	CAG expansion
SCA-7	3p14.1	Ataxin 7	CAG expansion
SCA-8	13q21	SCA-8	CTG expansion
SCA-10	22q13	SCA-10	ATTCT expansion
SCA-11	15q14-21.3	SCA-11	Unknown
SCA-12	5q32	PPP2R2B	CAG expansion
SCA-13	19q13.3-13.4	SCA-13	Unknown
SCA-14	19q13.4	SCA-14	Unknown
SCA-15	Reserved	SCA-15	
SCA-16	8q23-24.1	SCA-16	Unknown
SCA-17	6q27	TBP	CAG expansion
SCA-18	7q31-32	Unknown	Unknown
SCA-19	Reserved	Unknown	Unknown
SCA-21	7p21.3-15.1	Unknown	Unknown
SCA-22	Reserved	Unknown	Unknown
SCA-23	20p13-12.2	Unknown	Unknown
DRPLA	12p	Atrophin	CAG expansion
EA-1	12p	KCNA1	Point mutations
EA-2	19p	CACNA1	Point mutations

DRPLA = dentatorubral-pallidoluysian atrophy; EA = episodic ataxia;
MJD = Machado-Joseph disease; TBP = TATA-binding protein.

SPORADIC ATAXIAS

The term *sporadic ataxia* encompasses progressive cerebellar ataxias that clinically resemble inherited ataxias but have no definite genetic etiology.

Sporadic Cortical Cerebellar Atrophy

Sporadic cortical cerebellar atrophy usually has onset after age 50 years and results in a slowly progressive ataxia not associated with other neurological deficits. Brain MRI scans show isolated cerebellar atrophy.

Table 47.4: Distinctive phenotypical features of some dominant ataxias; in general, the various genotypes resemble each other closely

Phenotypical Feature	Disorders
Age at onset	Young adult: SCA-1, SCA-2, MJD; older adult: SCA-6; childhood onset frequent in SCA-7/DRPLA
Degree of anticipation	More in SCA-7, DRPLA
Benign course	SCA-6
Upper motor neuron signs	SCA-1, -7, -8, MJD; rare in SCA-2
Akinetic-rigid/ Parkinson's signs	MJD, SCA-2, SCA-17
Chorea	Prominent in DRPLA; late in SCA-2, -1, MJD
Action tremor	SCA-12, -16
Very slow saccades	Early in SCA-2, -7; late in SCA-1, MJD; never in SCA-6
Downbeat nystagmus	SCA-6, EA-2
Generalized areflexia	SCA-2, SCA-4, older adult-onset MJD
Visual loss	SCA-7
Seizures	SCA-10, early onset DRPLA, SCA-7

DRPLA = dentatorubral-pallidoluysian atrophy; EA = episodic ataxia; MJD = Machado-Joseph disease; SCA = spinocerebellar ataxia.

Sporadic Ataxia with Added Noncerebellar Deficits

The ataxia is slowly progressive ataxia and later joined by signs of corticospinal dysfunction, ophthalmoplegia, parkinsonian features, and autonomic failure. MRI scans show cerebellar and brainstem degeneration. The clinical picture merges with the olivopontocerebellar atrophy form of multiple system atrophy (MSA). Among patients with idiopathic progressive ataxia, one third will transition to probable MSA over 5–10 years. Median survival after such transition is only 3.5 years.

CLINICAL APPROACH TO PATIENTS WITH DEGENERATIVE ATAXIAS

A careful clinical approach to patients presenting with progressive ataxia allows accurate diagnosis and appropriate management. The age at onset, the tempo of progression, associated neurological and systemic signs, and the family history are all important in making a diagnosis. Imaging studies, especially MRI of the brain, allow the exclusion of nongenetic causes of ataxia. Diagnosis of those disorders in which characteristic morphological abnormalities underlie ataxia require other valuable laboratory studies including thyroid function, Vitamin E and Vitamin B_{12} levels, serology for syphilis, gliadin and anti-GAD antibodies, antibodies associated with paraneoplastic syndromes, and possibly CSF examination.

DNA testing is now available for FA, SCA-1, SCA-2, SCA-3, SCA-6, SCA-7, SCA-8, SCA-10, SCA-12, SCA-17, and denta-torubral-pallidoluysian atrophy. Gene testing is possible but not readily available for AT, ARSACS, AVED, AOA-1, and EA syndromes.

For a more detailed discussion, see Chapters 23 and 76 in Neurology in Clinical Practice, 4th edition.

Disorders of Bones, Joints, Ligaments, and Meninges

48

CRANIOCERVICAL DEFORMITIES

Occipitalization of the Atlas

Occipitalization of the atlas is a partial or complete fusion of the first cervical vertebra to the occiput. The anterior arch of the atlas may fuse to the lower end of the clivus or the posterior arch of the atlas may fuse to the occiput. The anomaly is often asymptomatic but may become symptomatic after trauma. The loss of movement between the occiput and atlas increases the stresses at the atlantoaxial joint, predisposing it to gradual degeneration or traumatic dislocation. Patients with occipitalization of the atlas may have associated anomalies, such as a Klippel-Feil anomaly, basilar impression, or Chiari malformation.

Basilar Impression

Basilar impression or *invagination* refers to abnormal cephalad position of the foramen magnum. Several radiological lines (Chamberlain, McGregor, McRae, digastric) and measurements are useful for diagnosis. Congenital basilar impression may occur in isolation or be associated with conditions such as achondroplasia, occipital dysplasia, Down syndrome, Hurler's syndrome, Klippel-Feil anomaly, and cleidocranial dysplasia. Some instances of basilar impression are genetic. Often, the skeletal anomaly is associated with anomalies of the neuraxis, including Chiari I or II malformation and syringomyelia. Basilar impression can cause compression of the brainstem or cerebellum or, rarely, vertebral artery compression, leading to vertebrobasilar ischemia. It is often asymptomatic, particularly when mild and unaccompanied by other anomalies. *Platybasia*, a straightening of the angle between the clivus and the floor of the anterior fossa, may accompany basilar impression.

Klippel-Feil Anomaly

Failure of normal segmentation of the cervical vertebrae between the third and eighth weeks of fetal development causes this anomaly. The anomaly can cause direct nerve root, cervical spinal cord, or vertebral or spinal artery compression. Neck pain is common. Hearing loss is the most common symptom of cranial neuropathy. Mirror movements of the hands may occur in children secondary to incomplete decussation of the pyramidal tracts. Associated abnormalities include scoliosis, Sprengel's deformity with unilateral shoulder elevation, hydrocephalus, syringomyelia, or syringobulbia. Most are neurologically normal.

Atlantoaxial Dislocation

Several congenital or acquired conditions disrupt the integrity of the atlantoaxial joint and cause dislocation (Table 48.1). In horizontal subluxation, C1 usually moves anteriorly to C2.

Table 48.1: Mechanisms of atlantoaxial dislocation

I. Congenital
    A. Os odontoideum (failure of the odontoid to fuse with the body of the axis)
        1. Isolated
        2. With connective tissue dysplasias (e.g., Down syndrome, pseudoachondroplasia, multiple epiphyseal dysplasia, spondyloepiphyseal dysplasia, Morquio's disease, Klippel-Feil anomaly, Conradi's syndrome)
    B. Hypoplastic dens
        1. With connective tissue dysplasia
        2. With incomplete segmentation (e.g., occipital assimilation of atlas, basilar invagination, incomplete segmentation of C2, C3, and so forth)
    C. Other anomalies of C2 (e.g., bifid dens, tripartite dens with os apicale, agenesis of all or part of dens)
    D. Laxity of the transverse atlantal ligament (e.g., Down syndrome)
II. Acquired
    E. Traumatic, acute or chronic un-united dens fracture
    F. Infectious
    G. Neoplastic (e.g., neurofibroma)
    H. Arthritic (e.g., in rheumatoid arthritis, ankylosing spondylitis, renal amyloidosis)
    I. Bone disease (e.g., vitamin D–resistant rickets and others associated with basilar invagination)

Patients with horizontal atlantoaxial joint subluxation are likely to compress their spinal cords if the diameter of the spinal canal at the level of the dens is less than 14 mm. Patients with congenital atlantoaxial dislocation may have associated abnormalities such as Chiari I malformation or diastematomyelia. Atlantoaxial subluxation occurs in patients with long-standing rheumatoid arthritis (RA). Patients with atlantoaxial subluxation may be asymptomatic but are vulnerable to spinal cord trauma during intubation or during whiplash injury. Patients with Down syndrome or chronic RA should have lateral flexion and extension cervical spine radiography performed before general anesthesia.

Arnold-Chiari Malformation

Abnormal extension of the cerebellar tonsils below the foramen magnum, sometimes accompanied by rostral displacement or extension of the medulla, characterizes the Chiari malformation. The discussion is in Chapter 35.

Hydromyelia and Syringomyelia

Hydromyelia

Hydromyelia is an abnormal dilatation of the central spinal canal, which usually communicates with the fourth ventricle. A syrinx is a cavity in the spinal cord (syringomyelia) or brainstem (syringobulbia). The cavity may connect to a dilatated central spinal canal. Most syringes are in the cervical spinal cord. Those developing from hydromyelia of the central canal are usually associated with Chiari I or II malformations, communicating hydrocephalus, or abnormalities at the craniocerebral junction.

Syringomyelia

The typical presentation of a syrinx is the combination of lower motor neuron signs at the level of the lesion and spinal long tract dysfunction below the level of the lesion. The clinical features vary with the size, location, and shape of the cavity. Common complaints include neck ache, headache, back pain, radicular pain, and areas of segmental dysesthesia. Magnetic resonance imaging (MRI) provides a complete evaluation of the cord and surrounding soft tissues.

Syringomyelia accompanies 25–60% of intramedullary spinal tumors; conversely, tumors cause 8–16% of syringes. The syrinx usually extends rostral from the tumor. Syringes sometimes develop as late sequelae of serious spinal cord trauma. Pain is often a prominent symptom. Any illness causing arachnoid inflammation can lead to formation of a noncommunicating syrinx. Causes other than trauma and tumors include spinal ischemic or hemorrhagic strokes, radiation necrosis, or transverse myelitis.

Simple myelotomy or shunting to the subarachnoid, peritoneal, or pleural cavity drains the cavity. Syrinx-associated Chiari I malformations improves after decompression of the malformation and dural grafting. Syringes extending from an intramedullary tumor regress after resection of the tumor without surgical drainage of the cavity. Syringes extending from an area of localized arachnoiditis regress after resection of the arachnoiditis.

Achondroplasia

Achondroplasia, the most common cause of abnormally short stature, is an autosomal dominant disorder of endochondral bone formation caused by a specific mutation of the fibroblast growth factor-3 gene. The diagnosis is confirmed by radiographic changes or by DNA testing. Neurological complications include hydrocephalus, compression at the foramen magnum, thoracolumbar kyphosis, sleep apnea, and spinal stenosis.

CONGENITAL SPINAL CORD DISORDERS

Spinal Dysraphism

Dysraphism refers to disorders that result from failure of closure of the neural tube. The discussion is in Chapter 35.

Tethered Cord Syndromes

Congenital abnormalities of the spinal cord or cauda equina can prevent normal cephalad movement of the conus medullaris during early life. The mechanism of progressive neurological dysfunction is traction on the cord or nerve roots. The most common neurological finding is unilateral lower motor neuron dysfunction in one leg. Sensory, upper motor neuron, or sphincter dysfunction occurs. Children may present with orthopedic foot deformities or scoliosis.

Diastematomyelia

Diastematomyelia is a congenital malformation characterized by sagittal division of a portion of the cord into two hemicords. The division is usually located in the lower thoracic or lumbar region.

Skin abnormalities, such as a tuft of hair at the level of the lesion, often are associated. If each hemicord is enclosed in its own arachnoid sheath, the sheathes are usually separated by a bony, cartilaginous, or fibrous spur and by dura in the cleft between the two portions of the cord. The spur tethers the spinal cord, leading to progressive neurological dysfunction. MRI or computed tomographic (CT) myelography confirms the diagnosis. Surgical therapy consists of attempts to free all structures tethering the cord.

SPINAL DEFORMITIES AND METABOLIC BONE DISEASE

Osteoporosis

Osteoporosis is mainly a disease of older women. The main complication is vertebral compression fractures in the thoracic and thoracolumbar spine. Although these may lead to kyphosis and loss of body height, most are painless. In younger men and women, acute posttraumatic compression fractures are more likely to be painful. The level of the compression is the center of pain and loss of spinal range of motion. Pain increases with activity, decreases with bed rest, and resolves slowly—sometimes incompletely. Compression fracture accompanied by myelopathy suggests the possibility of a metastatic vertebral lesion. Percutaneous vertebroplasty with polymethylmethacrylate decreases the duration of pain.

Osteogenesis Imperfecta

Osteogenesis imperfecta is an inherited connective tissue disorder characterized by brittle osteopenic bones and recurrent fractures. Four types vary in severity and associated findings such as short stature, blue sclera, hearing loss, scoliosis, and skeletal abnormalities. Potential neurological complications include communiccating hydrocephalus, basilar invagination, macrocephaly, skull fractures, and seizure disorder. The basilar invagination can lead to brainstem compression.

Osteomalacia and Rickets

Osteomalacia and rickets are conditions of deficient bone mineralization. Long bones usually are more involved than the spine. Spinal pain, kyphosis, and compression fractures can occur in osteomalacia, but compression of spinal cord or nerve roots is rare. Basilar impression occurs in patients with osteo-malacia.

Osteopetrosis

Osteopetrosis is a rare disease characterized by increased bone density caused by impaired bone resorption. Inheritance is either autosomal dominant or autosomal recessive. Osteopetrosis of the skull can cause cranial neuropathies, basilar impression, hydrocephalus, or syringomyelia. Osteopetrosis of the spine can contribute to spinal canal stenosis with secondary compressive myelopathy.

Paget's Disease

Paget's disease is a focal metabolic bone disease of excessive osteoclastic bony destruction and reactive osteoblastic activity. The incidence increases with age and varies among ethnic groups. The incidence in elderly northern Europeans is 5%. Men are more affected than women. The leading pathogenic hypothesis is a chronic viral infection of osteoclasts on a background of genetic susceptibility.

Clinical Features
When symptomatic, it causes symptoms by bone or joint distortion, fractures, compression of neurological tissue by calcification, hemorrhage, or focal ischemia caused by a vascular steal by the metabolically hyperactive bony tissue. It may also cause hypercalcemia, especially in patients confined to bed. Osteogenic sarcoma can develop in pagetic bone.

Paget's disease of the skull causes head enlargement, headache, and hearing loss. Disease of the cribriform plate disrupts olfaction. Optic neuropathy, trigeminal neuralgia, and hemifacial spasm can occur. Distortion of the posterior fossa or basilar invagination leads to brainstem or cerebellar compression, hydrocephalus, or syringomyelia. Symptomatic disease of the spine occurs most often in the lumbar region, where it causes mono-radiculopathies or a cauda equina syndrome. Myelopathy is more common with thoracic than cervical involvement.

Diagnosis
Characteristic findings on radiography establish the diagnosis. Osteolytic activity causes well-demarcated round patches of low bone density. Osteoblastic activity leads to thickening of cortical bone and a general increase in bone density, often with distortion of normal organization. Osteolytic and osteoblastic findings are often present together. Serum bone alkaline phosphatase

concentrations are elevated and are used to follow the response to treatment.

Treatment

Bisphosphonates are the treatment of choice. Other treatment options include calcitonin, plicamycin, or gallium nitrate. Within 1–2 weeks of treatment, bone pain improves, and serum alkaline phosphatase levels decrease. Some patients experience significant neurological improvement after treatment, but often delay of improvement is 1–3 months. Severe cord compression requires decompression. Patients with cranial neuropathy have less impressive responses to drug therapy. Those with hydrocephalus may benefit from ventricular shunting.

Scoliosis

Idiopathic scoliosis that develops during childhood, with or without kyphosis, is usually not associated with neurological abnormalities. Indications for spinal MRI include pain, progression suddenly or after spinal maturity, thoracic curvature to the right, or abnormal neurological examination findings. Only a small number have a syrinx or Chiari I malformation. Spinal cord compression is a rare complication of idiopathic scoliosis, especially in the absence of kyphosis. Congenital scoliosis, unlike idiopathic scoliosis, is usually associated with anomalous vertebrae and other developmental problems. Scoliosis is also caused by several neurological diseases (cerebral palsy, spinocerebellar degenerations, inherited neuropathies, myelopathies, spinal muscular atrophies, and genetic myopathies) and is the most common skeletal complication of neurofibromatosis type 1.

Diffuse Idiopathic Skeletal Hyperostosis

Diffuse idiopathic skeletal hyperostosis (*DISH, Forestier disease, ankylosing hyperostosis*) is a syndrome of excessive calcification that develops with aging. Men are more often affected than women. Spinal radiographs show "flowing" calcifications along the anterior and lateral portion of at least four contiguous vertebral bodies. Disc height is not lost, and radiographs are not typical of ankylosing spondylitis. Most patients are asymptomatic; some have spinal pain or limited spinal motion. Large anterior cervical calcifications can contribute to dysphagia, hoarseness, sleep apnea, or difficulty with intubation.

Ossification of the Posterior Longitudinal Ligaments or Ligamentum Flavum

Both ossification of the posterior longitudinal ligament anterior to the spinal canal and ossification of the ligamentum flavum are uncommon syndromes of acquired calcification. Either ligament can ossify in later life, independent of the usual processes of spondylosis and degenerative arthritis. Ossification of the posterior longitudinal ligament may be visible on lateral spinal radiography but is better seen by CT scan. Ossification of the posterior longitudinal ligament is most likely to be symptomatic in the cervical spine, where it contributes to cord compression.

The ligamentum flavum contributes by hypertrophy or ossification to spinal stenosis in the lower thoracic or lumbar spine, affecting the cord or cauda equina. Risk factors include trauma, hemochromatosis, calcium pyrophosphate deposition disease, diffuse idiopathic skeletal hyperostosis, ankylosing spondylitis, or ossification of the posterior longitudinal ligament.

DEGENERATIVE DISEASE OF THE SPINE

Spinal Osteoarthritis and Spondylosis

Routine spinal radiography shows spinal osteoarthritis in more than 90% of people by age 60 years. Involvement of the spinal facet joints results in joint narrowing, sclerosis, osteophyte formation, and degenerative disease of the intervertebral discs. The degeneration is visible on radiography as disc space narrowing and vertebral endplate sclerosis. It is the most common cause of compressive myelopathy or radiculopathy.

Cervical Spondylosis

Cervical osteoarthritis and spondylosis are an expected part of aging and are rarely attributable to specific activities or injuries. They have no established role in contributing to chronic neck pain or headache. Surgery is not a treatment of headache or neck ache in the absence of cervical radiculopathy or myelopathy.

Cervical Radiculopathy

Clinical Features
Symptoms often appear suddenly. Although acute trauma may cause disc herniation or nerve root contusion, trauma is not a factor in most cases. Disc herniation is the likely cause before age 45 years and neural foraminal stenosis by degenerative changes

afterwards. The typical feature is neck pain with radiation to an arm, made worse by coughing. Arm pain may increase with neck rotation and flexion to the side of the pain (*Spurling sign*). The C5, C6, and C7 roots are the ones most commonly involved in cervical spondylosis, because they are at the level of greatest mobility, where disc degeneration is greatest.

Diagnosis
MRI of the cervical spine usually identifies the nerve root compression. Cervical myelography followed by CT is sometimes more sensitive than MRI. However, cautious interpretation of all studies is required because degenerative abnormalities are common in the asymptomatic spine. Electromyography and nerve conduction studies can be useful in difficult diagnostic cases.

Treatment
Cervical radiculopathy usually improves over 4–8 weeks, regardless of treatment. Treatments such as nonsteroidal anti-inflammatory drugs and use of a soft cervical collar, physical therapy, or cervical traction give similar results. Surgical nerve root decompression is indicated when patients have intractable weakness or pain after conservative therapy. Anterior cervical discectomy is more widely used than posterior cervical laminectomy.

Cervical Spondylotic Myelopathy

Clinical Features
Myelopathy caused by compression of the cervical spinal cord by the changes of spondylosis usually develops insidiously. Sometimes, trauma precipitates myelopathy or progress occurs in a stepwise fashion. Typical findings are a combination of leg spasticity, arm weakness or clumsiness, and sensory changes in the arms, legs, or trunk. Sphincter dysfunction, if it occurs, is a late finding. Neck pain is not prominent, and neck range of motion may not be impaired. Some patients experience leg or trunk paresthesias induced by neck flexion. The natural history of cervical spondylotic myelopathy is variable. Some patients may have stable neurological deficit for many years without specific therapy, whereas others may have gradual or stepwise deterioration.

Diagnosis
MRI images the relation between the spinal canal and the spinal cord and provides detail such as secondary cord edema or gliosis.

Treatment
Some patients improve with treatments such as bed rest, soft collars, or immobilizing collars. Surgical decompression is the treatment of cervical spondylotic myelopathy. All treatment results are best when the neurological deficit is mild and present less than 6 months and when the patient is younger than 70 years.

Thoracic Spondylosis

Degenerative changes are less common in the thoracic than in the lumbar or cervical spine. Thoracic disc herniations are visible on MRI in many asymptomatic individuals. Thoracic disc herniations in the lower thoracic spine rarely cause cord or root compression and may regress spontaneously. Most cases of thoracic disc herniation occur between ages 30 and 60 years. Symptom development is insidious, without preceding trauma. Back pain is variable. Sphincter dysfunction is present in more severe cases. Thoracic MRI or CT confirms the diagnosis. Treatment is by surgical decompression.

Lumbar Spondylosis

Low Back Pain
The most common symptom is episodic low back pain that resolves in a few days. Several pain-sensitive structures in the lumbar region may be responsible. Specific localization is not valuable in planning therapy.

Spondylolysis and Spondylolisthesis

Spondylolisthesis is displacement of one lumbar vertebral body relative to an adjacent vertebral body. Spondylolysis, a discontinuity in the vertebral pars interarticularis that disrupts the normal stabilizing effect of the facet joints, is the underlying cause. Other causes of spondylolisthesis include congenital vertebral anomalies, degenerative spondylosis, and vertebral trauma. Spondylolysis occurs in 6% of the population and is usually asymptomatic. Spondylolisthesis is either painless or causes low back pain that may radiate to the buttocks. Spondylolytic spondylolisthesis is a common cause of back pain in adolescents. Advanced spondylolisthesis compresses nerve roots in the neuroforamina or causes lumbar canal stenosis.

Lumbar Radiculopathies

Three pain syndromes merit specific diagnostic consideration.

Monoradiculopathy

The features of lumbosacral monoradiculopathy caused by nerve root compression are unilateral leg pain (sciatica) radiating into the buttock and lateroposterior thigh, and sometimes paresthesias. Low back pain is usually present. Pain increases with movement, coughing, sneezing, or Valsalva maneuver and decreases with rest. Pain increases upon raising the straightened ipsilateral leg while the patient is supine or straightening the leg of the seated patient. The most commonly compressed nerve roots are L5, usually by L4-L5 disc herniation, or S1, usually by L5-S1 disc herniation. For L5 radiculopathy, the typical findings are medial foot and hallux pain, paresthesias of the medial dorsal foot, and weakness in the extensor hallucis longus, the ankle dorsiflexors, and peroneal muscles. S1 nerve root compression can lead to lateral foot pain and paresthesias, depressed ankle jerk, and weakness of peroneal muscles and less frequently of ankle plantar flexors. When the radiculopathy is mild, the patient may have no objective neurological deficit.

MRI allows visualization of the anatomical relations between the nerve roots and the surrounding tissues. Unfortunately, all spinal imaging modalities frequently show anatomical abnormalities that are not the cause of symptomatic nerve root dysfunction. Electromyography can aid in neurological localization by demonstrating neuropathic abnormalities in specific myotomes.

Low back pain and sciatica usually recover within 6 weeks with brief periods of bed rest, activity limitations as required by pain, and simple analgesics. Prolonged immobilization is detrimental. Consider surgical nerve root decompression for patients with progressive weakness or sensory loss or for those with severe pain that fails to improve after 6 weeks of bed rest. Chronic low back pain or repeated exacerbations of acute low back pain occur in a small number of patients. Back strengthening exercises, the avoidance of maneuvers that put strain on the lower back, and the judicious use of nonsteroidal anti-inflammatory drugs generally improve chronic low back pain. Most patients report excellent relief of neuropathic pain following surgery, but severe chronic pain develops in others (*failed back syndrome*). These patients require careful neurological evaluation to consider such problems as surgery performed at the wrong level, incomplete removal of extruded disc fragment or other matter compressing the nerve root, progression of spinal degeneration, postoperative arachnoiditis, and psychosocial issues interfering with recovery.

Acute Cauda Equina Syndrome

Acute cauda equina syndrome presents as low back and leg pain and neurological deficits caused by compression of multiple lumbosacral nerve roots. Particularly worrisome findings are sacral sensory loss or impaired function of the rectal and urinary sphincters. The cause is usually a large midline disc herniation, most often at L4-L5 or L5-S1. Urgent spinal imaging and decompressive surgery restore neurological function.

Lumbar Canal Stenosis

Lumbar canal stenosis results from anatomical changes that decrease the cross-sectional area of the spinal canal including congenitally small canal size, degenerative osteophytes, spondylolisthesis, facet joint hypertrophy, thickening of the ligamentum flavum, and disc herniation. It usually develops insidiously and rarely becomes symptomatic before age 40 years. Men are more often affected than women. The typical symptom of lumbar canal stenosis is *neurogenic intermittent claudication*: leg discomfort elicited by walking or by certain postures such as standing straight, which is relieved within minutes by stopping walking or changing posture. The pain may be anywhere in the legs or buttocks and may include numbness or paresthesias. Most patients do not have objective signs of nerve root dysfunction.

MRI is the diagnostic study of choice. Mild analgesics are satisfactory to manage patients with stable symptoms without progressive neurological deficits. Wide laminectomy of the stenosed spinal canal treats leg pain or progressive neurological deficits.

INFECTIOUS DISEASES OF THE SPINE

Pyogenic Vertebral Osteomyelitis and Spinal Epidural Abscess

Vertebral osteomyelitis is an uncommon condition that presents with focal spinal pain and tenderness. Epidural abscesses in the anterior spinal canal are more likely to be associated with osteomyelitis than those in the posterior canal. Abscesses in either location cause radiculopathic pain, compromise nerve root function, and compress the spinal cord. Some patients are afebrile at presentation, but nearly all have an elevated sedimentation rate. MRI of the involved area is sensitive for detecting vertebral body abnormalities and is particularly helpful to assess for epidural or paravertebral infection. The most common causative organism is *Staphylococcus aureus*. Polymicrobial infection is uncommon after hematogenous infection but can occur when the source is open trauma or contiguous spread from other tissues. Diabetes, alcoholism, immunosuppression, intravenous drug use, and spinal trauma are all risk factors. Long-term antibiotic therapy can be curative. Spinal instability may require surgical stabilization. Myelopathy is an indication for urgent surgical decompression.

Granulomatous Vertebral Osteomyelitis

Tuberculosis (TB) of the spine (Pott's disease) is the most common granulomatous spinal infection. The risk is highest in regions or populations where TB is endemic. Other organisms capable of causing granulomatous osteomyelitis include brucellosis, *Actinomyces,* and several varieties of fungi. Granulomatous spinal infection typically presents with insidious progression of back pain. The patient often has symptoms of systemic infection such as weight loss, fever, night sweats, or malaise.

Pott's disease usually presents with destruction of vertebral bodies. Routine spinal radiography results are usually abnormal by the time of diagnosis, and spinal deformity is a common complication. MRI assesses for contiguous abscess in the epidural or paraspinal spaces and evaluates possible nerve root or spinal cord compression. Delayed neurological compromise caused by infarction from endarteritis obliterans, delayed degenerative bony changes, or reactivation of infection may occur after apparently successful treatment of the infection. Treatment of vertebral TB requires long-term multiple drug antituberculous therapy. Spinal surgery corrects deformity and is required in cases of neurological compression.

INFLAMMATORY JOINT DISEASE

Rheumatoid Arthritis

Systemic Presentation

RA is a chronic, inflammatory, symmetrical destructive immune-mediated polyarthritis. Disease incidence in women is twice that of men. The cause of RA is unknown, but genetic factors are evident in familial cases, and susceptibility linkage exists to some human leukocyte antigen-DR (HLA-DR) types. The most commonly affected joints are the small joints of the hands and feet. Characteristic clinical findings are the basis of diagnosis.

Serological testing for rheumatoid factor supports the diagnosis when positive. Radiography shows juxta-articular demineralization or characteristic joint erosions in advanced cases.

Neurological Manifestations
Neurological complications of RA include carpal tunnel syndrome and other nerve entrapments, peripheral neuropathy, and myopathy. RA evolves to a rheumatoid vasculitis that causes ischemic mononeuritis, mononeuritis multiplex, and stroke. Headache and neck ache are common. Focal neurological dysfunction is rare and occurs late in the course. Progressive RA causes subluxation at the atlantoaxial joint. The earliest neurological sign is usually hyperreflexia. Vertical subluxation leads to spinal cord or brainstem compression and, rarely, to vertebral artery compression or injury. Neurological dysfunction from atlantoaxial subluxation occurs in patients already debilitated by their disease. Many do not regain neurological function after surgical stabilization of the subluxation. The 5-year survival of patients at this late stage of RA is perhaps 50%.

Inflammatory Spondyloarthropathies

Clinical Presentation
The inflammatory spondyloarthropathies include ankylosing spondylitis, reactive arthritis, psoriatic arthritis, and the arthritis of inflammatory bowel disease. The characteristics of ankylosing spondylitis are inflammatory low back pain, loss of spinal range of motion, and sacroiliitis. Characteristic of inflammatory lumbosacral spine disease is an insidious onset of low back pain lasting more than 3 months with prominent morning stiffness that improves with activity. Onset is before age 40 years, and a male gender bias exists. Other organ manifestations include uveitis, mucocutaneous lesions, peripheral arthritis, gastrointestinal disease, cardiac disease, and pathology at sites of insertion of ligament or tendon to bone.

Neurological Complications
The neurological complications of the inflammatory spondyloarthropathies occur after spinal disease is clinically advanced. Spinal complications include atlantoaxial joint subluxation, spinal fractures, vertebral destruction, spinal canal stenosis, and a cauda equina syndrome caused by lumbar arachnoid diverticula. Proximal weakness and atrophy, sometimes with mild elevations of serum creatine kinase, occur in advanced cases of spondylitis. In patients with psoriatic arthritis, the myopathy is occasionally painful. Patients with inflammatory spondyloarthropathies sometimes have mild elevations of cerebrospinal

fluid (CSF) protein with normal glucose concentration and cell counts.

Epidural Lipomatosis

Epidural lipomatosis is a non-neoplastic accumulation of fatty tissue in the thoracic or lumbar epidural space. It is a complication of chronic corticosteroid excess, obesity, or hypothyroidism. A typical patient has used corticosteroids for more than 6 months and is obese and cushingoid. Criteria for the diagnosis include: (1) history consistent with segmental spinal cord compression or nerve root compression, (2) epidural fat thickness greater than 7 mm in the region of compression, and (3) a body mass index greater than 27.5 kg/m^2. The compressive tissue regresses when corticosteroid doses decrease.

Chronic Adhesive Arachnoiditis

Chronic focal or diffuse inflammation of the spinal theca is termed *chronic spinal arachnoiditis* or *chronic adhesive arachnoiditis*. All layers of the meninges are involved and in its chronic stages may be fibrotic rather than inflammatory. An occasional late finding is calcification of the meninges (*arachnoiditis ossificans*). The symptoms can include local or radicular pain, radicular paresthesia, and, less commonly, motor loss or sphincter dysfunction. MRI establishes the diagnosis by showing clumping of nerve roots, nodules in the subarachnoid space, loculation of spinal fluid, and local areas of enhancement. Spinal fluid may show increased CSF protein concentration and mild to moderate mononuclear pleocytosis. Symptomatic pain control is the goal of treatment.

Recurrent Meningitis

Dural CSF leaks, parameningeal infections, and immunodeficiency are considerations in patients with recurrent attacks of acute bacterial meningitis. Systemic inflammatory diseases are rare causes. These include systemic lupus erythematosus, Sjögren's syndrome, Behçet's disease, Lyme disease, familial Mediterranean fever, and sarcoidosis. Table 48.2 lists conditions that produce the combination of chronic or recurrent meningitis and uveitis.

Fibromyalgia

Fibromyalgia, a syndrome defined by widespread musculoskeletal or soft tissue pain and multiple tender points, is part of the differential diagnosis of many patients with spinal pain.

Table 48.2: Causes of combined uveitis and meningitis

Acute multifocal placoid pigmentary epitheliopathy
Acute retinal necrosis
Behçet's syndrome
Human T-lymphotropic virus type 1 infection
Infection in immunocompromised host
Isolated central nervous system angiitis
Lyme disease
Primary central nervous system lymphoma
Sarcoid
Syphilis
Systemic lupus erythematosus
Vogt-Koyanagi-Harada syndrome

Source: Reprinted with permission from Rosenbaum, R. B., Campbell, S. M., & Rosenbaum, J. T. 1996, *Clinical Neurology of Rheumatic Diseases*, Butterworth–Heinemann, Boston.

To meet the classification criteria of the American College of Rheumatology, a patient must have tenderness to palpation at 11 or more of 18 specific points. Typically, patients have multiple symptoms including fatigue, stiffness, nonrestorative sleep, headaches, and mood disorders. Patients may have many symptoms of neurological import such as weakness, paresthesia, and dizziness but a normal neurological examination. The cause of most cases of fibromyalgia is unknown. Behavioral and biological factors both contribute to the clinical presentation of the syndrome. Treatment includes a supportive doctor–patient relationship, tricyclic antidepressants, aerobic exercise, and avoiding inactivity.

For a more detailed discussion, see Chapter 77 in Neurology in Clinical Practice, 4th edition.

Disorders of Upper and Lower Motor Neurons

49

The term *motor neuron disease* (MND) encompasses a spectrum of diseases characterized by degeneration of upper motor neurons (UMNs), lower motor neurons (LMNs), or both. In some MNDs, only UMNs are affected; others affect only the LMNs. *Amyotrophic lateral sclerosis* (ALS) is the combination of UMN and LMN involvement.

DISORDERS OF UPPER MOTOR NEURONS

Primary Lateral Sclerosis

Primary lateral sclerosis (PLS), an uncommon sporadic disease, may be an independent disease entity or a variant of ALS.

Clinical Features and Diagnosis
Onset is in the sixth decade. The major clinical feature is a slowly progressive paraparesis evolving over decades. The spastic paraparesis spreads to the upper limbs and eventually causes pseudobulbar palsy. Other features include cramps, fasciculations, and urinary urgency. PLS is a diagnosis of exclusion. Exclusion of LMN involvement by electromyography (EMG) is required to exclude ALS. Also to be excluded are other causes of a UMN syndrome such as structural abnormalities and myelopathies. Cervical spondylotic myelopathy and multiple sclerosis are the most common causes of a progressive UMN syndrome that presents like PLS. A positive family history should suggest familial spastic paraplegia or adrenomyeloneuropathy.

Treatment
No specific pharmacological therapies are available. However, antispasticity drugs such as baclofen and tizanidine provide symptomatic treatment. Botulinum toxin injections reduce adductor spasm. Severe spasticity sometimes requires the insertion of an intrathecal baclofen pump. Management of

pseudobulbar affect lability is with tricyclic antidepressants, selective serotonin reuptake inhibitors, and a combination of dextromethorphan and quinidine.

Hereditary Spastic Paraplegia

Hereditary spastic paraplegia (HSP) (or familial spastic paraparesis) is a genetically and clinically heterogeneous group of disorders. Genetic linkage studies of families around the world have mapped loci to several autosomal chromosomes and the X chromosome. Forty percent of all families link to an autosomal dominantly inherited locus on chromosome 2p22-21. More than 50 mutations affect the spastin gene. The exact role of spastin in the pathogenesis of HSP is undefined, but may disrupt axonal transport by disturbing the interaction of spastin with cellular tubulin.

Clinical Features

The clinical feature common to all cases is progressively worsening spasticity of the lower limbs with variable degrees of weakness. The most common mode of inheritance is autosomal dominant, but inheritance is also recessive or X linked. A broad division of the syndrome is into the *pure* and *complicated* forms. Patients with the pure form only develop leg spasticity. Those with the complicated form may also have optic neuropathy, deafness, ataxia, ichthyosis, amyotrophy, peripheral neuropathy, dementia, autoimmune hemolytic anemia and thrombocytopenia (*Evans' syndrome*), extrapyramidal dysfunction, mental retardation, and bladder dysfunction.

Diagnosis

The diagnosis of HSP requires evidence of a family history. When there is no family history, the differential diagnosis is the same as that for PLS.

Treatment

Treatment for HSP is limited to symptomatic interventions, supportive care to reduce spasticity, as in PLS, and orthotics such as canes, walkers, and wheelchairs.

HTLV-1–Associated Myelopathy or Tropical Spastic Paraparesis

Human T-lymphotropic virus-1 (HTLV-1) is a retrovirus that causes a chronic progressive myelopathy. HTLV-1–associated myelopathy (HAM) or tropical spastic paraparesis (TSP) is a chronic, insidiously progressive myelopathy that typically begins after age 30 years. In addition to slowly progressive spastic paraparesis, patients complain of lower extremity paresthesia, a painful sensory neuropathy, and bladder dysfunction. Some patients develop optic neuropathy and spinocerebellar ataxia. The definitive diagnosis requires HTLV-1–positive serology in blood and cerebrospinal fluid (CSF). The most sensitive and specific CSF detection involves a combination of polymerase chain reaction (PCR) amplification of viral DNA, together with evidence of an increased HTLV-1–specific antibody index and oligoclonal bands. No present antiviral agents effectively treat TSP/HAM, but plasmapheresis may provide partial benefit.

HTLV-2–Associated Myelopathy

HTLV-1 and HTLV-2 are antigenically distinct. The characteristics of HAM are spastic paraparesis, diffuse hyperreflexia, spastic bladder, and periventricular white matter changes on magnetic resonance imaging (MRI). Intravenous (IV) drug abusers presenting with spastic paraparesis are at high risk for infection.

Adrenomyeloneuropathy

Adrenomyeloneuropathy is a variant of adrenoleukodystrophy, an X-linked recessive disorder caused by mutations in the *ABCD1* gene on chromosome Xq28. Mutations in this gene lead to abnormal peroxisomal beta-oxidation, which results in the harmful accumulation of very-long-chain fatty acids (VLCFAs). The most common phenotype affects young boys between the ages of 4 and 8 years. They develop severe adrenal insufficiency, progressive cognitive deterioration, seizures, blindness, deafness, and spastic quadriparesis.

Clinical Features

In contrast to adrenoleukodystrophy, the characteristic feature of adrenomyeloneuropathy is a slowly progressive spastic paraparesis and mild polyneuropathy in adult men. Sensory symptoms, sphincter disturbances, and mild adrenal insufficiency may be present. Adult female carriers may develop a slowly progressive spastic paraparesis.

Diagnosis

Sural nerve biopsy specimens show loss of myelinated and unmyelinated axons with some degree of onion bulb formation. Nerve conduction studies and needle electrode examination reveal a predominantly axonal sensorimotor polyneuropathy with a lesser component of demyelination. An increased VLCFA concentration in plasma, red blood cells, or cultured skin fibroblasts confirms the diagnosis.

Plant Excitotoxins

Lathyrism
Lathyrism is an endemic toxic paraparesis resulting from the consumption of the chickling or grass pea (*Lathyrus sativus*). The toxic agent is β-N-oxalylamino-L-alanine, an excitatory amino acid. Onset is usually sudden. The legs feel heavy and weak. Walking difficulty can develop slowly over months. Prominent symmetrical spasticity and hyperreflexia in the legs are invariable. The history of toxic ingestion establishes the diagnosis. The level of disability sometimes improves after eliminating *L. sativus* from the diet.

Konzo
Konzo ("tied legs") is a toxic-nutritional disorder of cortical motor neurons caused by chronic dietary ingestion of a neurotoxin derived from flour made from short-soaked cassava roots. The disorder is endemic in protein-deficient communities. The neurotoxic effect of chronic cassava root ingestion derives from the liberation of cyanohydrins from flour, which then metabolize to thiocyanate. The clinical syndrome is similar to lathyrism.

DISORDERS OF LOWER MOTOR NEURON

Acute Poliomyelitis

The cause of poliomyelitis (acute anterior poliomyelitis) is a poliovirus. The mode of spread is by the fecal-oral route. Before the introduction of oral polio vaccine, epidemics of acute paralytic poliomyelitis were relatively common.

Clinical Features
A viremia occurs after a 3–6 day incubation period, during which approximately 90% of individuals remain asymptomatic. However, most of the remaining 10% develop an acute, flulike illness with cough, malaise, diarrhea, myalgia, headache, and fever. This self-limited, abortive polio usually lasts 2–3 days and an acute muscle weakness syndrome does not develop, although some patients may develop features of the postpolio syndrome many years later. A few develop self-limited aseptic meningitis. Fewer than 1% develop the acute paralytic syndrome, characterized by localized fasciculations, severe myalgia, hyperesthesia, and usually focal and asymmetrical paralysis. Weakness of the diaphragm and intercostal muscles causes respiratory distress. The leg muscles are most frequently affected and the bulbar muscles least often.

Physical examination reveals severe LMN-type muscle weakness with hypoactive or absent deep tendon reflexes, decreased muscle tone, and fasciculations. With time, disease muscle atrophy occurs. Objective signs of sensory loss are not characteristic. The risk of paralytic disease increases with patient age and viral virulence. Most patients with paralytic disease recover significant strength, but two thirds have some degree of functional impairment.

Laboratory Features

The CSF typically shows a pleocytosis, with polymorphonuclear cells predominating during the acute stages and lymphocytes predominating later in the disease. CSF protein concentrations are elevated. Identification of CSF poliovirus-specific immunoglobulin M (IgM) antibody confirms the diagnosis. Stool cultures are positive for poliovirus in nearly 90% of patients by the tenth day of illness. A fourfold or greater increase in antibody titer against poliovirus in sera provides further confirmation.

Treatment and Prevention

The treatment of acute paralytic poliomyelitis is supportive care. Most patients require hospitalization in an intensive care unit to optimize close monitoring of ventilatory and cardiovascular function. The best cure for polio is prevention. Two vaccines are available, the Sabin and the Salk. The Sabin trivalent oral polio vaccine contains all three live-attenuated serotypes of poliovirus and is almost 100% effective in preventing acute paralytic poliomyelitis. However, one in a million individuals receiving the vaccine will develop paralytic polio. Immunocompromised individuals and their household contacts should receive the inactivated Salk vaccine.

Progressive Postpoliomyelitis Muscular Atrophy

Many years after recovery from acute poliomyelitis, some patients experience progressive weakness. The incidence of progressive postpoliomyelitis muscular atrophy (PPMA) among polio survivors ranges from 28% to 64%. Patients with PPMA have recovered from acute poliomyelitis and the disease course has been stable for at least 10 years after the recovery. Table 49.1 lists the clinical features. A history of clinical stability for at least 10 years after recovery from acute poliomyelitis is an absolute prerequisite for considering the diagnosis of PPMA. No specific pharmacotherapy is available to treat PPMA. Management must focus on general supportive measures that preserve function.

Table 49.1: Characteristic features of progressive postpoliomyelitis muscular atrophy

Medical history
  Recovery from acute poliomyelitis
  A long stable course, at least 10 yr
Signs and symptoms
  Progressive weakness usually in previously affected muscles
  Accompanying overstress muscle pains and arthralgia
Laboratory studies
  EMG is helpful to identify evidence of previous polio infection
  None of tests is specific for PPMA
Diagnosis
  Exclusion of other treatable diseases
Treatment
  Symptomatic and supportive care

EMG = electromyography; PPMA = postpoliomyelitis muscular atrophy.

Multifocal Motor Neuropathy

Multifocal motor neuropathy (MMN) is a pure motor syndrome that develops in association with motor nerve fiber demyelination. The etiology is not established. Multifocal demyelination conduction block and elevated titers of antibodies against GM_1 gangliosides are associated.

Clinical Features
The age at onset is between 20 and 75 years and men are more often affected than women. Initial presentation is 1 or more years after onset of symptoms. The course then extends over many years. Although MMN is associated with disability, most patients remain in the workplace and uncomplicated MMN is generally not a fatal disorder. The characteristic findings are an asymmetrical, slowly progressive weakness that most commonly begins in the hands in the distribution of two or more individual peripheral nerves. MMN also affects the legs, often with slowly progressive footdrop. In early stages, the degree of muscle weakness exceeds the degree of muscle atrophy, indicative of a primarily demyelinating disorder rather than one of axon loss. The muscle stretch reflexes are usually preserved but diminished.

Diagnosis
Electrodiagnosis reveals the presence of focal conduction block along two or more motor nerve fibers. Some cases may have focal conduction slowing along segments of motor nerve rather than actual conduction block. High titers of serum anti-GM_1 antibodies support a diagnosis of MMN. CSF protein

concentration is usually within the normal range but may be modestly elevated.

Treatment
Neither plasma exchange nor corticosteroids are effective and may even worsen the condition. The treatment of choice is intravenous immune globulin (IVIG) prepared from pooled human immunoglobulin G (IgG). Cyclophosphamide treatment is also effective.

Benign Focal Amyotrophy

Other terms to describe benign focal amyotrophy are *monomelic amyotrophy* or *juvenile segmental muscular atrophy*. The etiology is unknown.

Clinical Features
The disease usually begins in adolescence or young adult life. The most common presentation is a slowly progressive, painless weakness and atrophy in one hand or forearm. The distribution of muscle weakness varies markedly, but a characteristic feature is that the condition remains limited to only a few myotomes in the affected limb. Tendon reflexes are normal except in muscles innervated by the involved cord segment; weal muscles have reduced or absent reflexes. UMN signs are not present. Also spared are the cranial nerves, pyramidal tracts, and the autonomic nervous system. Weakness and atrophy may progress steadily for the initial 2–3 years but stabilize within 5 years. An affected arm is three times more common than an affected leg.

Diagnosis
No pathognomonic diagnostic test exists. The main purpose is to exclude alternative diagnoses.

Treatment
Although not life threatening, it seriously impairs motor function in the involved limb. Supportive care consisting of physical and occupational therapy and effective use of assistive devices (splinting and braces) are the main treatment components.

Infantile and Juvenile Spinal Muscular Atrophy

The estimated incidence of infantile and juvenile spinal muscular atrophy (SMA) is 1 in 6,000–10,000 births. Inheritance is by autosomal recessive transmission. Autosomal dominant childhood SMA probably accounts for fewer than 2% of all childhood cases. X-linked SMA is associated with arthrogryposis and bone fractures. SMA is classified into three types based on the age at onset: SMA type 1 (infantile SMA or *Werdnig-Hoffmann disease*), SMA type 2 (intermediate SMA), and SMA type 3 (juvenile SMA or *Kugelberg-Welander disease*).

Genetics

All three types of autosomal recessive childhood SMA map to chromosome 5q11.2-5q13.3. The normal 5q region on each chromosome contains two inversely homologous copies of the survival motor neuron (*SMN*) gene, termed *SMN1* (telomeric) and *SMN2* (centromeric). The 5q region also contains the neuronal apoptosis inhibitory protein (*NAIP*) gene. *SMN1* is *the* SMA gene and the severity of SMA relates to the dosage of inherited SMN1. The SMN1 protein is functionally absent in 95–98% of cases, and small amounts are present in the remaining percentage. Although mutations in the *SMN1* gene produce the disease, the clinical phenotype relates to the expression of SMN2.

Clinical Features

SMA-1 (*infantile form; Werdnig-Hoffmann disease*): The disease begins within the first few months of life. Infants with SMA-1 never sit without support and die from respiratory failure and pneumonia before age 2 years. Symptoms include severe hypotonia, a weak cry, respiratory distress, and absent head control. External rotation of the thighs and flexion of the knees is the resting posture. Limb weakness is severe, generalized, and worse proximally. Tendon reflexes are usually absent and the sensory examination findings are normal. Contractures develop after several months of immobilization. Bulbar muscle weakness makes feeding laborious and eventually leads to aspiration pneumonia. Tongue fasciculations occur in half of affected infants. Facial muscles are mildly affected. Extraocular movements are always normal. Weakness of the intercostal muscles with preservation of diaphragmatic strength causes outward flaring of the lower ribcage.

SMA-2 (*intermediate form*): The onset of symptoms begins before 18 months. The symptoms may be present at birth, but delayed motor milestones are often the first clue to neurological impairment. A fine hand tremor is present. The distribution, pattern, and progression of weakness are similar to SMA-1, but the type 2 disease is milder and progresses more slowly. Most children roll over and sit unsupported but rarely achieve independent walking. The child becomes immobilized and wheelchair confined. Contractures of the hips and knees, clubfoot deformities, severe scoliosis, and dislocation of the hips may eventually develop. The long-term prognosis varies markedly; some die in childhood because of respiratory failure, but many others survive into the third or fourth decade of adulthood.

SMA-3, juvenile form (Kugelberg-Welander disease): Onset is after 18 months of age (usually between the ages of 5 and 15 years). The initial feature is difficulty in walking. The child develops a waddling gait with an exaggerated lumbar lordosis and trouble climbing stairs. The appearance suggests a limb-girdle muscular dystrophy. Weakness of the neck, shoulders, and arms develops, but weakness in the legs is always more severe. A fine action tremor is common. Absent tendon reflexes and a normal sensory examination is the rule. The clinical course is one of slowly progressive limb-girdle weakness with long periods of stability. The eventual degree of disability is unpredictable.

Diagnosis

No further workup is necessary if molecular genetic analysis identifies mutations in the *SMN* gene. In the absence of *SMN1* mutations, assay for the combination of a deleted *SMN* allele on one gene and a small mutation on the other. Not all SMAs are related to chromosome 5q region abnormalities; some cases are X linked or autosomal dominant and the genes have yet to be identified. Nongenetic tests to confirm the diagnosis are electrodiagnosis and muscle biopsy. Needle EMG indicates denervation and muscle histology shows a highly distinct pattern of grouped fascicular atrophy with hypertrophied type I fibers.

Treatment

No disease-specific pharmacotherapy is available for SMA. The management objectives include: (1) maintaining active mobility and independence as long as possible, (2) preventing the development of contractures and kyphoscoliosis, and (3) provision of mobility devices.

Fazio-Londe Disease (Progressive Bulbar Paresis of Childhood)

Fazio-Londe disease is a rare progressive facial and bulbar palsy. Affected children are normal at birth but develop progressive bulbar palsy (PBP) and eventual respiratory failure. Other motor neurons and extraocular motility are normal.

Adult-Onset Spinal Muscular Atrophy (SMA Type 4)

Onset is after age 20 years, usually in the mid-thirties. The course is relatively benign; few are wheelchair confined over a period of 20 years. Autosomal recessive inheritance accounts for 70% of adult-onset cases. Homozygous deletions in the *SMN1* gene are unusual, homozygous deletions of the *SMN2* gene are more common, and the remaining are autosomal dominant and are not linked to chromosome 5. Typical features are a slowly progressive limb-girdle weakness, leading associated with fasciculations. Muscle biopsy specimens and needle EMG findings are consistent with denervation. No specific pharmacotherapy is available.

Kennedy's Disease (X-Linked Recessive Bulbospinal Neuronopathy)

Kennedy's disease is an X-linked recessive SMA with bulbar involvement and gynecomastia. The molecular abnormality is a trinucleotide repeat on the androgen receptor gene located on the X chromosome. A greater number of repeats is associated with younger age at onset. Continuous androgen receptor function may be crucial to maintain normal motor neuron function throughout life.

Clinical Features
Affected males remain largely asymptomatic until after age 30 years. Prominent muscle cramps, muscle twitching, difficulty walking, and limb-girdle muscle weakness are characteristic symptoms. Dysarthria and dysphagia occur in fewer than half the patients. Tendon reflexes are absent, muscles are atrophied, and occasionally calves are hypertrophied. Coarse muscle fasciculations and hand tremor can be prominent. Facial and particularly perioral fasciculations are characteristic. Gynecomastia is a unique feature and occurs in up to 90% of patients. Endocrine abnormalities include testicular atrophy, feminization, and infertility in approximately 40% of patients. Female carriers may manifest late-onset bulbar dysfunction.

Diagnosis
Molecular genetic testing is diagnostic. Motor nerve conduction study results are generally normal and needle electrode examination shows prominent chronic denervation changes.

Treatment
Specific treatment is not available. Management is supportive and symptomatic.

Progressive Muscular Atrophy

Progressive muscular atrophy (PMA) is an ALS variant involving mainly LMNs.

Subacute Motor Neuronopathy in Lymphoproliferative Disorders

A subacute, progressive, and painless motor neuron syndrome may develop in patients who have Hodgkin's and non-Hodgkin's lymphoma with or without a paraproteinemia. Patchy, asymmetrical leg wasting is the initial feature. Neuropathology shows a loss of anterior horn cells and ventral root nerve fibers; some have evidence of inflammation in the anterior horns of the spinal cord. Twenty percent of patients have myeloma or macroglobulinemia.

Postirradiation Lower Motor Neuron Syndrome

Radiation directed to the lumbar paravertebral area for the treatment of testicular cancer can cause a pure LMN syndrome in the legs that appears many years after the irradiation. Sensory abnormalities and sphincter dysfunction are rare, and the electrodiagnostic findings are consistent with a disorder of the cauda equina. The disease usually progresses over the first few years after symptom onset but subsequently becomes arrested.

DISORDERS OF BOTH THE UPPER AND THE LOWER MOTOR NEURONS

Amyotrophic Lateral Sclerosis

ALS is a progressive neurodegenerative disorder of undetermined etiology that primarily affects the motor neuron cell population. Most patients die of respiratory failure. Several variants are recognized. Included in this group are PLS, PBP, and PMA. Between 5% and 10% of cases of ALS are familial rather than sporadic, with the most common inheritance pattern being autosomal dominant. The incidence is estimated at 1 to 3 per 100,000 and the prevalence varies from 6 to 8 per 100,000.

ALS occurs as early as the second decade of life, but the most common onset is in the patient's early sixties. It is rare in those older than 85 years. The mean disease duration from symptom onset to death is approximately 3 years, although some patients live for more than a decade.

Etiology
Viral infection, immune system disturbances, exogenous toxins, and hormonal disturbances are suggested factors, but none are proven. The role of glutamate excitotoxicity and free radical injury is subject to active investigation.

Clinical Features

Muscle weakness in ALS usually begins in a focal area, first spreading to contiguous muscles in the same region before involvement of another region. Onset of muscle weakness is more common in the arms than the legs. In 25% of patients, weakness begins in bulbar-innervated muscles. Respiratory muscle onset is rare. Symptoms of muscle weakness vary, depending on which motor function is impaired. Fasciculations are an uncommon presenting feature but develop in almost all cases soon after onset. Muscle cramps are common and often precede other symptoms by many months.

Natural History

Estimates are that up to 40% of anterior horn cell motor neurons are lost before the clinical detection of motor abnormalities. Once the clinical phase is evident, decline is linear. The characteristic pattern of spread is to adjacent parts. When onset is in one arm, spread is often first to the contralateral side, then the ipsilateral leg, the contralateral leg, and finally the bulbar region. Onset in the leg often follows a similar pattern, with final involvement of the bulbar region. Bulbar-onset ALS tends to spread to the hand first, with spread to thoracic myotomes, and then the legs. Overall, the pattern suggests that rostral-caudal involvement is faster than caudal-rostral spread. During the course of the disease, transitory improvement, plateaus, or sudden worsening occur, but spontaneous improvement is rare.

Prognosis

The median duration of ALS ranges from 23 to 52 months and the mean duration is from 27 to 43 months. Only 25% of patients survive 5 years and fewer than 16% survive beyond 10 years. Factors that influence the prognosis of ALS include the age at onset, clinical type, and duration from onset to the time of diagnosis. In general, younger patients and a prolonged duration between onset and diagnosis indicate a better prognosis.

Diagnosis

The basis for the diagnosis of definite ALS is the history and clinical examination, after excluding other possible causes. The EDX examination is a valuable tool in the investigation of ALS and its variants. It serves as an adjunct to the clinical examination and is particularly useful in determining the presence or extent of LMN disease. The needle electrode examination characteristically reveals a combination of acute (positive sharp waves and fibrillation potentials) and chronic (neurogenic firing pattern with evidence of increased amplitude and duration, and polyphasic motor unit potentials) changes in a widespread distribution that is not in keeping with any single root or peripheral nerve distribution. Fasciculation potentials are expected and their absence should prompt an investigation for another disorder. Denervation potentials are observed in a certain topographical distribution, and ideally should be carried out in at least three of the four regions of the neuraxis (bulbar, cervical, thoracic, and lumbosacral).

Clinical evidence of both UMN and LMN signs in three or more regions is *definite ALS*. *Probable ALS* is the diagnosis in those with UMN and LMN signs in two regions. *Possible ALS* implies that a patient either has UMN and LMN signs in one region only or has UMN signs alone in two regions.

Treatment
The first step in the management of ALS is to present the diagnosis in a compassionate yet informative manner. The decision-making process must include the patient and/or the family. It is important to discuss issues such as advance directives and issues regarding terminal care. Riluzole is the first specific drug for the treatment of ALS. The survival benefit is modest and is disproportionately beneficial in bulbar-onset disease. The median prolongation of survival is only 2 months. However, others report survival benefits of up to 20 months. Riluzole appears to maintain patients in a milder state of disease for a longer period. The cost of the drug (approximately $8000–$9000 per year) is the main factor in whether patients elect to take riluzole. Table 49.2 summarizes specific pharmacological and nonpharmacological symptomatic treatments.

The care of patients with ALS has become increasingly complex. Many patients are cared for by a multidisciplinary team rather than by a single treating physician. The team often consists of neurologists, a nurse coordinator, physical therapists, occupational therapists, dietitians, speech pathologists, and social workers. Pulmonary specialists and other health professionals should also be available.

Familial Amyotrophic Lateral Sclerosis

Between 5% and 10% of all ALS cases are familial, and most are inherited in an autosomal dominant pattern. It is possible that the true frequency of familial ALS (FALS) is underestimated. ALS1 is a form of late-onset motor neuron disorder that accounts for 15–20% of all cases of FALS and is associated with mutations in the gene that encodes copper/zinc superoxide dismutase 1 (SOD1) located on chromosome 21q21. ALS2 is a

Table 49.2: Symptomatic treatment in amyotrophic lateral sclerosis

Symptoms	Pharmacotherapy	Other Therapy
Fatigue	Pyridostigmine bromide	Energy conservation
	Antidepressants	Work modification
	Amantadine hydrochloride	Assistive devices
Spasticity	Baclofen	Physical therapy
	Tizanidine	Range-of-motion exercises
	Dantrolene sodium	
	Diazepam	
Cramps	Quinine sulfate	Massage
	Baclofen	Physical therapy
	Vitamin E	
Fasciculations	Carbamazepine	Assurance
Sialorrhea	Anticholinergic drugs	Mechanical cleaning
Thick mucinous saliva	Beta blocker	None
Pseudobulbar laughing or crying	TCA	
	SSRI	
	l-dopa/carbidopa	
	Lithium	
Secretion and expectoration	Dextromethorphan	Hydration
	Organidin	Moist air; aspiration devices; insufflator/exsufflator

Condition	Medication	Other treatment
Aspiration	Cisapride	Modified food consistency Tracheostomy Modified laryngectomy and tracheal diversion
Joint pains	Anti-inflammatory drugs Analgesics TCAs	Range-of-motion exercises Heat
Depression	SSRI	Counseling
Insomnia	Zolpidem tartrate Lorazepam Opioids	Support group meetings; psychiatry
Respiratory failure	Bronchodilators Morphine sulfate	Hospital bed Nocturnal noninvasive ventilator IPPB Noninvasive ventilation; permanent ventilation Exercise
Constipation	Increase oral liquid Metamucil Dulcored suppositories Lactulose and other laxative	

IPPB = intermittent positive pressure breathing; SSRI = selective serotonin reuptake inhibitor; TCA = tricyclic antidepressant.

rare, recessively inherited disorder mapped to a gene on chromosome 2q33. Transmission of ALS4 and ALS5 is as autosomal recessive traits, and ALS4 and ALS5 map to chromosomes 9q21-q22 and 15q15-q22, respectively. A large European family with an adult-onset autosomal dominant ALS linked to chromosome 18q21 is *ALS3*. *ALS3* also denotes familial cases not yet linked to a chromosomal locus or associated with an inherited genetic mutation.

Adult Hexosaminidase-A Deficiency

Adult hexosaminidase-A deficiency is an autosomal recessively inherited late-onset GM_2 gangliosidosis. The cause of all three subtypes is an abnormal accumulation of GM_2 ganglioside in neurons as a result of a deficiency in the activity of the lysosomal enzyme. The adult form may present as slowly progressive proximal weakness. In some, severe cramps may present in association with muscle weakness, mimicking SMA. In others, however, a combination of dysarthria, spasticity, and LMN signs resembles ALS.

Triple A Syndrome

Triple A syndrome (AAAS) (Allgrove syndrome) is a rare autosomal recessive disorder that derives its name from the combination of *a*chalasia, *a*lacrima, and *a*drenocorticotrophic insufficiency. The *AAAS* gene is located on chromosome 12q13 and encodes a ubiquitous protein called aladin, which, when expressed in the neuroendocrine system, may be important in regulation of the cell cycle, cell signaling intracellular transport, and the cell cytoskeleton. The syndrome includes mental retardation, optic atrophy, and seizures.

Disinhibition-Dementia-Parkinsonism-Amyotrophy Complex

Disinhibition-dementia-parkinsonism-amyotrophy complex is an autosomal dominant progressive neurodegenerative disease described in a large Irish American family. The clinical features are disinhibited behavior (excessive eating and inappropriate sexual behavior), personality changes, dementia, parkinsonian manifestations, and amyotrophy with fasciculations.

For a more detailed discussion, see Chapter 80 in Neurology in Clinical Practice, 4th edition.

Disorders of the Nerve Roots and Plexuses

50

DISORDERS OF NERVE ROOTS

The clinical features of nerve root disorders are radicular pain and paresthesias. Dermatomal sensory loss, myotomal weakness, and segmental diminished tendon reflex activity occur at the segmental level subserved by the nerve root. Polyradicular syndromes resemble a polyneuropathy or a progressive muscular atrophy. Increased cerebrospinal fluid (CSF) protein concentration and pleocytosis, the presence of positive sharp waves and fibrillation potentials in the paraspinal muscles, and magnetic resonance imaging (MRI) evidence of nerve root compromise or enhancement favor nerve root disease.

Traumatic Nerve Root Avulsions

Clinical Features
The nerve roots are the weakest point in the nerve root–spinal nerve–plexus complex and severe traction may cause nerve root avulsion from the spinal cord. Ventral roots are more vulnerable to avulsion than dorsal roots.

Most root avulsions occur in the cervical region and cause two distinct clinical syndromes. *Erb's palsy* is paralysis of C5- and C6-innervated muscles. The arm hangs at the side internally rotated and extended at the elbow. Motorcycle accidents are the most common cause, followed by difficult vertex deliveries. *Klumpke's palsy* is paralysis of C8 and T1 muscles. The hand muscles innervated by the C8 and T1 roots are weak and wasted. The result is a claw hand deformity. Many motorcycle accidents involve all of the roots. Flaccid paralysis and complete anesthesia develop in the myotomes and dermatomes served by ventral and dorsal roots, respectively.

The usual cause of Erb's palsy is a sudden and severe increase in the angle between the neck and shoulder. Transmission of the generated stress is along the upper portion of the brachial plexus to the C5 and C6 roots. C5 root avulsion results in complete paralysis of the rhomboids and spinates and a varying degree of weakness of the deltoid, biceps, brachioradialis, and serratus anterior. Motorcycle accidents are the most common cause, followed by difficult vertex deliveries with pulling of the head to deliver the after-coming shoulder and from breech position with downward pulling of the arm to deliver the after-coming head.

Diagnosis
The electromyographic (EMG) finding of cervical paraspinal fibrillation potentials supports the diagnosis of root avulsion. Contrast-enhanced MRI studies of the cervical paraspinal muscles show severe atrophy are accurate indicators of root avulsion injuries. Abnormal enhancement occurs in the multifidus muscle. Intraspinal neuroimaging using postmyelographic computed tomography (CT) or MRI demonstrates an outpouching of the dura filled with contrast or CSF at the level of the avulsed root. MRI usually shows an outpouching of the dura filled with contrast or CSF at the level of the avulsed root. Postmyelographic CT with 1–3 mm axial slices provides the most accurate diagnosis.

Treatment
The surgical treatment of avulsion injuries is an area of active ongoing investigation, with the promise that restoring continuity between spinal cord and nerve roots may recover function. Complete paralysis of a limb may indicate amputation. With less profound injuries, muscle and tendon transplants are sometimes used. Coagulation of the dorsal root entry zone treats the intractable pain associated with cervical root avulsion injuries.

Disc Herniation

Chapter 48 discuses the radiculopathies caused by the herniation of cervical and lumbar intervertebral discs.

Diabetic Polyradiculoneuropathy

Symmetrical polyneuropathies and *asymmetrical focal* or *multifocal disorders* are the two major groups of diabetic neuropathies. The latter are exemplified by the cranial mononeuropathies and the thoracoabdominal and lumbosacral polyradiculoneuropathies. They often coexist in an individual patient.

Clinical Features

Rapid-onset pain and paresthesias are the initial features of thoracic root involvement in the abdominal and chest wall. The pain is severe and described as burning, sharp, aching, or throbbing. Heightened sensitivity to light touch over affected regions is associated with patches of sensory loss on the anterior, lateral, or posterior aspects of the trunk and unilateral abdominal swelling because of localized weakness of the abdominal wall muscles.

Diabetic lumbosacral polyradiculoneuropathy (*diabetic amyotrophy*) tends to affect patients in the sixth or seventh decade of life who are known to have non–insulin-dependent diabetes of several years' duration. It involves the upper lumbar roots, especially the anterior thighs, with pain, dysesthesia, and weakness. Onset is usually abrupt, with symptoms developing over days to a couple of weeks. The early features are unilateral and include weakness of muscles supplied by the L2-L4 roots (the iliopsoas, quadriceps, and hip adductors), reduced or absent patellar tendon reflexes, and mild impairment of sensation over the anterior thigh. Later, the polyradiculoneuropathy evolves to involve proximal, distal, or contralateral muscles. The evolution may occur in a steady or a stepwise fashion. The time from onset to maximal involvement averages 6 months, with a range of 2–18 months.

Diagnosis

The erythrocyte sedimentation rate is usually normal. EMG shows evidence for a coexisting diabetic distal polyneuropathy in 75% of patients and may be the cause of a severe motor sensory polyneuropathy sometimes with features of a plexopathy. The CSF protein concentration is usually 120 mg/dl or higher.

Treatment

Improvement occurs spontaneously in most patients; the recovery phase ranges between 1 and 18 months, with a mean of 6 months. The goal of therapy is pain relief. Tricyclics, especially nortriptyline, selective serotonin reuptake inhibitors, anticonvulsants, clonazepam, baclofen, clonidine, mexiletine, intravenous lidocaine, and topical capsaicin may have a role separately or in combination. Immunotherapy may be beneficial.

Neoplastic Polyradiculopathy (Neoplastic Meningitis)

Neoplasms that spread to the leptomeninges are solid tumors (carcinoma of the breast, lung, and melanoma), non-Hodgkin's lymphomas, and intravascular lymphomatosis. Most neoplastic polyradiculopathies occur in patients with known underlying malignancy.

Clinical Features

The clinical features of neoplastic polyradiculopathy include radicular pain, dermatomal sensory loss, areflexia, and weakness of the lower motor neuron type. Often, the distribution of the sensory and motor deficits is widespread and simulates a severe sensorimotor polyneuropathy. Associated features from meningeal infiltration are nuchal rigidity, confusion, and cranial polyneuropathies.

Diagnosis

Examination of the CSF shows a pleocytosis, elevated protein and decreased glucose concentrations, and often tumor cells. A sensitive electrophysiological indicator of nerve root involvement is a prolonged F-wave latency or absent F responses, which should raise the suspicion of leptomeningeal metastases. Spinal MRI shows abnormalities in half of patients.

Treatment

Standard therapy for neoplastic meningitis includes radiotherapy to sites of symptomatic disease, intrathecal chemotherapy (methotrexate, thiotepa, and cytosine arabinoside), and optimal treatment of the underlying malignancy. A complication of aggressive treatment is a necrotizing leukoencephalopathy that becomes symptomatic months after treatment with radiation and intrathecal methotrexate.

Infectious Radiculopathy

Infectious radiculopathy most often occurs in patients with syphilis (tabes dorsalis), acquired immunodeficiency syndrome infected with cytomegalovirus, Lyme disease, and herpes zoster (see Chapter 28). Acquired demyelinating polyradiculoneuropathies (Guillain-Barré syndrome and chronic inflammatory demyelinating polyradiculoneuropathy) are postinfectious radiculopathies and are discussed in Chapter 51.

Acquired Disorders of the Dorsal Root Ganglia

The dorsal root ganglia (DRG) are selectively vulnerable to several malignant and nonmalignant conditions that produce a sensory neuronopathy syndrome. The loss of large- and small-diameter dorsal root ganglion cells explains the clinical features. The best example is *subacute sensory neuropathy* (or neuronopathy), a paraneoplastic disorder that develops over weeks to months. Ataxia and hyperalgesia, with preserved muscle strength, characterize the clinical features (see Chapter 27).

Other causes of DRG neuronopathy include hereditary, toxic, and autoimmune disorders. The main features of hereditary sensory neuropathies are chronicity, acrodystrophic ulcerations, fractures, bouts of osteomyelitis, and lack of paresthesias. Pyridoxine abuse and cisplatin neurotoxicity are generally easily recognized. A sensory neuronopathy syndrome has also been associated with elevated titers of an autoantibody that reacts with the GD_{1b} ganglioside, present on the surface of neurons in the DRG.

RADICULOPATHIES SIMULATING MOTOR NEURON DISEASE

Disorders of the motor roots may have clinical features that resemble motor neuron diseases (see Chapter 49). This possibility becomes a consideration in patients when clinical features of lower motor neuron involvement are associated with a monoclonal gammopathy.

DISORDERS OF THE BRACHIAL PLEXUS

Clinical Features and Diagnosis

Neurological Examination
The usual patterns of involvement are of the entire plexus, the upper trunk, or the lower trunk. Partial plexopathies caused by selective cord lesions are uncommon. A complete plexopathy causes weakness, sensory loss, and loss of tendon reflexes in the segments served by C5 and T1. Lesions of the upper trunk involve C5 and C6, and lesions of the lower trunk involve C8 and T1. Posterior cord lesions produce weakness in radial nerve–and axillary nerve–innervated muscles, with sensory loss in the distributions of the posterior cutaneous nerve of the forearm and the radial and axillary nerves. Lateral cord injuries produce weakness in muscles supplied by the musculocutaneous nerve and the muscles of the median nerve supplied by the C6 and C7 roots (the pronator teres and flexor carpi radialis).

Electrodiagnostic Studies
The EMG is helpful in confirming the diagnosis of brachial plexopathy. Evidence for a neurogenic lesion (fibrillation potentials, positive sharp waves, and reduced motor unit recruitment)

in muscles innervated by at least two cervical segments involving at least two different peripheral nerves identifies the condition as a disorder of the plexus.

Radiological Studies
A lesion in the pulmonary apex or erosion of the head of the first and second rib or the transverse processes of C7 and T1 suggests that an apical lung (Pancoast's) tumor is responsible for a lower brachial plexopathy. CT and MRI of the brachial plexus are the imaging modalities of choice for detecting mass lesions of the plexus.

Traumatic Plexopathy

The general categories of brachial plexus injury are: (1) direct trauma, (2) secondary injury from damage to structures about the shoulder and neck, such as fractures of the clavicle and first rib, and (3) iatrogenic injury, usually seen as a nerve block complication. Supraclavicular injuries are more common, are more severe, and have a worse prognosis than infraclavicular injuries.

Early Management
The ultimate objective is to restore as much neurological function as possible. In open injuries, immediate operative intervention is necessary to save the patient's life. Damage may have occurred to great vessels in the neck and to the lung. During surgery, one assesses the degree of plexus injury for later repair. Sharply transected portions of the plexus undergo primary repair. Most plexus elements show partial recovery when primarily repaired, whereas only half show partial recovery when repaired secondarily.

Long-Term Management
In the absence of root avulsion, assessing spontaneous recovery requires months of observation before contemplating brachial plexus exploration. During the observation period, regular passive range-of-motion exercises to the joints prevent contractures. If the plexus elements are in continuity, return of normal strength and sensation is expected. If the axons degenerate, the main factor limiting return of function is the distance the regenerating axon sprouts must traverse before making contact with end organs. Recommend plexus exploration if little improvement occurs after 2–4 months for open injuries or 4–5 months for stretch injuries. The surgeon must determine whether an injured length of plexus that appears to be in continuity actually contains regenerating axons by intraoperative electrical nerve stimulation. Intraoperative motor evoked potentials are

helpful in assessing the functional state of anterior motor roots and motor fibers.

NEUROGENIC THORACIC OUTLET SYNDROME

Clinical Features

Neurogenic thoracic outlet syndrome is a rare entity. Most patients are young adult women. Pain and tingling on the inner side of the arm are the initial features. Slowly progressive wasting and weakness of the hand muscles follow. Atrophy of the hand muscle is greatest in the hypothenar eminence. Mild atrophy and weakness in the forearm muscles sometimes occur. Sensory loss is present along the inner side of the forearm.

Diagnosis

Cervical spine radiographs disclose small, bilateral cervical ribs or enlarged down-curving C7 transverse processes. MRI of the brachial plexus reveals deviation or distortion of nerves or blood vessels. EMG shows a mildly reduced ulnar motor response and reduced ulnar sensory amplitude. The needle study typically reveals features of chronic axon loss with mild fibrillation potential activity in C8- and T1-innervated muscles. The clinical and EMG findings point to a lesion of the lower trunk of the brachial plexus. In most patients, a fibrous band extends from the tip of a rudimentary cervical rib to the scalene tubercle of the first rib.

Treatment

Surgical division of the fibrous band usually relieves pain and paresthesias and arrests muscle wasting and weakness, but return of muscle bulk and strength is unlikely.

METASTATIC AND RADIATION-INDUCED BRACHIAL PLEXOPATHY IN PATIENTS WITH CANCER

Damage to the brachial plexus in patients with cancer is usually secondary to either metastatic plexopathy or radiation-induced injury. Lung and breast carcinomas are the tumors that most frequently metastasize to the brachial plexus; lymphoma, sarcoma, and melanoma are less common. The main feature is severe pain that is generally located in the shoulder girdle and radiates to the elbow, medial portion of the forearm, and fourth and fifth digits of the hand. The main differential diagnosis is with radiation plexopathy, which is not painful. Cervical CT-myelography or MRI is usually diagnostic.

Radiation-induced plexopathy is unlikely to occur if the dose is less than 6000 cGy. With larger doses, the interval between the end of radiation therapy and the onset of symptoms and signs of radiation plexopathy ranges from 3 months to 26 years, with a mean interval of approximately 6 years. Weakness is usually most prominent in muscles innervated by branches of the upper trunk, but the entire limb may be involved. In women with radiation plexopathy following treatment for carcinoma of the breast, progressive weakness resulted in loss of hand function in 90% of patients.

Idiopathic Brachial Plexopathy

Idiopathic brachial plexopathy is an immune-mediated disorder that occurs mainly in adults. An upper respiratory tract infection, a flulike illness, or a tetanus toxoid immunization precedes half of cases.

Clinical Features
The initial feature is the abrupt onset of intense, unilateral arm pain, usually located in the shoulder. It is sharp, stabbing, throbbing, or aching, and generally lasts from hours to a week before gradually abating. Lessening of pain is associated with evolving weakness, which peaks 2 to 3 weeks after the onset of pain. Paresthesias occur in approximately one third of patients but do not correlate with the severity or extent of weakness.

Approximately half of patients have weakness in muscles of the shoulder girdle, one third have weakness referable to both upper and lower parts of the plexus, and approximately 15% have evidence for lower plexus involvement alone. Most diffuse plexus lesions are incomplete because there is sparing of one or more muscles in the same root distribution. One third of cases are bilateral, but few are symmetrical. Unilateral or bilateral diaphragmatic paralysis occurs in very few patients.

Diagnosis
Cervical radiculopathy is the main differential diagnostic consideration. It is unusual, however, for radicular pain to subside as weakness is increasing. The results of cervical paraspinal needle EMG performed several weeks after the onset of pain should be normal in brachial plexus neuropathy but should

show increased insertional activity and fibrillation potentials in cervical radiculopathy.

Management
A 10-day course of corticosteroids may be beneficial in some patients. Arm and neck movements often aggravate pain, so immobilization of the arm in a sling is helpful. With the onset of paralysis, range-of-motion exercises help prevent contractures. Thirty-six percent recover by the end of the first year, 75% by the end of 2 years, and 89% by the end of 3 years without treatment.

Disorders of the Lumbosacral Plexus

Clinical Features
Lumbar plexopathy produces weakness, sensory loss, and reflex changes in segments L2-L4, resulting in weakness and sensory loss in obturator- and femoral-innervated territories. Sacral plexopathy causes the same abnormalities in segments L5-S3, causing weakness and sensory loss in the gluteal (motor only), peroneal, and tibial nerve territories.

Electrodiagnostic Studies
Needle EMG differentiates plexopathies from radiculopathies. A plexopathy is confirmed if needle EMG discloses denervation potentials and reduced recruitment in muscles innervated by at least two lumbosacral segmental levels and involving at least two peripheral nerves. EMG also determines whether a lumbosacral plexopathy is associated with a polyneuropathy. Myokymic discharges point to the diagnosis of radiation plexopathy.

Radiological Studies
MRI identifies individual plexal components. Normal MRI results make a structural plexopathy very unlikely.

Differential Diagnosis
The differential diagnosis of lumbosacral plexopathy includes spinal root disorders, anterior horn cell disorders, and myopathic conditions. Radiculopathies are usually painful, and the distribution of the pain follows a predictable radicular distribution. Weakness involves several muscles supplied by the same root, and EMG shows paraspinal muscle involvement.

Anterior horn cell disorders give rise to painless, progressive weakness with atrophy and fasciculation in the absence of sensory loss. Myopathies are rarely confused with lumbosacral plexopathy.

Structural Lumbosacral Plexopathy

Hematoma

Patients with hemophilia and those receiving anticoagulants are at risk of developing hemorrhage into the iliopsoas muscle. Two anatomical syndromes are associated. In one, only the femoral nerve is affected. In the other, the obturator and lateral femoral cutaneous nerves are involved. Retroperitoneal hematoma causes pain in the groin that radiates to the thigh and leg and is associated with paresthesias and weakness. Large hemorrhages are palpable as a mass in the lower abdominal quadrant. A bruise appears in the inguinal area or femoral canal several days later. Recovery is usually satisfactory; only 15% show no improvement.

Abscess

Psoas abscess is a common complication of tuberculosis, but lumbar plexopathy and femoral neuropathy are rare. Acute, nontuberculous psoas infection rarely produces nerve compression. Lumbar plexopathy is a complication of pelvic hydatidosis, caused by the tapeworm *Echinococcus granulosus*.

Aneurysm

Back and abdominal pain is an early feature of abdominal aortic aneurysms. An expanding abdominal aortic aneurysm compresses the iliohypogastric or ilioinguinal nerve, leading to pain that radiates into the lower abdomen and inguinal areas. Pressure on the genitofemoral nerve produces pain in the inguinal area, testicle, and anterior thigh. Compression of nerve trunks L5-S2, which lie directly posterior to the hypogastric artery, may cause sciatica.

Abdominal aortic aneurysm hemorrhage produces prominent neurological problems because of the retroperitoneal location of the hemorrhage. A large retroperitoneal hematoma injures the femoral and obturator nerves and even branches of the sacral plexus. Rupture of a hypogastric or common iliac artery aneurysm extends into the pelvis, compressing the L5 through S2 nerve trunk. Early recognition of an aneurysm is important because the mortality rate for operation on unruptured aneurysms is 5–7%, as compared to 35–40% for symptomatic ruptured aneurysms.

Trauma

Sacral fractures or sacroiliac joint separation accounts for most traumatic lumbosacral plexus injuries. The remainder are secondary to fractures of the pelvis, acetabulum, or femur and to surgery on the proximal femur and hip joint. Leg weakness is often incorrectly attributed to traumatic mononeuropathy involving the femoral or sciatic nerves rather than lumbosacral plexopathy. Conservative measures are the most appropriate way to manage posttraumatic injuries. More than two thirds of patients show good or moderate recovery after 18 months.

Pregnancy

The fetal head may compress the mother's lumbosacral trunk during the second stage of labor (see Chapter 56).

Neoplasia

The lumbosacral plexus may be damaged by tumors that invade the plexus either by direct extension from intra-abdominal neoplasm or by metastases. Most are unilateral. CT or MRI usually establishes the diagnosis.

Nonstructural Lumbosacral Plexopathy

Radiation Plexopathy

The initial feature of radiation plexopathy is slowly progressive, painless weakness. The latent interval between radiation and the onset of neurological manifestations is between 1 and 31 years (median of 5 years), with no consistent relationship between the duration of the symptom-free interval and the amount of radiation. Radiation plexopathy is gradually progressive and results in significant or severe disability. CT and MRI findings of the abdomen and pelvis are normal. Needle EMG discloses paraspinal fibrillation potentials in 50% of patients. Almost 60% of patients have myokymic discharges, an uncommon feature in neoplastic plexopathy.

Vasculitis

Vasculitic neuropathy is usually associated with mononeuritis multiplex but can also cause a painful lumbosacral plexopathy.

Idiopathic Lumbosacral Plexopathy

Lumbosacral plexopathy occurs in the absence of a recognizable underlying disorder. Similar to idiopathic brachial plexus neuropathy, pain is the initial feature. Weakness follows within days. EMG discloses a patchy pattern of denervation in the distribution of part or all of the lumbosacral plexus, but the paraspinal muscles are spared, indicating that the process does not affect the lumbosacral roots. Immunomodulating therapy may be beneficial.

For a more detailed discussion, see Chapter 80 in Neurology in Clinical Practice, 4th edition.

Disorders of Peripheral Nerves | *51*

CLINICAL APPROACH TO DISORDERS OF PERIPHERAL NERVES

Pathological Processes Involving Peripheral Nerves

Despite the large number of causes of neuropathy, the peripheral nerve has only four pathological reactions to physical or metabolic insults: (1) wallerian degeneration, which is the response to axonal interruption, (2) axonal degeneration or axonopathy, (3) primary neuronal (perikaryal) degeneration or neuronopathy, and (4) segmental demyelination. The patient's symptoms, the type and pattern of distribution of signs, and the nerve conduction study results provide information about the underlying pathological changes.

Diagnostic Clues from the History

The symptoms of neuropathic disorders fall under the general headings motor, sensory, or autonomic disturbances. Muscle cramps, fasciculations, myokymia, and tremor are positive manifestations of motor nerve dysfunction. Motor symptoms in polyneuropathies produce early distal toe-extensor and ankle-extensor weakness. Positive sensory symptoms include prickling, searing, burning, and tight bandlike sensations. *Paresthesias* are unpleasant sensations arising spontaneously without apparent stimulus. Paresthesias are four times more common in acquired than in inherited neuropathies. *Allodynia* is the perception of nonpainful stimuli as painful. *Hyperalgesia* is painful hypersensitivity to noxious stimuli. Neuropathic pain is a cardinal feature of many neuropathies. Neuropathic pain often has a deep, burning, or drawing character that may be associated with jabbing or shooting pains and typically increases during periods of rest. Some neuropathies have prominent autonomic symptoms. Orthostatic lightheadedness, fainting spells, reduced or excessive sweating, heat intolerance, and bladder, bowel, and sexual dysfunction suggest autonomic dysfunction. Symptoms suggestive of gastroparesis include anorexia, early satiety, nausea, and vomiting. The tempo of disease (acute, subacute, or chronic) and the course (monophasic, progressive, or relapsing) narrow diagnostic possibilities.

Diagnostic Clues from the Examination

Mononeuropathy means focal involvement of a single nerve and implies a local process. Direct trauma, compression or entrapment, vascular lesions, and neoplastic infiltration are the most common causes. Electrophysiological studies provide precise localization of the lesion. *Multiple mononeuropathy* or *mononeuropathy multiplex* signifies simultaneous or sequential damage to multiple noncontiguous nerves. Electrodiagnostic studies ascertain whether the primary pathological process is axonal degeneration or segmental demyelination. Distal motor and sensory deficits and distal attenuation of reflexes characterize a *polyneuropathy*. Motor weakness is greater in extensor muscles than in corresponding flexors. *Motor deficits* dominate the clinical picture in acute and chronic inflammatory demyelinating neuropathies and hereditary motor and sensory neuropathies. Asymmetrical weakness without sensory loss suggests motor neuron disease or multifocal motor neuropathy with conduction block.

Predominant sensory involvement may be a feature of neuropathies caused by diabetes, carcinoma, Sjögren's syndrome, dysproteinemia, acquired immunodeficiency syndrome (AIDS), Vitamin B_{12} deficiency, celiac disease, intoxications with cisplatin, thalidomide, or pyridoxine, and inherited and idiopathic sensory neuropathies. *Autonomic dysfunction* of clinical importance is seen in association with specific acute (e.g., Guillain-Barré syndrome [GBS]) or chronic (e.g., amyloid and diabetic) sensorimotor polyneuropathies (Table 51.1).

Laboratory Studies

Carefully performed electrodiagnostic studies adapted to the particular clinical situation play a key role in the evaluation by (1) confirming the presence of neuropathy, (2) providing precise localization of focal nerve lesions, and (3) giving information about the nature of the underlying nerve pathology. Nerve biopsy is informative only when performed in centers with established experience with the technique. Nerve biopsy is essential for diagnosis in relatively few disorders (Table 51.2).

Table 51.1: Neuropathies with autonomic nervous system involvement

Acute
Acute panautonomic neuropathy (idiopathic, paraneoplastic)
Guillain-Barré syndrome
Porphyria
Toxic: vincristine, vacor
Chronic
Diabetes mellitus
Amyloid neuropathy (familial and primary)
Paraneoplastic sensory neuronopathy (malignant inflammatory sensory polyganglionopathy)
Human immunodeficiency virus–related autonomic neuropathy
Hereditary sensory and autonomic neuropathy

Table 51.2: Indications for nerve biopsy

Nerve biopsy results show diagnostic abnormalities
Vasculitis*
Amyloidosis*
Sarcoidosis*
Hansen's disease (leprosy)
Giant axonal neuropathy
Polyglucosan body disease
Tumor infiltration
Nerve biopsy results show suggestive abnormalities
Charcot-Marie-Tooth disease types 1 and 3
Chronic inflammatory demyelinating polyradiculoneuropathy
Paraproteinemic neuropathy (immunoglobulin M monoclonal gammopathy with anti–myelin-associated glycoprotein antibody)

*Consider combined nerve and muscle biopsies.

Approximately one third of patients report unpleasant sensory symptoms at the biopsy site after 1 year.

It is important to screen for monoclonal proteins in all patients with chronic undiagnosed neuropathy, particularly those older than 60 years. Several serum autoantibodies with reactivity to various components of peripheral nerve are associated with peripheral neuropathy syndromes. Table 51.3 lists those of greatest clinical utility. Several molecular genetic tests for inherited neuropathies are available for the diagnosis of genetic neuropathies.

Table 51.3: Neuropathies associated with serum autoantibodies

Autoantibody	Disease (% Positive)
Antibodies against gangliosides	
GM$_1$ (polyclonal IgM)	Multifocal motor neuropathy (70%)
GM$_1$, GD1a (polyclonal IgG)	Guillain-Barré syndrome (30%)
GQ1b (polyclonal IgG)	Miller Fisher variant (>95%)
Antibodies against glycoproteins	
Myelin-associated glycoprotein (monoclonal IgM)	IgM monoclonal gammopathy of undetermined significance neuropathy (50%)
Antibodies against RNA-binding proteins	
Anti-Hu, antineuronal nuclear antibody 1	Malignant inflammatory polyganglionopathy (>95%)

Ig = immunoglobulin.

CHRONIC IDIOPATHIC AXONAL POLYNEUROPATHY

Acquired idiopathic chronic sensorimotor and sensory neuropathies are common in individuals older than 50 years. The clinical features are either mixed sensorimotor or pure sensory. Symptoms are tingling, prickling, numbness or burning of the feet, and stiffness of the toes. Examination reveals loss of pinprick, loss of vibratory sensation in the feet, absent ankle reflexes, and mild toe-extensor weakness. Nerve conduction and nerve biopsy studies are compatible with a length-dependent axonal neuropathy. Idiopathic small-fiber neuropathy presents with painful, burning feet, with or without numbness. Both idiopathic sensorimotor and sensory polyneuropathies pursue a very slow progressive course or reach a stable plateau. Even after more than 10 years, severe disability does not occur and ambulation is independent.

PAIN IN PERIPHERAL NEUROPATHY

Pain is a cardinal symptom of peripheral nerve disorders. Neuropathic pain occurs spontaneously or is provoked by noxious or non-noxious stimuli. *Hyperalgesia* is an increased pain response to noxious stimuli. *Allodynia* is the sensation of pain elicited by

Table 51.4: Peripheral neuropathies frequently associated with pain

Diabetic neuropathies
  Painful symmetrical polyneuropathy
  Asymmetrical polyradiculoplexopathy
  Truncal mononeuropathy
  Brachial and lumbosacral plexopathy
Idiopathic distal small-fiber neuropathy
Guillain-Barré syndrome
Vasculitic neuropathy (sometimes)
Toxic neuropathies (sometimes)
  Arsenic, thallium
  Alcohol
  Vincristine, cisplatin
  Dideoxynucleosides
Amyloid neuropathies: primary and familial
Paraneoplastic sensory neuronopathy
Sjögren's syndrome
Human immunodeficiency virus–related distal symmetrical
  polyneuropathy
Uremic neuropathy
Fabry's disease
Hereditary sensory autonomic neuropathy

non-noxious stimuli. Table 51.4 lists peripheral neuropathies in which neuropathic pain is an initial symptom.

Management of Neuropathic Pain

Regardless of the underlying cause, the management to alleviate neuropathic pain is identical for all painful neuropathies. Symptomatic treatment of neuropathic pain seldom provides complete relief. Simple analgesics (aspirin, acetaminophen, and certain nonsteroidal anti-inflammatory drugs) are rarely beneficial. Most patients require tricyclic antidepressants, anticonvulsants, sodium-channel blockers, opioids and non-narcotic analgesics, and topical agents (see Chapter 57).

ENTRAPMENT NEUROPATHIES

An entrapment neuropathy is a focal neuropathy caused by restriction or mechanical distortion of a nerve. Compression, constriction, angulation, or stretching may injure nerves at vulnerable anatomical sites (Tables 51.5 and 51.6). The

Table 51.5: Entrapment neuropathies of upper limbs

Nerve	Site of Compression	Predisposing Factors	Major Clinical Features
Median	Wrist (carpal tunnel syndrome)	Tenosynovitis, arthritis, etc.	Paresthesia, pain, thenar atrophy
	Anterior interosseous	Strenuous exercise, trauma	Abnormal pinch sign, normal sensation
	Elbow (pronator teres syndrome)	Repetitive elbow motions	Tenderness of pronator teres, sensory loss
Ulnar	Elbow (cubital tunnel syndrome)	Elbow leaning, trauma	Clawing and sensory loss of fourth and fifth fingers
	Guyon's canal	Mechanics, cyclists	Hypothenar atrophy, variable sensory loss
Radial	Axilla	Crutches	Wristdrop, triceps involved, sensory loss
	Spiral groove	Abnormal sleep postures	Wristdrop, sensory loss
	Posterior interosseous	Elbow synovitis	Paresis of finger extensors, radial wrist deviation
	Superficial sensory branch (cheiralgia paresthetica)	Wrist bands, hand cuffs	Paresthesias in dorsum of hand
Suprascapular	Suprascapular notch	Blunt trauma	Atrophy of supraspinatus and infraspinatus muscles
Dorsal scapular	Scalene muscle	Trauma	Winging of scapula on arm abduction
Lower trunk of the brachial plexus or C8/T1 roots	Thoracic outlet	Cervical rib, enlarged C7 transverse process	Atrophy of intrinsic hand muscles, paresthesias of hand and forearm

Table 51.6: Entrapment neuropathies of lower limbs

Nerve	Site of Compression	Predisposing Factors	Major Clinical Features
Sciatic	Sciatic notch	Endometriosis, intramuscular injections	Pain down thigh, footdrop, absent ankle jerk
	Hip	Fracture dislocations	
	Piriformis muscle		
	Popliteal fossa	Popliteal Baker's cyst	Footdrop, weak evertors, sensory loss in dorsum of foot
Fibular	Fibular neck	Leg crossing, squatting	Footdrop
Posterior tibial	Anterior compartment	Muscle edema	Sensory loss over sole of foot
	Medial malleolus (tarsal tunnel syndrome)	Ankle fracture, tenosynovitis	
Femoral	Inguinal ligament	Lithotomy position	Weak knee extension, absent knee jerk
Lateral femoral cutaneous	Inguinal ligament (meralgia paresthetica)	Tight clothing, weight gain, utility belts	Sensory loss in lateral thigh
Ilioinguinal	Abdominal wall	Trauma, surgical incision	Direct hernia, sensory loss in the iliac crest, crural area
Obturator	Obturator canal	Tumor, surgery, pelvic fracture	Sensory loss in medial thigh, weak hip adduction

double-crush syndrome refers to focal compression of proximal nerve fibers, altering axoplasmic transport to render the distal nerve more susceptible to symptomatic entrapment neuropathy.

HEREDITARY NEUROPATHIES

The hereditary neuropathies constitute a complex group of diseases that frequently share insidious onset and indolent course over years to decades. Several disorders have a known metabolic defect (familial amyloid neuropathies, Refsum's disease, Fabry's disease, porphyria, and hypolipoproteinemias). For other inherited neuropathies, classification depends on clinical phenotype, mode of inheritance, and class of neurons predominantly affected. These conditions include hereditary motor neuropathy or spinal muscular atrophy, hereditary motor and sensory neuropathy (HMSN), and hereditary sensory and autonomic neuropathy (HSAN). Major advances in understanding the molecular basis of inherited neuropathies have come from identifying chromosomal loci or causative genes for a given disease phenotype.

Charcot-Marie-Tooth Disease (Hereditary Motor and Sensory Neuropathy)

Charcot-Marie-Tooth (CMT) disease is the most common inherited neuropathy. Electrophysiological studies allows a separation into two main groups: (1) the hypertrophic or demyelinating form of CMT disease (CMT1, also HMSN type I) and (2) the axonal form of CMT disease (CMT2, or HMSN type II), in which motor nerve conduction velocities (NCVs) are normal or near normal. In addition to CMT types 1 and 2, there are rare cases of severe demyelinating neuropathy with onset in early childhood. These are called *Dejerine-Sottas disease*. Both CMT1 and CMT2 display autosomal dominant inheritance. DNA-based diagnosis is available for almost all forms.

Charcot-Marie-Tooth Disease Type 1
Onset of CMT1 is in the first or second decade of life. Initial features are foot deformity and difficulties running or walking secondary to symmetrical weakness and wasting in the intrinsic foot, peroneal, and anterior tibial muscles. Similar involvement of the hands develops later in two thirds of patients. Inspection reveals pes cavus and hammer toes in nearly 75% of adult patients, mild kyphosis in approximately 10%, and enlarged, hypertrophic peripheral nerves in 25%. Absent ankle tendon reflexes are universal. Absent or reduced knee and upper limb

reflexes follow. Diminished vibration sense and light touch in feet and hands is common. Few patients have an essential or postural upper limb tremor. Motor nerve conduction studies show uniform slowing by more than 25% of the lower limits of normal in all nerves.

Charcot-Marie-Tooth Disease Type 2
Clinical symptoms of CMT2 begin in the second decade of life or later. Foot and spinal deformities are less prominent. The clinical features closely resemble those of CMT1 except for lack of peripheral nerve enlargement and less common arm involvement and tremor. A subgroup of severely affected patients, designated CMT2C, develop vocal cord, intercostal, and diaphragmatic muscle weakness. Respiratory failure shortens life expectancy. Motor NCVs are normal or mildly reduced.

X-linked Charcot-Marie-Tooth Disease
X-linked CMT (CMTX) disease is phenotypically similar to CMT1 except that affected men have severe symptoms and affected females have a mild neuropathy or are asymptomatic. No male-to-male transmission occurs. NCVs in men show significant slowing, whereas in women the slowing parallels the loss of compound motor action potential (CMAP) amplitude. Brainstem auditory evoked responses are often abnormal.

Charcot-Marie-Tooth Disease Type 3
CMT type 3 (CMT3), or Dejerine-Sottas disease, is an uncommon progressive hypertrophic neuropathy with onset in childhood. Clinical features include delayed motor development, proximal weakness, global areflexia, enlarged peripheral nerves, and severe disability. Most cases are sporadic or result from a new dominant mutation. Motor NCVs are less than 10 m per second. The cerebrospinal fluid (CSF) protein concentration is typically increased. Cases of congenital hypomyelination neuropathy probably represent a variant of CMT3.

Charcot-Marie-Tooth Disease Type 4
CMT type 4 (CMT4) is an autosomal recessive neuropathy characterized by onset in early childhood and progressive weakness, leading to inability to walk in adolescence. NCVs are slow (20–30 m per second); CSF protein concentration is normal. Nerve biopsy shows loss of myelinated fibers, hypomyelination, and onion bulbs.

Complex Forms of Charcot-Marie-Tooth Disease
Several families with peroneal muscular atrophy exhibit additional features such as optic atrophy, pigmentary retinal degeneration, deafness, and spastic paraparesis.

Molecular Advances of Charcot-Marie-Tooth Disease and Related Disorders

Most patients with CMT1 have DNA rearrangements on chromosome 17.11.2 as the molecular mechanism of their disease. Table 51.7 lists the mode of inheritance and the chromosomal locus or causative genes.

Treatment and Management

The rates of progression of CMT1 and CMT2 are slow, disability occurs relatively late, and life span may be normal. Management is mainly symptomatic and includes provision of proper foot care, ankle-foot orthoses, and avoidance of neurotoxic drugs.

Hereditary Neuropathy with Liability to Pressure Palsies

Hereditary neuropathy with liability to pressure palsies (HNPP) is an autosomal dominant disorder of peripheral nerves leading to increased susceptibility to mechanical traction or compression. The presenting feature is recurrent isolated mononeuropathies, typically affecting, in order of decreasing frequency, the common peroneal, ulnar, brachial plexus, radial, and median nerves. Painless brachial plexus neuropathy occurs in one third of patients. The initial episode usually occurs before age 30 years. Attacks are sudden in onset, painless, and usually provoked by compression, slight traction, or other minor trauma. Complete recovery follows within days or weeks. Nerve conduction studies in patients with HNPP associated with PMP-22 deletion typically consist of prolonged distal motor latencies with only mild slowing of forearm segments of median and ulnar nerves, focal slowing of ulnar and fibular nerves at compression sites, and diffuse reduction of sensory nerve action potential (SNAP) amplitudes.

Molecular diagnosis of the 17p11.2 deletion is available and replaced nerve biopsy for diagnosis. The primary treatment strategy is to prevent nerve injury by avoiding pressure damage.

Giant Axonal Neuropathy

Giant axonal neuropathy (GAN) is a rare autosomal recessive multisystem disorder of intermediate filaments affecting the peripheral nervous system (PNS) and central nervous system (CNS). GAN presents as a slowly progressive axonal sensorimotor neuropathy in early childhood and leads to death by late adolescence. Most affected children have tightly curled hair and distal leg weakness. Some develop a peculiar gait disturbance with a tendency to walk on the inner edges of the feet. With disease

Table 51.7: Molecular genetic classification of Charcot-Marie-Tooth disease and related disorders (2002)

Disorder	Locus	Gene	Mechanism	Testing Available
CMT1				
CMT1A	17p11.2	PMP-22	Duplication>pm	Yes
CMT1B	1q22–q23	PMZ	pm	Yes
CMT1C	16p13.1	LITAF	pm	—
CMT1D	10q21	EGR2	pm	Yes
CMTX				
CMTX1	Xq13.1	Cx32	pm	Yes
CMTX2	Xq24	?	?	—
CMT2				
CMT2A	1p35	KIF1Bβ	pm	—
CMT2B	3q13–q22	?	?	—
CMT2C	12q24	?	?	—
CMT2D	7p15	?	?	—
CMT2E	8p21	NF-L	pm	Yes
CMT2P$_0$	1q22	PMZ	pm	Yes
HNPP	17p11.2	PMP22	Deletion>pm	Yes
DSS				
	1q22–q23	PMZ	pm	Yes
	17p11.2	PMP22	pm	Yes
	10q21–q22	EGR2	pm	Yes
AR CMT				
CMT4A	8q21	GDAP1	pm	—
CMT4B	11q22	MTMR2	pm	—
CMT4C	5q23–q33	?	?	—
CMT4D	8q24	NDRG1	pm	Yes
CMT4E	10q21–q22	EGR2	pm	Yes
CMT4F	19q13	Periaxin	pm	—

AR = autosomal recessive; CMT = Charcot-Marie-Tooth disease; CMTX = X-linked CMT; Cx32 = connexin-32; DSS = Dejerine-Sottas syndrome; EGR2 = early growth response 2 gene; GDAP1 = ganglioside-induced differentiation–associated protein 1; HNPP = hereditary neuropathy with liability to pressure palsies; KIF1Bβ = microtubule motor KIF1Bβ; LITAF gene = lipopolysaccharide-induced tumor necrosis factor-α factor; MTMR2 = myotubularin-related protein 2; NDRG1 = N-myc downstream regulated gene 1; NF-L = neurofilament light chain gene; pm = point mutations; PMP-22 = peripheral myelin protein-22; PMZ = myelin protein zero gene.

progression, evidence of CNS involvement occurs, including optic atrophy, nystagmus, cerebellar ataxia, upper motor neuron signs, intellectual decline, and abnormal visual, auditory, and somatosensory evoked potentials.

Hereditary Sensory and Autonomic Neuropathy

HSAN is a group of neuropathies characterized by prominent sensory loss with autonomic features but without significant motor involvement. These neuropathies are divided into five main groups based on inheritance, clinical features, and populations of sensory neurons affected (Table 51.8). Complications are preventable by avoiding trauma to the insensitive distal limb segments.

Familial Amyloid Polyneuropathy

Familial amyloid polyneuropathy (FAP) is a group of autosomal dominant disorders characterized by the extracellular deposition of amyloid in peripheral nerves and other organs. Amyloid is a fibrillar protein. Clinical presentation was the traditional basis for classification. The basis of modern classification is protein composition and molecular genetics (Table 51.9).

Porphyric Neuropathy

Inactivation of one of a pair of allelic genes that encode for an enzyme of the heme biosynthetic pathway causes the porphyrias. These dominantly inherited disorders include acute intermittent porphyria (AIP), variegate porphyria (VP), and hereditary coproporphyria (HCP). The inheritance of a fourth disorder, referred to as plumboporphyria, is as an autosomal recessive trait. More than 90 mutations in the PBG deaminase gene decrease enzyme activity and cause AIP. These partial enzyme defects remain latent until precipitating factors trigger acute attacks. Precipitating factors include certain inducing drugs, the menstrual cycle, alcohol, hormones, and fasting, either intentional or during an intercurrent illness.

Clinical Features of the Acute Porphyric Attack

The manifestations of the acute attack are identical regardless of the specific type of hepatic porphyria. Dysfunction of the autonomic nervous system, the PNS, and the CNS explains the clinical symptoms. Porphyric attacks first occur during the third and fourth decades of life and are five times more common and severe in women than men. The presenting symptoms are abdominal pain, nausea, vomiting, and severe constipation. Other manifestations are tachycardia, labile hypertension, orthostatic hypotension, and difficulty with micturition. Rarely do patients progress to develop the more ominous motor neuropathy or CNS involvement. Onset of the predominantly motor neuropathy is subacute. Generalized, proximal, or

Table 51.8: Hereditary sensory and autonomic neuropathies

Disease	Inheritance	Locus	Gene	Clinical Features
HSAN I(HSN I)	AD	9q22	SPTLC1*	Small > large MF sensory loss, distal weakness, onset in second to fourth decade
HSAN II	AR	?	?	Pansensory loss in infancy
HSAN III (FD)	AR	9q31	IKBKAP*	Sensory loss, autonomic dysregulation, absent tears, fungiform tongue papillae
HSAN IV	AR	1q21	TRKA/NGF receptor	Insensitivity to pain, anhidrosis at birth, nl SNAPs
HSAN V	AR	?	?	Insensitivity to pain at birth, nl SNAPs, absent small MF

AD = autosomal dominant; AR = autosomal recessive; FD = familial dysautonomia; IKBKAP = IKAP, the protein encoded by IKBKAP gene is a member of the human elongator complex; HSAN = hereditary sensory and autonomic neuropathies; MF = myelinated fibers; nl SNAP = normal sensory nerve action potential; SPTLC1 = SPTLC1 encodes serine palmitoyltransferase long chain 1; TRKA/NGF = TRKA encodes for the high affinity NGF (nerve growth factor) receptor
*Molecular gene testing is clinically available.

Table 51.9: Familial amyloid neuropathies

Aberrant Protein	Type	Decade of Onset	Neuropathy	Associated Lesions
TTR	FAP I	Third through fifth	Sensorimotor neuropathy, autonomic neuropathy	Heart, kidney
TTR	FAP II	Fourth through fifth	Carpal tunnel syndrome	Heart
Apolipoprotein A1	FAP III	Third through fourth	Sensorimotor neuropathy	Kidney, peptic ulcers
Gelsolin	FAP IV	Third	Cranial	Corneal lattice dystrophy

FAP = familial amyloid polyneuropathy; TTR = transthyretin.

asymmetrical muscle weakness develops over days or weeks. Weakness of the proximal arm muscles precedes distal weakness. The rate of improvement varies.

Laboratory Studies
The biochemical hallmark of the porphyric attack is the marked elevation of PBG and ALA in blood and urine.

Treatment and Management
The treatment of patients with acute hepatic porphyria involves three important steps: (1) prevention of attacks, (2) attempts to repress hepatic δ-ALA synthase activity, thereby reducing porphyrin production, and (3) supportive care. A high-carbohydrate diet orally or by nasogastric feeding (at least 400 g daily or the equivalence of glucose or levulose infusions) results in reduced porphyrin precursor production. Persistent symptoms or neurological deficits that progress for 24 hours after carbohydrate loading are indications for treatment with hematin (a hydroxide of heme).

INFLAMMATORY DEMYELINATING POLYRADICULONEUROPATHIES

Inflammatory demyelinating polyradiculoneuropathies are acquired immune-mediated disorders. Two major groups exist: (1) an acute inflammatory demyelinating polyradiculoneuropathy called the GBS and (2) chronic inflammatory demyelinating polyradiculoneuropathy (CIDP). In GBS, the maximal deficits develop over days (maximum 28 days), followed by a plateau phase and gradual recovery. Chronic forms pursue either a slowly progressive or a relapsing course.

Acute Inflammatory Demyelinating Polyradiculoneuropathy (Guillain-Barré Syndrome)

Clinical Features
GBS is a nonseasonal illness that affects persons of all ages. Approximately two thirds of patients report a preceding event, most frequently an upper respiratory or gastrointestinal tract infection, surgery, or immunization 1–4 weeks before the onset of neurological symptoms. The agent responsible for the prodromal illness frequently remains unidentified. The most common identifiable bacterial organism linked to GBS and particularly its axonal forms is *Campylobacter jejuni*. Patients may initially have paresthesia, sensory symptoms with weakness, or weakness

alone. The symmetrical weakness of the lower limbs ascends proximally over hours to several days to involve arm, facial, and oropharyngeal muscles, and in severe cases respiratory muscles. Less often, weakness may begin in proximal nerve– or cranial nerve–innervated muscles. Its severity varies from mild involvement, in which patients are still capable of walking unassisted, to quadriplegia. Hyporeflexia and areflexia are invariable features, although they may be missing early in the course of the disease. By definition progression ends by 1–4 weeks into the illness; if it continues longer, the condition is termed either *subacute inflammatory demyelinating polyradiculoneuropathy* if progression continues for 4–10 weeks or *CIDP* if there is chronic progression or multiple relapses.

Laboratory Studies
Cerebrospinal fluid (CSF) examination and serial electrophysiological studies are critical for confirming the diagnosis of GBS. In the first week of neurological symptoms, the CSF protein concentration may be normal but then becomes elevated on subsequent examinations. In 10% of cases, the CSF protein concentration remains normal throughout the illness. Abnormalities of electrophysiological studies reflect an evolving picture of multifocal demyelination associated with secondary axonal degeneration. The most common electrophysiological abnormalities include prolonged distal motor and F-wave latencies, absent or impersistent F waves, conduction block, reduction in distal CMAP amplitudes with or without temporal dispersion, and slowing of motor NCVs.

Treatment
Observe patients with rapidly worsening acute GBS in the hospital until the maximum extent of progression is established. Supportive care in intensive care units (ICUs) and the prevention of complications, of which respiratory failure and autonomic dysfunction are the most important, provide the best chance for a favorable outcome. Plasma exchange and high-dose intravenous immune globulin (IVIG) infusions are equally effective in shortening the course of disease.

Chronic Inflammatory Demyelinating Polyradiculoneuropathy

The major differences between CIDP and GBS are in the time course and their response to corticosteroids. CIDP has a more protracted clinical course, is rarely associated with preceding infections, has an association with human lymphocyte antigens, and responds to corticosteroid therapy. Two patterns of temporal evolution of CIDP exist. More than 60% of patients show a continuous or stepwise progressive course over months to years, whereas one third have a relapsing course with partial or complete recovery between recurrences.

Clinical Features
The peak incidence is in the fifth and sixth decades of life. Most patients have symmetrical motor and sensory involvement. Weakness must be present for at least 2 months. Proximal limb weakness is almost as severe as distal limb weakness. All limbs are weak; the legs are more severely affected. Generalized hyporeflexia or areflexia is the rule. Sensory symptoms in a stocking-glove distribution (numbness or tingling) implicating large-fiber involvement occur frequently, whereas pain is uncommon. Children differ from adults by a more precipitous onset and more prominent gait abnormalities.

Laboratory Studies
Table 51.10 lists the laboratory studies that support the diagnosis of CIDP.

Treatment
Prednisone, plasmapheresis, and IVIG are equally effective in CIDP and are the mainstays of treatment.

Prognosis
In contrast to the good prognosis in GBS, CIDP tends to be associated with prolonged neurological disability and is less likely to have spontaneous remissions.

Multifocal Motor Neuropathy with Conduction Block

Multifocal motor neuropathy is either a distinct nosological entity or a multifocal motor variant of CIDP.

Clinical Features
The disorder is more common in men and mainly affects young adults, two thirds being 45 years or younger. Progressive, asymmetrical, predominantly distal limb weakness and atrophy develop over months to years. Arm weakness is more common than leg weakness. Wristdrop, grip weakness, and footdrop are the most common presenting features. Muscle cramps and fasciculations are common. Profound weakness in muscles with normal bulk or focal weakness in the distribution of individual nerves rather than in a spinal segmental pattern provides clues that should alert the clinician to suspect this disorder. Cranial nerve involvement is unusual. Tendon reflexes are depressed or absent. Upper motor neuron signs are absent. Objective sensory

Table 51.10: Diagnostic criteria for chronic inflammatory demyelinating polyradiculoneuropathy

I. Mandatory clinical criteria
  Progressive or relapsing muscle weakness for 2 months or longer
  Symmetrical proximal and distal weakness in upper or lower extremities
  Hyporeflexia or areflexia
II. Mandatory laboratory criteria
  Nerve conduction studies with features of demyelination (motor nerve conduction <70% of lower limit of normal)
  Cerebrospinal fluid protein level >45 mg/dL, cell count <10/µl
  Sural nerve biopsy with features of demyelination and remyelination including myelinated fiber loss and perivascular inflammation
III. Mandatory exclusion criteria
  Evidence of relevant systemic disease or toxic exposure
  Family history of neuropathy
  Nerve biopsy findings incompatible with diagnosis
IV. Diagnostic categories
  A. Definite: Mandatory inclusion and exclusion criteria and all laboratory criteria
  B. Probable: Mandatory inclusion and exclusion criteria and 2 of 3 laboratory criteria
  C. Possible: Mandatory inclusion and exclusion criteria and 1 of 3 laboratory criteria

Source: Adapted from Cornblath, D. R., Asbury, A. K., Albers, J. W., et al. 1991, "Research criteria for diagnosis of chronic inflammatory demyelinating polyneuropathy (CIDP)," *Neurology,* vol. 41, pp. 617–618.

deficits are absent. The course is slowly or less often stepwise progressive over months to years.

Laboratory Studies
The diagnosis depends on electrophysiological studies demonstrating persistent focal motor conduction block in one or more motor nerves at sites not prone to compression. Additional features of multifocal motor demyelination are usually present in nerve segments without conduction block, including motor conduction slowing, temporal dispersion, and prolonged F-wave and distal motor latencies. Only motor axons show the block. SNAPs and sensory conduction are preserved. The CSF protein concentration is frequently normal, although moderately increased protein levels (<100 mg/dl) occur in one third of patients. Anti-GM$_1$ antibodies are neither specific nor required

for the diagnosis of multifocal motor neuropathy but are a marker for the disease.

Treatment
In contrast to CIDP, prednisone or plasma exchange have little or no benefit. Treatment with IVIG is the preferred treatment. IVIG (0.4 g/kg of body weight per day for 5 consecutive days) benefits 70% of patients. Improvement begins within 3 weeks of treatment but lasts only for weeks to months. Continue treatment with IVIG every 1–8 weeks in patients who have a functionally meaningful response.

PERIPHERAL NEUROPATHIES ASSOCIATED WITH MONOCLONAL PROTEINS

Monoclonal Gammopathy of Undetermined Significance

Approximately 10% of patients with idiopathic peripheral neuropathy have an associated monoclonal gammopathy—a sixfold increase over the general population. Finding an M protein among patients with neuropathy may lead to the discovery of underlying disorder. Two thirds of patients with a monoclonal protein have no detectable underlying disease and have a monoclonal gammopathy of undetermined significance (MGUS). The risk of progression of MGUS to a malignant plasma cell proliferative disorder is about 1% per year. Approximately 5% of patients with MGUS have an associated polyneuropathy.

Clinical Features
The neuropathies associated with different heavy-chain classes are similar. The median age at onset is in the sixth decade of life and progression is slow. A distal symmetrical sensorimotor polyneuropathy is typical. Cranial nerves and autonomic functions are preserved. Muscle stretch reflexes are usually absent. A predominantly sensory neuropathy occurs in 20% of patients.

Laboratory Features
Electrophysiological studies show evidence of demyelination or both demyelination and axonal degeneration. In half of patients with immunoglobulin M (IgM) MGUS neuropathy, the IgM monoclonal protein has reactivity against myelin-associated glycoprotein (MAG). About 15% of patients with IgM MGUS neuropathy have autoantibodies directed against gangliosides. The underlying mechanism of nerve fiber damage in MGUS neuropathy is unknown but is believed to be immune mediated.

Treatment

The optimal treatment of MGUS neuropathy is not established. Patients with minor deficits and indolent course are not treated. Patients with progressive, disabling neuropathy caused by IgM MGUS with or without anti-MAG reactivity may respond to aggressive immune interventions aimed at lowering the IgM level. This may be achieved by intermittent courses of oral cyclophosphamide (300 mg/m^2 of body surface daily for 4 days) combined with prednisone (40 mg/m^2 of body surface daily for 5 days) given at 4-week intervals for 6 months.

Waldenström's Macroglobulinemia

The characteristic features of Waldenström's macroglobulinemia (WM) are proliferation of malignant lymphocytoid cells in bone marrow and lymph nodes that secrete an IgM monoclonal spike of more than 3 g/dl. WM typically affects elderly men; systemic symptoms of fatigue, anemia, bleeding, and hyperviscosity dominate. Peripheral neuropathy occurs in approximately one third of patients with WM and is a chronic, symmetrical, predominantly sensory polyneuropathy similar to that associated with nonmalignant IgM M proteins. Other presentations include pure sensory or pure motor neuropathies, multiple mononeuropathies associated with cryoglobulins, and typical amyloid neuropathy. Fifty percent of patients with WM have anti-MAG reactivity. Patients with positive anti-MAG antibodies have slowed motor NCVs and prolonged distal latencies consistent with demyelination. Patients with demyelinating polyneuropathy may respond to chemotherapy, plasmapheresis, or both, but the response appears to be less consistent than in IgM MGUS-related neuropathy.

Multiple Myeloma

Polyneuropathy occurs in approximately 5% of patients with multiple myeloma. Most patients present with mild distal sensorimotor polyneuropathy. A pure sensory neuropathy also occurs. Painful dysesthesias, preferential involvement of small-fiber sensory modalities, autonomic dysfunction, and carpal tunnel syndrome suggest amyloid neuropathy. Rectal or sural nerve biopsy specimens identify patients with amyloidosis. Nerve conduction and sural nerve biopsy study results are consistent with an axonal process with loss of myelinated fibers. Treatment of the underlying myeloma may sometimes improve the neuropathy.

Osteosclerotic Myeloma and POEMS Syndrome

Osteosclerotic myeloma is a rare complication of myeloma and is usually associated with peripheral neuropathy that resembles CIDP. The neuropathy of osteosclerotic myeloma is different from that associated with multiple myeloma in several aspects: It occurs at an earlier age and mostly in men; it is a demyelinating, predominantly motor neuropathy with slow motor NCVs and elevated CSF protein levels, usually in excess of 100 mg/dl. Ninety percent of cases have an M protein. It responds to irradiation or excision of the isolated plasmacytoma. It is associated with systemic manifestations referred to as *Crow-Fukase* or *POEMS syndrome* (polyneuropathy, organomegaly, endocrinopathy, M protein, and skin changes). Treatment of patients with solitary lesions includes tumoricidal irradiation, complete surgical extirpation, or both. Patients with multiple bone lesions receive radiation combined with prednisone and melphalan. High-dose chemotherapy with autologous blood stem-cell support is another option for patients with multifocal bone lesions or diffuse bone marrow plasmacytic infiltration.

Cryoglobulinemia

Cryoglobulins are classified into three groups: Type I includes monoclonal immunoglobulins that are associated with myeloma, macroglobulinemia, and other lymphoproliferative disorders; type II consists of a mixture of a monoclonal protein, usually IgM-κ with antirheumatoid factor activity, and polyclonal immunoglobulin G (IgG); and type III includes polyclonal IgM and IgG. The prevalence of peripheral neuropathy varies from 37% to 57%. The most common presentation is a painful sensory or sensorimotor polyneuropathy or less often mononeuropathy multiplex. Patients with biopsy-proven vasculitis and progressive neurological deficits require immunosuppression with either oral or intravenous cyclophosphamide or corticosteroids.

Primary Systemic Amyloidosis

Systemic amyloidoses are multisystem disorders caused by extracellular deposition of insoluble fibrillar proteins. Primary amyloidosis usually occurs after age 40 years. The male-to-female ratio is 2:1. The initial symptoms are fatigue and weight loss, followed by dysfunction of specific organ involvement. The organs most commonly affected, either individually or together, are the kidney, heart, liver, and the autonomic nervous system and the PNS. Peripheral neuropathy occurs in 15–35%

of patients and is the presenting feature in 10%. Most patients develop features of autonomic dysfunction, including postural hypotension, impotence, gastrointestinal disturbances, impaired sweating, and loss of bladder control.

Electrodiagnostic studies show changes of axonal neuropathy, with low-amplitude or absent SNAPs, low-amplitude CMAPs, but preserved motor NCVs. Ninety percent of patients have monoclonal proteins or light chains. Histological demonstration of amyloid deposition in tissues establishes the diagnosis. The prognosis in primary amyloidosis is poor, with a median survival of less than 18 months.

NEUROPATHIES ASSOCIATED WITH SYSTEMIC DISORDERS

Chapter 24 discusses the neuropathies associated with many systemic disorders. Chapter 27 discusses the neuropathies associated with cancer, Chapter 28 the neuropathies associated with infectious disease, and Chapter 32 the neuropathies associated with deficiency diseases.

Critical Illness Polyneuropathy

Critical illness polyneuropathy is a common problem in ICUs. It is a major cause of difficulty in weaning patients from the respirator after excluding cardiac and pulmonary causes. Most patients have generalized flaccid weakness with depressed tendon reflexes. Pain or paresthesias are not features of critical illness neuropathy. At least 50% of critically ill patients admitted to ICUs with sepsis and multiple organ failure for at least 2 weeks have electrodiagnostic features of an axonal neuropathy. Nerve conduction studies reveal a distal axonal neuropathy with reduced CMAP and SNAP amplitudes, in conjunction with fibrillation potentials and decreased motor unit potentials on electromyography. CSF is usually normal. Critical illness myopathy is difficult to distinguish clinically from its neuropathic counterpart.

For a more detailed discussion, see Chapter 82 in Neurology in Clinical Practice, 4th edition.

Disorders of the Autonomic Nervous System

52

PRIMARY AUTONOMIC FAILURE

Disorders of primary autonomic failure (PAF) are those in which the cause is unknown. Most are *chronic autonomic failure syndromes*. Table 52.1 outlines the clinical features of PAF.

Chronic Autonomic Failure

Both the sympathetic and the parasympathetic systems fail. The clinical categories include: (1) autonomic failure and no other neurological features (idiopathic orthostatic hypotension) and (2) autonomic failure associated with other neurological abnormalities (Shy-Drager syndrome and multiple system atrophy [MSA]). MSA is defined as a sporadic, progressive disorder characterized by autonomic dysfunction, parkinsonism, and ataxia in any combination. Additional neurological features are the basis for the subtypes of MSA. The parkinsonian or striatonigral degeneration form has parkinsonian features associated with striatonigral degeneration and loss of pigmented cells in the substantia nigra and locus ceruleus. The cerebellar or olivopontocerebellar atrophy form has cerebellar features, with or without pyramidal signs. Atrophy of the cerebellum, olives, and pons is associated. The mixed or multiple form has features of combined extrapyramidal, cerebellar, and pyramidal dysfunction. Approximately 20% of patients have the parkinsonian form, 20% have the cerebellar form, and 60% have the multiple form.

In the different parkinsonian syndromes (other than MSA), the extent and degree of autonomic dysfunction relates to the underlying diagnosis. Cardiovascular autonomic failure is an exclusionary feature in progressive supranuclear palsy. In dementia with Lewy bodies, orthostatic hypotension and autonomic failure may be severe and an early manifestation,

Table 52.1: Clinical Features in Primary Chronic Autonomic Failure

Cardiovascular: postural (orthostatic) hypotension

Sudomotor: anhidrosis, heat intolerance

Gastrointestinal: constipation, occasionally diarrhea, oropharyngeal dysphagia

Renal and urinary bladder: nocturia, frequency, urgency, retention, incontinence

Sexual: erectile and ejaculatory failure in the male

Ocular: anisocoria, Horner's syndrome

Respiratory: stridor, involuntary inspiratory gasps, apneic episodes

Other neurological deficits: parkinsonian and cerebellar or pyramidal features

Source: Adapted with permission from Mathias, C. J. & Bannister, R., eds, 2002, *Autonomic Failure. A Textbook of Disorders of the Autonomic Nervous System*, 4th ed, Oxford, Oxford University Press.

even before the onset of parkinsonian features. Autonomic deficits occur in patients with the Guam parkinsonian-dementia complex, the Machado-Joseph syndrome, and Wilson's disease.

In PAF, the evidence favors a distal lesion involving the intermediolateral cell mass in the thoracolumbar regions and the paravertebral ganglia. The disorder usually is not progressive. In MSA, clinical presentations vary and the disorder is progressive. The clinical course, the *in vivo* neuroimaging data, and neuropathological data indicate that MSA is a single disorder. The reasons for selective initial involvement, sparing of certain areas, and possible interaction with genetic and environmental factors are not determined.

Acute and Subacute Dysautonomias

In the Guillain-Barré syndrome, autonomic disorders range from hyperactivity to failure. The cardiovascular changes range from hypertension and tachycardia to hypotension and bradycardia. The axonal and demyelinating forms are different. Autonomic disturbances contribute to both morbidity and mortality.

SECONDARY AUTONOMIC DYSFUNCTION

The pathological changes of secondary autonomic dysfunction depend on the causative or associated disease or disorder.

Cerebral

Autonomic failure may result from specific lesions, especially in the brainstem. Posterior fossa tumors and syringobulbia may cause postural hypotension by ischemia or destruction of brainstem cardiovascular centers. Demyelination or plaque formation in multiple sclerosis causes a variety of autonomic defects of cerebral origin, although it is difficult to exclude a spinal contribution. Autonomic failure in the elderly may be largely central, because of widespread neuronal degeneration. Some cerebral disorders cause a pathological increase in autonomic activity.

Cushing-sensitive areas may raise blood pressure by increasing sympathetic activity. In tetanus, hypertension may result from increased sensitivity of brainstem centers through retrograde spread of tetanus toxin along the nerve fibers. In fatal familial insomnia, a prion disease predominantly involving the thalamus, autonomic dysfunction includes an increase in blood pressure, heart rate, lacrimation, salivation, sweating, and body temperature, along with altered hormonal circadian rhythms in the presence of intact target organ function.

Spinal Cord

Damage to the spinal cord by trauma, transverse myelitis, syringomyelia, or spinal cord tumors may disturb or sever connections between the brain and the thoracolumbar sympathetic and sacral parasympathetic outflow. Activated spinal reflexes through unaffected areas in the cord below the lesion result in abnormal peripheral autonomic activity.

Peripheral

Peripheral autonomic dysfunction is associated with several diseases and syndromes. It may involve a specific afferent pathway, only efferent pathways, or both. Autonomic dysfunction occurs in familial amyloid polyneuropathy, paraneoplastic syndromes, acquired immunodeficiency syndrome, neuroectodermal syndromes, and neuroblastomas.

NEURALLY MEDIATED SYNCOPE

Neurally mediated syncope is a disorder in which intermittent dysfunction affects the autonomic nervous system. This dysfunction results in bradycardia caused by increased parasympathetic cardiac activity and hypotension caused by withdrawal of sympathetic vasoconstrictor tone. It probably accounts for a substantial proportion of recurrent syncope and presyncope, after excluding cardiac and other causes. Situational syncope occurs in weightlifters and during micturition, defecation, or laughing.

For a more detailed discussion, see Chapter 83 in Neurology in Clinical Practice, 4th edition.

Disorders of
Neuromuscular
Transmission

53

MYASTHENIA GRAVIS

Clinical Features

Patients seek medical attention for specific muscle weakness or dysfunction and not for generalized fatigue. Ptosis and diplopia are the initial features in two thirds of affected individuals and are usually present within 2 years. Difficulty chewing, swallowing, or talking is the initial symptom in 15% of patients, and limb weakness in 10%. The initial weakness is rarely limited to single muscle groups. Weakness typically fluctuates during the day, usually being least in the morning and worse as the day progresses, especially after prolonged use of affected muscles.

Weakness remains restricted to the ocular muscles in approximately 40% of cases. Maximum weakness occurs during the first year in two thirds of patients. Before corticosteroids were used for treatment, approximately one third of patients improved spontaneously, one third became worse, and one third died of the disease. Four stages are recognized. During the *early phase*, spontaneous improvement is common and symptoms fluctuate; this is followed by an *active phase*, during which symptoms become progressively severe for several years. The active stage is followed by an *inactive stage*, in which fluctuations in strength are attributable to fatigue, intercurrent illness, or other identifiable factors. After 15–20 years, the weakness may become fixed, and the most severely involved muscles are frequently atrophic (*burnt-out stage*). In about 20% of patients, weakness remains purely ocular. Treatment significantly modifies the course.

Factors that worsen myasthenic symptoms are emotional upset, systemic illness (especially viral respiratory infections), hypothyroidism or hyperthyroidism, pregnancy, the menstrual cycle, drugs affecting neuromuscular transmission, and increases in body temperature. Repetitively assess strength during maximum effort and again after brief periods of rest when examining patients with known or suspected myasthenia gravis (MG). Ocular and oropharyngeal muscle function testing best demonstrates the strength fluctuations. Tendon reflexes are normal in weak muscles.

Pathophysiology

MG is an immune-mediated disease of the acetylcholine receptor (AChR) complex. Circulating antibodies directed against the AChR are often present, but their role in the pathophysiology is not fully understood. MG is not transmitted by mendelian inheritance, but a genetic predisposition to developing MG and other immune-mediated disorders exists within families.

Ten percent of patients with MG have a thymic tumor (thymoma), and 70% have hyperplastic changes (germinal centers) that indicate an active immune response. The frequency of thymoma is 20% when symptoms begin between the ages of 30 and 60 years. Most thymomas are benign, well differentiated, and encapsulated and completely removed at surgery. Usually associated with thymoma is more severe disease, higher levels of AChR antibodies, and more severe electromyographic (EMG) abnormalities.

Diagnostic Procedures

Edrophonium Chloride (Tensilon) Test
Weakness caused by abnormal neuromuscular transmission characteristically improves after intravenous administration of edrophonium chloride. The test is most reliable when the patient has ptosis, paralytic strabismus, or nasal speech. Improved strength after edrophonium chloride administration is not unique to MG. The maximum dose is 0.15 mg/kg injected intravenously, not to exceed 10 mg. Ten percent of the total dose is given first as a test of excessive responsiveness, and additional 30% increments are then injected and the response to each increment is monitored for 60 seconds. Subsequent injections are 3 and 5 mg. If improvement occurs within 60 seconds after any dose, no further injections are given. In children, the total dose is 0.15 mg/kg.

Antibodies Against Acetylcholine Receptors
Eighty percent of patients with acquired generalized myasthenia and 55% with ocular myasthenia have serum antibodies that bind human AChR. The serum concentration of AChR antibody varies widely and does not predict the severity of disease.

Approximately 10% of patients who lack binding antibodies have antibodies that either block the AChR or modulate its turnover in tissue culture. Virtually all patients with MG and thymoma have elevated AChR-binding antibodies and many have high concentrations of AChR-modulating and antistriated muscle antibodies.

Electromyography

The following are practice recommendations of the American Association of Electrodiagnostic Medicine regarding the use of EMG in MG.

Repetitive nerve stimulation (RNS) of a nerve supplying a symptomatic muscle should be performed. Abnormality in MG is considered to be a reproducible 10% decrement in amplitude when comparing the first stimulus to the fourth or fifth, which is found in at least one muscle. Anticholinesterase medications should be withheld 12 hours before testing, if this can be done safely.

If RNS is abnormal and there is a high suspicion for a neuromuscular junction (NMJ) disorder, single-fiber EMG (SFEMG) of at least one symptomatic muscle should be performed. If SFEMG findings in one muscle are normal and clinical suspicion for an NMJ disorder is high, a second muscle should be studied.

As an option, if the patient has very mild or solely ocular symptoms and it is believed the RNS will be normal, or if the discomfort associated with RNS prevents completion of RNS, SFEMG testing may be performed in place of RNS as the initial NMJ test. In laboratories with SFEMG capability, SFEMG may be performed as the initial test for disorders of neuromuscular transmission because it is more sensitive than RNS. Routine needle EMG and nerve conduction studies may be necessary to exclude disorders other than MG or Lambert-Eaton myasthenic syndrome (LEMS).

Treatment

All recommended regimens are empirical because controlled clinical trials of medical or surgical modality are lacking. Although the response to treatment may be difficult to assess because the severity of symptoms fluctuates and spontaneous remissions occur, treatment and control of symptoms of MG with modern therapy is generally very successful.

Cholinesterase Inhibitors

Cholinesterase (ChE) inhibitors provide symptomatic relief by retarding the enzymatic hydrolysis of acetylcholine (ACh) at

Table 53.1: Equivalent doses of anticholinesterase drugs

	Route and Dose (mg)			
	Oral	*Intra-muscular*	*Intra-venous*	*Syrup*
Neostigmine bromide (Prostigmin Bromide)	15			
Neostigmine methylsulfate (Prostigmin Methylsulfate)		1.5	0.5	
Pyridostigmine bromide (Mestinon Bromide)	60	2.0	0.7	60 mg/ 5 ml
Mestinon Timespan	90–180			
Ambenonium chloride (Mytelase Chloride)	5			

Note: These values are approximations only. Appropriate doses should be determined for each patient based on the clinical response.

cholinergic synapses. ACh accumulates at the NMJ and its action is prolonged. The therapeutic effect is variable, but strength rarely returns to normal. Pyridostigmine and neostigmine are the most commonly used inhibitors. Pyridostigmine generally is preferred because it has a lower frequency of gastrointestinal side effects. The initial oral dose in adults is 30–60 mg q6–8h. Equivalent dosages of these drugs are listed in Table 53.1. In infants and children, the initial oral dose of pyridostigmine is 1.0 mg/kg and the initial dose of neostigmine is 0.3 mg/kg. No fixed dosage schedule suits all patients.

Thymectomy
A prospective, controlled study has never demonstrated the efficacy of thymectomy as a treatment for immune-mediated myasthenia. Based on review of existing studies, the Quality Standards Subcommittee of the American Academy of Neurology concluded that for patients with nonthymomatous auto-immune MG, thymectomy is recommended as an option to increase the probability of remission or improvement. The preferred surgical approach is transthoracic. The presence or level of AChR antibodies should not influence the decision to recommend thymectomy.

Corticosteroids
Marked improvement or complete relief of symptoms occurs in more than 75% of patients treated with prednisone, and some improvement occurs in most of the rest. Much of the

improvement occurs in the first 6–8 weeks. Treatment begins with a daily dose of 1.5–2.0 mg/kg per day. When sustained improvement occurs, usually within 2 weeks, the dosing changes to an alternate-day schedule and then is gradually decreased monthly to the lowest dose necessary to maintain improvement, usually less than 20 mg every other day (qod). If weakness returns during the taper, further reductions will cause even greater weakness. At this point, the prednisone dose should be increased, another immunosuppressant added, or both. Most patients who respond well to prednisone weaken after stopping the drug, but maintain strength on 5–10 mg qod. Indefinite treatment is required.

Approximately one third of patients become weaker temporarily after starting prednisone, usually within the first 7–10 days and lasting for up to 6 days. ChE inhibitors usually manage the weakness. Patients with oropharyngeal weakness or respiratory insufficiency before treatment should first undergo plasma exchange to prevent or reduce the severity of corticosteroid-induced exacerbations and to produce a more rapid response.

The major disadvantages of chronic corticosteroid therapy are the side effects. The severity and frequency of adverse reactions increase after more than 1 month of continuous high daily doses. Most side effects are minimal at doses of less than 20 mg qod.

Immunosuppressant Drugs
Several immunosuppressant drugs are effective in MG (Table 53.2). Azathioprine is the most frequently used. It reverses

---

Table 53.2: Immunosuppressant drugs in myasthenia gravis

Azathioprine
  Onset action: 4–8 mo
  Common side effects: allergic reaction ("flulike syndrome")
  Less common side effects: hepatic toxicity, leukopenia
Cyclosporine A
  Onset action: 2–3 mo
  Common side effects: renal toxicity, hypertension, multiple
  potential drug interactions
Cyclophosphamide
  Onset action: variable
  Common side effects: leukopenia, hair loss, cystitis
Mycophenolate mofetil
  Onset action: 2–4 weeks
  Common side effects: diarrhea, mild leukopenia

symptoms in most patients after a 4–8 month delay. The initial dose is 50 mg daily, increased in 50-mg increments every 7 days to a total of 150–200 mg per day. Improvement continues as long as the drug is given, but symptoms usually recur 2–3 months after stopping the drug.

Cyclosporine (CYA) provides improvement in most patients, with or without concurrent use of corticosteroids. The initial dose is 5–6 mg/kg per day, in two divided doses. After 1 month, dose adjustments are required to produce a trough serum CYA concentration of 75–150 ng/ml and a serum creatinine of less than 150% of pretreatment values. Serum creatinine is measured at least every 2–3 months.

Cyclophosphamide (CP), given intravenously in monthly, pulsed doses, is used in severe, generalized, refractory MG. The initial dose is 500 mg/m^2 and is subsequently titrated according to changes in strength and side effects. Oral CP is also effective at doses of 150–200 mg per day, to a total of 5–10 g, as required to relieve symptoms. Alopecia is the major side effect.

Mycophenolate mofetil (MM) (CellCept) has a role as a corticosteroid-sparing agent and as adjunctive therapy in refractory MG. The usual dose is 2 g a day, in two divided doses. Improvement may occur as early as 2 weeks and usually within 2 months. The most common side effect is diarrhea, which is managed by altering the dose schedule. The risk of leukopenia requires periodic blood counts, especially after beginning therapy.

Plasma Exchange
Plasma exchange is used as a short-term intervention for patients with sudden worsening of myasthenic symptoms, to improve strength before surgery, concomitantly with starting high-dose corticosteroids, and as a chronic intermittent treatment for patients who are refractory to all other treatments. The clinical response determines the need for plasma exchange and its frequency of use.

Intravenous Immune Globulin
The indications for intravenous immune globulin (IVIG) are similar to those for plasma exchange. A transitory favorable response to 2 g/kg of IVIG infused over 2–5 days occurs in almost all patients. The common adverse effects of IVIG relate to the rate of infusion and include headaches, chills, and fever. Pretreatment with acetaminophen and diphenhydramine reduces adverse reactions.

Treatment Plan

Ocular Myasthenia
Start with ChE inhibitors. If the response is unsatisfactory, prednisone is justified if ptosis or diplopia impairs function.

Generalized Myasthenia, Onset before Age 60
Consider thymectomy and pretreat with high-dose daily prednisone, plasma exchange, or both preoperatively in patients with oropharyngeal or respiratory muscle weakness to minimize the risks of surgery. Prednisone is the treatment of choice.

Generalized Myasthenia, Onset after Age 60
ChE inhibitors are the initial treatment. Add azathioprine or prednisone if the response is unsatisfactory. For a more rapid response, high-dose daily prednisone is the first drug, with or without plasma exchange or IVIG.

Thymoma
Thymectomy is indicated in all patients with thymoma. Medical treatment is then the same as that for patients without thymoma.

Juvenile Myasthenia Gravis
Juvenile myasthenia is the onset of immune-mediated MG before age 20 years. Twenty percent of children with juvenile MG and almost 50% of those with onset before puberty are seronegative. ChE inhibitors are the primary treatment because the rate of spontaneous remission is high. Recommend thymectomy if drugs fail to prevent disability or progressive weakness.

Seronegative Myasthenia Gravis
The treatment of seronegative MG (SN-MG) is the same as that for seropositive patients. Genetic myasthenia is a consideration in all childhood-onset SN-MG cases.

Special Situations

Myasthenic or Cholinergic Crisis
Myasthenic crisis is respiratory failure from disease. Patients in myasthenic crisis who previously had well-compensated respiratory function usually have a definable precipitating event, such as infection, surgery, or rapid tapering of immunosuppression. Cholinergic crisis is respiratory failure from overdose of ChE inhibitors. Respiratory failure of any cause is a medical emergency and requires prompt intubation and ventilatory support.

Anesthetic Management
As a rule, local or spinal anesthesia is preferred over inhalation anesthesia. Use neuromuscular-blocking agents sparingly, if at all.

Transitory Neonatal Myasthenia

A transitory form of MG affects 10–20% of newborns whose mothers have immune-mediated MG. The severity of symptoms in the newborn does not correlate with the severity of symptoms in the mother. After the birth of one child with transitory neonatal MG (TNMG), subsequent pregnancies are likely to have the same result. Affected newborns are hypotonic and feed poorly during the first 3 days. Symptoms usually last less than 2 weeks but may continue for as long as 12 weeks. The mechanism of TNMG is uncertain. Affected and unaffected newborns have equally high antibody concentrations. Assess all children of myasthenic mothers for TNMG. Edrophonium or RNS establishes the diagnosis. Affected newborns require symptomatic treatment with ChE inhibitors if swallowing or breathing is impaired. Consider plasma exchange in newborns with respiratory weakness.

D-*Penicillamine–Induced Myasthenia Gravis*

D-Penicillamine is used to treat rheumatoid arthritis, Wilson's disease, and cystinuria. Patients treated with D-penicillamine for several months may develop a myasthenic syndrome that disappears after stopping the drug. D-Penicillamine–induced myasthenia is usually mild and often restricted to the ocular muscles. The response to ChE inhibitors, characteristic EMG abnormalities, and serum AChR antibodies establishes the diagnosis.

GENETIC MYASTHENIC SYNDROMES

Genetic forms of myasthenia are not immune mediated. They are a heterogeneous group of disorders caused by several abnormalities of neuromuscular transmission. Symptoms are typically present at birth or early childhood but may begin in young adult life. The response to edrophonium chloride and characteristic EMG findings confirm abnormal neuromuscular transmission. The onset of myasthenic symptoms at birth is always genetic, with the exception of the transitory neonatal form. The transmission of all genetic forms of myasthenia is by autosomal recessive inheritance, except *slow-channel syndrome*, transmitted as an autosomal dominant trait. Myasthenia that begins in infancy or childhood may be genetic or acquired.

Congenital Myasthenia

Congenital myasthenia is a clinical term that encompasses several genetic neuromuscular defects. Overall, a 2:1 male predominance exists.

Clinical Features

Children with congenital myasthenia develop ophthalmoparesis and ptosis during infancy. Mild facial paresis may be present as well. Ophthalmoplegia is often incomplete at onset but progresses to complete paralysis during infancy or childhood. Some children develop generalized fatigue and weakness, but limb weakness is usually mild compared to ophthalmoplegia. Respiratory distress is unusual.

Diagnosis

Suspect congenital myasthenia in any newborn or infant with ptosis or ophthalmoparesis. Subcutaneous injection of edrophonium usually produces a transitory improvement in ocular motility. A decremental response to RNS is found in some limb muscles, but proximal limb or facial muscles are tested if hand muscles show a normal response. SFEMG shows increased jitter.

Treatment

ChE inhibitors improve limb muscle weakness in many forms of congenital genetic myasthenia and may be effective even when edrophonium is not. Ocular muscle weakness is less responsive to ChE inhibitors. The weakness in some children responds to a combination of pyridostigmine and 3,4-diaminopyridine (DAP). DAP is available only as an investigational new drug in the United States.

Congenital Myasthenic Syndrome with Episodic Apnea (Familial Infantile Myasthenia)

Congenital myasthenic syndrome with episodic apnea (familial infantile myasthenia) has characteristic clinical and electrophysiological features that differ from other congenital myasthenic syndromes.

Clinical Features

Generalized hypotonia is present at birth. Repeated episodes of life-threatening apnea and feeding difficulty complicate the neonatal course. Assisted ventilation is often required. Arthrogryposis may be present. Ocular muscle function is usually normal. Within weeks after birth, the child becomes stronger and ultimately breathes unassisted. However, episodes of life-threatening apnea occur repeatedly throughout infancy and childhood, even into adult life. A history of sudden infant death syndrome in siblings is common. The correct diagnosis may be unsuspected until a second affected child is born.

Diagnosis

Edrophonium usually improves both weakness and respiratory distress. A decremental response to RNS is present in weak muscles and occurs in strong muscles after exhausting the muscle by several minutes of RNS. Abnormal resynthesis and repackaging of ACh in the motor nerve is demonstrable in some patients.

Treatment
ChE inhibitors improve strength in most affected children, but sudden episodes of respiratory distress occur with intercurrent illness. As the patients get older, strength improves, attacks of respiratory distress become less frequent, and the need for medication decreases. Symptomatic improvement occurs when DAP is given with pyridostigmine.

Slow-Channel Congenital Myasthenic Syndrome

The transmission of slow-channel congenital myasthenic syndrome is by autosomal dominant inheritance, and a family history of similar illness is common.

Clinical Features
Onset of symptoms always occurs after infancy and may present as late as the third decade. Slowly progressive weakness selectively involves the arm, leg, neck, and facial muscles. Unlike other myasthenic syndromes, atrophy of symptomatic muscles is expected.

Diagnosis
A decremental response is present. Repetitive discharges are seen after nerve stimulation, similar to those seen in ChE inhibitor toxicity or congenital deficiency of endplate acetylcholinesterase. The underlying defect is a prolonged open time of the ACh channel.

Treatment
ChE inhibitors, thymectomy, and immunosuppression are not effective treatments. Quinidine sulfate and fluoxetine may improve strength.

Lambert-Eaton Myasthenic Syndrome

LEMS is a presynaptic abnormality of ACh release. The probable mechanism in most, if not all, patients is an immune-mediated process directed against the voltage-gated calcium channels on nerve terminals.

Clinical Features

LEMS usually begins after age 40 years. Males and females are equally affected. Approximately one half of patients with LEMS have an underlying malignancy; 80% of these have small cell lung cancer. The main feature is weakness, and sometimes pain, of proximal muscles, especially in the legs. Oropharyngeal and ocular muscles may be mildly affected. Strength may improve initially after exercise and then decrease with sustained activity. Tendon reflexes, although diminished or absent, are often enhanced by repeated muscle contraction or repeated tapping of the tendon.

Diagnosis

Edrophonium chloride does not improve strength to the degree seen in MG. EMG confirms the diagnosis of LEMS. The characteristic findings are a reduced compound motor action potential (CMAP) size that is further reduced in response to RNS at frequencies between 1 and 5 Hz. CMAP size doubles in response to repetitive stimulation at 20–50 Hz and shows a transitory increase in size after brief maximum voluntary contraction. Virtually all patients with LEMS have a decrementing response to 3-Hz stimulation in a hand or foot muscle, and almost all have low CMAP size in some muscles.

Treatment

Initial treatment is directed at the underlying malignancy, and weakness may improve after effective cancer therapy. Some patients require no further treatment for the neuromuscular defect. The following treatment plan is a general guide that should be modified to suit specific situations. Pyridostigmine, 30–60 mg every 6 hours, should be tried for several days. Oral 3,4-DAP, 5–25 mg three to four times a day, improves strength and autonomic symptoms in most patients with LEMS. The response to DAP is enhanced by the concomitant use of pyridostigmine, 30–60 mg three or four times a day. In patients with severe weakness, plasma exchange or IVIG may be used first and prednisone and azathioprine added after improvement begins. Repeated courses of treatment may be needed to maintain improvement.

The long-term prognosis in LEMS is determined by the response to cancer therapy. In patients without cancer, immunosuppression produces improvement in many patients, but most require substantial and continuing doses of immunosuppressive medications.

DRUGS THAT ADVERSELY AFFECT MYASTHENIA GRAVIS AND LAMBERT-EATON MYASTHENIC SYNDROME

Drugs that compromise neuromuscular transmission make patients with MG or LEMS weaker. Avoiding such drugs is

Table 53.3: Drug alert for patients with myasthenia gravis or Lambert-Eaton myasthenic syndrome

1. Interferon-α, botulinum toxin, and D-penicillamine should never be used in myasthenic patients.
2. The following drugs produce worsening of myasthenic weakness in most patients who receive them. Use with caution and monitor patient for exacerbation of myasthenic symptoms.
   Succinylcholine, D-tubocurarine, or other neuromuscular-blocking agents
   Quinine, quinidine, and procainamide
   Aminoglycoside antibiotics, particularly gentamicin, kanamycin, neomycin, and streptomycin
   Beta blockers (systemic and ocular preparations): propranolol, timolol maleate eyedrops
   Calcium-channel blockers
   Magnesium salts (including laxatives and antacids with high Mg^{2+} concentrations)
   Iodinated contrast agents
3. Many other drugs are reported to exacerbate the weakness in some patients with myasthenia gravis. All patients with myasthenia gravis should be observed for increased weakness whenever a new medication is started. An up-to-date reference document for such adverse interactions is maintained on the Web site of the Myasthenia Gravis Foundation of America (www.myasthenia.org/drugs/reference.htm).

not always possible. Table 53.3 lists potentially hazardous drugs.

BOTULISM

A toxin produced by the anaerobic bacterium *Clostridium botulinum* causes botulism by blocking the release of ACh from the motor nerve terminal (see Chapter 28).

OTHER CAUSES OF ABNORMAL NEUROMUSCULAR TRANSMISSION

The NMJ is uniquely sensitive to the effects of neurotoxins. These are discussed in Chapter 33.

For a more detailed discussion, see Chapter 84 in Neurology in Clinical Practice, 4th edition.

Disorders of Skeletal Muscle | *54*

Striated muscle is the tissue that converts chemical energy into mechanical energy. The component processes include: (1) excitation and contraction occurring in the muscle membranes, (2) the contractile mechanism, (3) structural supporting elements that allow muscle to withstand mechanical stress, and (4) the energy system that supports the activity and integrity of the other three systems. Chapter 39 discusses abnormalities in the membrane ion channels involved in muscle excitation (channelopathies).

MUSCULAR DYSTROPHIES

The muscular dystrophies are a group of hereditary muscle disorders that occur at all ages and with all degrees of severity. For the most part, the underlying molecular abnormalities in the dystrophies involve structural proteins (Table 54.1). The structural proteins include dystrophin, the sarcoglycans, and laminin. These constitute a vital structural mechanism linking the contractile proteins with the extracellular supporting structures.

Dystrophin Deficiency (Duchenne's Muscular Dystrophy, Becker's Muscular Dystrophy, and Atypical Forms)

Progressive destruction of muscle results from an absence or deficiency of dystrophin. The responsible gene is located on the short arm of the X chromosome at locus Xp21. Approximately two thirds of cases are associated with a detectable deletion or duplication of segments within the gene. The others are presumably caused by point mutations too small to be detected

Table 54.1: Molecular defects of muscular dystrophies

Disease	Chromosome	Protein
DMD/BMD	Xp21	Dystrophin
EDMD	Xq28	Emerin
Myotonic dystrophy	19q13.2	Myotonin protein kinase
Myotonic dystrophy type 2/PROMM	3q	ZNF9
FSHD	4q35	?
Oculopharyngeal dystrophy	14q	Polyalanine binding protein 2 (PABP2)
Bethlem myopathy 1	21q22.3	Collagen type VI (α-1 or α-2 subunits)
Bethlem myopathy 2	2q37	Collagen type VI (α-6 subunit)
LGMD 1A	5q22-31	Myotilin
LGMD 1B with cardiopathy/autosomal dominant EDMD	1q11-12	Nuclear lamin A/C
LGMD 1C	3p25	Caveolin-3
LGMD 2A	15q15	Calpain-3
LGMD 2B/Miyoshi's myopathy	2p13	Dysferlin
LGMD 2C	13q13	γ-Sarcoglycan
LGMD 2D	17q21	α-Sarcoglycan

LGMD 2E	4q12	β-Sarcoglycan
LGMD 2F	5q33	δ-Sarcoglycan
LGMD 2G	17q11-12	Telethonin
LGMD 2H	9q31-q33	TRIM32
LGMD 2I	19q13.3	Fukutin-related protein, *FKRP1*
Congenital muscular dystrophy (CMD)		
Merosin-negative classic type	6q21-22	Merosin (α-2 subunit)
Merosin-positive integrin deficiency	12q13	α-7 Integrin
Merosin-positive FRRP deficiency	19q13.3	Fukutin-related protein, *FKRP1*
Fukuyama type	9q31-33	Fukutin
Walker-Warburg syndrome	9q31-33	?
Muscle-eye-brain disease	1p32-p34	POMGnT1
CMD with rigid spine syndrome	1p35-36	Selenoprotein 1

DMD = Duchenne's muscular dystrophy; BMD = Becker's muscular dystrophy; EDMD = Emery-Dreifuss muscular dystrophy; PROMM = proximal myotonic myopathy; FSHD = facioscapulohumeral muscular dystrophy; LGMD = limb-girdle muscular dystrophy; POMGnT1 = *O*-mannose-β-1,2-*N*-acetylglucosaminyl transferase; ZNF9 = zinc finger 9.

using standard techniques. In-frame deletions are usually associated with the severe Duchenne variety of the disease (Duchenne's muscular dystrophy [DMD]), whereas the latter may cause the milder Becker's variant (Becker's muscular dystrophy [BMD]).

Duchenne's Muscular Dystrophy

In DMD, affected males are normal at birth. During the second year, the clumsiness of toddlers persists, the hands are used to help push off from the floor (Gowers' sign), and the calf muscles become firm and rubbery. During the next 2–3 years, affected children do not run or jump properly. The iliotibial bands and the heel cords become tight, and the child walks on his toes. Labored stair climbing and sudden falls occur by age 6 years. At 8–10 years of age, stair climbing and standing from the floor cease, and distance movement requires a wheelchair. Contractures of the hips, knees, and ankles become severe when the relatively untreated child spends much of the day in the wheelchair. The progression of disability depends largely on the parental and medical care provided. With prednisone therapy, bracing, reconstructive surgery, and physiotherapy, the average age at wheelchair confinement is 12.2 years. Degeneration and fibrosis of the posterolateral wall of the left ventricle characterizes the cardiac involvement. Death is secondary to either respiratory failure or the cardiomyopathy that is relatively resistant to treatment.

Demonstrating a deletion in the dystrophin gene is the simplest test to confirm the diagnosis. Muscle biopsy establishes the absence of dystrophin in the 30% of children who fail to show a deletion. The primary aim of physical therapy is to keep the joints as loose as possible. The appropriate use of bracing combined with surgery can delay progression to wheelchair bound by 2 years. Spinal stabilization prevents progressive scoliosis. Prednisone is the only drug that improves muscle strength and function.

Becker's Muscular Dystrophy

BMD shares all the characteristics of the severe form but has a milder course. The first signs of weakness usually appear in the first decade, although the onset of symptoms is sometimes delayed until the fourth decade or later. The muscular hypertrophy, contractures, and pattern of weakness are similar to that seen in DMD. However, these boys continue to walk independently past the age of 15 years and may not have to use a wheelchair until the third decade.

Autosomal Dominant Limb-Girdle Muscular Dystrophies (LGMD-1)

LGMD-1A (Myotilin Deficiency)

The onset of LGMD-1A is during the second and third decades. Proximal arm weakness is greater than leg weakness. Some patients have distal arm and leg weakness as well as facial and pharyngeal weakness. Serum creatine kinase (CK) concentrations can be normal or moderately elevated. Rimmed vacuoles within muscle fibers are seen in histological preparations.

LGMD-1B (Lamin A/C Deficiency)

LGMD-1B is allelic, with the disorder previous reported as autosomal dominant Emery-Dreifuss muscular dystrophy (EDMD). Limb-girdle weakness is the presenting feature in some patients, and humeral-peroneal weakness and early contractions are the initial features in others. Cardiomyopathy and severe conduction defects and arrhythmias may occur. Fatal arrhythmias are common and pacemakers are often needed. Serum CK concentrations may be normal or elevated 25-fold. Muscle histology shows dystrophic features and rare rimmed vacuoles.

LGMD-1C (Caveolin-3 Deficiency)

LGMD-1C is a rare myopathy characterized by childhood-onset proximal weakness greater in the legs than the arms and exertional myalgia. The clinical phenotype is heterogeneous. Some families have distal weakness and others have the syndrome of autosomal dominant rippling muscle disease. Serum CK concentrations are increased 3–25 times normal. Some patients have increased serum CK concentrations and no weakness.

LGMD-2A (Calpain-3 Deficiency)

LGMD-2A, an autosomal recessive LGMD that was first described in an inbred population on Reunion Island in the Indian Ocean, is worldwide in distribution and accounts for 25% of dystrophies with normal dystrophin and sarcoglycan. The onset is in childhood or early adult life. Most cases have a slowly progressive course with loss of ambulation in adult life. In more severe forms, weakness first occurs in the hips and then the shoulders. The facial muscles and the neck flexors and extensors are strong. Scapular winging is characterized by a jutting backward of the entire medial scapular border. The posterior thigh muscles are weaker than the knee extensors, and the rectus abdominis muscles are weak early in the course. The serum CK concentration is markedly elevated early but then decreases and may normalize.

LGMD-2B (Dysferlin Deficiency)

Mutations in the gene encoding for dysferlin lead to at least two phenotypes. One is a limb-girdle pattern of weakness (LGMD-2B), and the other is weakness and atrophy of the calf muscles (Miyoshi myopathy). Some patients have earlier involvement of the anterior tibial muscles. Among patients with dysferlinopathy, 8% have a distal myopathy, 8% have LGMD, and 6% have asymptomatic elevations of serum CK. Onset is in adolescence or early adult life. Progression is usually slow but variable. Some lose the ability to walk in the second decade, although others walk until late in life. Clinical variability in the pattern of weakness and disease progression may exist within the same family. Serum CK concentrations are elevated 35–200 times normal. Immunostaining and immunoblot confirm the diagnosis.

LGMD Types 2C, 2D, 2E, and 2F (Sarcoglycan Deficiencies)

Four sarcoglycans expressed in muscle are associated with different forms of autosomal recessive LGMD-2. The cause is mutations in the genes for γ-sarcoglycan, α-sarcoglycan, β-sarcoglycan, and δ-sarcoglycan, respectively. The sarcoglycans are tightly knit; absence of one often causes absence of others. This is particularly true of α-sarcoglycan, making it both useful and misleading as a screening tool. The sarcoglycanopathies account for more than 10% of patients with an LGMD syndrome and positive dystrophin. All sarcoglycanopathies have the same features at onset: trunk and limb weakness, a serum CK concentration of 1000 IU/L and higher, and calf hypertrophy. Facial strength is good and cardiac findings are not prominent.

LGMD-2G (Telethonin Deficiency)

LGMD-2G is a rare form of muscular dystrophy that may be associated with either proximal or distal weakness. Mean age at onset is 12.5 years. Legs are weaker than arms and the quadriceps and anterior tibial muscles are significantly weak. Serum CK concentrations are elevated 3–17 times normal.

LGMD-2H

The age at onset of LGMD-2H is 8–27 years and ambulation is not lost until the fourth decade. Serum CK concentrations range from 250 to more than 3000 IU/L.

LGMD-2I

Despite only 17 known affected kinships, phenotypic variation is considerable. The age at symptom onset of LGMD-2I ranges from birth to the fourth decade. The clinical course can be similar to a congenital muscular dystrophy (CMD) or a mild BMD. Severe cardiomyopathy may develop. Serum CK concentrations are elevated 10–30 times normal in children but may be normal in adults.

Congenital Muscular Dystrophies

The CMDs are a group of disorders that usually present at birth as severe hypotonia and weakness of the trunk and limbs. All are autosomal recessive traits and some cause central nervous system dysfunction. Joint contractures are prominent, particularly in the legs. Mental retardation may be present. In many infants, magnetic resonance imaging (MRI) shows a striking increase in T2-weighted signal in the cerebral white matter. Among the several CMD forms, the ones best characterized are classic or occidental CMD, Fukuyama-type muscular dystrophy, Walker-Warburg disease, and muscle-eye-brain disease of Santavuori.

Laminin-α₂ (Merosin) Deficiency
The essential features of merosinopathy are severe weakness of the trunk and limbs and hypotonia at birth. The extraocular and facial muscles are usually spared. Contractures of the feet and hips are prominent. Intelligence is often normal. The incidence of epilepsy is 12–20%. MRI of the brain often reveals increased signal in the white matter on T2-weighted images. For the most part, affected children are severely disabled and many are dependent lifelong.

Other Forms of Classic CMD Type 1
Some children with phenotypes identical to CMD type 1 have no abnormality in the laminin-α₂ gene. Muscle symptoms are milder, and with time sufficient function is regained to support independent walking. These myopathies progress more slowly than merosin-negative CMD, and many of the patients survive to adult life.

Fukuyama-type Muscular Dystrophy
Affected newborns usually have normal strength. Some are floppy. Joint contractures of the hip, knee, and ankles are present in 70% by age 3 months. Mental retardation is often so severe that speech never develops. Convulsions, either major motor seizures or staring spells, are common. The skull is asymmetrical and weakness is diffuse, sometimes involving the face and neck. Affected children are completely dependent and never attain any degree of unsupervised activity. The muscle disease is moderately or slowly progressive, and survival into early adult life is common. Brain MRI shows white matter abnormalities, which disappear with time. Malformations of gyral formation include agyria, pachygyria, and microgyria.

Walker-Warburg Syndrome and Muscle-Eye-Brain Disease
The combination of muscular dystrophy, lissencephaly, cerebellar malformations, and severe retinal and eye malformations characterizes the Walker-Warburg syndrome and muscle-eye-brain disease. Both disorders are more severe than Fukayama congenital muscular disorder (FCMD). Walker-Warburg is a catastrophic disease, causing death within the first 2 years of life. The eye changes are more severe in Walker-Warburg disease than in muscle-eye-brain disease. Characteristic findings are microphthalmia, colobomas, congenital cataracts and glaucoma, corneal opacities, retinal dysplasia and nonattachment, hypoplastic vitreus, and optic atrophy. In muscle-eye-brain disease, high myopia and possibly a preretinal membrane or gliosis occur, but not severe structural eye abnormalities. MRI in Walker-Warburg syndrome shows hydrocephalus, aqueductal stenosis, cerebellar and pontine hypoplasia, Dandy-Walker malformations, and an agyric or pachygyric cobblestone cortex. T1-weighted images show diffuse decreased white matter signal; T2-weighted images show myelination defects. In muscle-eye-brain disease, the cortical changes are milder and the white matter changes less diffuse. Whether Walker-Warburg disease and FCMD are genetically distinct is uncertain.

Other Regional Forms of Muscular Dystrophies

X-Linked Emery-Dreifuss Dystrophy (Emerin Deficiency)
The inheritance of the most common form of EDMD is by X-linked recessive disease. The main features are wasting and weakness of the upper arms, shoulders, and anterior compartment muscles of the legs. Contractures of the elbows, the posterior neck, the paraspinal muscles, and the Achilles' tendon occur early in the course. Severe elbow contractures occur during childhood. EDMD is slowly progressive. Cardiac complications are common. Atrial paralysis causes a conduction block that results in sudden death. The atria become electrically inexcitable and the heart responds only to ventricular pacing. Ventricular myocardial disease with ventricular failure also occurs. DNA studies confirm the diagnosis.

Facioscapulohumeral Dystrophy
The inheritance of facioscapulohumeral dystrophy (FSHD) is as an autosomal dominant trait. Anticipation occurs, age at onset is younger, and severity of illness is greater with successive generations. Some patients may have only mild facial weakness, whereas others have total paralysis of the face and severe weakness of other muscles, causing wheelchair confinement

during childhood. The most common age at presentation is adolescence. Weakness of the shoulder muscles affects scapular fixation. The deltoid muscle remains strong even late in the course. The biceps and triceps muscles are weak, but the forearm muscles are less involved. Weakness of the hip flexors and the quadriceps is common. The ankle dorsiflexors are often weak, although plantar-flexor strength is preserved.

DNA studies reliably establish the diagnosis. The treatment of FSHD is supportive.

Scapuloperoneal Syndromes

Weakness of the muscles of the shoulder and the anterior compartment of the lower leg are early symptoms of several diseases. Some forms of scapuloperoneal dystrophy relate to the FSHD genetic site, but others do not. The inheritance of scapuloperoneal muscular dystrophy may be as an autosomal dominant trait or as an X-linked recessive trait.

Oculopharyngeal Muscular Dystrophy

Oculopharyngeal muscular dystrophy (OPMD) usually begins in the fifth or sixth decade of life. Eye muscle weakness and ptosis are the initial features. The severity of extraocular palsies is variable, but ptosis is a constant feature. Difficulty swallowing occurs concomitant with or shortly after the development of ocular symptoms. Facial and proximal limb weakness is common in the late stages. The definitive diagnosis relies on DNA testing of the genetic abnormality. Treatment is supportive.

Distal Muscular Dystrophies/Distal Myopathies

Miyoshi Myopathy

Miyoshi myopathy is linked to mutations in the gene encoding the sarcolemmal protein, dysferlin, and was discussed with the limb-girdle dystrophies (LGMD-2B).

Welander's Myopathy

Inheritance of Welander's myopathy is as an autosomal dominant trait. The initial symptoms begin between 40 and 60 years of age. Weakness begins in the hands and later causes footdrop. Careful evaluation may show mild distal hypesthesia and temperature sensation loss associated with some loss of small myelinated fibers. Muscle histology shows myopathic features and the rimmed vacuoles that are characteristic of other distal myopathies. The serum CK concentration is normal or slightly elevated.

Markesbery-Griggs-Udd Myopathy
Transmission is as an autosomal dominant trait. Footdrop secondary to weakness in the anterior tibial muscles characterizes the myopathy. Onset is typically after age 35 years. Eventually, wristdrop and fingerdrop develop because of extensor compartment weakness of the forearms. Proximal limb muscles are rarely involved. The serum CK concentration is normal or slightly elevated. Muscle histology demonstrates myopathic features and rimmed vacuoles.

Nonaka Myopathy, Autosomal Recessive Hereditary Inclusion Body Myopathy
The phenotype is similar to Markesbery-Griggs-Udd myopathy. Weakness initially involves the anterior tibial muscles in the legs and extensor muscles of the forearm. Inheritance is as an autosomal recessive trait with onset before age 30 years. Kinships with Nonaka myopathy and those with autosomal recessive inclusion body myopathy are allelic.

Laing Distal Myopathy
Laing distal myopathy is a distinct autosomal dominant distal myopathy that has weakness of the anterior tibial muscle groups and the neck flexors. Onset is in childhood or early adult life. Serum CK concentrations are normal or slightly elevated and the electromyogram (EMG) has a myopathic pattern.

Myotonic Dystrophies

Myotonic Dystrophy Type 1
Muscle wasting and weakness, myotonia, and multisystem abnormalities characterize myotonic dystrophy type 1 (DM-1). Inheritance is as an autosomal dominant trait. The incidence is 1 per 8000 live births. A mutation causes CTG trinucleotide repeats. The size of the expansion correlates with severity of disease. Newborns with severe congenital DM have very large expansions (>750 repeats). Mothers with more than 100 repeats are at greater risk of having a child with the severe infantile form than mothers with a smaller expansion. The severity of DM-1 ranges from no symptoms, early cataracts, or mild weakness in some adults to profound mental retardation and severe weakness in children. The more typical picture is hand weakness and often footdrop beginning in early adolescence. Accentuating a rather long face with a mournful expression is hollowing of the temples secondary to masseter and temporalis atrophy. In the fully developed disease, ptosis is present and the mouth is slack and tented. Weakness is not limited to distal muscles; shoulder, hip,

and leg weakness may be prominent. Percussion and grip myotonia are present.

Cardiac disease complicates DM-1. Ventricular arrhythmia or complete heart block occurs early and can cause sudden death. Excessive daytime somnolence is common. Several other organs are commonly involved. Cataracts are almost universal by slit-lamp examination. Disturbances of endocrine function involve the thyroid, pancreas, hypothalamus, and gonads. Testicular atrophy, with disappearance of the seminiferous tubules, leads to progressive infertility in males. Females may develop habitual abortion and menstrual irregularities. DNA analysis is the definitive test for myotonic dystrophy. Supportive treatment includes the use of ankle-foot orthoses to treat footdrop and medications to ease myotonia.

Congenital Myotonic Dystrophy
Congenital myotonic dystrophy expresses itself in newborns of myotonic mothers. Extreme hypotonia, respiratory insufficiency, facial paralysis, failure to thrive, and feeding difficulty are the main features. Frequent respiratory tract infections that develop into pneumonia are common. Affected newborns have a large increase in the trinucleotide repeat region. This occurs with maternal transmission, particularly if the mother has a sizable expansion.

Myotonic Dystrophy Type 2 or Proximal Myotonic Myopathy
Whereas DM-1 has a predilection for the distal muscles, patients with proximal myotonic myopathy (PROMM) have greater stiffness, pain, and weakness in proximal than distal muscles. Transmission is also by autosomal dominant inheritance. Cataracts are part of the phenotype, but gonadal atrophy and cardiac conduction defects are much less common than in DM-1. Hyperintense areas on T2-weighted MRI images in the cerebral white matter and progressive deafness occur. The prognosis is relatively good. The mutations are expanded CCTG repeats.

METABOLIC MYOPATHIES

Any disturbance in the biochemical pathways that supports adenosine triphosphate (ATP) levels in muscle inevitably results in exercise intolerance. One common symptom is muscle fatigue, but other symptoms include muscle pain and sometimes muscle cramps. Normally functioning muscle has safety mechanisms that prevent exercise to the point of muscle destruction. When a patient with a metabolic myopathy exercises, muscle pain develops, followed by a muscle contracture in which the muscle is hard, swollen, and tender. This may be associated with the release of myoglobin into the blood and urine.

Disorders of Carbohydrate Metabolism

Myophosphorylase Deficiency

The defect is an absence of myophosphorylase activity. Phosphorylase exists in two forms: phosphorylase-a, the active tetramer, and phosphorylase-b, an inactive dimer. Conversion of the inactive form to the active form is catalyzed by phosphorylase-b kinase, which itself is activated by a protein kinase under the control of cyclic adenosine monophosphate (cAMP). Both phosphorylase deficiencies cause exercise intolerance and are inherited as autosomal recessive traits.

Children with the disorder are unable to keep up with peers. During adolescence, fatigue and pain begin within the first few minutes of strenuous exercise. Continued exercise causes painful muscle contractions and myoglobinuria. If exercise is continued, pain develops within the muscle, which at first is deep and aching but gives way to the rapid development of a painful contracture. The muscle contracture may last for several hours. It is different from a muscle cramp on two counts: The EMG is electrically silent, and the duration of the contracture is far longer than that of a physiological cramp, which disappears after a few minutes at most. Another aspect of McArdle disease is the development of the second-wind phenomenon. If, with the onset of fatigue, the patient slows down but does not stop, the abnormal sensation may disappear, and thereafter the muscle may function more normally. A simple diagnostic clinical test is the exercise forearm test (previously ischemic exercise test). During exercise, the normal response is a threefold to fourfold increase in lactic acid and ammonia. In phosphorylase deficiency, ammonia concentrations rise but not lactic acid concentrations. Definitive diagnosis requires showing the enzyme deficiency in muscle.

Phosphofructokinase Deficiency

Phosphofructokinase (PFK) is the enzyme that converts fructose-6-phosphate to fructose-1,6-diphosphate and is a step in the glycolytic chain downstream from that activated by phosphorylase. Inheritance of PFK deficiency is as an autosomal recessive trait. Heterozygotes have decreased but not absent levels of enzyme activity. PFK deficiency is almost identical clinically to phosphorylase deficiency, although the second-wind phenomenon is uncommon. Most attacks are associated with nausea, vomiting, and muscle pain. A mild hemolytic anemia and gall bladder pigment stones may be associated.

Phosphoglycerate Kinase Deficiency

Phosphoglycerate kinase is involved in another step in the glycolytic pathway. Muscle deficiency produces a predictable picture very similar to that of phosphorylase deficiency. Venous lactate concentrations do not rise after exercise, as expected.

Phosphoglycerate Mutase Deficiency

Patients with an absence of phosphoglycerate mutase have attacks of muscle pain and myoglobinuria and, in one case, typical attacks of gouty arthritis. Exercise testing shows some elevation of lactate, but not to the concentrations usually seen in the other disorders of glycogen metabolism.

Treatment of the Glycolytic Disorders

No effective treatment for glycolytic disorders is available. Counsel the patient to avoid situations that might precipitate myoglobinuria. Graded exercise on a treadmill can train the patient to recognize how to slow down with the first onset of symptoms and then resume exercise in small increments.

Disorders of Lipid Metabolism

Carnitine Palmitoyltransferase Deficiency

Although exercise does not require fatty acids at the beginning, they become increasingly important after 20–30 minutes of endurance exercise, and after an hour they are the major energy supplier. Therefore defects in lipid metabolism cause symptoms after sustained activity. Carnitine palmitoyltransferase (CPT) is the enzyme that links carnitine to long-chain fatty acids for transport across the mitochondrial membrane (CPT-I). It is also responsible for unhooking carnitine when the complex reaches the other side of the membrane (CPT-II). CPT-II deficiency is one of the more common biochemical abnormalities in muscle. Inheritance is as an autosomal recessive trait.

The typical patient is a young adult male who experiences a first bout of weakness and myoglobinuria after strenuous exercise. Many have experienced brief episodes of myalgia as children. Attacks of myoglobinuria in CPT deficiency are more severe than those occurring in disorders of glycolysis, with a greater tendency to cause renal damage. Cold exposure and the fasting state predispose to attacks. The serum CK concentration and muscle biopsy results are normal unless the patient has had a recent attack. Biochemical analysis of muscle reveals the CPT deficiency.

Carnitine Deficiency Myopathy

Carnitine deficiency causes a failure in the production of energy for metabolism and the storage of triglycerides. The primary genetic defect is transmitted by autosomal recessive inheritance. The clinical features may be restricted to skeletal muscle or may include systemic symptoms that resemble Reye's syndrome. The most common clinical picture in muscle carnitine deficiency is a slowly progressive weakness on which sudden exacerbations or a fluctuating course is superimposed. Fatigue and exercise-related pains occur but do not constitute major complaints; myoglobinuria is almost never a problem. The weakness is usually proximal, and the symptoms begin during childhood or early teenage life. Facial and bulbar weakness occurs.

The treatment of carnitine deficiency by replacing L-carnitine is not uniformly successful. Approximately 2–4 g per day has been given to adults in divided doses, with the equivalent of 100 mg/kg in infants and children. No serious adverse effects are seen, although patients find L-carnitine unpleasant to take because of accompanying nausea and a fishy odor of the sweat.

Disorder of Abnormal Nucleotide Metabolism

Myoadenylate Deaminase Deficiency

Approximately 1–2% of the population has a deficiency of the enzyme myoadenylate deaminase (AMP deaminase [AMPDA]). The disorder is inherited as an autosomal recessive trait. The enzyme plays a role in supporting ATP levels by acting in conjunction with adenylate kinase. Early studies suggested that AMPDA deficiency caused myalgia. However, most people with AMPDA deficiency are asymptomatic and have no symptoms of exercise intolerance.

Mitochondrial Myopathies

Several defects in respiratory chain function cause mitochondrial myopathies. They are generally part of multiple organ dysfunction syndromes. Most present with central nervous system dysfunction and are discussed in Chapter 38. Histochemistry of affected muscle usually shows ragged-red fibers, whereas unaffected muscle in the same patient may be normal. Assay of mitochondrial enzyme activity and mutational analysis of the mitochondrial DNA can be performed to confirm the diagnosis.

Congenital Myopathies

The congenital myopathies comprise a group of developmental neuromuscular disorders. Their clinical features are present at birth. Diagnosis relies solely on the characteristic muscle histological findings. Several of these disorders are nonprogressive or only slowly progressive and therefore are not classified as dystrophies.

Central Core Disease

Central core disease is inherited as an autosomal dominant trait. Sporadic cases occur. The responsible gene is on chromosome 19q13.1. The mutation causes a disturbance in the ryanodine receptor and is allelic to the mutation in malignant hyperthermia. Malignant hyperthermia and central core disease coexist in some families. The newborn is floppy, and congenital hip dislocation is common. Motor milestones are delayed in infancy, and children are clumsy later. Strength is decreased, but disability is unusual. Tendon reflexes are diminished in many children and normal in others. Skeletal deformities are unusual. A rare, severe form of central core disease results in wheelchair confinement and profound kyphoscoliosis that requires surgical stabilization.

The EMG shows nonspecific myopathic changes, and the serum concentration of CK is usually normal. Muscle biopsy discloses type 1 fiber predominance and central cores in almost every fiber. The central cores are tightly packed and poorly organized myofibrils that react intensely to adenosine triphosphatase (ATPase) but not to many of the oxidative histochemical reactions. Specific treatment is not available, although bracing may correct a footdrop deformity. Any family in whom central core disease has been found should be advised about the possibility of malignant hyperthermia because this is a potentially fatal complication.

Nemaline Myopathy

The diagnosis of nemaline myopathy is based on the presence of small, rodlike particles in the muscle fibers. The disorder is genetically heterogeneic. The gene for the autosomal dominant form is on chromosome 1q21-q23 and the autosomal recessive is associated with mutations in the genes on chromosome 19q13. Both autosomal dominant and recessive cases are associated with mutations on chromosome 1q42.1.

The clinical picture of nemaline myopathy is heterogeneous. The most common syndrome includes infantile hypotonia, followed by diffuse limb weakness in childhood. Mild weakness occurs in the face and bulbar muscles. The face is long and narrow with a jaw that is prognathous or short. The feet are often high arched and kyphoscoliosis is common. The weakness is usually non-progressive. Other syndromes of nemaline myopathy are late-onset proximal weakness and fatal respiratory failure in the newborn.

EMG shows nonspecific myopathic changes and the serum CK concentration is normal or mildly elevated. Muscle histology shows nemaline rods, type 1 fiber predominance and selective atrophy, and type 2B fiber deficiency. The rods appear as small rodlike particles in muscle fibers when the fibers are stained with modified trichrome. Electron microscopy shows that the rods originate in the Z disc and exhibit structural continuity with the thin filament.

Centronuclear or Myotubular Myopathy

Myotubular myopathy can be inherited as an autosomal recessive or as an X-linked recessive (Xq28) trait. The autosomal recessive form causes delayed motor milestones and weakness in childhood, including ptosis, extraocular weakness, and facial weakness. Electrical or clinical seizures are often associated. The X-linked form is uniformly fatal in the newborn because of respiratory failure. Weakness is diffuse and severe and affects the face, neck, and extraocular muscles. The EMG shows myopathic units, and the serum CK concentration is normal or mildly elevated. Muscle histology shows variability in fiber size, most of which are small. In the center of many fibers is a large, plump nucleus, resembling the myotube stage of muscle development. With the oxidative enzyme reaction, many of the fibers have a darkly staining central spot; with the ATPase reaction, almost all the fibers have a pale-staining area that runs through the middle of the fiber. Treatment of the milder illness is supportive and includes anticonvulsant therapy. Treatment is not available for the X-linked form.

Congenital Fiber-type Disproportion

Congenital fiber-type disproportion is inherited as an autosomal dominant trait in approximately 40% of cases. This disorder may represent nemaline myopathy without rods. Affected infants are hypotonic at birth and have diffuse, mild weakness in child-hood. The face and neck muscles may be involved. Contractures of the ankle tendon are common, as are respiratory disturbances during the first 2 years. EMG shows myopathic potentials but no evidence of muscle membrane instability. The serum CK concentration may be normal to slightly elevated. The muscle biopsy is diagnostic. A marked size disproportion exists between the type 2 and type 1 fibers. Type 1 fibers are small, but there are many of them.

Myofibrillar Myopathy

Myofibrillar myopathy (MFM) is characterized by the pathological finding of myofibrillar disruption on electron microscopy and excessive desmin accumulation in muscle fibers on immunostain. A spectrum of clinical phenotypes exists. Most develop weakness between 25 and 45 years of age, but onset can begin in infancy or late adulthood. Either cardiac or skeletal muscle involvement dominates the clinical picture. Distal limb weakness affects the arms or the legs. The cardiomyopathy may manifest as arrhythmias or conduction defects, as well as congestive heart failure. Serum CK concentration is normal or only slightly increased. Muscle histology demonstrates variability in fiber size, increased central nuclei, and occasionally type 1 fiber predominance. The two main types of lesions are hyaline structures and nonhyaline lesions. Both contain desmin and numerous other proteins.

INFLAMMATORY MYOPATHIES

Polymyositis, dermatomyositis, and inclusion body myositis are the three most common inflammatory diseases seen by clinicians.

Dermatomyositis

Dermatomyositis is an illness in which weakness is associated with a characteristic skin rash. It is the common form of myositis occurring in childhood through middle adult life. Adult cases are often associated with an underlying malignancy. The rash usually occurs with onset of muscle weakness, although it may develop during the course of the disease. It is characteristically a purplish discoloration of the skin over the cheeks and eyelids—often in a butterfly distribution—that blanches with applied pressure. Another area that may be affected is a V-shaped distribution on the chest below the neck. The rash may spread widely over the body. The skin over the elbows, knees, and knuckles is particularly prone to develop a reddened, indurated appearance.

The weakness is proximal and symmetrical. One third of patients have pain. The illness often follows a relapsing and remitting course, but occasionally is monophasic even to the point of recovering spontaneously without treatment. The serum CK concentrations are usually elevated in dermatomyositis but can be normal early or in patients with a very indolent course. Serum CK levels do not necessarily reflect activity of the disease. EMG demonstrates a combination of myopathic features and indications of muscle hyperirritability. Perifascicular atrophy is the characteristic histological feature on muscle biopsy. This feature is seen in dermatomyositis but not in polymyositis.

The principles of treatment in dermatomyositis are the same as those for polymyositis.

Polymyositis

Polymyositis is an acute or subacute illness that typically occurs in adults. Cases of polymyositis occurring in infants and children are most likely to represent muscular dystrophies with inflammation. Polymyositis is an acute or subacute illness that occurs at all ages and causes widespread weakness that is more proximal than distal. The incidence peaks from age 40 to 60 years. It is slightly more common in women than in men, as are other autoimmune diseases. The weakness is not characteristic and may be confused with some limb-girdle muscular dystrophies. Severe muscle pain is not associated. Tendon reflexes are decreased or absent. Other organ involvement is characterized by Raynaud's phenomenon, cardiac conduction defects, cardiomyopathy, interstitial pneumonitis, and delayed gastric and esophageal emptying.

The diagnostic studies in polymyositis are similar to those in dermatomyositis, with serum CK concentrations, serum antibodies, EMG, and muscle biopsy as the mainstay. Serum CK concentrations may be quite markedly elevated during the course of the illness. Polymyositis is a cell-mediated disorder, the immune attack being directed against some unknown antigen(s) on the muscle fibers. The inflammatory cells are composed of predominantly T lymphocytes (CD8 > CD4) and macrophages. The cytotoxic T cells are seen to surround and invade nonnecrotic muscle fibers.

General agreement exists that polymyositis and dermatomyositis should be treated with corticosteroids, other immunosuppression, or a combination of both. Daily prednisone is used in the early stages in doses of up to 1.5 mg/kg or with a maximum of 100 mg. After 2–4 weeks, prednisone is switched to alternate-day therapy. In extremely weak patients or those with systemic involvement, a slower taper by 10 mg per week to an alternate-day regimen is recommended. When significant improvement has occurred, the prednisone dose is decreased by 5 mg every 2–3 weeks. Once the patient is down to 20 mg every other day, further reduction continues in steps of 2.5 mg.

Patients who do not respond are treated with other immunosuppressants. Most neurologists use azathioprine as their second-line agent. Unfortunately, it often takes 9 months or longer to see an effect from azathioprine. High-dose intravenous pooled human immune globulin (2 g/kg per day over 2–5 days) is effective in patients with dermatomyositis. The improvement occurs by the second or third treatment in most patients but must be repeated at intervals. Many prefer methotrexate as the second drug after or with prednisone because it works within 2–3 months. Methotrexate is usually administered orally at a dose of 7.5 mg per week and is gradually increased as necessary up to 20 mg per week.

Inclusion Body Myositis

Inclusion body myositis is the most common myopathy in patients older than 50 years. Inclusion body myositis is much more common in men than women. The disease weakens the distal muscles of the arms and legs. The deep finger flexors (particularly of the ulnar two fingers), including the flexor pollicis longus, and wrist flexors are affected quite early and are almost always more involved than the wrist and finger extensors. In the legs, the quadriceps and anterior tibial muscles are affected early. The disease generally has a chronic progressive course and is relatively unresponsive to prednisone and other immunosuppressive agents. The diagnosis is suspected based on the clinical features and is confirmed on muscle biopsy. The muscle biopsy demonstrates endomysial inflammation, increased variation in fiber size with fiber hypertrophy, and macrophage invasion of non-necrotic muscle fibers similar to polymyositis. In addition, muscle fibers contain rimmed vacuoles. The structures have a sharply demarcated vacuole, around which is a rim of altered tissue that stains red with the trichrome stain. Eosinophilic inclusions are present in the nuclei and adjacent cytoplasm. Congo red demonstrates amyloid deposits in the vacuolated muscle fibers. Unfortunately, because of sampling error, the biopsy is not definitively diagnostic 20–30% of the time.

Polymyalgia Rheumatica

Polymyalgia rheumatica is mainly a disorder of women older than 55 years. The main feature is proximal muscle pain that affects the arms more commonly than the legs. The pain is worse in the morning and on movement of the limbs. Chronic malaise, pyrexia, night sweats, and weight loss may be associated. Weakness is not present on examination. Temporal arteritis is a complicating condition in approximately one fourth of patients.

The serum CK concentration and the EMG findings are normal, and muscle histology shows only type II fiber atrophy. The sedimentation rate is elevated, often greater than 70 mm per hour, and is essential in the diagnosis. Daily prednisone is the treatment of choice. Symptoms may resolve within hours to days. The initial dose is 30–50 mg per day. After 2 months, the dose can be lowered, but treatment must be continued for at least 2 years.

For a more detailed discussion, see Chapter 85 in Neurology in Clinical Practice, 4th edition.

Neurological Problems of the Newborn

55

NEONATAL SEIZURES

Diagnosis

Table 55.1 is a classification of the common types of neonatal seizures. They are not specific for cause, but some occur more frequently with certain conditions. Tonic seizures occur in up to 50% of premature newborns with severe intraventricular hemorrhage. Focal clonic seizures in the term newborn are usually associated with focal cerebral infarction or traumatic injury, such as cerebral contusion.

Distinguishing Seizures from Nonconvulsive Movements
Subtle seizures often fail to show epileptiform discharges concomitant with the movement; the abnormal movements may be brainstem release phenomena rather than seizures. Epileptiform discharges rarely accompany tonic extensor posturing in newborns with severe intraventricular hemorrhage and anticonvulsant therapy is not useful. A normal electroencephalogram (EEG) distinguishes benign neonatal sleep myoclonus, which occurs in healthy newborns, from myoclonic seizures. Jitteriness, an exaggerated startle response, is often confused with clonic seizures, especially because both jitteriness and clonic seizures occur in conditions such as hypoxic-ischemic or metabolic encephalopathies and in drug withdrawal. The absence of associated ocular movements and the presence of stimulus sensitivity are characteristic of jitteriness. The predominant movement is tremor that stops with passive flexion of the affected limb.

Determination of the Underlying Cause
Table 55.2 summarizes the main causes of neonatal seizures and age at onset.

Table 55.1: Types of neonatal seizures

Neonatal Seizure Types	Clinical Manifestations	Age Distribution
Subtle	Eye deviation, blinking, fixed stare Repetitive mouth and tongue movements Apnea Pedaling, tonic posturing of limbs	Premature and term
Tonic: focal or generalized	Tonic extension of limbs Tonic flexion of upper limbs, extension of legs	Primarily premature
Clonic: multifocal or focal	Multifocal, clonic, synchronous, or asynchronous limb movements Nonordered progression Localized clonic limb movements Consciousness often preserved	Primarily term
Myoclonic: focal, multifocal, or generalized	Single or several synchronous flexion jerks of upper more than lower limbs	Rare

Table 55.2: Major causes of neonatal seizures: clinical features and outcome

Cause	Most Common Age at Onset	Relative Incidence Premature	Full-Term	Outcome (% of Normal Development)
Hypoxic-ischemic encephalopathy	<3 days	+++	+++	50
Intracranial hemorrhage				
Intraventricular hemorrhage	<3 days	++		<10
Primary subarachnoid hemorrhage	<1 day	+		90
Hypoglycemia	<2 days		+	50
Hypocalcemia				
Early-onset	23 days	+	++	50
Late-onset	>7 days		++	100
Intracranial infection				
Bacterial meningitis	>3 days	++	++	50
Intrauterine viral	>3 days	++	++	<10
Developmental defects	Variable	++	++	0
Drug withdrawal	<3 days	+	+	Unknown

Note: +++ = most common; ++ = less common; + = least common.
Source: Reprinted with permission from Volpe, J. J. 2000, *Neurology of the Newborn*, 4th ed., WB Saunders, Philadelphia.

Management

Neonatal seizures require urgent treatment. Once adequate ventilation and perfusion are established, the blood glucose concentration is measured. The administration of 10% dextrose (2 ml/kg) is indicated when the glucose concentration is less than 20 mg/dl in premature newborns or less than 30 mg/dl in full-term newborns. In the absence of hypoglycemia, immediate treatment with anticonvulsant medications is indicated (Table 55.3). Phenobarbital alone controls seizures in most newborns. Intravenous fosphenytoin is useful if seizures continue. In newborns, the oral absorption of phenytoin is poor. Intravenous therapy is the only effective route. Discontinue phenobarbital before hospital discharge if seizures have stopped and EEG findings are normal. Phenobarbital has potential deleterious effects on brain development, and maintenance therapy should continue for the briefest possible time.

HYPOXIC-ISCHEMIC BRAIN INJURY IN THE TERM NEWBORN

Diagnosis

Hypoxic-ischemic encephalopathy (HIE) in full-term newborns is mainly an antepartum and intrapartum event. The history of maternal risk factors and abnormalities of labor and delivery requires careful documentation. The clinical features of HIE are determined by the severity and timing of the insult. Acute total asphyxia may cause disproportionate injury to thalamus and brainstem nuclei, whereas prolonged partial asphyxia causes injury principally to cerebral cortex and subcortical white matter.

Clinical Features

The initial features of severe HIE are depressed level of consciousness, periodic breathing, hypotonia, and seizures (Table 55.4). An apparent increase in alertness may occur between 12 and 24 hours of age; however, seizures worsen and apnea may be noted. Between 24 and 72 hours of age, the level of consciousness deteriorates and brainstem abnormalities may become prominent. After 72 hours, infants who survive show continued although diminishing stupor, abnormal tone, and brainstem dysfunction with disturbances of sucking and swallowing. Severe HIE results in mental retardation, seizures, and spastic quadriparesis. Mild HIE is common. Increased

Table 55.3: Treatment of neonatal seizures

I. Ensure adequate ventilation and perfusion
II. Begin therapy for specific metabolic disturbances (if present)

	Acute therapy	Maintenance therapy
Hypoglycemia: glucose (10% solution)	2 ml/kg IV (0.2 g/kg)	Up to 8 mg/kg/min IV
Hypocalcemia: calcium gluconate (5% solution)	4 ml/kg IV (Note: monitor cardiac rhythm)	500 mg/kg/24 hr PO
Hypomagnesemia: magnesium sulfate (50% solution)	0.2 ml/kg IM	0.2 ml/kg/24 hr IM
Pyridoxine deficiency: pyridoxine	50–100 mg IV	100 mg PO daily for 2 wk

III. Begin anticonvulsant therapy

	Acute therapy	Maintenance therapy (begin 12 hr after loading dose)
Phenobarbital	20 mg/kg IV if necessary, additional 5–25 mg/kg IV in 5 mg/kg aliquots (Note: monitor blood pressure and respiration)	4–6 mg/kg/24 hr IV/IM/PO
Phenytoin*	2 doses of 10 mg/kg IV, diluted in normal saline (Note: monitor cardiac rate and rhythm)	5–10 mg/kg/24 hr IV
Lorazepam	0.05–0.10 mg/kg IV	

*Fosphenytoin may be the preferred form of phenytoin.
IV = intravenous; IM = intramuscular; PO = orally.

Table 55.4: Clinical features of severe hypoxic-ischemic encephalopathy

Clinical Features	Time After Insult			
	0–12 hr	12–24 hr	24–72 hr	72 hr
Seizures	++	+++	++	±
Increased intracranial pressure (full-term)		±	+++	
Stupor/coma	+++	++	+++	++
Apnea	+ (periodic breathing)	++	+++	+
Abnormal pupil/oculomotor responses		±	++	
Hypotonia	+++	+++	+++	++
Limb weakness	++	++	++	++
Proximal, upper > lower (term)	±	±	±	+
Hemiparesis	±	±	±	
Lower limbs (premature)	±			
Electroencephalographic features	Amplitude (suppression) frequency	Periodic pattern, ± multifocal sharp activity	Prominent periodic pattern + more voltage suppression	isoelectric pattern

Note: − = absent; ± = possibly present; + = present; ++ = more common; +++ = most common.

irritability, exaggerated Moro's and tendon reflexes, and sympathetic over-reactivity characterize mild HIE. Recovery is usually complete within 2 days, and no long-term sequelae occur.

Management

Optimal management begins *in utero* by measures to prevent hypoxic-ischemic injury. Early identification of fetuses at risk allows serial monitoring and consideration for cesarean delivery when signs of fetal distress persist. An asphyxiated newborn requires immediate treatment to prevent additional hypoxic-ischemic cerebral injury. This includes close attention to ventilation, perfusion, and blood glucose concentrations, control of seizures, and maintenance of perfusion and function of other affected organs, including the heart, liver, kidneys, and those of the gastrointestinal tract. Uncorrected metabolic derangements may worsen the cerebral injury.

Computed tomography (CT) in the full-term newborn and ultrasound (US) in the premature newborn are valuable for locating and quantitating cerebral injury. The maximum severity of acute HIE injury at term is seen as decreased attenuation on CT between 3 and 5 days. Magnetic resonance imaging (MRI) accomplishes a more precise anatomical delineation of brain injury later.

HEMORRHAGIC AND HYPOXIC-ISCHEMIC BRAIN INJURY IN THE PREMATURE NEWBORN

HIE in the premature newborn affects predominantly the periventricular regions, resulting in periventricular leukoencephalopathy (PVL). This results in spastic diplegia, quadriplegia, or visual impairment because the corticospinal tracts and optic radiations are involved. More severe injury may affect the cerebral cortex, resulting in microcephaly and cognitive impairment. Periventricular-intraventricular hemorrhage (PIVH) occurs in 20% of premature newborns of birth weight less than 1500 g. PIVH occurs on the first day in 50% and by the fourth day in 90%. It originates from rupture of small vessels in the subependymal germinal matrix. Approximately 80% of germinal matrix hemorrhages extend into the ventricular system. Hemorrhagic lesions in the cerebral parenchyma accompany severe germinal hemorrhages. These are usually unilateral and are probably hemorrhagic venous infarctions of the periventricular region.

Diagnosis

PVL is not diagnosable by clinical features at birth, but is demonstrable by US. US is routine in all newborns born at less than 32 weeks of gestation and in older premature newborns who show decreased states of consciousness, apnea, seizures, or hypotonia. Severe hemorrhage may be associated with the systemic abnormalities of metabolic acidosis, hypotension, bradycardia, and abnormal glucose and water homeostasis. After the neonatal period, CT or MRI shows the areas of PVL.

Management

The primary management strategy for PIVH is the prevention of premature delivery. Muscle paralysis with pancuronium bromide in ventilated premature newborns has an established role in reducing the frequency and severity of PIVH by stabilizing fluctuations of cerebral blood flow velocity. The role of other agents is less well established.

Newborns with PIVH require serial US for early diagnosis of posthemorrhagic hydrocephalus (PHH). Factors that influence the management of PHH are the rate of progression, the ventricular size, and the intracranial pressure. In approximately 50% of cases, ventriculomegaly arrests or resolves spontaneously, usually within 4 weeks. The definitive treatment is placement of a ventriculoperitoneal shunt, but this must wait for clearing of the ventricular blood. Temporizing measures include serial lumbar punctures, external ventriculostomy or ventricular catheter with subcutaneous reservoir to remove cerebrospinal fluid (CSF), and drugs that reduce CSF production, such as osmotic agents (isosorbide and glycerol), carbonic-anhydrase inhibitors, and diuretics (acetazolamide and furosemide). In cases of rapidly progressive hydrocephalus, ventriculoperitoneal shunt placement is required despite the morbidity associated with shunt placement in small, premature infants.

Prognosis

The prognosis after PIVH relates to the severity of hemorrhage and to the concomitant HIE. Germinal matrix hemorrhage alone is rarely a cause of significant neurological morbidity. Blood in the ventricles also has a relatively good prognosis unless ventricular dilatation occurs. Newborns with severe ventricular dilatation and intraparenchymal hemorrhage may die in the neonatal period, and most survivors develop PHH.

INTRAVENTRICULAR HEMORRHAGE IN THE TERM NEWBORN

Although intraventricular hemorrhage (IVH) primarily occurs in premature newborns, it also occurs in otherwise healthy full-term newborns. Hypoxia and trauma are factors in approximately 50% of cases. The sites of origin of IVH are more variable in the full-term newborn and include residual germinal matrix (2%), choroid plexus (1.1%), vascular malformations, tumor, or hemorrhagic venous infarction of the thalamus. The latter type usually presents at several days or weeks of age.

The diagnosis and management of IVH and its complications in the full-term newborn are similar to those described for premature newborns. Neuroimaging confirms the clinical suspicion of IVH. Long-term neurological sequelae occur in more than 50% of cases. Half will develop posthemorrhagic hydrocephalus, which requires shunt placement and an additional 20% develop ventricular dilatation.

INFECTIONS OF THE CENTRAL NERVOUS SYSTEM

Bacterial infections of the central nervous system (CNS) in the newborn include bacterial meningitis, epidural and subdural empyema, and brain abscess.

Neonatal Meningitis

Bacterial meningitis is more common in premature than in full-term infants. The acquisition of "early-onset" disease, within the first postpartum day, is from the birth canal. The organisms are group B streptococci, *Escherichia coli*, and *Listeria monocytogenes*. The acquisition of "late-onset" disease, after several days, is from the mother or other contacts. The causes include the organisms listed earlier, as well as *Staphylococcus* or *Pseudomonas aeruginosa*. Early diagnosis and treatment is critical. Lumbar puncture is essential for diagnosis.

Management
Mothers with positive rectal or genital cultures for group B streptococcus or other major risk factors for neonatal sepsis are treated with intravenous ampicillin during labor. Empirical treatment of a neonate with bacterial meningitis of unknown cause is the intravenous combination of ampicillin,

an aminoglycoside, and cefotaxime. Ventriculitis commonly causes hydrocephalus. Treatment of meningitic hydrocephalus is external ventricular drainage, often with a reservoir for intermittent draining of CSF and instillation of antibiotics if active infection is present. Most newborns require a permanent ventriculoperitoneal shunt after eradication of the infection.

Cerebral abscess is a rare complication of neonatal meningitis. It occurs most frequently with *Citrobacter* infection but may also occur after other virulent gram-negative infections or, rarely, gram-positive organisms. Abscess is suspected when newborns with increased intracranial pressure respond poorly to treatment. Brain imaging confirms the diagnosis. The duration of antibiotic therapy is prolonged, and surgical exploration and drainage are the treatments of choice. The mortality is approximately 15%, and survivors often have major neurological impairment.

Prognosis
Overall, mortality is between 20% and 30% but is highest for gram-negative infections. Permanent neurological sequelae occur in 30–50% of survivors and include hydrocephalus, cerebral palsy, epilepsy, intellectual deficits, and deafness.

Viral and Parasitic Infections

The name *TORCH syndrome* is a means to remember the major nonbacterial neonatal infections *t*oxoplasmosis, *o*thers (such as syphilis), *r*ubella, *c*ytomegalovirus (CMV) infection, and *h*erpes simplex. All of the TORCH infections occur during pregnancy by transplacental inoculation, except for herpes simplex contracted by passage of the fetus through an infected birth canal. Although most newborns with TORCH syndromes have clinical features of disease in the first month, symptom onset can be delayed until infancy and childhood.

Congenital Rubella
Despite a greatly diminished incidence of congenital rubella infection by use of rubella vaccination, it remains a significant problem in many parts of the world. The congenital rubella syndrome occurs when the fetal infection occurs before 20 weeks of gestation. The clinical features include low birth weight, jaundice, hepatosplenomegaly, petechial rash, congenital heart disease, cataracts, sensorineural deafness, microcephaly, bone lesions, and thrombocytopenia. Less severely affected infants appear normal at birth and later show features of neurological and ocular defects, deafness, and congenital heart disease. Infected infants are highly infectious, may shed virus

for several years, and are a hazard to nonimmune women. Virus culture of urine confirms the diagnosis. Antiviral treatment is unavailable.

Cytomegalovirus

CMV is the most common congenital viral infection. It results either from primary maternal infection or from reactivation of maternal virus. Most newborns with congenital CMV are asymptomatic. A few have hepatosplenomegaly, jaundice, petechiae, microcephaly, periventricular calcifications, chorioretinitis, and blindness. In symptomatic cases, virus can be cultured from throat swabs or urine, and CMV-specific immunoglobulin M (IgM) is present in serum. Specific therapy with a 3-month course of ganciclovir may provide clinical benefit for symptomatic newborns. Supportive therapy involves control of seizures. Most asymptomatic newborns with congenital CMV infection develop normally. However, some develop impaired intellectual function, deafness, microcephaly, chorioretinitis, ataxia, and seizures. Mortality in symptomatic newborns is 20–30%, and most survivors have severe neurological sequelae.

Herpes Simplex

Neonatal herpes simplex infection may present as localized orocutaneous or ophthalmic disease, localized disease of the CNS, such as meningitis, or disseminated disease with hepatosplenomegaly, severe disseminated intravascular coagulation, renal failure, and meningoencephalitis. Studies of the CSF are usually consistent with viral meningoencephalitis. Polymerase chain reaction (PCR) assay is the best technique to identify the virus rapidly in CSF. CT or MRI, especially diffusion-weighted MRI, is useful for delineating the extent and severity of brain injury. In full-term newborns, initiate a 14-day course of acyclovir (30 mg/kg per day in evenly divided doses every 8 hours) even before knowing the results of PCR. Reduce dosages in premature infants and infants who have impaired renal function. Acyclovir may improve outcome but is not as effective as in postnatally acquired infection.

Human Immunodeficiency Virus

An increasing number of newborns are seropositive for human immunodeficiency virus (HIV). Transmission may occur *in utero*, during labor and delivery, or postnatally by breastfeeding. Most infected newborns, although asymptomatic at birth, later develop opportunistic systemic infections (CMV, *Pneumocystis*) and dementia with cerebral atrophy, and acquired microcephaly caused by viral infection of the brain. A program of prenatal, perinatal, and postnatal therapy with zidovudine may reduce the risk of maternal-fetal transmission. Elective cesarean section and avoidance of breast-feeding may also reduce transmission.

Toxoplasmosis

Toxoplasmosis is a transplacentally acquired parasitic infection. Infection causes extensive necrosis and calcification of the cerebral cortex and periventricular tissue. Periaqueductal infection obstructs CSF flow and causes hydrocephalus. Cataracts and microphthalmia are the main eye abnormalities. Other organs that may be involved are the liver, bone marrow, lungs, muscles, and myocardium. Antibody screening for neonatal infection may suggest congenital toxoplasmosis, but test results for toxoplasma-specific IgM often are negative. Examination of the CSF may show lymphocytosis, high protein content, and trophozoites. Skull radiography, CT, and US reveal diffuse intracerebral calcifications. Treatment of the infected mother and her infant during the first year is with piramycin, pyrimethamine, and sulfadiazine with folinic acid. In cases of severe meningoencephalitis, corticosteroids may be considered. Approximately one third of infected infants are symptomatic, and their mortality is 25%. Most survivors have significant neurological sequelae. The prognosis is favorable in asymptomatic newborns.

MECHANICAL TRAUMA

Intracranial Hemorrhage

Intracranial hemorrhages other than PIVHs are usually associated with traumatic delivery or a bleeding diathesis. CT visualizes hemorrhages better than US. Subdural hemorrhage results from laceration of major veins and sinuses, usually from excessive molding of the head. Convexity subdural hematoma, especially if associated with midline shift, requires decompression by craniotomy or subdural tap. Subarachnoid hemorrhage is also of venous origin but is usually self-limited, originating from small vessels in the leptomeningeal plexus or bridging veins within the subarachnoid space. They are often asymptomatic or associated with seizures. The CSF is uniformly blood stained or xanthochromic. In the absence of severe trauma or HIE, the outcome is normal in 90% of cases.

Extracranial Hemorrhage

Caput succedaneum is superficial bleeding between the skin and the epicranial aponeurosis, subgaleal hemorrhage is located between the aponeurosis and the periosteum of the skull, and cephalohematoma occurs in the deepest plane between the periosteum and cranial bones. Extracranial hemorrhage rarely requires intervention, except for subgaleal hemorrhage, in which the amount of acute blood loss may cause shock.

Skull Fractures

Linear skull fractures are usually parietal. Bony continuity is lost without depression. Depressed skull fractures buckle inward without loss of continuity, like a depression in a ping-pong ball (ping-pong fracture). Occipital diastasis is not an actual fracture but rather a traumatic separation of the squamous and lateral parts of the occipital bones that is usually associated with breech delivery.

CT shows the relation of depressed bone to the cerebral surface and a linear fracture beneath a cephalohematoma. Occipital diastasis may be associated with posterior fossa subdural hemorrhage, cerebellar contusion, and brainstem compression without hemorrhage or contusion. In the absence of intracranial lesions, treatment is required only when a depressed fracture impinges on the brain.

Spinal Cord Injury

The causes of spinal cord injury are excessive torsion or traction. Seventy-five percent of spinal cord injuries occur during breech delivery and involve principally the lower cervical and upper thoracic regions, whereas injuries during vertex delivery more commonly involve the upper and midcervical cord. The usual cause of injuries of the lower thoracic and lumbar spinal cord is vascular occlusion secondary to umbilical artery catheterization or air embolus from peripheral intravenous injection. Newborns with high cervical lesions are stillborn or die quickly from respiratory failure. Lower cervical–upper thoracic lesions cause urinary retention, hypotonia, weakness, and areflexia of all limbs, evolving subsequently to spastic paraplegia or quadriplegia. The distinguishing features of cord injuries from neuromuscular disorders and brain injuries are a distinct sensory level of response to pinprick, urinary retention, and a patulous anus.

Cesarean delivery of all fetuses with a hyperextended head minimizes spinal cord injury in breech position. The clinical features are the basis for diagnosis of spinal cord injury. The use of high-dose corticosteroids in controlled trials in spinal cord injury have not been done in the pediatric age-group.

Traumatic Injury to the Peripheral Nervous System

Facial Paralysis

Facial paralysis is uncommon and more often occurs by *in utero* compression of the facial nerve against the sacral promontory than by the pressure of forceps blades during delivery. Most cases recover within weeks or months. Facial paralysis and asymmetrical crying facies secondary to congenital aplasia of the depressor angularis oris muscle must be distinguished.

Brachial Plexus Injury

Brachial plexus injuries usually occur in large newborns who are difficult to deliver. The upper roots of the brachial plexus are always involved. Injury of the third to fifth cervical roots causes diaphragmatic paralysis. The basis for diagnosis is the neurological examination. If the affected arm is painful, immobilize the arm across the upper abdomen for 1 week before initiating passive range-of-motion exercises. Improved arm function within 2 weeks is a favorable prognostic sign. Most recover by 12 months. In infants with no evidence of spontaneous recovery at 4 months, surgical reconstruction of the plexus is a consideration.

EFFECTS OF DRUGS AND TOXINS

The consequences of fetal exposure to medications and toxins may be teratogenic or cause passive addiction. Table 55.5 lists the major adverse effects of the most commonly used neuroactive agents taken during pregnancy.

Passive addiction occurs in most newborns of mothers who use drugs that affect the CNS during pregnancy. The clinical features of addiction and withdrawal are similar for most drugs, but the time of withdrawal differs according to the elimination half-life for the specific drug. The initial features of withdrawal in infants include jitteriness, irritability, and disturbances of sleep-wake patterns, shrill cry, and frantic sucking. Later features are gastrointestinal disturbances, such as poor feeding, vomiting, and diarrhea. Less common symptoms include sneezing, tachypnea, and excessive sweating. Fever and seizures are uncommon and suggest the possibility of sepsis or other serious neonatal disorders.

Table 55.5: Major adverse effects of neuroactive drugs administered during pregnancy

Neuroactive Drugs	Passive Addiction	Known Teratogenic	Neonatal Seizures	Intrauterine Growth Retardation	Coagulation Disorders (Neonatal Intracranial Hemorrhage)
Alcohol	+	+	+	+	
Heroin/methadone	+		+ (methadone)	+	
Cocaine	+	+	?	+	
Benzodiazepines	+		+		
Tricyclic antidepressants	+				
Hydroxyzine (Atarax)	+				
Ethchlorvynol (Placidyl)	+		+		
Propoxyphene (Darvon)	+				
Pentazocine (Talwin)	+		+		
"T's and blues" (pentazocine, tripelennamine)	+				
Codeine	+				
Hydantoins		+ + +			
Barbiturates	+ +		+ (short-acting)		+ + +
Primidone	+ +	+			
Valproate		+		±	
Oxazolidine derivatives (trimethadione)				+	

Note: + = present; – = not present; ± = possibly present.

Therapy consists of managing respiratory complications, infection, dehydration, and metabolic derangements. In addition, severe and persistent irritability, vomiting, and diarrhea may require treatment with paregoric, phenobarbital, chlorpromazine, or diazepam.

For a more detailed discussion, see Chapter 86 in Neurology in Clinical Practice, 4th edition.

Neurological Problems of Pregnancy

56

NEUROLOGICAL COMPLICATIONS OF CONTRACEPTION

The use of oral contraceptive agents containing more than 80 μg of estrogen increases the incidence of stroke. Agents containing less than 50 μg of estrogen in nondiabetic, nonhypertensive patients pose no additional risk. Anticonvulsants do not affect efficacy or dose of medroxyprogesterone, but unwanted pregnancies with levonorgestrel use have occurred in women taking phenytoin or carbamazepine. Estrogen-containing oral contraceptive agents may worsen chronic inflammatory demyelinating polyneuropathy (CIDP), unmask systemic lupus erythematosus, worsen migraine, and produce chorea in patients with antiphospholipid antibody syndrome.

HEADACHE

The most common headache during pregnancy is tension type, often symptomatic of depression and situational stresses. Tension headaches may presage postpartum depression. Simple analgesics treat occasional tension headache. Recurrent tension headaches warrant psychological assessment and prophylaxis with a tricyclic antidepressant such as amitriptyline. Amitriptyline use is not linked to birth defects. However, avoid regular use of aspirin and benzodiazepines.

Pregnancy affects migraine favorably in 80% of cases. During pregnancy and lactation, ergotamine is contraindicated. No data are available on the safety of the triptans. The treatment of occasional migraine attacks is with antihistaminic antiemetics and analgesics. The treatment of frequently recurring migraine is propranolol or calcium-channel blockers. Valproic acid causes fetal malformations and is not to be used during pregnancy. During pregnancy, discontinue the use of propranolol, atenolol, and other beta blockers or reduce the dose to the lowest effective dose. When prophylactic therapy is required, the benefit of metoprolol, propranolol, or verapamil may outweigh risks. Lithium is teratogenic in animals and therefore should be avoided in humans. Naproxen sodium is relatively safe throughout pregnancy but is safest when used during the first two trimesters. Metoclopramide, acetaminophen, and meperidine do not increase fetal risk and may be beneficial.

NEUROMUSCULAR DISORDERS

Leg Cramps

One fourth of women experience muscle cramps each morning on initiating movement during the last trimester of pregnancy. Salt depletion, hypokalemia, and other metabolic conditions aggravate cramping. Magnesium lactate or magnesium citrate tablets (122 mg in the morning and 244 mg in the evening) considerably improve symptoms in approximately 80% of patients. Oral calcium carbonate or gluconate, 500 mg three or four times a day, may also provide relief. Placebo is similarly effective in 40%.

Restless Legs

Approximately 10–30% of women develop restless legs syndrome during the last trimester of pregnancy. The irresistible urge for the legs to fidget begins 30 minutes after lying down. Excessive caffeine ingestion and anemia aggravate restless legs. Oral folic acid supplementation (500 mg daily) decreases the frequency of restless legs. Walking about and taking a hot shower before retiring may lengthen the latent period enough to allow women to fall asleep. For severe restless legs during pregnancy, carbidopa/L-dopa 25 mg/100 mg may be preferable to other agents. A single bedtime dose may be effective for both restless legs and periodic movements of sleep and has low teratogenic potential.

Myasthenia Gravis

During pregnancy, approximately equal proportions of myasthenic women improve, stay the same, or worsen. The course during one pregnancy does not predict that during subsequent pregnancies. Abortion does not induce a remission. Approximately half weaken during the puerperium. At least 12% of infants born to myasthenic women develop transitory neonatal myasthenia gravis and require close monitoring for at least 4 days.

Pregnancy does not significantly alter the usual management of myasthenia gravis. Insufficient data are available on the safety of intravenous immune globulin (IVIG) during pregnancy. Permit breast-feeding but avoid treatment with cyclosporine and azathioprine. Both are in breast milk and carry immunosuppressive risks and tumorigenic potential. Corticosteroids also are in breast milk but in small amounts. Large doses of anticholinesterase drugs taken by the mother may lead to gastrointestinal upset in the breast-fed newborn.

Myopathies

Myotonic Dystrophy
Myotonia, whether part of myotonic dystrophy or myotonia congenita, often increases during the second half of pregnancy. Ineffective uterine contractions, premature labor, and breech presentation frequently complicate labor. Oxytocin can stimulate the myotonic uterus to increased contraction. Regional anesthesia is preferred over general anesthesia. After delivery, hypotonic uterine dysfunction results in an increased risk of retained placenta and postpartum hemorrhage. One half of the children inherit the disorder and may have severe impairment at birth.

Inflammatory Myopathy
Pregnancy worsens or activates polymyositis and dermatomyositis. Manifestations of collagen vascular disease commonly associated with myositis may complicate pregnancy. More than one half of fetuses die, but surviving infants thrive. Immunosuppressive treatment is advisable for gravid women.

Neuropathies

Bell's Palsy
Facial nerve palsy is three to four times more common during pregnancy and the puerperium. The prognosis for recovery of facial nerve function is worse when the palsy occurs during pregnancy. Some researchers find an increased frequency of toxemia in patients with gestational facial palsy. Herpes simplex virus type 1 is the cause of most facial palsies, and far less frequently, varicella zoster. Pharmacological therapy of Bell's palsy during pregnancy remains controversial. No reports on

efficacy of therapy with prednisone and acyclovir during pregnancy are available. Individually, the drugs pose low risk.

Carpal Tunnel Syndrome
Approximately one fifth of pregnant women complain of nocturnal hand paresthesias, primarily in the last trimester. A few have a median neuropathy. Pregnant women with carpal tunnel syndrome can expect their symptoms to regress after delivery.

Meralgia Paresthetica
The expanding abdominal wall and the increased lordosis of pregnancy stretch the lateral femoral cutaneous nerve to the thigh as it penetrates the tensor fascia lata or at the inguinal ligament. This unilateral or bilateral affliction of late pregnancy resolves within 3 months postpartum.

Acute Polyradiculoneuropathy (Guillain-Barré Syndrome)
Pregnancy does not affect the frequency or course of acute polyradiculoneuropathy. Infants of a mother without complications are born healthy. Some recommend fluid loading before plasmapheresis to prevent hypotension. Others suggest avoiding tocolytics in the presence of autonomic instability. Intravenous human immunoglobulin is safe for use during pregnancy.

Chronic Inflammatory Demyelinating Polyneuropathy
CIDP is three times more likely to relapse during the last trimester and puerperium than in the absence of pregnancy. Infants are unaffected. Corticosteroids, plasmapheresis, and IVIG treat exacerbations during pregnancy. Oral contraceptives can worsen CIDP.

Gestational Polyneuropathy
Distal symmetrical neuropathy affects malnourished women. Presumably, thiamine and possibly other nutrients are deficient in these patients. The acute presentation of symmetrical neuropathy and Wernicke's encephalopathy (see later discussion) in the third and fourth months may be secondary to the thiamine deficiency associated with hyperemesis gravidarum.

Maternal Obstetric Palsy
Peripheral nerves are occasionally the objects of intrapartum compressive trauma by the fetal head, the application of forceps, and improperly positioned leg holders. Craniopelvic disproportion, dystocia, prolonged labor, and primigravida status contribute to these injuries. Unilateral lumbosacral plexus injury is most common. Most maternal obstetric palsies recover within 6 weeks.

CEREBRAL DISORDERS

Wernicke's Encephalopathy

More than three fourths of women experience nausea and vomiting during pregnancy, most commonly between 6 and 16 weeks of gestation. The diagnosis of *hyperemesis gravidarum* describes severe vomiting resulting in weight loss or metabolic derangement requiring intravenous therapy. Apathy, drowsiness, memory loss, catatonia, ophthalmoplegia, nystagmus, ataxia, optic neuritis, and papilledema may result, typically between 14 and 20 weeks of gestation. Death or severe morbidity results when this condition is not treated. Only one half of women with this condition deliver normal children.

Chorea Gravidarum

Chorea of any cause beginning in pregnancy is chorea gravidarum. Chorea commonly presents during the second to fifth month of pregnancy and less commonly postpartum. Subtle, sometimes severe, cognitive change may accompany the chorea. Usually, this condition resolves spontaneously within weeks to months, often shortly after delivery. Choice of therapy depends on the severity of the disorder and other accompanying clinical manifestations.

Multiple Sclerosis

Uncomplicated multiple sclerosis has no apparent effect on fertility, pregnancy, labor, delivery, and the rate of spontaneous abortions, congenital malformations, or stillbirths. Oral contraceptive agents do not affect the incidence of multiple sclerosis. Studies of glatiramer acetate, interferon-β-1a, and interferon-β-1b during pregnancy are not available. Mitoxantrone causes fetal damage in animals, so it should not be used during pregnancy.

Brain Tumors

Most brain tumors present in the second half of pregnancy. Surgery for supratentorial malignant gliomas and many infratentorial tumors occurs during pregnancy. Meningiomas have estrogen receptors, which may explain their frequent enlargement during pregnancy. Spinal hemangiomas are more likely to rupture during gestation. Symptoms of meningioma, vascular tumors, and acoustic neuromas may remit postpartum. Because brainstem herniation can occur during labor, delivery is by cesarian section. Indications for premature interruption of pregnancy include increasing intracranial pressure and visual failure caused by papilledema. Malignant tumors, or tumors threatening compression of vital brain structures, usually require surgery during pregnancy. Some benign tumors can wait several weeks postpartum to observe for spontaneous improvements. Delivery for most women with brain tumors is by cesarean section. Corticosteroids reduce symptoms of brain tumors but cause fetal hypoadrenalism. Delay teratogenic chemotherapy until after delivery.

Pituitary Tumors

Women with untreated hyperprolactinemia often are anovulatory and infertile. Treatment with dopamine agonists restores ovulation in 90% of patients. During pregnancy, medical therapy focuses on preventing complications of tumor growth. Bromocriptine reduces prolactinoma size usually within 6 weeks to 6 months but suppresses lactation. Women with macroadenomas are advised to have trans-sphenoidal surgery before attempting pregnancy or to receive bromocriptine therapy during pregnancy. Usually, women with pituitary tumors deliver vaginally.

Idiopathic Intracranial Hypertension (Pseudotumor Cerebri)

Idiopathic intracranial hypertension (IIH) usually worsens with pregnancy. IIH develops during the fourteenth gestational week and disappears after 1–3 months, but it sometimes persists until the early puerperium. Some authors advise a delay in pregnancy until all signs and symptoms of pre-existing IIH abate. The value of terminating pregnancy is unknown, so it is not indicated. Frequent checks of optic fundi, visual acuity, and visual fields monitor the condition and the results of treatment. Most physicians advise moderation in diet to reduce weight gain. Two-week courses of corticosteroids treat vision loss. A course of four to six serial lumbar punctures are performed weekly before advising optic nerve sheath fenestration or lumboperitoneal shunt.

Human studies are inadequate to determine the efficacy or teratogenic potential of acetazolamide. It has treated IIH during many pregnancies productive of healthy infants. Some physicians recommend restricting its use until after 20 weeks of gestation.

EPILEPSY AND ITS TREATMENTS

Maternal Considerations

Women with epilepsy have approximately 15% fewer children than expected. The fewer seizures occur in the 9 months before conception, the lower the risk of worsening during the pregnancy. Women who have at least one seizure a month before pregnancy have more seizures during pregnancy. Approximately one fourth of women experience an increase in seizure frequency during gestation. Elevated seizure frequency may result from lowered levels of circulating unbound antiepileptic drugs (AEDs). Convulsive seizures during pregnancy can result in blunt trauma to the mother. Trauma is the leading nonobstetrical cause of maternal death in women with epilepsy, but the frequency is very low.

Fetal Considerations

Nearly 90% of epileptic women deliver healthy babies. However, an increased risk exists of miscarriage, stillbirth, prematurity, developmental delay, and major malformations. Maternal seizures, AEDs, and socioeconomic, genetic, and psychological aspects of epilepsy affect outcome. Consensus among neurologists is that maternal seizures probably are more dangerous than AEDs. In general, use of a single AED increases the risk of congenital malformations to 4–8%. Researchers find a 5.5% frequency of malformations with two anticonvulsant drugs, 11% with three anticonvulsant drugs, and 23% with four AEDs. Pregnant women may be reassured that after an uncomplicated seizure during the first trimester current data do not indicate increased risk of malformation to their fetus.

Valproic acid increases the risk of neural tube defects and other malformations 3-fold to 20-fold, to approximately 1–2%, and its teratogenic effects are dose related. Carbamazepine also is associated with neural tube defects, with a frequency of 0.5–1.0%.

Common Advice and Management Strategy

Evaluate the need for AED therapy before conception. Monotherapy at the lowest effective dose is preferred. Monitor AED levels more frequently during gestation and the postpartum period and adjust dosage as indicated. Manage pregnant women with epilepsy who present to the neurologist already taking AEDs on an individual basis. During pregnancy, and particularly once the period of organogenesis has passed, changes in medications are likely to cause more harm than good.

Occasionally, seizures present for the first time during pregnancy. Pregnancy has little effect on the use of diagnostic examinations and treatment considerations. The most common causes of seizures during childbearing years include idiopathic epilepsy, trauma, congenital defects, neoplasms, meningitis, intracerebral hemorrhage, and drug or alcohol toxicity. Zonisamide, lamotrigine, and oxcarbazepine are classified as unsafe to use while breastfeeding, although the safety of other newer AEDs remains uncertain.

CEREBROVASCULAR DISEASE

Arteriovenous Malformations

No specific therapeutic course is best for women with known arteriovenous malformations (AVMs) planning pregnancy. The additional risk of hemorrhage during pregnancy is uncertain. Multiple pregnancies do not increase the rate of hemorrhage. Women whose AVMs are repaired surgically can undergo vaginal delivery. Recommend cesarean section for incompletely repaired or partially treated previously ruptured AVMs.

Intracranial Hemorrhage

Intracerebral hemorrhage occurs twice as often during pregnancy and almost 30 times more often during the 6 weeks postpartum. Almost half of hemorrhages are associated with eclampsia and preeclampsia. In one third, no specific cause is determined. Mode of delivery does not affect outcome and epidural anesthesia is satisfactory for vaginal delivery. Hemorrhage from aneurysms and vascular malformations accounts for 25–35% of intracranial hemorrhages. Management strategies are generally the same as those applied outside of pregnancy. Mode of delivery did not affect outcome in the studies available.

Ischemic Stroke

Pregestational stroke has no effect on outcome. Stroke during one pregnancy is not a risk factor for stroke in subsequent pregnancies, except for women with systemic lupus erythematosus or antiphospholipid antibody syndrome. Women with conditions predisposing to stroke, such as emboligenic cardiac disease and coagulopathies, are at increased risk. Heparin is the anticoagulant of choice. Heparin does not cross the placenta and is not associated with teratogenic effects. Warfarin is teratogenic, with highest risk during the period of 7–12 weeks of gestation. Magnetic resonance imaging (MRI) is the modality of choice to image the brain. No study or clinical observation has detailed harmful effects on mother or child. Aspirin at low doses (60–150 mg per day) is safe in the second and third trimesters. Clopidogrel and ticlopidine are of unknown safety and efficacy during pregnancy.

Cardiac Disease

Mechanical prosthetic heart valves have the highest embolization rates. Risk of thromboembolism of some mechanical valve prostheses during pregnancy is 25–35%. Aortic or mitral valvular location, the presence of atrial fibrillation, left atrial size or thrombus, and previous thromboembolic episodes influence some recommendations for anticoagulation. The teratogenic effects of warfarin are maximal during the first 6–12 weeks of gestation and are associated with fetal loss, congenital malformations, and mental and physical disability. Approximately 30% of living progeny suffer the "fetal warfarin syndrome," including nasal hypoplasia/stippled epiphyses, limb hypoplasia, low birth weight, hearing loss, and ophthalmic anomalies. Unfractionated heparin and low-molecular-weight heparin (LMWH) do not cross the placenta and reduce frequency of heparin-induced thrombocytopenia, osteoporosis, and bleeding complications. No blood test is required to monitor its safety. The frequency of cerebral embolism associated with chronic atrial fibrillation during pregnancy is 2–10%. When atrial fibrillation is associated with cardiac disease, physicians recommend anticoagulation throughout gestation, commonly with high-dose subcutaneous heparin.

Antiphospholipid Antibody Syndrome

Women with circulating antiphospholipid antibodies and without a history of pregnancy loss do not require treatment to prevent stroke during pregnancy. A combination of low-dose aspirin and LMWH during pregnancy is current practice in the United Kingdom for women with antiphospholipid antibodies and a history of fetal loss after 16 weeks of gestation, intra-uterine growth retardation, early onset preeclampsia, placental abruption, or stillbirth.

Postpartum Stroke

Such patients present with puerperal focal neurological signs and symptoms, often with headaches, and have hypertension without edema or proteinuria. Brain MRI depicts ischemia primarily in the parieto-occipital region, and angiography shows vasospasm. The course often is benign. Cases that include reversible headache, altered sensorium, seizures, or visual loss without hemorrhage belong in the category "reversible posterior leukoencephalopathy syndrome."

Cerebral Venous Thrombosis

Aseptic thrombosis of the cerebral venous system presents with puerperal headache worsening over several days, a change in behavior or personality, convulsive seizures, and neurological deficits. Initial symptoms generally begin 1 day to 4 weeks postpartum and peak in frequency 7–14 days postpartum. Cerebral venous thrombosis is associated with hypercoagulable states, infection, sickle cell disease, dehydration, and ulcerative colitis, in addition to gestation. Differential diagnoses include eclampsia, meningitis, and cerebral mass. Brain MRI with magnetic resonance venography detects occlusion of major sinuses with high sensitivity, but when smaller veins are involved detection may be more difficult.

ECLAMPTIC ENCEPHALOPATHY

Preeclampsia (toxemia gravidarum) and eclampsia remain the principal causes of maternal perinatal morbidity and death. The characteristic preeclamptic syndrome includes edema, proteinuria, and hypertension after 20 weeks of gestation. Eclampsia is epileptic seizures in the setting of preeclampsia. Eclamptic seizures may precede the clinical triad of preeclampsia. Preeclampsia develops in approximately 4–8% of the pregnancies. Eclampsia accounts for nearly one fourth of cerebral infarcts in pregnancy and puerperium. Short intervals between pregnancies reduce the risk of preeclampsia. Parental magnesium sulfate treats severe preeclampsia and eclampsia. The mechanism of action remains unclear.

For a more detailed discussion, see Chapter 87 in Neurology in Clinical Practice, 4th edition.

Principles of Pain Management | *57*

PAIN MECHANISMS

Nociceptive Pain

The acute pain of tissue injury is either somatic or visceral pain based on differences in character. Somatic pain is clearly localized and sharp or dull in character. Visceral pain localizes poorly and is cramping, spasmodic, or aching in character. Chronic pain is similar to acute pain in the same region, but the consequences of modulation of nociceptive transmission and the affective components of pain are more important than the acute pain. Depression, sleep disorders, and the sequelae of disuse (e.g., muscle atrophy and limited joint mobility) contribute to the disability of chronic pain disorders.

Although nociceptive pain usually arises from localized tissue injury, the distribution of perceived pain does not always identify the source. Tissue injury occurring at one site may be felt as arising from another (*referred pain*). Common examples of referred pain are listed in Table 57.1. In addition to the convergence of visceral and somatic input at the spinal level, other possible mechanisms of referred pain include innervation of two structures by different branches of the same nociceptive afferent fiber and changes in the receptive field of thalamic neurons.

Neuropathic and Deafferentation Pain

Pain is an important consequence of direct injury to peripheral nerves; common examples are nerve and nerve root compression syndromes, acute and chronic pain after nerve transection, neuritis in association with infectious and inflammatory lesions (e.g., herpes zoster), and diffuse polyneuropathies.

Neuropathic pain is the consequence of direct injury to peripheral nerves. It has several qualities. A common form is sharp, lancinating pain that is brief but very intense or shocklike and

Table 57.1: Common referred pain syndromes

Pain Location	Segmental Distribution	Causes
Frontal or vertex headache	Trigeminal nerve	Traction, inflammation, or other lesions involving the supratentorial meninges
Ear pain	Glossopharyngeal and vagus nerves	Tumor, abscess, or inflammatory lesion in the oropharynx or hypopharynx
Right shoulder pain	Phrenic nerve (C3–C5)	Cholecystitis or diaphragmatic irritation
Left chest/arm pain	T1–T4	Cardiac ischemia
Left upper abdominal wall pain	T8	Gastric diseases
Middle and lower abdominal wall pain	T10–T11	Small intestine and colon disorders
Testicle/inguinal region pain	T12–L2	Renal or perirenal abscess or tumor
Knee pain	L3–L4	Pelvic, acetabular, and femoral head disorders

well localized. Typically, the pain radiates in a pattern suggesting a dermatomal or peripheral nerve distribution. A *trigger zone* may exist, where stimulation of a specific area elicits intense shocklike pains. A superimposed burning pain is common, which light stimulation exacerbates out of proportion to the stimulus intensity. A slight breeze or movement of a sheet over the skin is sufficient to produce exquisite pain in patients with painful neuropathies.

Complex Regional Pain Syndromes

The term *causalgia* was used for a syndrome of severe progressive distal limb pain with swelling, changes in color and temperature, atrophy, and loss of use following a major nerve trunk injury. A similar syndrome that often follows minor trauma was termed *reflex sympathetic dystrophy* (RSD). These entities are now called: (1) *complex regional pain syndrome* (CRPS) type I (formerly *RSD*) and (2) CRPS type II (formerly *causalgia*). They are three times more common in women than men, and the age at for most patients is early to middle adulthood. The primary feature is distal pain, with the hand more frequently involved than the foot. The pain has neuropathic qualities and with time spreads proximally. In CRPS type II, the pain begins within days of the injury and is severe from the start. In CRPS type I, weeks or months may elapse before the development of pain, which tends to progress more gradually.

The clinical criteria for the diagnosis of CPRS type I include: (1) an initiating, noxious event, or cause of immobilization, (2) continuing pain, allodynia, or hyperalgesia with which the pain is disproportionate to any inciting event, (3) evidence at some time of edema, changes in blood flow, or abnormal pseudomotor activity in the region of pain, and (4) the absence of conditions that would otherwise account for the degree of pain and dysfunction.

The treatment of the CRPSs is only partially successful. A trial of regional sympathetic blockade is still recommended as part of the early management. Physical therapy and analgesics including nonsteroidal anti-inflammatory drugs (NSAIDs) and agents for neuropathic pain such as gabapentin are also common in the early management of CRPS. Opioid analgesics add substantially to pain control for some patients. Other treatment modalities include implanted spinal cord stimulators, spinal cord stimulation, physical therapy, sympathetic blockade, and transcutaneous electrical nerve stimulation (TENS). Contracture and dystonia contribute to the pain and disability of CRPS type I.

Intrathecal baclofen markedly reduces dystonia and improves function in the affected limb. Botulinum toxin reduces dystonia and pain.

Idiopathic and Psychogenic Pain

Pain that occurs in the absence of a definable cause of nociceptor activation and lacking any mechanism of neuropathic generation is often categorized as idiopathic or psychogenic. Idiopathic pain problems are not all psychogenic, but many people with idiopathic chronic pain develop psychological factors that promote or sustain the pain problem. Tension-type headache and fibromyalgia fall into this category. These factors should be explored as potential avenues of therapy. Feigning illness, such as chronic pain for the purpose of obtaining an obvious, often tangible, secondary gain, is *malingering*.

Unexplained pain is an uncommon presenting complaint of a major psychiatric disorder. Occasionally, somatic delusions that include pain occur as part of depression and resolve with antidepressant therapy. Headache is the most common pain complaint in patients with depression. Conversely, depression is relatively common among patients with chronic pain.

APPROACH TO THE PATIENT WITH PAIN

Acute Pain

The useful features that characterize a new pain complaint are location, character, mode of onset, factors that aggravate and relieve pain, and concurrent features, such as fever, dyspnea, nausea, and others. The relationship between the severity of pain and the patient's emotional response and attributed disability must be assessed. Prior medical problems often explain current pain syndromes. The initial examination is mainly directed by the location of the pain. Maneuvers that elicit or relieve pain should be duplicated.

Even with rigorous investigation, the pathophysiological basis of many pain complaints cannot be established. The attribution of a new pain complaint to a psychiatric disorder requires the rigorous exclusion of other causes.

Chronic Pain

Pain that lasts months or longer, without a defined cause and of sufficient severity to interfere with normal daily activities, is a relatively common and difficult problem. Several central nervous system (CNS) disorders can produce chronic pain syndromes that pose difficult diagnostic problems (e.g., multiple sclerosis, thalamic tumors, or infarcts). Psychological factors are usually important, and a multidisciplinary approach to pain control that includes pharmacological, behavioral, and psychological management is often needed.

PHARMACOLOGICAL APPROACHES TO PAIN MANAGEMENT

The escalating analgesic approach is applicable to the patient with a defined lesion that produces persistent somatic nociceptive pain, such as patients with cancer, but this approach is also a useful framework for other persistent or chronic pain problems. The main points are (1) the titration of analgesics in relation to the severity of the pain, (2) the use of regularly scheduled as opposed to "as-needed" dosing for persistent pain, and (3) the use of adjuvant medications, whose actions are not primarily analgesic, to improve the efficacy of the principal analgesics.

NSAIDs are used first. If pain control is not achieved, a low-potency opiate or adjuvant agents such as tricyclics are added. If pain persists, opiate analgesics are used while continuing adjuvant agents. Alternative routes of analgesic administration (i.e., intravenous and epidural) and surgical approaches are reserved for specialized situations in which pain control cannot be achieved or maintained with the first steps of the approach.

Placebo Therapy and Pain Relief

Thirty percent of patients enrolled in placebo-controlled trials respond to placebo. The response rate in psychogenic and nociceptive pain is the same. Therefore a placebo response is not a diagnostic test for psychogenic pain or malingering. The mechanism of placebo action is probably central modulation of nociceptive input.

Nonopioid Analgesics

The nonopioid analgesics include acetaminophen and NSAIDs (Table 57.2), and are indicated for mild to moderate nociceptive pain and are particularly useful in the treatment of pain originating in bone and joints, but are generally not useful in the management of neuropathic pain syndromes. NSAIDs are also anti-inflammatory and antipyretic. They may be combined

Table 57.2: Selected nonopioid analgesics

Class	Drug	Half-Life (in hrs)	Dose Range	Major Toxicities
Paraminophenol derivative	Acetaminophen	3	650–1000 mg q4–6h	Hepatotoxicity with high doses
Salicylates (carboxylic acids)	Aspirin	0.5	650–1000 mg q4–6h	GI, including dyspepsia, gastritis, ulceration Increased bleeding time CNS toxicity at high doses Hypersensitivity reaction (may occur with all NSAIDs) No antiplatelet effects
	Diflunisal (Dolobid)	13	500–750 mg q12h	GI toxicity less common than aspirin
	Choline magnesium trisalicylate (Trilisate)	215	1000–1500 mg q8–12h	No antiplatelet effects
Nonselective COX-1 and COX-2 inhibitors Propionic acids	Ibuprofen (Motrin)	2	400–1000 mg q6–8h	GI toxicity, may be less common than with acetic acid NSAIDs Renal toxicity, particularly in combination with diuretics

	Drug		Dose	Comments
Acetic acids	Naproxen (Naprosyn)	14	250–500 mg q12h	May aggravate hypertension; CNS toxicities include dizziness, headache, drowsiness, fatigue; Similar to ibuprofen
	Indomethacin (Indocin)	45	25–50 mg q8–12h	GI toxicity; CNS toxicity, particularly headache; Renal toxicity, particularly with triamterene
	Sulindac (Clinoril)	14	150–200 mg q12h	May produce hyperkalemia; GI and CNS effects are less common than with indomethacin; may have less renal toxicity
	Ketorolac (Toradol)	47	15–30 mg IM or 10 mg PO q6h	GI toxicity; for short-term therapy only
Enolic acid	Piroxicam (Feldene)	57	20–40 mg daily	GI toxicity
Fenamic acid	Mefenamic acid (Meclomen)	2	100–250 mg q6–8h	For short-term use only; GI toxicity and diarrhea
COX-2 inhibitors	Celecoxib (Celebrex)	11	100–200 mg BID	No antiplatelet effects; possibly fewer GI side effects than nonselective COX-1 and COX-2 inhibitors

Continued

Table 57.2: (continued)

Class	Drug	Half-Life (in hrs)	Dose Range	Major Toxicities
	Rofecoxib (Vioxx)	17	12.5–25 mg daily	No antiplatelet effects; possibly fewer GI side effects than nonselective COX-1 and COX-2 inhibitors
	Valdecoxib (Bextra)	8	10–20 mg daily	No antiplatelet effects; possibly fewer GI side effects than nonselective COX-1 and COX-2 inhibitors

CNS = central nervous system; GI = gastrointestinal; NSAIDs = nonsteroidal anti-inflammatory drugs.

with opiates for more severe pains, and their use is not associated with tolerance or physical dependence. Progressive increments beyond a certain dosage often fail to provide improved pain control (the *ceiling effect*).

Opioid Analgesics

Opioids are divided into the mild and strong analgesics, based on their relative potency (Table 57.3). This distinction is arbitrary, and potency alone is not a good indicator of efficacy. Chronic opioid use is associated with *physical dependence*, in which a typical pattern of symptoms develops after rapid withdrawal, including irritability, chills, salivation, diaphoresis, and abdominal discomfort with nausea and vomiting. The time course and severity of the withdrawal are a function of the potency of the opioid and its half-life. *Psychological dependence* may develop. Addictive behaviors include craving, drug seeking, and other maladaptive behaviors. Studies of medical patients receiving narcotics indicate that the risk of dependence is less than 1%. The greatest risk of psychological dependence occurs in patients with a history of drug abuse and in those with a family history of addiction.

The most common regimen is to start with a mild-potency opioid analgesic, codeine, hydrocodone, or oxycodone, often combined with acetaminophen, on a 4–6 hour dosing schedule. For persistent and chronic pain symptoms, regularly scheduled dosing with supplemental dosing for breakthrough pain is more effective than as-needed dosing. The dose is increased until pain is controlled or toxicities occur. Using short-acting opioids, titration can be achieved in hours to days, unlike using NSAIDs, which may require weeks. Incremental dosing changes of less than 25% seldom produce significantly improved pain control for patients on chronic opioid therapy. During initial titration, however, larger increments often produce nausea, dysphoria, or sedation. Unlike the NSAIDs, opioid analgesics do not have a ceiling effect.

Adjuvant Medications Useful in Pain Management

Other drugs that are not primarily analgesics but that are used to improve pain control are anticonvulsants, tricyclic antidepressants, benzodiazepines, stimulants, corticosteroids, topical capsaicin, and anesthetics.

Table 57.3: Commonly used opioid analgesics

Drug	Half-Life	Dose Equianalgesic to Morphine 10 mg IM		Typical Dosage	Comments
		IM	PO		
Mild					
Codeine	3 hrs	120	200	30–60 mg PO q4–6h	Often coadministered with acetaminophen Nausea, constipation, and dysphoria common Often useful when codeine is not well tolerated
Oxycodone (+ acetaminophen = Percocet) (+ aspirin = Percodan)	2–3 hrs		30	5 mg PO q4–6h	Same as oxycodone
Hydrocodone (+acetaminophen = Lortab or Vicodin)	4 hrs		30	2.5–7.5 mg PO q4–6h	
Propoxyphene (Darvon)	6–12 hrs		150–200	65 mg PO q4h	Active metabolite (norpropoxyphene) with long half-life (30–36 hrs)
Meperidine (Demerol)	2 hrs	75	300	50–100 mg IM	Encephalopathy, myoclonus, and seizures due to metabolite (normeperidine) limit chronic use Contraindicated in patients taking monoamine oxidase inhibitors

Strong

					Comments
Morphine	2–3 hrs	10	30–60	2–10 mg IM/IV 30–60 mg PO q4h	With chronic use the IM:PO ratio falls from 1:6 to 1:3 Available in slow-release preparation (MS Contin)
Hydromorphone (Dilaudid)	2–3 hrs	1.5	7.5	1–4 mg PO q4h	Good choice for chronic therapy due to high potency and short half-life
Pentazocine (Talwin)	2–3 hrs	60	180	50–100 mg PO q4h	Mixed agonist-antagonist Ceiling effect for analgesia May precipitate withdrawal in opioid-dependent patients Encephalopathy with dose escalation
Methadone (Dolophine)	15–30 hrs	10	20	10–20 mg PO q4–8h	Duration of analgesia is highly variable, often only 4–8 hrs Long half-life leads to drug accumulation and prolonged CNS toxicity

Continued

Table 57.3: (continued)

Drug	Half-Life	Dose Equianalgesic to Morphine 10 mg IM		Typical Dosage	Comments
		IM	PO		
Levorphanol (Levo-Dromoran)	12–16 hrs	2 mg	4 mg	2–4 mg PO q4h	Like methadone
Fentanyl transdermal (Duragesic)	3–12 hrs when given IV	*	*	25–100 µg/hr transdermal patch every 3 days	CNS toxicities like morphine Slow onset with peak concentration at 24–72 hrs Reservoir effect leads to prolonged toxicity Slow titration

CNS = central nervous system.
*Dose equivalence is not well defined, but the ratio of fentanyl (transdermal) to parenteral morphine is approximately 1:30.

NONPHARMACOLOGICAL APPROACHES TO PAIN MANAGEMENT

Ablative Procedures

Regional Nerve Blockade
Nerve blocks with local anesthetics such as lidocaine are used to manage transitory, severe, localized pain. An example is epidural blockade for obstetric procedures. Epidural blockade is particularly useful when the pain is localized to one or two dermatomal segments on the trunk. Phenol can be injected to produce permanent neurolysis in patients with cancer who are expected to survive less than 1 year. Sympathetic blockade is an important component in the treatment of causalgia and related disorders. It usually is accomplished by serial blocks with local anesthetics and occasionally by neurolytic blockade. The use of temporary blockade and neurolysis is limited by their nonselective effect on all nerve fibers.

Peripheral Surgical Approaches
The use of peripheral nerve and dorsal nerve root transection is generally confined to patients with well-localized or truly segmental truncal pain syndromes that have responded to nerve blockade. Sympathetic ganglionectomy is occasionally performed in patients with causalgia and related syndromes who benefit only transiently from sympathetic blockade.

Central Surgical Approaches

The most common central ablative surgical procedure for pain management is anterolateral spinal cordotomy with surgical transection of the lateral spinothalamic tract. The best candidates are patients with cancer with unilateral somatic, nociceptive pain in one leg or the trunk. A patient whose life expectancy is 12 months or longer is not appropriate because the analgesic benefit declines with time, and painful dysesthesia is a late complication. Pituitary ablation is used to treat pain from disseminated bone metastases of hormonally sensitive cancers (i.e., breast and prostatic carcinoma). Other targets for ablative pain-control procedures include the periaqueductal gray, trigeminal nucleus, thalamus, primary sensory cortex, frontal lobes, and portions of the limbic system, such as the cingulate gyrus.

Pituitary ablation is used primarily to treat pain from disseminated bone metastases of hormonally sensitive cancers (i.e., breast and prostatic carcinoma). It is usually performed by alcohol instillation via a transsphenoidal approach.

Modulating Procedures

The concept that nociceptive input can be reduced by peripheral stimulation is fundamental to the gate theory of pain transmission. In practice, this is accomplished most often by electrical stimulation using a TENS device. Placebo effect contributes substantially to the analgesic efficacy of TENS, although some studies of postoperative pain indicate benefit greater than that obtained with sham stimulation. The combination of percutaneous electrical stimulation using acupuncture-like needles for electrodes is useful for patients with chronic low back pain.

For a more detailed discussion, see Chapter 51 in Neurology in Clinical Practice, 4th edition.

INDEX

Page numbers followed by "t" refer to tables.